Endoscopic Surgery of the Orbit

Endoscopic Surgery of the Orbit

Raj Sindwani, MD, FACS, FRCS(C)

Vice Chairman and Section Head
Rhinology, Sinus & Skull Base Surgery | Head and Neck Institute
Co-Director | Minimally Invasive Cranial Base & Pituitary Surgery Program
Rosa Ella Burkhardt Brain Tumor & Neuro-Oncology Center
Vice Chair of Enterprise Surgical Operations | Cleveland Clinic
Cleveland, Ohio

ELSEVIER

Elsevier
3251 Riverport Lane
St. Louis, Missouri 63043

ENDOSCOPIC SURGERY OF THE ORBIT ISBN: 978-0-323-61329-3

Library of Congress Control Number: 2020933845

Content Strategist: Jessica L. McCool
Content Development Manager: Meghan B. Andress
Publishing Services Manager: Shereen Jameel
Senior Project Manager: Umarani Natarajan
Design Direction: Bridget Hoette

Printed in China

Last digit is the print number: 9 8 7 6 5 4 3 2 1

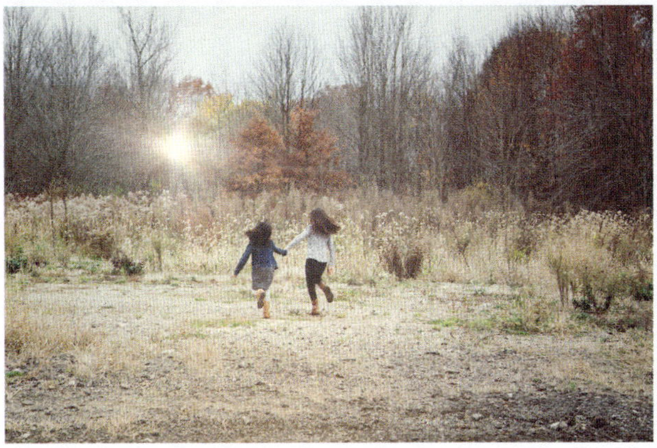

This book is dedicated to my daughters, Sienna and Sasha,
whose mere presence makes me want to be a better person and make our world a better place.
Girls, always remember that your place in the world is wherever *and* whatever *you want it to be.*
The fact that this book now exists in physical form is a testament to the love,
support, and countless sacrifices of several people in my life—most notably my parents and my wife,
Sangeeta—who, first, convinced me that I really could do anything that I put my mind to,
and then, second, provided me the runway to do it.

Raj Sindwani, MD, FACS, FRCS(C)

Preface

This textbook is as unique as the evolving field of endoscopic orbital surgery. More than any other sphere, contemporary approaches to the orbit and skull base are the epitome of multidisciplinary care and the "team of teams" approach to problem-solving. These approaches take exquisite advantage of the anatomic reality that the sinonasal tract is largely an air-filled column of bony cells that can readily be removed without consequence. At their core, the advantages of endoscopic approaches to the orbit closely parallel the advantages that we now routinely leverage during endoscopic skull base techniques—namely, direct-line access to pathology in hard-to-reach areas of the head that we are able to manage through the nose with minimal retraction on sensitive neurovascular structures.

With concurrent improvement in office examination techniques and imaging technology, clinicians with an interest in disorders affecting the orbit are often able to achieve increased precision in preoperative diagnosis and offer their patients more refined, and in some cases less invasive, treatment options. Minimally invasive orbital techniques offer the promise of a more streamlined approach to comprehensive patient care, improved patient satisfaction and experience, and superior outcomes.

The modern era of endoscopic surgery of the orbit has witnessed an unparalleled partnership between the specialties of otolaryngology and ophthalmology. Beyond even this core dyad, however, the complex nature of endoscopic orbital surgery requires a cohesive, multidisciplinary team consisting of otolaryngologists, ophthalmologists, neurosurgeons, endocrinologists, medical and radiation oncologists, and radiologists and pathologists. In addition to providing expertise and perspectives from these various specialties, *Endoscopic Surgery of the Orbit* (1st edition) also highlights the two-surgeon, multihanded surgical techniques that have ushered in a new era in managing complex pathologies involving the orbit and skull base.

Infused with the knowledge and wisdom of global thought leaders, it was my mission to provide a comprehensive resource that could serve as an authoritative text to practitioners performing endoscopic orbital procedures and caring for these patients. I am immensely grateful to my distinguished colleagues and friends for their contributions to this important project; your time and dedication are very much appreciated.

It is my sincere hope that readers find this work informative, thought-provoking, entertaining, and inspiring.

Raj Sindwani, MD, FACS, FRCS(C)

Biography

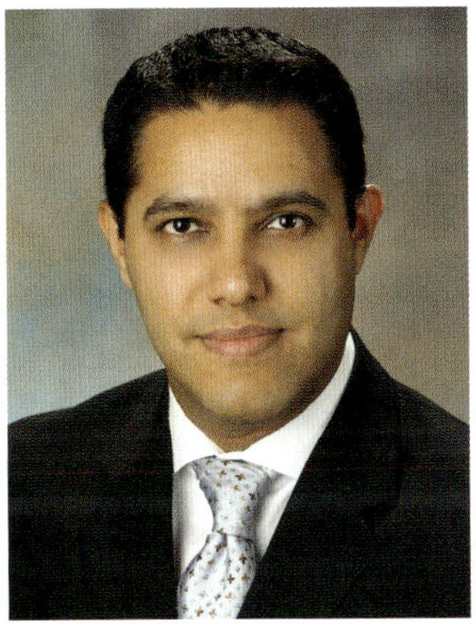

Raj Sindwani, MD, FACS, FRCS(C)

Dr. Sindwani is vice chairman and head of the Section of Rhinology, Sinus & Skull Base Surgery of the Head & Neck Institute at the Cleveland Clinic. He is also co-director of the Minimally Invasive Cranial Base and Pituitary Program of the Rose Ella Burkhardt Brain Tumor and Neuro-Oncology Center. He has held several important leadership roles at the Cleveland Clinic and is currently vice chairman of Enterprise Surgical Operations. In this role, he and his team champion procedural and surgical safety and quality while working to address access, efficiency, and service-line development across the Cleveland Clinic health system. He also serves as president-elect of the medical staff and is a member of the Cleveland Clinic Board of Governors.

Dr. Sindwani is presently the editor-in-chief of the *American Journal of Rhinology & Allergy* and past editor-in-chief of the *Year Book of Otolaryngology.* He serves on several high-impact editorial and scientific advisory boards and has trained many fellows and residents. He is an established authority on the medical and surgical management of conditions affecting the sinuses, orbit, and skull base and has pioneered endoscopic surgical approaches to these regions. He has published extensively in the field and has lectured at many institutions, instructional courses, and scientific symposia around the world.

Contents

Video Contents

Contributors

Omar H. Ahmed, MD
Fellow, Rhinology and Cranial Base Surgery
Department of Otolaryngology
University of Pittsburgh Medical Center
Pittsburgh, PA, United States

Shaheryar F. Ansari, MD
Fellow, Pacific Neuroscience Institute
John Wayne Cancer Institute
Providence's Saint John's Health Center
Santa Monica, CA, United States

Leopold Arko IV, MD
Minimally Invasive Endoscopic Skull Base Fellow
Department of Neurological Surgery
Weill Cornell Medical College
New York Presbyterian Hospital
New York, NY, United States

Catherine Banks, MD, FRACS
Fellow/Clinical Instructor in Rhinology and Skull Base Surgery
Department of Otolaryngology
Massachusetts Eye and Ear Infirmary
Harvard Medical School
Boston, MA, United States

Garni Barkhoudarian, MD, PhD
Associate Professor
Department of Neuroscience and Neurosurgery
John Wayne Cancer Institute
Santa Monica, CA, United States

Federico Biglioli, MD
Professor and Chair
Maxillofacial Surgery Unit
Santi Paolo e Carlo Hospital, Università degli Studi di Milano
Milan, Italy

Benjamin S. Bleier, MD
Associate Professor
Director of Endoscopic Skull Base Surgery
Co-Director Center for Thyroid Eye
Disease and Orbital Surgery
Department of Otolaryngology – Head and Neck Surgery
Massachusetts Eye and Ear Infirmary
Harvard Medical School
Boston, MA, United States

Kofi Boahene, MD
Professor
Department of Otolaryngology – Head and Neck Surgery
Johns Hopkins
Baltimore, MD, United States

Hamid Borghei-Ravazi, MD
Assistant Professor
Department of Neurosurgery
Cleveland Clinic Florida
Weston, FL, United States

Zachary J. Cappello, MD
Otolaryngologist
Charlotte Eye, Ear, Nose, and Throat Associates
Charlotte, NC, United States

Anais L. Carniciu, MD
Department of Ophthalmology
University Hospitals Cleveland Medical Center
Case Western Reserve University School of Medicine
Cleveland, OH, United States

Ricardo L. Carrau, MD
Professor
Departments of Otolaryngology – Head and Neck Surgery
Neurological Surgery, and Communication Sciences and Disorders
The Ohio State University
Columbus, OH, United States

Matthew Cassidy, CNIM
Intraoperative Neuromonitoring Workleader
Intraoperative Neuromonitoring
Cleveland Clinic Foundation
Cleveland, OH, United States

Rakesh Chandra, MD
Professor
Department of Otolaryngology
Vanderbilt University Medical Center
Nashville, TN, United States

Chandala Chitguppi, MD
Fellow, Division of Rhinology and Skull Base Surgery
Department of Otolaryngology and Head and Neck Surgery
Thomas Jefferson University
Philadelphia, PA, United States

Brian H. Chon, MD
Oculofacial Plastic Surgery
Cleveland Clinic Foundation, Cole Eye Institute
Cleveland, OH, United States

Giacomo Colletti, MD
Staff Physician
Maxillofacial Surgery Unit
Santi Paolo e Carlo Hospital, Università degli Studi di Milano
Milan, Italy

Gustavo Coy, MD
Mr.
São Paulo ENT & Skull Base Center
Edmundo Vasconcelos Hospital
São Paulo, Brazil

Iacopo Dallan, MD
Unit of Otolaryngology, Audiology and Phoniatrics
University of Pisa
Pisa, Italy

Jackson Deere, BS
Medical Student
School of Medicine
University of Texas Southwestern Medical Center
Dallas, TX, United States

Nora Dewart, BSc(Hon)
Department of Otolaryngology – Head and Neck Surgery
University of Toronto
Toronto, ON, Canada

Eric M. Dowling, MD
Resident Physician
Department of Otorhinolaryngology – Head and Neck Surgery
Mayo Clinic
Rochester, MN, United States

Charles S. Ebert, Jr., MD, MPH
Associate Professor
Department of Otolaryngology – Head and Neck Surgery
UNC School of Medicine
University of North Carolina
Chapel Hill, NC, United States

Jean Anderson Eloy, MD, FACS, FARS
Professor and Vice Chair
Departments of Otolaryngology – Head and Neck Surgery, Neurological Surgery, Ophthalmology and Visual Science
Rutgers New Jersey Medical School
Newark, NJ, United States

James J. Evans, MD
Professor
Department of Neurological Surgery and Otolaryngology
Thomas Jefferson University Hospital
Philadelphia, PA, United States

Nicole I. Farber, MD
Resident
Department of Otolaryngology
Rutgers New Jersey Medical School
Newark, NJ, United States

Nyssa Fox Farrell, MD
Fellow
Department of Otolaryngology – Head and Neck Surgery
Oregon Health & Science University
Portland, OR, United States

Judd H. Fastenberg, MD
Fellow, Division of Rhinology and Skull Base Surgery
Department of Otolaryngology – Head and Neck Surgery
Thomas Jefferson University
Philadelphia, PA, United States

Giovanni Felisati, MD
Professor and Chair
Otorhinolaryngology Unit and Head and Neck Department
Santi Paolo e Carlo Hospital, Università degli Studi di Milano
Milan, Italy

Juan C. Fernandez-Miranda, MD
Professor
Department of Neurosurgery
Surgical Director
Brain Tumor, Skull Base and Pituitary Centers
Stanford University
Stanford, CA, United States

Paul A. Gardner, MD
Associate Professor
Departments of Neurological Surgery and Otolaryngology
University of Pittsburgh School of Medicine
Co-Director
Center for Cranial Base Surgery
University of Pittsburgh Medical Center
Pittsburgh, PA, United States

Inbal Gazit, MD
Department of Ophthalmology
Assaf Harofeh Medical Center
Tzrifin, Isreal

Christos Georgalas, MD, PhD, MRCS (England), DLO, FRCS (ORL-HNS)
Consultant and Otolaryngologist – Head and Neck Surgeon Director of Endoscopic Skull Base Center
Hygeia Hospital
Athens, Greece
Professor of Surgery
St. George's Medical School at Nicosia University Program
Nicosia, Greece

Kyle J. Godfrey, MD
Division of Ophthalmic Plastic, Reconstructive, and Orbital Surgery
Department of Ophthalmology
Weill Cornell Medical College
New York, NY, United States;
Division of Oculoplastic and Orbital Surgery
Department of Ophthalmology
Harkness Eye Institute
Columbia University Medical Center
New York, NY, United States

Ezequiel Goldschmidt, MD, PhD
Intra-Residency Fellow, Open and Endoscopic Cranial Base Surgery
Department of Neurosurgery
University of Pittsburgh
Pittsburgh, PA, United States

Jessica W. Grayson, MD
Rhinology and Skull Base Research Group
Applied Medical Research Centre
University of New South Wales
Australian School of Advanced Medicine Macquarie University
Sydney, Australia

Ashleigh A. Halderman, MD
Assistant Professor
Department of Otolaryngology – Head and Neck Surgery
University of Texas Southwestern Medical Center
Dallas, Texas, United States

John F. Hardesty, MD
Department of Ophthalmology and Visual Sciences
Washington University School of Medicine
St. Louis, MO, United States

Morris E. Hartstein, MD, FACS
Director, Ophthalmic Plastic and Reconstructive Surgery
Department of Ophthalmology
Assaf Harofeh Medical Center
Zerfin, Israel
Clinical Associate Professor
Department of Ophthalmology
Saint Louis University
St. Louis, MO, United States

Richard J. Harvey, MD, PhD
Professor
Rhinology and Skull Base Surgery, Applied Medical Research Centre
University of New South Wales
Sydney, Australia
Professor
Faculty of Medicine and Health Science
Macquarie University
Sydney, Australia

Stephen C. Hernandez, MD
Assistant Professor
LSU School of Medicine
New Orleans, LA, United States

Eric Hink, MD
Associate Professor
Departments of Otolyngology – Head and Neck Surgery and Ophthalmology
University of Colorado School of Medicine
Aurora, CO, United States

John Bryan Holds, MD, FACS
Ophthalmic Plastic and Cosmetic Surgery, Inc.
Des Peres, MO, United States
Departments of Ophthalmology and Otolaryngology – Head and Neck Surgery
Saint Louis University
St. Louis, MO, United States

Wayne D. Hsueh, MD
Assistant Professor
Department of Otolaryngology – Head and Neck Surgery
Center for Skull Base and Pituitary Surgery
Neurological Institute of New Jersey
Rutgers New Jersey Medical School
Newark, NJ, United States

Catherine J. Hwang, MD
Oculofacial Plastic Surgery
Cleveland Clinic Foundation
Cole Eye Institute
Cleveland, OH, United States

Christopher Karakasis, MD
Associate Staff
Division of Neuroradiology
Cleveland Clinic
Cleveland, OH, United States
Assistant Professor
Diagnostic Radiology
Lerner College of Medicine of Case Western Reserve University
Cleveland, OH, United States

Michael Kazim, MD
Division of Oculoplastic and Orbital Surgery
Department of Ophthalmology
Harkness Eye Institute
Columbia University Medical Center
New York, NY, United States

Daniel F. Kelly, MD
Director, Pacific Neuroscience Institute
Department of Neurosurgery
Pacific Neuroscience Institute
Santa Monica, CA, United States

Kathleen M. Kelly, MD
Resident Physician
Department of Otolaryngology – Head and Neck Surgery
UT Southwestern Medical Center
Dallas, TX, United States

Adam J. Kimple, MD, PhD
Assistant Professor
Otolaryngology – Head and Neck Surgery
UNC School of Medicine
University of North Carolina at Chapel Hill
Chapel Hill, NC, United States

Todd T. Kingdom, MD
Professor
Departments of Otolyngology – Head and Neck Surgery and Ophthalmology
University of Colorado School of Medicine
Aurora, CO, United States

Courtney Lynn Kraus, MD
Department of Ophthalmology
Johns Hopkins University
Baltimore, MD, United States

Howard Kraus, MD
Professor of Surgery
Director of Eye, Ear & Skull Base Center
John Wayne Cancer Institute
Providence Saint John's Health Center
Santa Monica, CA

Varun R. Kshettry, MD
Physician
Department of Neurosurgery
Cleveland Clinic
Cleveland, OH, United States

Edward C. Kuan, MD, MBA
Assistant Professor
Department of Otolaryngology – Head and Neck Surgery
University of California, Irvine
Irvine, CA, United States

Andrew P. Lane, MD
Professor
Department of Otolaryngology – Head and Neck Surgery
Johns Hopkins University School of Medicine
Baltimore, MD, United States

Donald Charles Lanza, MD, MS
Director
Rhinology & Skull Base Surgery
Sinus and Nasal Institute of Florida Foundation
St. Petersbrug, FL, United States

Victoria S. Lee, MD
Assistant Professor
Department of Otolaryngology – Head and Neck Surgery
University of Illinois at Chicago College of Medicine
Chicago, IL, United States

Riccardo Lenzi, MD, PhD
Consultant Otorhinolaryngologist
Azienda USL, Toscana, Nord Ovest
Unit of Otorhinolaryngology
Apuane Hospital
Massa, Italy

James K. Liu, MD, FACS, FAANS
Professor
Departments of Otolaryngology – Head and Neck Surgery and Neurological Surgery
Center for Skull Base and Pituitary Surgery
Neurological Institute of New Jersey
Rutgers New Jersey Medical School
Newark, NJ, United States

Lisa D. Lystad, MD
Neuro-Ophthalmology
Cole Eye
Cleveland Clinic Foundation
Cleveland, OH, United States

Robi Nicolas Maamari, MD
Ophthalmic Plastic and Cosmetic Surgery, Inc.
Des Peres, MO, United States;
Department of Ophthalmology and Visual Sciences Oculoplastics fellow
Washington University School of Medicine
St. Louis, MI, United States

João Mangussi-Gomes, MD
São Paulo ENT & Skull Base Center
Edmundo Vasconcelos Hospital
São Paulo, Brazil

Ralph B. Metson, MD
Professor
Department of Otolaryngology – Head and Neck Surgery
Massachusetts Eye and Ear
Harvard Medical School
Boston, MA, United States

Kapil Mishra, MD
Resident Physician
Department of Ophthalmology
Wilmer Eye Institute
Johns Hopkins Hospital
Baltimore, MD, United States

Ron Mitchell, MD
Professor and Chief
Department of Otolaryngology – Head and Neck Surgery
School of Medicine
University of Texas Southwestern Medical Center
Dallas, TX, United States

Kris S. Moe, MD, FACS
Professor and Chief, Division of Facial Plastic Surgery
Departments of Otolaryngology and Neurological Surgery
University of Washington School of Medicine
Seattle, WA, United States

Luca Muscatello, MD
Azienda USL Toscana Nord Ovest
Unit of Otorhinolaryngology
Apuane Hospital
Massa, Italy

Dileep Nair, MD
Section Head of Adult Epilepsy
Epilepsy Center
Cleveland Clinic
Cleveland, OH, United States

John Nguyen, MD
Associate Professor
Fellowship Director
Ophthalmic Plastic & Reconstructive Surgery
Department of Ophthalmology & Visual Sciences
West Virginia University
Morgantown, WV, United States

Leah Novinger, MD, PhD
Resident
Department of Otolaryngology – Head and Neck Surgery
Indiana University School of Medicine
Indianapolis, IN, United States

Gurston G. Nyquist, MD
Associate Professor
Division of Rhinology and Skull Base Surgery
Department of Otolaryngology and Neurological Surgery
Thomas Jefferson University Hospital
Philadelphia, PA, United States

Lior Or, MD
Department of Ophthalmology
Assaf Harofeh Medical Center
Tzrifin, Israel

James N. Palmer, MD
Professor of Otorhinolaryngology
Division of Rhinology
Department of Otorhinolaryngology – Head and Neck Surgery
University of Pennsylvania
Philadelphia, PA, United States

Julian D. Perry, MD
Oculofacial Plastic Surgery
Cleveland Clinic Foundation, Cole Eye Institute
Cleveland, OH, United States

Anastasia Piniara, MD, MSc
Consultant and Otolaryngologist – Head and Neck Surgeon
Hygeia Hospital
Athens, Greece

Daniel M. Prevedello, MD
Professor
Department of Neurological Surgery
The Ohio State University
Columbus, OH, United States

Mindy R. Rabinowitz, MD
Assistant Professor
Division of Rhinology and Skull Base Surgery
Department of Otolaryngology and Neurological Surgery
Thomas Jefferson University
Philadelphia, PA, United States

Hassan Ramadan, MD
Professor and Chairman
Department of Otolaryngology
West Virginia University
Morgantown, WV, United States

Pablo F. Recinos, MD
Section Head, Skull Base Surgery
Department of Neurosurgery
Brain Tumor and Neuro-Oncology Center
Cleveland Clinic
Cleveland, OH, United States

Roxana Y. Rivera, MD
Director, Oculoplastic and Orbital Surgery Service
University Hospitals Cleveland Medical Center
Assistant Professor of Ophthalmology
Case Western Reserve University School of Medicine
Cleveland, OH, United States

Marc R. Rosen, MD
Professor, Division of Rhinology and Skull Base Surgery
Department of Otolaryngology and Neurological Surgery
Thomas Jefferson University Hospital
Philadelphia, PA, United States

Christopher R. Roxbury, MD
Assistant Professor
Division of Otolaryngology – Head and Neck Surgery
University of Chicago
Chicago, IL, United States

Paul Ruggieri, MD
Chief
Division of Neuroradiology
Cleveland Clinic
Cleveland, OH, United States

Charles Saadeh, MD
Resident
Department of Otolaryngology – Head and Neck Surgery
School of Medicine
University of Texas Southwestern Medical Center
Dallas, TX, United States

Raymond Sacks, MD
Rhinology and Skull Base Research Group
Applied Medical Research Centre
University of New South Wales;
Australian School of Advanced Medicine
Macquarie University;
Department of Otolaryngology
University of Sydney
Sydney, Australia

Soumya Sagar, MBBS
Clinical Research Fellow
Department of Neurosurgery
Brain Tumor and Neuro-Oncology Center
Cleveland Clinic
Cleveland, OH, United States

Alberto Maria Saibene, MD, MA
Staff Physician
Otorhinolaryngology Unit
Santi Paolo e Carlo Hospital
Università degli Studi di Milano
Milan, Italy

Griffin D. Santarelli, MD
Assistant Professor
Barrow Neurological Institute
Phoenix, AZ, United States

Jamie Lea Schaefer, MD
Fellow
Department of Ophthalmology & Visual Sciences
West Virginia University
Morgantown, WV, United States

Theodore H. Schwartz, MD
Professor of Neurosurgery, Otolaryngologiy, Neurology and Neuroscience
Department of Neurological Surgery
Weill Cornell Medical College
New York Presbyterian Hospital
New York, NY, United States

Rajeev D. Sen, MD
Resident
Department of Neurological Surgery
University of Washington School of Medicine
Seattle, WA, United States

Gopi Shah, MD
Assistant Professor
Department of Otolaryngology – Head and Neck Surgery
Division of Pediatric Otolaryngology
School of Medicine and Children's Medical Center
University of Texas
Southwestern Medical Center
Dallas, TX, United States

Raj Sindwani, MD, FACS, FRCS(C)
Vice Chairman and Section Head
Rhinology, Sinus & Skull Base Surgery
Head and Neck Institute
Co-Director
Minimally Invasive Cranial Base & Pituitary Surgery Program
Rosa Ella Burkhardt Brain Tumor & Neuro-Oncology Center
Vice Chair of Enterprise Surgical Operations
Cleveland Clinic
Cleveland, OH, United States

Arun D. Singh, MD
Cole Eye Institute
Professor of Ophthalmology
Director, Ophthalmic Oncology
Cleveland Clinic Foundation
Cleveland, OH, United States

Carl H. Snyderman, MD, MBA
Professor
Departments of Otolaryngology and Neurological Surgery
University of Pittsburgh School of Medicine
Pittsburgh, PA, United States
Co-Director
Center for Cranial Base Surgery
University of Pittsburgh Medical Center
Pittsburgh, PA, United States

Aldo C. Stamm, MD, PhD
São Paulo, ENT & Skull Base Center
Edmundo Vasconcelos Hospital
São Paulo, Brazil

Heinz Stammberger, MD (Deceased)
Professor
Department of General Otorhinolaryngology, Head and Neck Surgery
Medical University of Graz
Graz, Austria

Janalee K. Stokken, MD
Assistant Professor
Department of Otorhinolaryngology – Head and Neck Surgery
Mayo Clinic
Rochester, MN, United States

Eric Succar, MD
Instructor
Department of Otolaryngology
Vanderbilt University Medical Center
Nashville, TN, United States

Peter F. Svider, MD
Department of Otolaryngology – Head and Neck Surgery
Rutgers New Jersey Medical School
Newark, NJ, United States

Luisam Tarrats, MD, JD
Director
Department of Rhinology and Skull Base Surgery
La Clínica de Rinosinusitis, LLC
Cayey, Puerto Rico
Assistant Professor
Department of Otolaryngology – Head and Neck Surgery
University of Puerto Rico
San Juan, Puerto Rico

Brian D. Thorp, MD
Assistant Professor
Department of Otolaryngology – Head and Neck Surgery
UNC Medical School
University of North Carolina at Chapel Hill
Chapel Hill, NC, United States

Jonathan Y. Ting, MD, MS, MBA
Interim Chair
Department of Otolaryngology – Head and Neck Surgery
Indiana University School of Medicine
Indianapolis, IN, United States

Peter Valentin Tomazic, MD, PhD
Associate Professor
Department of General Otorhinolaryngology – Head and Neck Surgery
Medical University of Graz
Graz, Austria

Kyle K. VanKoevering, MD
Assistant Professor, Cranial Base Surgery
Otolaryngology – Head and Neck Surgery
University of Michigan
Ann Arbor, MI, United States

Erich Vyskocil, MD
Department of Otorhinolaryngology Head and Neck Surgery
Medical University of Vienna
Vienna, Austria

Eric W. Wang, MD
Associate Professor
Departments of Otolaryngology, Neurological Surgery and Ophthalmology
Director of Education, Center for Cranial Base Surgery
University of Pittsburgh Medical Center
Pittsburgh, PA, United States

Ian J. Witterick, MD, MSc, FRCSC
Professor and Chair
Department of Otorhinolaryngology – Head and Neck Surgery
University of Toronto
Toronto, ON, Canada

Peter J. Wormald, MD, FAHMS, FRACS, FRCS(Ed), FCS(SA), MBChB
Professor Otolaryngology Head and Neck Surgery
Professor Skull Base Surgery
Department of Otolaryngology Heads and Neck Surgery
University of Adelaide
Adelaide, Australia

Habib Zalzal, MD
Physician
Otolaryngology
West Virginia University
Morgantown, WV, United States

Adam M. Zanation, MD
Associate Professor
Department of Otolaryngology – Head and Neck Surgery
UNC School of Medicine
University of North Carolina at Chapel Hill
Chapel Hill, NC, United States

PART 1

Perspectives and Evolution in Techniques

1

Endoscopic Orbital Surgery: The Rhinologist's Perspective

RALPH B. METSON, MD

The specialties of otolaryngology and ophthalmology are separated by little more than the width of the lamina papyracea. This paper-thin bone that forms the boundary between the orbital and sinonasal cavities serves as a metaphor for the aligned interests of two specialties whose practitioners often find themselves operating in close anatomic proximity. Indeed, cooperative surgical endeavors between otolaryngologists and ophthalmologists have risen rapidly since the introduction of nasal endoscopes to treat patients with orbital disorders.

Endoscopic Dacryocystorhinostomy

Before the endoscopic age, attempts to surgically treat orbital disease through a transnasal approach were often fraught with poor visualization and poor outcome. The best documented attempt to perform a dacryocystorhinostomy (DCR) through the nose was described in 1921 by Harris P. Mosher, who then served as chairman of the Department of Otology and Laryngology at Harvard Medical School.[1] Using a headlight and nasal speculum, he described the drainage of pus from the infected lacrimal sacs of 12 patients. Although this intranasal approach avoided the need for a facial incision, a postoperative orbital infection developed in one patient who almost lost her eye, prompting Mosher to abandon the procedure in favor of a combined external-intranasal approach. In his words, "Where light is possible it is folly to work in the dark. The best surgery is done by sight." For the next 70 years, DCRs were performed almost exclusively in an external manner through a medial canthal incision, and largely by ophthalmologists.

With the advent of small-diameter, high-resolution nasal endoscopes for sinus surgery in the mid-1980s, a renewed interest developed in the possibility of accessing orbital pathology through the nose. Otolaryngologists found themselves routinely operating in the vicinity of the lacrimal sac as they cleared disease from adjacent ethmoid air cells under excellent visualization. While doing so, the potential to readily access the medial orbital structures via a transnasal approach became readily apparent, and early reports in the literature supported the concept.[2]

In 1989, I was approached by Daniel Townsend, an ophthalmologist at Massachusetts Eye and Ear Infirmary, who had recently performed an external DCR on a 52 year-old woman, only to have her troublesome tearing return 3 months later. When I examined the patient in the office with a nasal endoscope, a dense scar band could be seen overlying the region of the lacrimal sac along the lateral nasal wall. She appeared to be an ideal candidate to revisit Mosher's intranasal DCR approach, this time with the necessary "light" and visualization to perform a safe and effective surgery.

The trip to the operating room proved to be a fruitful one. The ophthalmologist passed lacrimal probes through the canaliculi to localize the obstructed lacrimal sac while I resected the scar tissue and made a wide opening around the probes into the sac. The patient tolerated the 90-minute procedure well, and her epiphora has not returned in more than 30 years.

The early success of endoscopic DCR led to its relatively rapid adoption by other surgeons at our hospital and across the country. The benefits of avoiding a facial incision and reducing patient morbidity offered by endoscopic DCR were obvious. However, not so obvious at the time were the subtleties of patient selection and surgical technique that affected clinical outcome.

One such example was the use of surgical lasers, which were quite popular at the time, for the performance of endoscopic DCR.[3] Although laser fibers could be passed through either the tear duct or nose to remove bone overlying the lacrimal sac, their use led to postoperative scar formation and restenosis. Laser endoscopic DCR had a success rate of 78% compared with a rate of more than 90% for conventional DCR. Because of these early setbacks, endoscopic DCR lost favor among many ophthalmologists who continued to perform conventional external DCR. Nevertheless, with increasing clinical experience, the performance of endoscopic DCR was refined and its adoption grew worldwide. Numerous reports over the past decade have described the safety and efficacy of this technique with results comparable to those of external DCR.[4]

Key Concepts and Lessons Learned

Over the past 30 years, personal experience supported by evidenced-based studies has taught me many lessons regarding the performance of endoscopic DCR. These lessons have been reinforced by the more than two dozen referring ophthalmologists with whom I have shared this journey. The following list enumerates some of the lessons learned.

1. **The benefits of a team approach.** Patients who undergo endoscopic DCR are best served when their care is provided by both an ophthalmologist and otolaryngologist. The complementary skill sets of these specialists allows for optimal treatment of these patients, including preoperative irrigation of the lacrimal

apparatus, intraoperative intubation of the canaliculi, and postoperative debridement of the surgical site.

2. **Starting with revision cases.** When learning to perform endoscopic DCRs, keep in mind that revision cases are usually easier than primary ones, because the thick bone overlying the sac has already been removed. In addition, ophthalmologists are more likely to refer one of their patients in whom external DCR with recurrent epiphora has failed. Such initial cases often lead to happy patients and a happy referring ophthalmologist.
3. **Adequate exposure of the lacrimal sac**. The technique used to remove thick bone overlying the lacrimal sac—drill, rongeur, ultrasonic aspirator—is not nearly as important as the location and amount of bone removed. The important thing is to remove the thick bone anterior to the maxillary line to provide adequate exposure of the entire medial sac wall.
4. **Placement of lacrimal stents.** Although placement of a stent through the newly created internal lacrimal ostium at the conclusion of endoscopic DCR may not be necessary in most cases, doing so has low patient morbidity and may help with postoperative debridement and healing.
5. **Visualization of the internal common punctum at the conclusion of surgery.** The goal of endoscopic DCR is nasalization of the internal common punctum. This punctum is visible as the opening through which the lacrimal stent enters the lateral sac wall. If this punctum is visible at the conclusion of surgery, the chances are high for a successful surgical outcome.
6. **Performance of septoplasty at time of endoscopic DCR.** If a superior septal deflection limits access to the region of the lacrimal sac, the practitioner should have a low threshold for performing septoplasty immediately before endoscopic DCR. Adequate visualization and exposure are key to safe and effective endoscopic surgery.
7. **Postoperative debridement.** Removal of tissue and debris from the surgical site under endoscopic guidance 1 week after surgery is just as important after DCR as it is after sinus surgery. Movement of the lacrimal stent with blinking as seen on endoscopy at the time of debridement suggests patent tear flow and is a positive prognostic sign for successful surgery.
8. **Intranasal causes of DCR failure.** The most common causes of DCR failure, whether performed through an endoscopic or external approach, are due to intranasal pathology. Such pathology, including adhesions and obstructing turbinates, can be readily visualized on postoperative endoscopic examination and addressed at the time of revision endoscopic DCR.

Endoscopic Orbital Decompression

Not long after the successful introduction of endoscopic DCR, sinus surgeons began to consider other possibilities for transnasal treatment of orbital pathology. At the completion of routine ethmoidectomy for chronic rhinosinusitis, the skeletonized lamina papyracea was in full view, yet its penetration was assiduously avoided for fear of exposing orbital fat and causing injury to intraorbital structures.

Those of us who trained in otolaryngology before the endoscopic era were familiar with the Walsh-Ogura transantral approach for treatment of patients with exophthalmos from Graves' disease.[5] Surgery started with a transoral incision to open the maxillary and ethmoid sinuses. The bony orbital floor and lamina papyracea were then removed, resulting in orbital decompression with immediate reduction in proptosis. But could similar surgery be performed through an endoscope? The answer came in 1990 when David Kennedy and his ophthalmologic colleague, Neil Miller, at Johns Hopkins described the successful treatment of eight patients with Graves' orbitopathy using an endoscopic technique.[6] Two of the patients underwent simultaneous Walsh-Ogura procedures to verify that adequate bone had been removed endoscopically along the orbital floor.

Later that year, I was approached by John Shore, an innovative ophthalmologist at Massachusetts Eye and Ear, who had a 38-year-old patient with a severe case of Graves' orbitopathy. He was particularly concerned about impending vision loss in this individual who had already had a vision-threatening corneal abrasion and was in need of a thorough decompression, including the region of the orbital apex, which can be difficult to visualize through a conventional approach.

When we took this first patient to the operating room, the ophthalmologist was amazed at the excellent visualization in the region of the orbital apex afforded by the endoscope. After removal of the entire lamina papyracea, I incised the periorbita in a posterior-to-anterior direction, resulting in immediate prolapse of orbital fat and reduction in the patient's proptosis. A tense orbit was now soft, and the referring physician was now sold on the advantages of an endoscopic approach to the medial orbit. A week after surgery, the patient's exophthalmos was 8 mm less than its preoperative level, but he did not have the postoperative facial swelling, numbness, and ecchymosis associated with nonendoscopic approaches to the orbit. The enhanced visualization and reduced patient morbidity afforded by the approach to the medial orbit led to a rapid growth in the number of endoscopic decompressions performed nationwide during the 1990s.[7]

Within the first 5 years of performing orbital decompressions, however, an unanticipated problem became evident: development of new-onset diplopia that was difficult for the strabismus surgeons to correct. We had known for many years that double vision was an expected sequela to orbital decompression in many patients, but the severity and incidence of the diplopia was troubling. An analysis of our results suggested that the problem was due to the thoroughness of medial orbital decompression when performed with endoscopic instrumentation compared with conventional transantral or transorbital approaches. Removal of the entire lamina papyracea and periorbita resulted in a greater prolapse of orbital fat and herniation of the medial rectus muscle into the sinonasal cavities than occurred with conventional approaches. This finding was particularly apparent in patients who had undergone only medial decompression without a concurrent lateral decompression.

Similar findings were reported by other authors who recommended the use of a "balanced decompression" technique with concurrent medial and lateral decompressions at the same operative setting.[8] This balanced decompression resulted in a significantly lower incidence of postoperative diplopia. It made sense that the lateral decompression relieved inward pressure on the orbital contents, resulting in less medial displacement of the orbital contents, including the medial rectus muscle, and thereby caused less double vision. Balanced decompressions are now performed on the majority of patients with Graves' disease in my practice who require surgical decompression. Only those with relatively mild proptosis and no optic neuropathy undergo medial decompression alone.

Another procedure developed to reduce the incidence of postoperative diplopia in patients with Graves' orbitopathy is known as the "orbital sling" technique. A 10-mm wide strip of the periorbita overlying the medial rectus muscle is preserved to prevent medial displacement of the muscle during surgery. Orbital fat is free to herniate above and below the fascial sling, providing adequate decompression of the orbital contents. When a balanced technique is used in the majority of patients, supplemented by the use of an orbital sling in select patients, the results of endoscopic orbital decompression are comparable to those of transantral and transorbital techniques, including the degree of decompression achieved and relatively low incidence of postoperative complications.[9,10]

Unlike endoscopic DCR, ophthalmologists gravitated relatively quickly to the concept of endoscopic orbital decompression. They realized the obvious advantages of endoscopic instrumentation for such surgery, including better visualization along the skull base and a more complete removal of the lamina papyracea than could be achieved with conventional approaches. The majority of orbital decompressions performed today use a team approach. It is common for the ororhinolaryngologist to perform the medial portion of the decompression while the ophthalmologist follows with the lateral decompression.

Key Concepts and Lessons Learned

Specific techniques used for orbital decompression are dependent on the individual patient's pathology and the surgeon's preferences. Nevertheless, personal experience over the past three decades, combined with evidenced-based studies, has led to a general set of principles that I apply in the treatment of patients requiring endoscopic orbital decompression:

1. **Endoscopic orbital decompression is only the first step in the rehabilitation of many patients with Graves' orbitopathy.** Once the proptosis has been successfully reduced, a series of additional surgical procedures performed by the ophthalmologist are often necessary to achieve the desired degree of normal function and appearance. These procedures may include lowering the position of the upper eyelid, which is often elevated in Graves' disease, and strabismus surgery to address any residual diplopia.
2. **A balanced decompression decreases the incidence of postoperative diplopia.** Postoperative diplopia is an expected sequela, not a complication, of endoscopic orbital decompression in many patients. Nevertheless, the incidence of double vision can be reduced by the performance of concurrent medial and lateral orbital decompression in the same operative setting.
3. **The use of an orbital sling technique can further decrease the incidence of postoperative diplopia in select patients.** Preservation of a 10-mm wide strip of the periorbita overlying the medial rectus muscle helps to stabilize the muscle position and function, particularly in patients without preexisting diplopia.
4. **Patients who present with optic neuropathy should have complete removal of lamina papyracea in the region of the orbital apex.** Decompression of the orbital apex region effectively removes pressure on the optic nerve and leads to improved vision in many patients with visual loss from optic neuropathy.
5. **Preserve the anterior, not posterior, inframedial orbital strut (IOS).** The anterior portion of the IOS (located anterior to the maxillary ostium) is routinely left in place during endoscopic medial orbital decompression. Preservation of the posterior portion of IOS makes decompression technically more difficult and alters postoperative diplopia only to the degree that it reduces the degree of orbital decompression.
6. **Revision orbital decompression is beneficial in select patients.** In cases of persistent or recurrent proptosis after decompression surgery, removal of any remaining bone along the medial orbit wall or floor may result in the additional desired degree of decompression.

Endoscopic Optic Nerve Decompression

Endoscopic optic nerve decompression is a natural extension of orbital decompression. Bone removal along the posterior orbit is continued into the sphenoid sinus following the optic canal as it courses along the lateral sphenoid wall. In the 1990s, a relatively large number of optic nerve decompressions were performed on patients who lost vision after head trauma, particularly during motor vehicle accidents. There was much debate at the time as to the best surgical approach to use to decompress the optic nerve in patients who lost vision after head trauma—endoscopic, open, transorbital, or transcranial. The debate ended when high-dose steroids were found to be just as effective as surgical decompression of the optic canal in these patients.[10]

Most individuals who present with optic neuropathy as a component of Graves' orbitopathy do very well after endoscopic orbital decompression alone. Provided adequate bone is removed to decompress the region of the orbital apex, their neuropathy, including the associated color blindness and visual field loss, usually resolves. Some ophthalmologists, however, do favor decompression of the optic canal at time of endoscopic orbital decompression in patients with severe optic neuropathy.

Endoscopic optic nerve decompression remains an excellent procedure in those patients whose visual loss is due to compression of the optic nerve within the sphenoid sinus from neoplasms, such as meningiomas, or osseous lesions, such as fibrous dysplasia. Experience has shown that unroofing the bony canal in the affected area is sufficient to restore vision in most cases. Incision of the optic nerve sheath is not necessary.[10]

Endoscopic Resection of Orbital Tumors

The inferior and medial rectus muscles are routinely exposed during endoscopic orbital decompression. Manipulation of these muscles to gain access to the intraconal region of the orbit was a natural extension of this surgical approach. Successful endoscopic removal of tumors of the medial orbit has been described by a number of authors.[11] Most of the early experience was with resection of orbital hemangiomas, which are not only the most common intraorbital tumor encountered but also are well encapsulated, facilitating their dissection from surrounding orbital contents. As experience with these techniques has advanced, the size, location, and pathology of orbital tumors successfully resected through an endoscopic approach have also advanced.

Future Directions

The history of endoscopic orbital surgery over the past 30 years reflects a natural progression of surgical exploration: from superficial to deep, from medial to lateral. As both the techniques and technologies associated with endoscopic orbital surgery advance, so too will the indications, extent, and success of these procedures. I foresee the day when otolaryngologists will work with ophthalmologists to perform surgery on extraocular muscles—retrieval of lost muscles during strabismus surgery, and remodeling of diseased muscles from Graves' disease. Endoscopic instrumentation also has potential benefits in the field of neuroophthalmology—placement of retinal and optic nerve implants, fenestration of the optic nerve for treatment of patients with visual loss from intracranial hypertension, and decompression of the optic nerve in patients with ischemic neuropathy.

Conclusion

The fields of otolaryngology and ophthalmology were once a single specialty. The advent of endoscopic techniques to treat patients with orbital disorders has served to foster the collaborative efforts of surgeons in these two specialties once again. With the growing use of endoscopic instrumentation to treat orbital disease, the future of endoscopic orbital surgery is a bright one, enabling surgeons and their patients to truly "see the light."

References

1. Mosher, H. P. (1921). Re-establishing intranasal drainage of the lacrymal sac. *Laryngoscope*, *31*, 492–512.
2. McDonogh, M., & Meiring, J. H. (1989). Endoscopic transnasal dacryocystorhinostomy. *Journal of Laryngology and Otology*, *103*(6), 585–587.
3. Metson, R., Wong, J. J., & Puliafito, C. A. (1994). Endoscopic laser dacryocystostomy. *Laryngoscope*, *104*(8 Pt 1), 269–274.
4. Kingdom, T. T., Barham, H. P., & Durairaj, V. D. (2019). Long-term outcomes after endoscopic dacryocystorhinostomy without mucosal flap preservation. *Laryngoscope*. https://doi.org/10.1002/lary.27989.
5. Walsh, T. E., & Ogura, J. H. (1957). Transnasal orbital decompression for malignant exophthalmos. *Laryngoscope*, *67*(6). 544–568.
6. Kennedy, D. W., Goldstein, M. L., Miller, N. R., & Zinreich, S. J. (1990). Endoscopic transnasal orbital decompression. *Archives of Otolaryngology–Head Neck Surgery*, *116*(3), 275–282.
7. Metson, R., Dallow, R. L., & Shore, J. W. (1994). Endoscopic orbital decompression. *Laryngoscope*, *104*(8 Pt 1), 950–957.
8. Kacker, A., Kazim, M., Murphy, M., Trokel, S., & Close, L. G. (2003). "Balanced" orbital decompression for severe Graves' orbitopathy: technique and treatment algorithm. *Otolaryngology–Head Neck Surgery*, *128*(2), 228–235.
9. Yao, W. C., Sedaghat, A. R., Yadav, P., Fay, A., & Metson, R. (2016). Orbital decompression in the endoscopic age: The modified inferomedial orbital structure. *Otolaryngology–Head Neck. Surgery*, *154*(5), 963–969.
10. Pletcher, S. D., Sindwani, R., & Metson, R. (2006). Endoscopic orbital and optic nerve decompression. *Otolaryngologic Clinics of North America*, *39*(5), 943–958.
11. McKinney, K. A., Snyderman, C. H., Carrau, R. L., Germanwala, A. V., Prevedello, D. M., Stefko, S. T., et al. (2010). Seeing the light: Endoscopic endonasal intraconal orbital tumor surgery. *Otolaryngology–Head Neck Surgery*, *143*(5), 600–701.

2

Endoscopic Orbital Surgery: The Ophthalmologists' Perspective: Formation of the Ophthalmology-Otolaryngology Team

ROBI NICOLAS MAAMARI, MD, JOHN F. HARDESTY, MD, AND JOHN BRYAN HOLDS, MD, FACS

Endoscopic orbital surgery has rapidly established itself as a highly evolving multidisciplinary surgical field, relying on the expertise and technical skills of ophthalmologists and otolaryngologists. In 1978, Norris and Cleasby first described the use of the endoscope for orbital surgery in the ophthalmic literature.[1] Three years later, in 1981, they reported a 15-patient case series describing their experience using a transorbital endoscopic approach for orbital trauma evaluation, foreign body removal, and tumor biopsy.[2] The adoption of transorbital endoscopic surgery by the ophthalmic community was limited owing to risks of irrigation-related intraorbital pressure elevation, tissue edema, and compressive injury. As a result, most ophthalmologists and oculofacial surgeons use endoscopic techniques mainly when performing endoscopic dacryocystorhinostomies (Fig. 2.1) and endoscopic brow lifts.

In contrast, the introduction of endoscopic surgery in the field of otolaryngology has revolutionized the treatment of sinus and allergic disease. The widespread use of the endoscopic transnasal approach has resulted in rapid development and implementation of technological innovations. These advances have led to an expansion of the clinical utility of the transnasal endoscopic approach, with a variety of applications addressing pathology and disease in the adjacent anatomic regions, including the skull base and orbit.

In particular, there has been a tremendous increase in the otolaryngology literature describing the endoscopic transnasal orbital decompression technique in the management of thyroid eye disease and compressive optic neuropathy. In 1990, Kennedy et al. introduced the transnasal endoscopic approach for orbital decompression.[3] In this study, they reported a mean improvement in Hertel exophthalmometry measurements of 4.7 mm in five patients after medial and inferior wall decompression using this transnasal endoscopic technique. Since then, several modifications to this approach have been described to improve outcomes and decrease complication risks. For example, the incidence of new-onset diplopia in early reports of endoscopic decompressions occurred in up to 45% of cases.[4] However, preservation of the inferomedial orbital bone strut in endoscopic orbital decompression has resulted in a tremendous reduction in new-onset postoperative diplopia.[5] Aside from the improvement in patient outcomes, this modification highlights the importance of an established interdisciplinary relationship and collaboration between the oculoplastic surgery and otolaryngology fields, as this technique was adopted from the work described by Goldberg, Shorr, and Cohen in the oculoplastic surgery literature in 1992.[6] The anatomic expertise of both fields has improved our understanding of the orbital strut and suspensory ligament complex and the sinus anatomy to preserve the position of the globe after endoscopic surgery. Furthermore, the preservation of a strip of the periorbita medial to the medial rectus muscle has also been introduced to limit medial rectus muscle prolapse into the ethmoid cavity.[7] This "orbital sling" technique is an additional modification that can be used to improve the versatility of the transnasal endoscopic approach for orbital decompression.

The growing use of the endoscopic approach for orbital decompressions in the surgical management of thyroid eye disease has fostered a strong relationship between the ophthalmologist and otolaryngologist. In 1993, one author (J.B.H.) began a collaborative relationship for orbital decompression to achieve a lower risk of complications and improve patient care and safety. In 1999, Graham and Carter described the combined-approach orbital decompression as a safe, efficient, and efficacious joint service procedure, wherein the otolaryngologist performed the

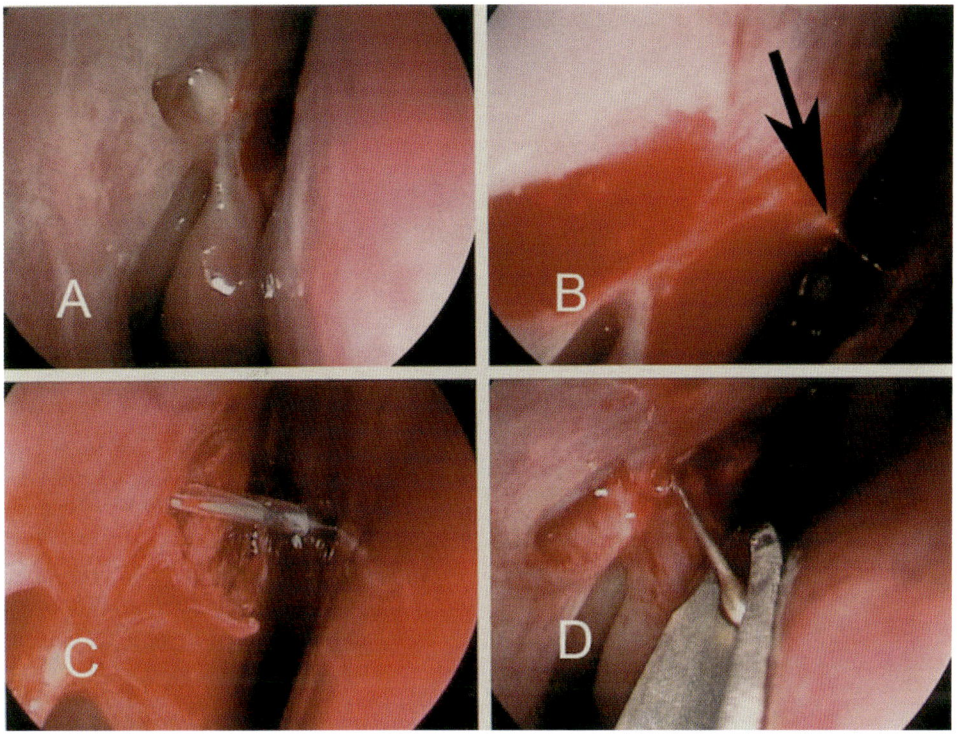

• **Fig. 2.1** Endoscopic transnasal surgical techniques largely developed in otolaryngology have been adopted by ophthalmologists and oculofacial surgeons for lacrimal and orbital surgery. Images from an endoscopic revision dacryoycystorhinostomy show (A) the nonfunctional lacrimal ostium; (B) a sharp dilator (*arrow*) penetrating at the site of the proposed ostium; (C) a balloon catheter about to be inflated to ensure an adequate opening after the removal of some mucosa; (D) retrieval of the Crawford lacrimal stents with a nasal groove director.

endoscopic medial wall decompression and the ophthalmologist completed the external, transorbital inferior, and lateral wall decompressions.[8] This collaborative effort leverages the advantageous features of each approach. The endoscopic approach provides improved visualization of the posterior medial wall, limiting the potential for surgical optic nerve injury and maximizing the extent of decompression at the orbital apex. These advantages are of particular importance in cases requiring decompression for progressive thyroid disease–related optic neuropathy. The external, transconjunctival, and lateral canthal approach provides direct visualization of the infraorbital nerve to enable extensive inferior wall decompression, both medial and lateral to the infraorbital nerve. Additionally, the simultaneous three-wall decompression facilitates maximal reduction in exophthalmos in a single operation, while also reducing the incidence of postoperative diplopia owing to the balancing effect when both the medial and lateral walls are decompressed.[9]

The remarkable advances in endoscopy in the past decades have introduced additional team-based surgical opportunities for the otolaryngologist and ophthalmologists. Specifically, several recent studies have highlighted the benefits of a combined procedure with complex posterior and apical orbital masses.[10–12] Curragh, Halliday, and Selva described the potential utility of a dual-route technique wherein the orbital apical mass is accessed via a transnasal endoscopic approach and a transcaruncular orbitotomy is simultaneously used to assist in manipulation and removal of the mass.[13] Additionally, they describe the advantageous incorporation of an external transconjunctival disinsertion of the medial rectus muscle to increase endoscopic exposure during orbital biopsies and excisions, which can be reinserted at the conclusion of the procedure.

Surgical navigation and localization is an area of rapid progress and evolution that enhances patient safety and surgical outcomes. These systems also play an integral role in robotic surgery. Initially used in neurosurgery and otolaryngology for localization in areas of critical anatomy or to allow for small incision approaches, these systems have been adopted in ophthalmology and oculofacial surgery to enhance patient safety (Fig. 2.2). Several reports in the ophthalmic plastic surgery literature highlight the utility of stereotactic image guidance systems as adjunctive tools in orbital tumor excisions and orbital decompressions.[14,15]

Through the development of these innovative surgical approaches and techniques, we are establishing and solidifying an evolving relationship between the fields of ophthalmology and otolaryngology. As a result, we may observe a transition in the standard of care and surgical management of a subset of orbital and apical tumors, with improved patient outcomes based on a collaborative practice that relies on the otolaryngologist's familiarity of sinus anatomy and the ophthalmologist's structural expertise in the intraorbital anatomic relationships.

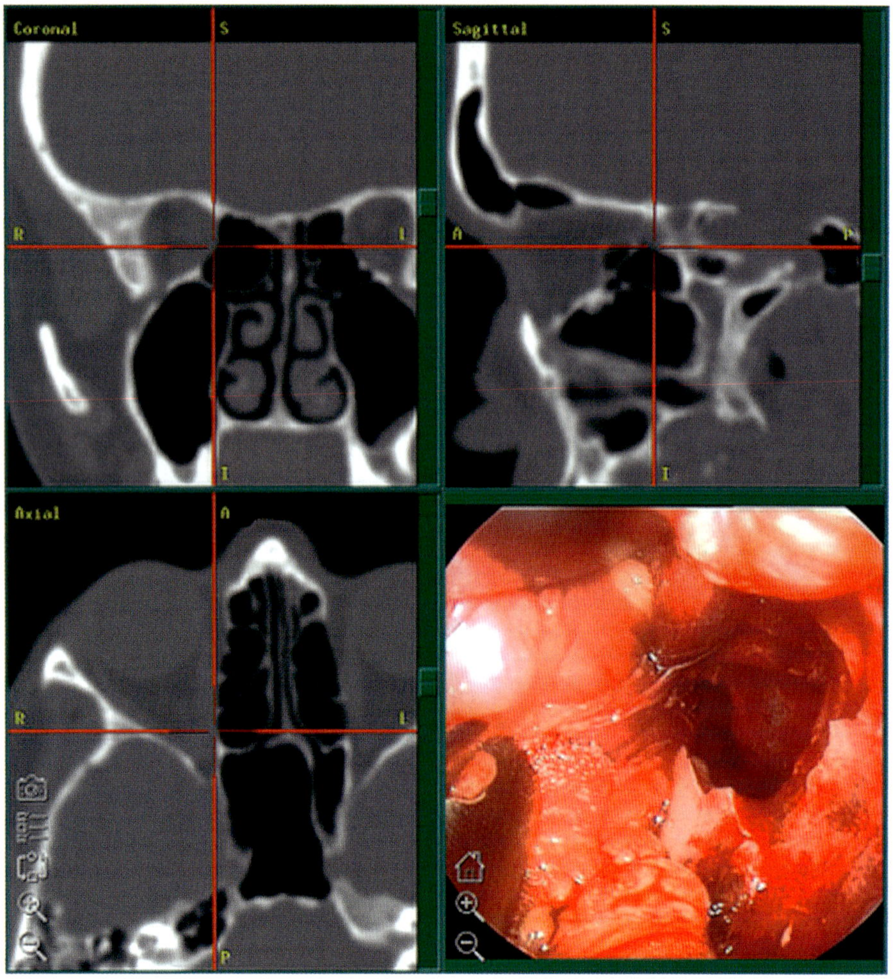

• **Fig. 2.2** Endoscopic visualization through the orbit and sinus (bottom right) and a stereotactic localization system (top left, coronal; top right, sagittal; bottom left, axial) are used to enhance patient safety in the resection of an apical orbital tumor between the medial rectus muscle and the optic nerve.

References

1. Norris, J. L., & Cleasby, G. W. (1978). An endoscope for ophthalmology. *American Journal of Ophthalmology, 85*(3), 420–422. https://doi.org/10.1016/S0002-9394(14)77741-4.
2. Norms, J. L., & Cleasby, G. W. (1981). Endoscopic orbital surgery. *American Journal of Ophthalmology, 91*(2), 249–252. https://doi.org/10.1016/0002-9394(81)90183-5.
3. Kennedy, D. W., Goodstein, M. L., Miller, N. R., & Zinreich, S. J. (1990). Endoscopic transnasal orbital decompression. *Archives of Otolaryngology–Head and Neck Surgery, 116*(3), 275–282. https://doi.org/10.1001/archotol.1990.01870030039006.
4. Yao, W. C., Sedaghat, A. R., Yadav, P., Fay, A., & Metson, R. (2016). Orbital decompression in the endoscopic age: The modified inferomedial orbital strut. *Otolaryngology–Head and Neck Surgery, 154*(5), 963–969. https://doi.org/10.1177/0194599816630722.
5. Wehrmann, D., & Antisdel, J. L. (2016). An update on endoscopic orbital decompression. *Current Opinion in Otolaryngology & Head and Neck Surgery, 25*(1), 73–78. https://doi.org/10.1097/MOO.0000000000000326.
6. Goldberg, R. A., Shorr, N., & Cohen, M. S. (1992). The medical orbital strut in the prevention of postdecompression dystopia in dysthyroid ophthalmopathy. *Ophthalmic Plastic and Reconstructive Surgery, 8*(1), 32–34.
7. Metson, R., & Samaha, M. (2002). Reduction of diplopia following endoscopic orbital decompression: The orbital sling technique. *Laryngoscope, 112*(10), 1753–1757. https://doi.org/10.1097/00005537-200210000-00008.
8. Graham, S. M., & Carter, K. D. (1999). Combined-approach orbital decompresion for thyroid-related orbitopathy. *Clinical Otolaryngology and Allied Sciences, 24*(2), 109–113. https://doi.org/10.1046/j.1365-2273.1999.00219.x.
9. Hernández-García, E., San-Román, J. J., González, R., Nogueira, A., Genol, I., Stoica, B., et al. (2017). Balanced (endoscopic medial and transcutaneous lateral) orbital decompression in Graves' orbitopathy. *Acta Oto-Laryngologica, 137*(11), 1183–1187. https://doi.org/10.1080/00016489.2017.1354394.
10. Stokken, J., Gumber, D., Antisdel, J., & Sindwani, R. (2016). Endoscopic surgery of the orbital apex: Outcomes and emerging techniques. *Laryngoscope, 126*(1), 20–24. https://doi.org/10.1002/lary.25539.

11. Sun, M. T., Wu, W., Yan, W., Tu, Y., & Selva, D. (2017). Endoscopic endonasal-assisted resection of orbital schwannoma. *Ophthalmic Plastic and Reconstructive Surgery*, *33*, S121–S124. https://doi.org/10.1097/IOP.0000000000000528.
12. Yao, W. C., & Bleier, B. S. (2016). Endoscopic management of orbital tumors. *Current Opinion in Otolaryngology & Head and Neck Surgery*, *24*(1), 57–62. https://doi.org/10.1097/MOO.0000000000000215.
13. Curragh, D. S., Halliday, L., & Selva, D. (2018). Endonasal approach to orbital pathology. *Ophthalmic Plastic and Reconstructive Surgery*, *34*(5), 422–427. https://doi.org/10.1097/IOP.0000000000001180.
14. Ali, M. J., Naik, M. N., Kaliki, S., & Dave, T. V. (2016). Interactive navigation-guided ophthalmic plastic surgery: The usefulness of computed tomography angiographic image guidance. *Ophthalmic Plastic and Reconstructive Surgery*, *32*(5), 393–398. https://doi.org/10.1097/IOP.0000000000000736.
15. Lee, K. Y. C., Ang, B. T., Ng, I., & Looi, A. (2009). Stereotaxy for surgical navigation in orbital surgery. *Ophthalmic Plastic and Reconstructive Surgery*, *25*(4), 300–302. https://doi.org/10.1097/IOP.0b013e3181ab6795.

3

Endoscopic Orbital Surgery: The Neurosurgeon's Perspective

LEOPOLD ARKO IV, MD AND THEODORE H. SCHWARTZ, MD

Neurosurgical approaches to the orbit are often done with the aid of ophthalmologist or otolaryngologist, to address intraorbital lesions invading intracranial spaces or, more recently, to gain skull base exposure. Dandy first reported use of a frontotemporal craniotomy to resect lesions from the orbit that then grew intracranial.[1] The approach Dandy described has now evolved into the skull base workhorse approaches now commonly used for lesions of the orbit as well as anterior and middle cranial fossa. The development by Yasargil of the pterional craniotomy allowed for easy exposure of lesions in the anterior and middle fossa.[2] Orbital pathology along the lateral edge of the orbit and the superior orbital fissure could be approached from the traditional version of this exposure. Later addition of a supraorbital craniotomy[3] to the pterional approach created the orbitozygomatic craniotomy, which allowed for further exposure of the orbit.[4,5] The purpose of the orbital removal with this exposure was not only to treat intraorbital pathology but to gain skull base exposure regardless of orbital involvement. Lesions of the superolateral area of the orbit as well as lesions extending into the anterior and middle cranial fossa could safely be resected from this approach. However, there are downsides of traditional craniotomies, including a large scar, temporalis atrophy, cerebrospinal fluid leak (CSF), and infection.

Subfrontal craniotomies are another commonly used approach to lesions of the orbit and anterior cranial fossa. These approaches usually include a variation of a bicoronal incision with removal of a portion of the frontal bar bilaterally or unilaterally depending on the pathology.[6] Subfrontal retraction then allows for views of the superior orbit along with extended views of the superolateral or superomedial orbit. The required cranial exposure and retraction of a bifrontal craniotomy can be extensive. Therefore attempts have also been made to decrease the amount of craniotomy needed to expose the anterior fossa. One of these more minimal approaches includes the supraorbital craniotomy, which allows for anterior fossa exposure while minimizing frontal lobe retraction. Visualization offered with the supraorbital craniotomy has greatly been expanded with use of the endoscope and combining the supraorbital approach with endonasal approaches.[7]

Endoscopic endonasal approaches were developed in the late 1990s by Jho, first for approaches to sellar pathology.[8] Later, expanded approaches were able to expose the inferomedial orbital apex as well as the anterior cranial fossa.[9] The first attempt to use the endoscope through the orbit was completed in the 1980s, but this technique was not advanced because of the lack of high-quality imaging and navigational capability.[10] The potential of transorbital surgery as a corridor to intracranial pathology would not be advanced again until 2010.[11] This transorbital corridor was developed in large part because of the tools developed for endonasal approaches, the advancement in imaging, and neuronavigation. The use of the endoscope allowed for small orbital craniotomies with more direct routes to surgical pathology of the anterior and middle cranial fossa, leading to minimization of brain retraction. Transorbital approaches have now opened the orbit as an extensive intracranial corridor.

Transorbital Approaches

Transorbital approaches have a classification based on the surgical target. Orbital endoscopic surgery is for access to the orbit and optic nerve within the orbit; transorbital endoscopic surgery or transorbital neuroendoscopic surgery (TONES) is for targeting intracranial pathology.[12] These approaches offer a corridor to the lateral aspect of the anterior and middle fossa, as opposed to the direct approach to the central anterior fossa provided by endoscopic endonasal approaches. The choice of transorbital approach depends on the targeted anatomical region. Endoscopic orbital approaches include the superior eyelid crease approach (SLC), the precaruncular approach (PC), lateral retrocanthal approach (LRC), and preseptal lower eyelid (PS) approach (Fig. 3.1).[11,12] All these approaches have been tested in both clinical and preclinical settings for different pathologies.

Superior Eyelid Crease Approach

The SLC approach involves a superior eyelid incision with careful dissection along the superior orbital rim.[11] Initial clinical use of this exposure was used to repair CSF leaks, fractures, and orbital compression as described by Moe et al.[11,13,14](Table 3.1). With this exposure, a large portion of the superior and lateral orbit can be visualized. With drilling of the posterior orbit, the anterior and middle cranial fossa can be reached through this exposure. The SLC approach limits include the superomedial limit defined by the superior orbital fissure, the inferior limit defined by the inferior orbital fissure, and the lateral limit defined by the temporalis muscle (Fig. 3.2).[15] Preclinical cadaver studies have thoroughly evaluated the potential of this approach (Table 3.2). The first use of this approach for intracranial pathology was described as a theoretical approach for an amygdalohippocampectomy. By drilling of the orbit adjacent to the inferior orbital fissure, the temporal pole was exposed and intradural exposure of the mesial temporal lobe was completed.[16] Further cadaver studies have shown that the lateral cavernous sinus, including the cavernous carotid, gasserian

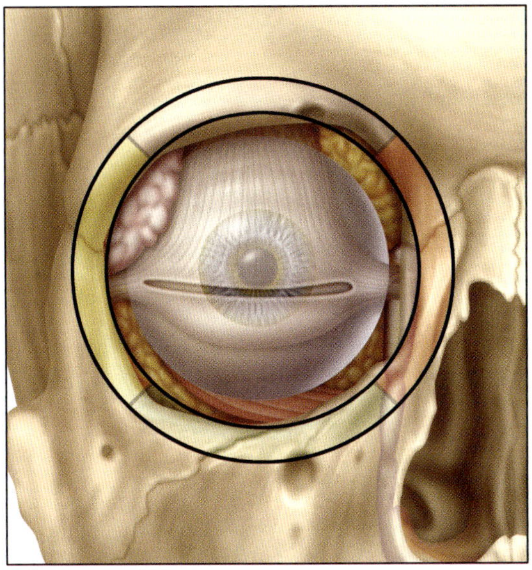

• **Fig. 3.1** Overview of four quadrants of the orbit. The superior quadrant is the area covered by the superior eyelid crease approach. The lateral quadrant (*yellow*) is covered by the lateral retrocanthal approach with some overlap with the superior eyelid crease. The inferior quadrant is covered by the preseptal lower eyelid approach. The medial quadrant (*red*) is covered by the precaruncular approach.

ganglion, ophthalmic division of trigeminal nerve (V1), maxillarydivision of trigeminal nerve (V2), and mandibular nerves division of trigeminal nerve (V3), could all be reached through the SLC approach by more lateral dissection along the orbital rim.[17-19] Using a combination of the SLC and endonasal approach, an almost 360-degree decompression of the optic nerve could be completed.[20,21] The sylvian fissure has also been dissected through this

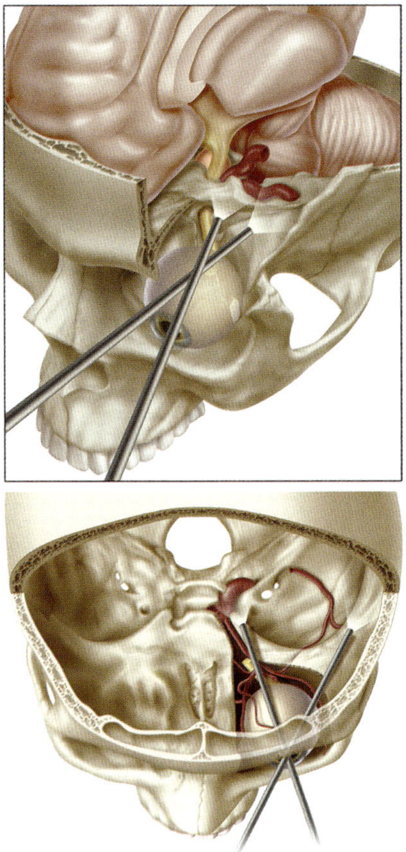

• **Fig. 3.2** Basic view provided by the superior eyelid approach. The upper panel is a lateral oblique view and the lower panel is an overhead view.

TABLE 3.1 Clinical Use of Endoscopic Transorbital Approaches

Author	Year	Approach	Pathology Treated	No. of Cases	Type of Multiport Access
Moe et al.[11]	2010	SLC	CSF leak, frontal sinus mucocele, decompression of orbit	9	—
		LRC	Decompression of orbit apex, CSF leak repair	2	—
		PC	Tumor debulking, CSF leak repair, foreign body removal	10	—
		PS	Decompression orbit apex, CSF leak repair, metastatic squamous cell debulking	2	—
Moe et al.[13]	2011	SLC	CSF leak, orbital wall fractures, frontal sinus fracture	6	—
		LRC	CSF leak, orbital wall fracture	1	—
		PC	CSF leak, orbital wall fracture	5	—
		PS	CSF leak, orbital wall fracture	1	—
Lim et al.[27]	2012	SLC	Orbital abscess, epidural abscess, frontal sinus mucopyocele	9	—
		PC	Orbital apex syndrome, orbital abscess, fronto-orbital mucocele,	4	—
Raza et al.[38]	2012	PC	CSF leak repair, Paget disease, adjunct juvenile angiofibroma, and esthesioneuroblastoma resection	6	Endonasal
Rajappa et al.[26]	2014	SLC	Epidural abscess	1	—
Bly et al.[25]	2014	SLC	Tension pneumocephalus	1	Endonasal

(*Continued*)

TABLE 3.1 Clinical Use of Endoscopic Transorbital Approaches—cont'd

Author	Year	Approach	Pathology Treated	No. of Cases	Type of Multiport Access
Dallan et al.[28]	2015	SLC	Adjunct resection spheno-orbital meningioma	3	Endonasal
		PS	Malignant schwannoma	1	—
Tham et al.[29]	2015	SLC	Fibrous dysplasia of orbit and ethmoid	1	Endonasal
Chen[27]	2015	SLC	Amygdalohippocampectomy	2	—
Ramakrishna et al.[14]	2016	SLC	CSF leak repair, mucocele resection, orbital hematoma evacuation, evacuation of mucopyocele, optic nerve decompression, orbital fracture repair, sinonasal melanoma resection, fibroxanthoma resection, frontal sinus fracture repair	13	—
		SLC/PS	CSF leak repair, ORIF orbit fracture, epidural abscess drainage	6	—
		LRC	Esthesioneuroblastoma resection, melanoma resection, CSF leak repair	4	—
		PC	CSF leak repair, esthesioneuroblastoma resection, meningocele repair, osteoma resection, orbital fracture repair, osteoblastoma resection, fibrous dysplasia resection, squamous cell carcinoma resection, encephalocele resection, meningioma resection	17	—
Almeida[15]	2017	SLC	Resection spheno-orbital meningioma	2	—
Kong[31]	2018	SLC	Spheno-orbital meningioma, osteosarcoma, plasmacytoma, sebaceous gland carcinoma, intraconal schwannoma, cystic teratoma, and fibrous dysplasia resection	18	—

CSF, cerebrospinal fluid; *LRC*, lateral retrocanthal; *ORIF*, open reduction with internal fixation; *PC*, precaruncular; *PS*, preseptal lower eyelid; *SLC*, superior eyelid crease.

TABLE 3.2 Progression of Preclinical studies for Transorbital Endoscopic Approaches

Author	Year	Approach	Focus of Investigation
Ciporen et al.[35]	20107	PC, endonasal	Sella region, pituitary gland
Bly et al.[17]	2014	LRC	Sella region, MCF, and GG
Chen et al.[16]	2014	SLC/LRC	Amygdalohippocampectomy
Ciporen[37]	2016	PC, endonasal	Cavernous carotid
Ferrari et al.[39]	2016	PS	MCF, GG, V2, V3
Almeida et al.[22]	2017	SLC	MCA, sylvian fissure, crural cistern
Ciporen et al.[36]	2017	PC, endonasal	posterior circulation arterial clipping
Dallan et al.[18]	2017	SLC	Cavernous sinus
Di Somma et al.[21]	2017	SLC, endonasal	Optic nerve decompression by SLC
Di Somma et al.[20]	2017	SLC	Surgical freedom, optic nerve decompression open versus combined
Priddy et al.[19]	2017	SLC	MCF, GG, V2, V3
Di Somma et al.[23]	2018	SLC	Sylvian fissure, MCF
D Somma et al.[24]	2018	SLC	MCF, petrous apex, GG
Noiphithak et al.[32]	2018	LRC	MCF, petrous apex, GG

GG, gasserian ganglion; *LRC*, lateral retrocanthal; *MCA*, middle cerebral artery; *MCF*, middle cranial fossa; *PC*, precaruncular; *PS*, preseptal lower eyelid; *SLC*, superior eyelid crease; *V2*, maxillary division of trigeminal nerve; *V3*, mandibular division of trigeminal nerve.

route with exposure of the middle cerebral artery.[22,23] More posterior exposure of the middle cranial fossa has also allowed for dissection and drilling of the petrous apex with the ability to visualize the cerebellopontine angle and internal auditory canal.[24]

Despite multiple preclinical studies showing theoretical exposures and applications, practical clinical use of the SLC approach has remained limited. The first clinical cases used the SLC approach to repair CSF leaks, drain cerebral abscesses, decompress pneumocephalus, and repair orbital fractures.[a] Decompression of the optic nerve and repair of difficult CSF leaks from trauma remain the most clinically used applications of the SLC approach. Because of the trajectory, SLC is particularly helpful in repair of

[a]References 11, 13, 14, 25, 26, 27.

anterior cranial fossa CSF leaks originating from the orbital roof, as well as CSF leaks from the frontal sinus.[11,13,14] Orbital abscesses and cranial epidural abscesses have also been a common target of the SLC approach. In one case report, the SLC approach was chosen for a patient with a prior cranioplasty after bifrontal craniotomies and an isolated supraorbital epidural abscess. Because of the localized approach, the epidural abscess was able to be evacuated without hardware removal.[26] One of the first reported nontraumatic applications of the SLC approach was a successful completion of two amygdalohippocampectomies.[27] Tumor resection transorbitally with the SLC approach was first described by Dallan et al., who reported its use in three spheno-orbital meningioma cases. In these cases, subtotal resection was accomplished using the SLC approach in conjunction with transpterygoid and transmaxillary approaches for local control.[29] Separate groups have also used the SLC approach as both a solo and combined approach for multiple types of mass lesions. Indications for SLC approach have included biopsy and resection of fibrous dysplasia,[30] resection of sinonasal melanoma,[14] and resection of fibroxanthoma.[14] SLC as a solo approach was used by Almeida et al. for resection of two spheno-orbital meningiomas in patients with predominantly hyperostosis and proptosis. By using the SLC approach to drill out the bone of the hyperostotic orbital roof and lateral wall, the proptosis cold be relieved, even though gross total resection was not possible.[15] The SLC approach is the most widely used transorbital approach in the literature. It was the approach chosen in the largest cohort of patients with mass lesions treated using the transorbital route.[31] This cohort consisted of a total of 18 patients. Twelve of the patients had a diagnosis of spheno-orbital meningioma, and the other patients had diagnoses of osteosarcoma, plasmacytoma, sebaceous gland carcinoma, intraconal schwannoma, cystic teratoma, and fibrous dysplasia. Several of the tumors also had an intradural component, which was resected and the dural defect was repaired using a double-button technique.[31] Only two of the patients with resections had a temporary CSF leak, but no long-term CSF leaks were reported.

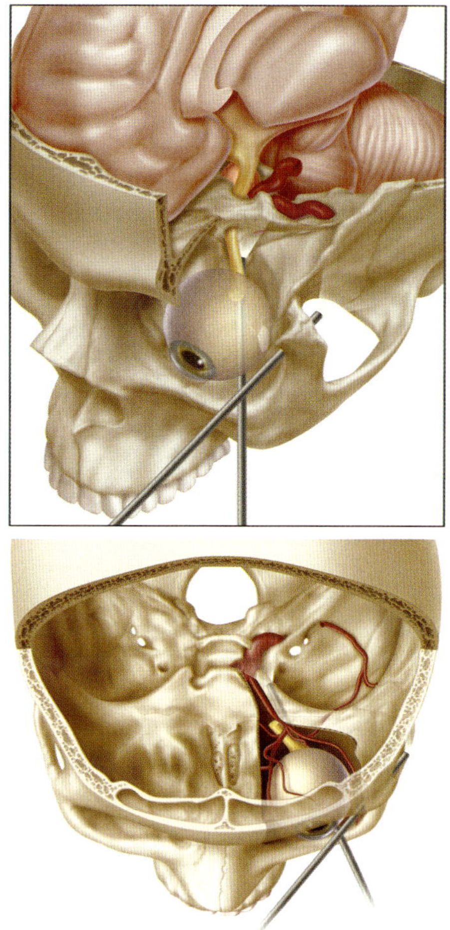

• **Fig. 3.3** Basic view provided by the lateral retrocanthal approach. The upper panel is a lateral oblique view and the lower panel is an overhead view.

Lateral Retrocanthal Approach

The lateral retrocanthal (LRC) approach avoids a cutaneous incision by instead incising the lateral conjunctiva. Further dissection and orbitotomy can provide access to the middle cranial fossa, the infratemporal fossa, and the lateral cavernous sinus. The advantage of the LRC approach over the SLC approach is the elimination of a skin incision and preservation of the eyelid support system.[31] However, the retrocanthal incision can limit the amount of orbital dissection. Initial cadaver studies using the LRC approach allowed for exposure of the middle cranial fossa and lateral cavernous sinus without the need to remove the lateral orbital rim (Fig. 3.3).[17] Later studies predicted that with the lateral orbital removal and lateral retrocanthal dissection an amygdalohippocampectomy might be feasible, but this was never tried in clinical practice.[16] Instead, the SLC approach was chosen to complete the first transorbital amygdalohippocampectomies.[27] The LRC approach has also been modified to allow exposure of the lateral orbital rim with removal of the orbital rim. This was modified by extending the LRC incision into the lateral skin crease. With the lateral orbital rim removed, the authors found more surgical freedom when approaching the petrous apex through the orbit.[33]

Clinically, the LRC approach was first used to repair both CSF leaks and orbital wall fractures.[11,13] Tumor resection has been limited through the LRC approach, likely owing to the limited surgical access. Ramakrishna et al. used the LRC approach to resect a metastatic dysplastic melanoma along the infraorbital nerve. In addition, an esthesioneuroblastoma that invaded into the orbit was also resected using the LRC approach in combination with an endoscopic endonasal approach.[14]

Precaruncular Approach

The PC approach provides medial access to the orbit with an avascular plane.[34] Through this access, both the anterior and posterior ethmoidal arteries as well as the orbital apex can be visualized.[11] With additional removal of the lamina papyracea, views of the pituitary gland and sella turcica can be obtained (Fig. 3.4). In a cadaver comparison, the PC approach provided a shorter working distance to the pituitary gland, optic chiasm, and cavernous internal carotid artery (ICA) than the transnasal approach.[35] Combining the PC with the endonasal approach provided better visualization of the parasellar area. In addition, this combination was shown in cadavers to allow for simulated clipping of the basilar artery tip[36] and cavernous carotid.[37] Clinically the PC approach was found to be useful with repair of CSF leaks,[11,13,14] orbital fractures,[11,13,14] and meningoceles.[11,37] The PC approach was the first TONES approach used to resect a mass lesion. Moe et al. used it to decompress cystic carcinoma by using a bilateral PC approach.[11] Raza et al. also used this as a solo approach to decompress Paget disease. They also combined the PC approach with the endonasal route to resect juvenile angiofibroma and esthesioneuroblastoma.[38]

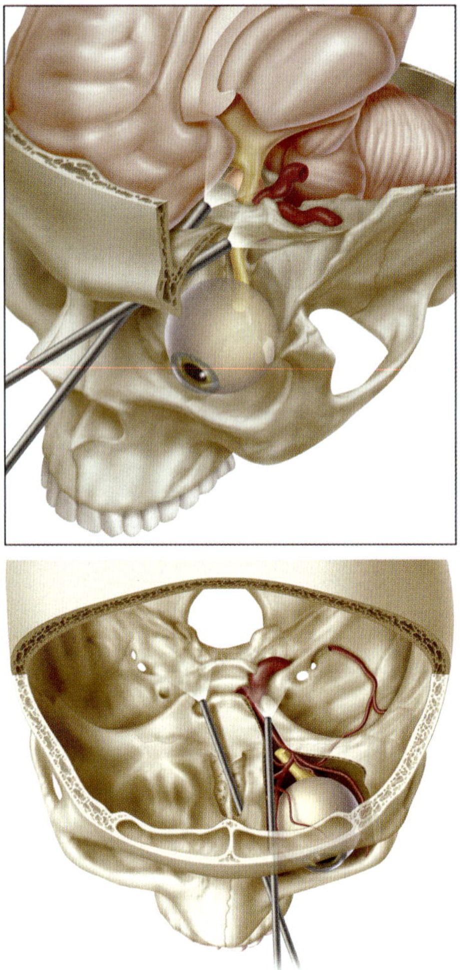

• **Fig. 3.4** Basic view provided by the precaruncular approach. The upper panel is a lateral oblique view and lower panel is an overhead view.

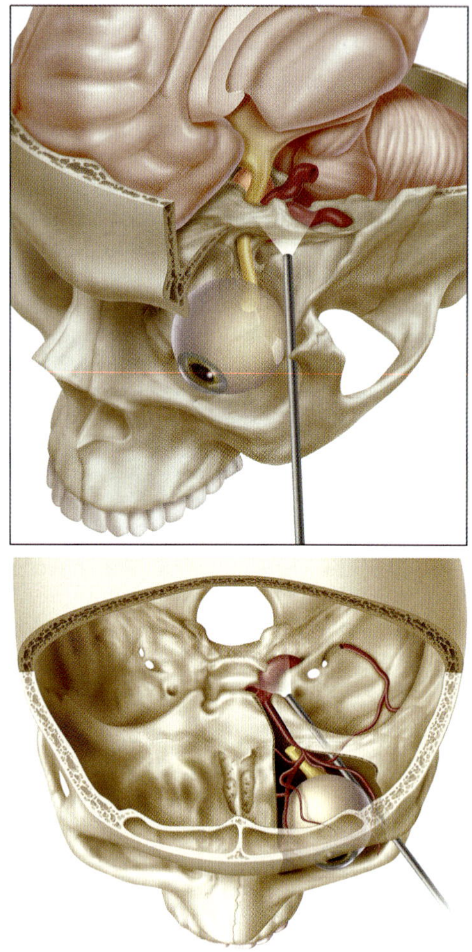

• **Fig. 3.5** Basic view provided by the preseptal lower eyelid approach. The upper panel is a lateral oblique and the lower panel is an overhead view.

The largest clinical experience with the TONES surgery was published by Ramakrishna et al. A total of 17 procedures were performed through the PCA approach in this series, making it the most used approach of this series. Of the 17 procedures performed via the PC approach, 7 of the approaches were a combined PC and transnasal approach. In this series, several mass lesions such as osteoblastoma and osteoma were resected in addition to repairs of CSF leaks, fractures, and mucoceles.[14]

Preseptal Lower Eyelid Approach

The PS approach is completed through the lower eyelid without a skin incision. Periosteal dissection then exposes the inferior orbital fissure laterally and can be combined with the LRC or PC approach to expose lateral and medial targets, respectively. In addition, the infraorbital nerve is exposed along the inferior orbital floor (Fig. 3.5).[11] Preclinical studies, although done through a skin incision, have shown that the PS approach can expose the floor of the middle cranial fossa and can be expanded more inferiorly to expose the infratemporal fossa. Through the inferior orbital access, Ferrari et al. were able to expose four major corridors: one to the Meckel cave, one to the carotid foramen, one to the petrous apex, and one to the intradural portion of the anterior temporal lobe.[39] Clinical application of the PS approach has been limited comparison with the SLC, LRC, and PC approaches. The PS approach was used mostly as a solo approach to repair CSF leaks and orbital fractures.[11,13] This was the first reported TONES approach used to debulk a tumor by Moe et al. in 2010.[11] In this series they excised a portion of the infraorbital nerve that was invaded by metastatic squamous cell carcinoma.[11] More recent studies have used the PS approach only in combination with other approaches. Ramakrishna et al. described using a combined SLC/PS approach to repair CSF leaks, open reduction with internal fixation of orbital fractures, and to drain epidural abscesses. Endonasal transmaxillary approach with the PS approach was also used to resect a malignant lesion of V2, which included intranasal and pterygopalatine growth.[14]

Conclusion

Neurosurgical use of an orbital corridor has greatly advanced with the use of the endoscope. Tools and techniques used with the recent explosion of endonasal approaches are in large part the reason for this progression. The transorbital approach has proven effective in exposure of anterior and middle cranial fossa lesions with the possibility of exposing posterior fossa lesions through the petrous apex. Transorbital approaches have been used successfully in the treatment of CSF leaks, orbital fractures, frontal sinus fractures, meningoceles, and encephaloceles. In addition, more groups are using these approaches for resection of mass lesions. Transorbital approaches, when combined with other skull base approaches, provide minimally invasive but full access to lesions without a large cranial approach. Transorbital access remains a very large area of interest and growth for skull base surgeons.

References

1. Dandy, W. E. (1941). Results following the transcranial operative attack on orbital tumors. *Archives of Ophthalmology, 25*(2), 191–216.
2. Yasargil, M. G. (1984). *Microneurosurgery.* (Vol. 1). Stuttgart: Georg Thieme Verlag.
3. Jane, J. A., Park, T. S., Pobereskin, L. H., Winn, H. R., & Butler, A. B. (1982). The supraorbital approach: Technical note. *Neurosurgery, 11*(4), 537–542.
4. Al-Mefty, O. (1987). Supraorbital-pterional approach to skull base lesions. *Neurosurgery, 21*(4), 474–477.
5. Alaywan, M., & Sindou, M. (1990). Fronto-temporal approach with orbito-zygomatic removal: Surgical anatomy. *Acta Neurochir (Wien), 104*(3–4), 79–83.
6. Haines, S. J., Marentette, L. J., & Wirtschafter, J. D. (1992). Extended fronto-orbital approaches to the anterior cranial base: Variations on a theme. *Skull Base Surg, 2*(3), 134–141.
7. Banu, M. A., Mehta, A., Ottenhausen, M., Fraser, J. F., Patel, K. S., Szentirmai, O., et al. (2016). Endoscope-assisted endonasal versus supraorbital keyhole resection of olfactory groove meningiomas: Comparison and combination of 2 minimally invasive approaches. *J Neurosurg, 124*(3), 605–620.
8. Jho, H. D., Carrau, R. L., Ko, Y., & Daly, M. A. (1997). Endoscopic pituitary surgery: An early experience. *Surg Neurol, 47*(3), 213–222. discussion. 222–213.
9. Roth, J., Fraser, J. F., Singh, A., Bernardo, A., Anand, V. K., & Schwartz, T. H. (2011). Surgical approaches to the orbital apex: Comparison of endoscopic endonasal and transcranial approaches using a novel 3D endoscope. *Orbit, 30*(1), 43–48.
10. Norris, J. L., & Cleasby, G. W. (1981). Endoscopic orbital surgery. *Am J Ophthalmol, 91*(2), 249–252.
11. Moe, K. S., Bergeron, C. M., & Ellenbogen, R. G. (2010). Transorbital neuroendoscopic surgery. *Neurosurgery, 67*(3 Suppl Operative), 16–28.
12. Balakrishnan, K., & Moe, K. S. (2011). Applications and outcomes of orbital and transorbital endoscopic surgery. *Otolaryngol Head Neck Surg, 144*(5), 815–820.
13. Moe, K. S., Kim, L. J., & Bergeron, C. M. (2011). Transorbital endoscopic repair of cerebrospinal fluid leaks. *Laryngoscope, 121*(1), 13–30.
14. Ramakrishna, R., Kim, L. J., Bly, R. A., Moe, K., & Ferreira, M., Jr. (2016). Transorbital neuroendoscopic surgery for the treatment of skull base lesions. *J Clin Neurosci, 24*, 99–104.
15. Almeida, J. P., Omay, S. B., Shetty, S. R., Chen, Y. N., Ruiz-Trevino, A. S., Liang, B., et al. (2018). Transorbital endoscopic eyelid approach for resection of sphenoorbital meningiomas with predominant hyperostosis: report of 2 cases. *J Neurosurg, 128*(6), 1885–1895.
16. Chen, H. I., Bohman, L. E., Loevner, L. A., & Lucas, T. H. (2014). Transorbital endoscopic amygdalohippocampectomy: A feasibility investigation. *J Neurosurg, 120*(6), 1428–1436.
17. Bly, R. A., Ramakrishna, R., Ferreira, M., & Moe, K. S. (2014). Lateral transorbital neuroendoscopic approach to the lateral cavernous sinus. *J Neurol Surg B Skull Base, 75*(1), 11–17.
18. Dallan, I., Di Somma, A., Prats-Galino, A., Solari, D., Alobid, I., Turri-Zanoni, M., et al. (2017). Endoscopic transorbital route to the cavernous sinus through the meningo-orbital band: A descriptive anatomical study. *J Neurosurg, 127*(3), 622–629.
19. Priddy, B. H., Nunes, C. F., Beer-Furlan, A., Carrau, R., Dallan, I., & Prevedello, D. M. (2017). A side door to Meckel's cave: Anatomic feasibility study for the lateral transorbital approach. *Oper Neurosurg (Hagerstown), 13*(5), 614–621.
20. Di Somma, A., Andaluz, N., Gogela, S. L., Cavallo, L. M., Keller, J. T., Prats-Galino, A., et al. (2017). Surgical freedom evaluation during optic nerve decompression: Laboratory investigation. *World Neurosurg, 101*, 227–235.
21. Di Somma, A., Cavallo, L. M., de Notaris, M., Solari, D., Topczewski, T. E., Bernal-Sprekelsen, M., et al. (2017). Endoscopic endonasal medial-to-lateral and transorbital lateral-to-medial optic nerve decompression: An anatomical study with surgical implications. *J Neurosurg, 127*(1), 199–208.
22. Almeida, J. P., Ruiz-Trevino, A. S., Shetty, S. R., Omay, S. B., Anand, V. K., & Schwartz, T. H. (2017). Transorbital endoscopic approach for exposure of the sylvian fissure, middle cerebral artery and crural cistern: An anatomical study. *Acta Neurochir (Wien), 159*(10), 1893–1907.
23. Di Somma, A., Andaluz, N., Cavallo, L. M., Keller, J. T., Solari, D., Zimmer, L. A., et al. (2018). Supraorbital vs endo-orbital routes to the lateral skull base: A quantitative and qualitative anatomic study. *Operative Neurosurgery, 15*(5), 567–576.
24. Di Somma, A., Andaluz, N., Cavallo, L. M., Topczewski, T. E., Frio, F., Gerardi, R. M., et al. (2018). Endoscopic transorbital route to the petrous apex: A feasibility anatomic study. *Acta Neurochir (Wien), 160*(4), 707–720.
25. Bly, R. A., Morton, R. P., Kim, L. J., & Moe, K. S. (2014). Tension pneumocephalus after endoscopic sinus surgery: A technical report of multiportal endoscopic skull base repair. *Otolaryngol Head Neck Surg, 151*(6), 1081–1083.
26. Rajappa, P., Krass, J., Parakh, S., Spinelli, H. M., & Greenfield, J. P. (2014). An aesthetic approach to the anterior cranial fossa: The endoscopic transadnexal transorbital roof method. *Aesthetic Plast Surg, 38*(2), 399–403.
27. Lim, J. H., Sardesai, M. G., Ferreira, M., Jr., & Moe, K. S. (2012). Transorbital neuroendoscopic management of sinogenic complications involving the frontal sinus, orbit, and anterior cranial fossa. *J Neurol Surg B Skull Base, 73*(6), 394–400.
28. Chen, H. I., Bohman, L. E., Emery, L., Martinez-Lage, M., Richardson, A. G., & Davis, K. A. (2015). Lateral transorbital endoscopic access to the hippocampus, amygdala, and entorhinal cortex: Initial clinical experience. *ORL J Otorhinolaryngol Relat Spec, 77*(6), 321–332.
29. Dallan, I., Castelnuovo, P., Locatelli, D., Turri-Zanoni, M., AlQahtani, A., & Battaglia, P. (2015). Multiportal combined transorbital transnasal endoscopic approach for the management of selected skull base lesions: Preliminary experience. *World Neurosurg, 84*(1), 97–107.
30. Tham, T., Costantino, P., Bruni, M., Langer, D., Boockvar, J., & Singh, P. (2015). Multiportal combined transorbital and transnasal endoscopic resection of fibrous dysplasia. *J Neurol Surg Rep, 76*(2), e291–e296.
31. Kong, D. S., Young, S. M., Hong, C. K., Kim, Y. D., Hong, S. D., Choi, J. W., et al. (2018). Clinical and ophthalmological outcome of endoscopic transorbital surgery for cranioorbital tumors. *J Neurosurg*, 1–9. https://doi.org/10.3171/2018.3.JNS173233.
32. Moe, K. S., Jothi, S., Stern, R., & Gassner, H. G. (2007). Lateral retrocanthal orbitotomy: A minimally invasive, canthus-sparing approach. *Arch Facial Plast Surg, 9*(6), 419–426.
33. Noiphithak, R., Yanez-Siller, J. C., Revuelta Barbero, J. M., Otto, B. A., Carrau, R. L., & Prevedello, D. M. (2018). Quantitative analysis of the surgical exposure and surgical freedom between transcranial and transorbital endoscopic anterior petrosectomies to the posterior fossa. *J Neurosurg*, 1–9. https://doi.org/10.3171/2018.2.JNS172334.
34. Moe, K. S. (2003). The precaruncular approach to the medial orbit. *Arch Facial Plast Surg, 5*(6), 483–487.
35. Ciporen, J. N., Moe, K. S., Ramanathan, D., Lopez, S., Ledesma, E., Rostomily, R., & Sekhar, L. N. (2010). Multiportal endoscopic approaches to the central skull base: A cadaveric study. *World Neurosurg, 73*(6), 705–712.

36. Ciporen, J. N., Lucke-Wold, B., Dogan, A., Cetas, J., & Cameron, W. (2017). Endoscopic endonasal transclival approach versus dual transorbital port technique for clip application to the posterior circulation: A cadaveric anatomical and cerebral circulation simulation study. *J Neurol Surg B Skull Base, 78*(3), 235–244.
37. Ciporen, J., Lucke-Wold, B., Dogan, A., Cetas, J. S., & Cameron, W. E. (2016). Dual endoscopic endonasal transsphenoidal and precaruncular transorbital approaches for clipping of the cavernous carotid artery: A cadaveric simulation. *J Neurol Surg B Skull Base, 77*(6), 485–490.
38. Raza, S. M., Quinones-Hinojosa, A., Lim, M., & Boahene, K. D. (2013). The transconjunctival transorbital approach: A keyhole approach to the midline anterior skull base. *World Neurosurg, 80* (6), 864–871.
39. Ferrari, M., Schreiber, A., Mattavelli, D., Belotti, F., Rampinelli, V., Lancini, D., et al. (2016). The inferolateral transorbital endoscopic approach: A preclinical anatomic study. *World Neurosurg, 90*, 403–413.

PART 2

Evaluation, Anatomy, and Imaging

4

Surgical Anatomy of the Orbit, Including the Intraconal Space

ANASTASIA PINIARA, MD, MSc AND CHRISTOS GEORGALAS, MD, PhD, MRCS (ENGLAND), DLO, FRCS (ORL-HNS)

Anatomy of the Orbit

Orbital Cavity

The orbits are the bony spaces that divide the upper facial skeleton from the middle face. The bony walls of the orbit, a four-sided pyramid, consist of a mosaic of seven bones: the zygomatic bone laterally, the frontal bone superiorly, the sphenoid bone posteriorly, with its lesser and greater wing forming the optic canal and the superior orbital fissure, the orbital process of the palatine bone and the maxillary bone inferiorly, along with the lacrimal and ethmoid bone medially[1-5] (see Fig. 4.1).

The roof (superior wall) is thin and concave, formed primarily by the orbital plate of the frontal bone joining the lesser wing of sphenoid near the apex of the orbit. The supraorbital foramen for the supraorbital nerve and vessels is presented in the middle of the supraorbital rim (Table 4.1). The floor (inferior wall) is formed by the orbital surface of maxilla and zygomatic bone and the minute orbital process of palatine bone, separating the orbit from the maxillary sinus. It is traversed by the infraorbital groove that leads to the infraorbital foramen. The floor is separated from the lateral wall by the inferior orbital fissure, which connects the orbit with the pterygopalatine and infratemporal fossa (Fig. 4.2). The medial wall consists of contributions from the orbital plate of the ethmoid, the frontal process of maxilla, the lacrimal bone, and a small part of the body of the sphenoid. The extremely thin ethmoid air cells form a delicate bony structure known as the lamina papyracea, and the thinnest medial wall is perforated by the anterior and posterior ethmoid canal.

The lacrimal groove for the nasolacrimal duct is located anteriorly. The posterior portion leads to the superior orbital fissure, a dehiscence between the two wings of the sphenoid bone that provides a passage for orbital nerves and vessels and corresponds to the anterior wall of the cavernous sinus, representing a line of communication between the middle cerebral fossa and the orbit.[6] The summit or apex of the orbit precisely coincides with the bulging portion of the superior orbital fissure. Above and medially is the exocranial foramen of the optic canal, which gives passage to the optic nerve with its meningeal sheath and the ophthalmic artery, presenting a site of communication between the orbit and the anterior cranial fossa.

At a small bony protuberance of the sphenoidal wing, the common tendinous ring (tendon of Zinn) is attached. The ring encircles the optic foramen and the central portion of the superior orbital fissure. The lateral wall is formed by the frontal process of zygomatic bone in front and by the orbital plate of the greater wing of sphenoid in the posterior two-thirds. The bones meet at the zygomaticosphenoid suture. The lateral wall is the thickest and separates the orbit from the cerebral temporal fossa and the temporal muscle.[5]

Orbital Fascia or Periorbita

The periorbita forms the periosteum of the orbit. It is loosely attached to the orbital bony walls, except for suture lines, fissures, and foramens of the orbit. It expands forward up to the orbital rim, to which it is strongly attached, and then merges with the cranial periosteum. It also sends out extensions toward the peripheral tarsal rim to form the orbital septum, which delineates the orbit in front and separates the intraorbital fat from the orbicular muscle of the eye.[7] On the orbital surface of the optic canal and the medial aspect of the superior orbital fissure, the periorbita thickens, forming the tendinous attachments of the four rectus muscles, the levator palpebrae superioris and the superior oblique muscles, creating a tendinous ring known as the annulus of Zinn. Medially it is attached to the posterior lacrimal crest and forms the lacrimal sac. The periorbita thus surrounds the contents of the orbit, posteriorly expanding around the optic canal and superior orbital fissure, continuous with the optic nerve sheath, and then finally ends up united with the dura mater. Throughout, it is perforated by the various vessels and nerves of the orbit and closes the inferior orbital fissure (Fig. 4.3).

Orbital Contents

The orbit can be divided into two parts, an anterior part containing the globe and a posterior compartment filled with a fatty matrix, called the adipose body, providing a cushioning effect on the muscles, the vessels, and the nerves supplying the globe. The eyeball does not touch any of the walls but is suspended at a distance of 6 mm outside and 11 mm inside.[5] From the optic nerve to the sclerocorneal junction, the eyeball is covered by a two-layer fascia

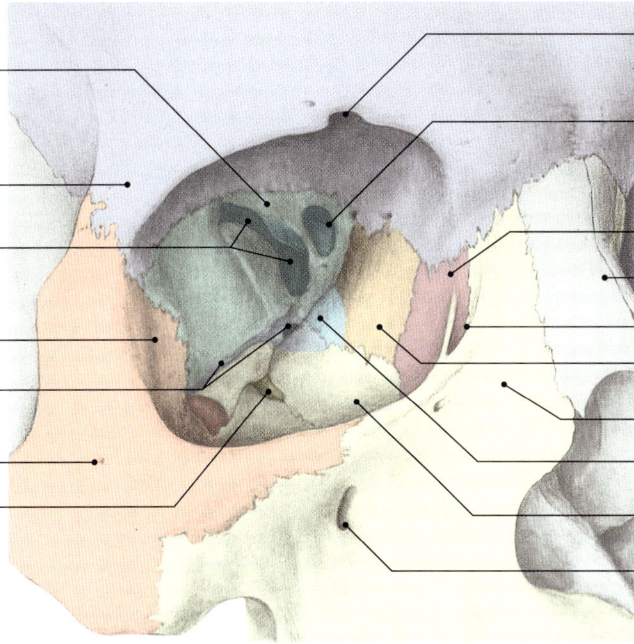

• **Fig. 4.1** Orbital bone anatomy. (Adapted from Paulsen, F., & Waschke T. [2019]. *Sobotta atlas of human anatomy* [Vol. 3] [15th ed., English]. Munich: Elsevier GmbH.)

TABLE 4.1 The Orbital Cavity

Foramina and Fissures	Contents
Supraorbital foramen	Supraorbital nerve (V1)
Infraorbital foramen	Infraorbital nerve (V2)
Superior orbital fissure	Oculomotor (II), trochlear (IV), abducens nerve (VI), opjthalmic branches (V1)
Inferior orbital fissure	Maxillary nerve branches (V2), zygomatic nerve, sphenopalatine ganglion branches, infraorbital artery and vein, inferior ophthalmic vein (leading to pterygoid plexus)
Optic canal	Optic nerve (II), ophthalmic artery
Ethmoidal canals	Anterior and posterior ethmoidal artery
*Annulus of Zinn	Superior division of cranial nerve III, nasociliary nerve (V1), sympathetic root of cervical ganglion, inferior division of cranial nerve III, cranial nerve VI, superior ophthalmic vein

*Annulus of Zinn: the common tendinous ring, not an anatomical bony foramen

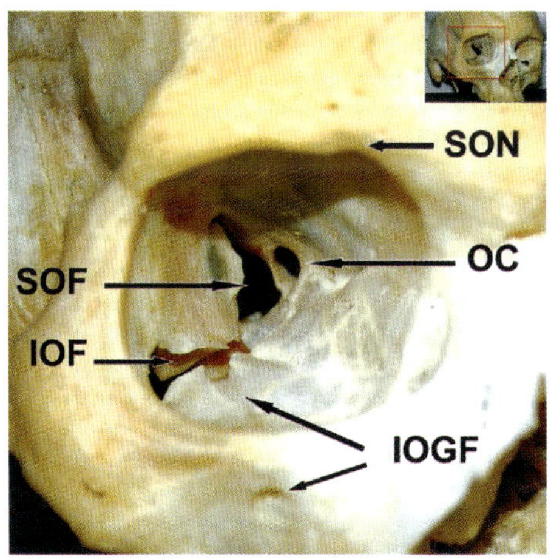

• **Fig. 4.2** Right orbital cavity: optic canal (*OC*), superior orbital fissure (*SOF*), inferior orbital fissure (*IOF*), infraorbital groove and foramen (*IOGF*), and supra orbital notch (*SON*). (From Hayek, G., Mercier, P. H., & Fournier, H. D. [2006]. Anatomy of the orbit and its surgical approach. In: Pickard, J. D., et al. [Eds.], *Advances and technical standards in neurosurgery* [Vol. 31] [pp. 36–55]. Vienna: Springer.)

(the Tenon capsule) with parietal and visceral sheets separating it from the orbital fatty tissue. There is a virtual space between the two sheets, known as the episcleral space, that forms a sort of lubricated joint system to facilitate the movements of the eye.

The fascia is merged with the capsule of the optic nerve posteriorly and with the sclera joining the cornea in the front. In its anterior part, it is perforated by the muscles of the eye. The fascia turns back over these muscles to create their aponeurotic sheath. The Lockwood ligament consists of dense connective tissue and is attached to muscles connected to the lower lid. It acts as a hammock supporting the undersurface of the globe; therefore any damage can cause lower eyelid ptosis.[8]

The orbital septum, also known as palpebral ligament, acts as the anterior soft-tissue boundary of the orbit. It extends from the tarsus to the orbital rim, where it gets attached to the bone and becomes the periorbita inside the orbit and the periosteum outside. The orbital septum is covered anteriorly by the preseptal orbicularis oculi muscle and is a consistent feature of both the upper and the lower eyelid, separating the orbital from the lid

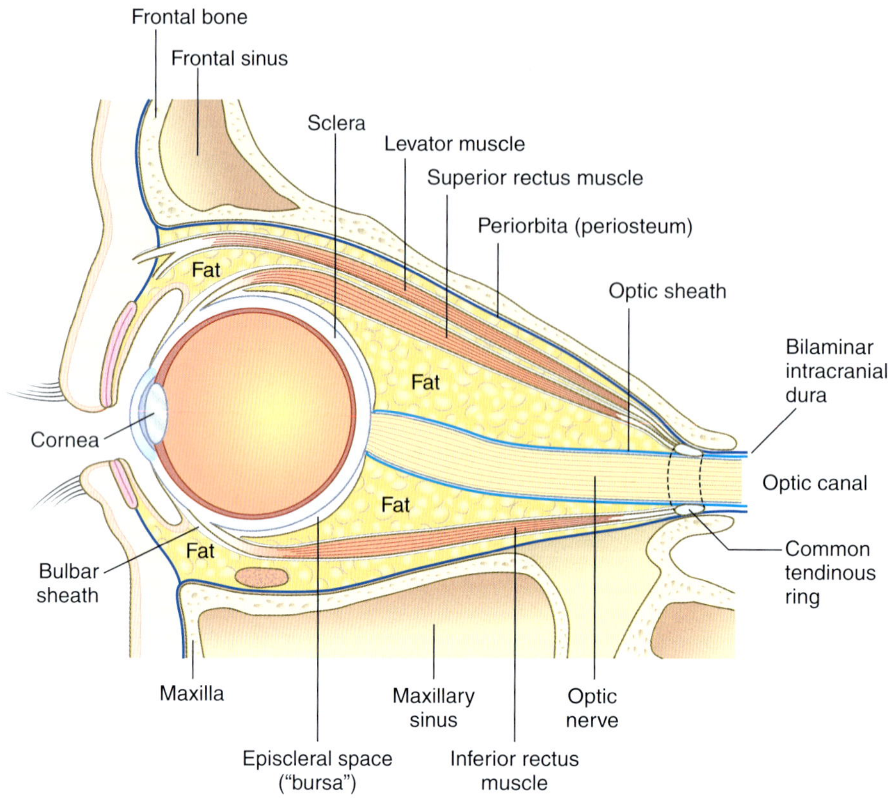

• **Fig. 4.3** Structures of the orbit. Periorbita: the periosteum that lines the orbital walls. Optic sheath: layer of the bilaminar intracranial dura around the optic nerve. Sclera: the tough whitish outer layer of the eyeball to which extraocular muscles attach. Episcleral space/bursa: outermost layer of sclera attached to Tenon's capsule. (Adapted from Robert F. Yellon, R. F., Timothy P. McBride, T. P., & Davis, H. W. [2007]. Otolaryngology. In: *Atlas of pediatric physical diagnosis* [5th Ed.]. St. Louis, MO: Mosby, Figure 23-57.)

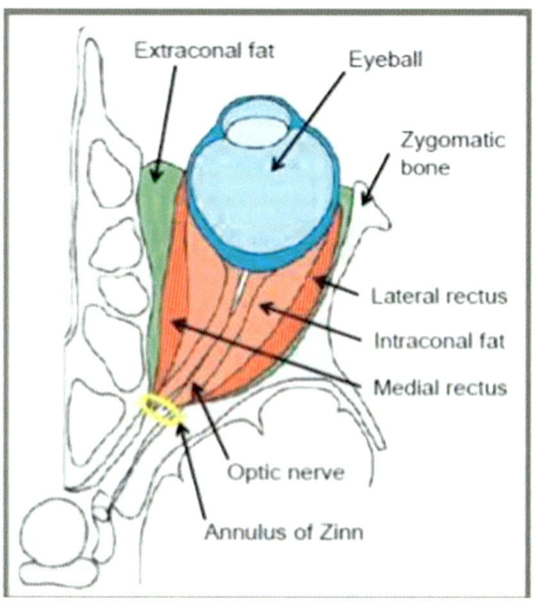

• **Fig. 4.4** Major anatomic orbital components, The eyeball (globe). The optic nerve. The medial and lateral rectus muscle. The Annulus of Zinn (the common tendinous ring). The intraconal and extraconal space and fat. (Adapted from W. S. Müller-Forell [Ed.] [2002]. *Imaging of orbital and visual pathway pathology.* New York, NY: Springer-Verlag. Reproduced with permission of Springer Science + Business Media.)

contents.[7] The orbital septum helps in differentiating orbital cellulitis (behind the septum) and periorbital cellulitis (in front of the septum). Its major purpose is to prevent the spread of infection as a physical barrier against pathogens. It also contains the extraconal fat that is prolapsing with age and is being reduced during blepharoplasty. Also, the annulus of Zinn, a tight fibrous ring, divides the superior orbital fissure into intraconal and extraconal spaces (Fig. 4.4).

Orbital Muscles

The orbit contains seven muscles, the superior palpebrae levator muscle and six other oculomotor muscles: four rectus muscles (superior, inferior, lateral, and medial) and two oblique muscles (superior and inferior)[5,9,10] (Fig. 4.5).

- The superior palpebrae levator originates above the optic canal, where it has a fine and tendinous form, and then broadens out with a triangular form running along the roof of the orbit on top of the superior rectus muscle. It terminates with an anterior tendon into a large fascia, which becomes inserted into the skin of the upper eyelid and upper tarsal plate. This muscle is innervated by the superior division of oculomotor nerve; by its elevating action it raises the upper eyelid, thus uncovering the cornea and portion of sclera, antagonizing the orbicularis oculi muscle, which is innervated by facial nerve. The deep surface of the levator aponeurosis also contains a layer of smooth muscle

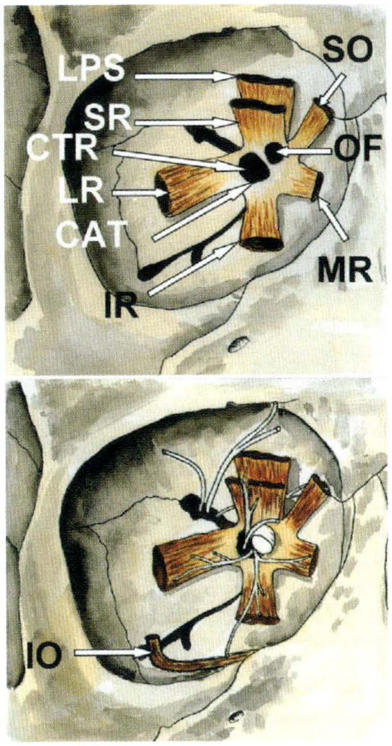

• **Fig. 4.5** Extraocular muscles on the right orbital cavity. Common annular tendon (*CAT*), common tendinous ring (*CTR*), optic foramen (*OF*), levator palpebrae superior muscle (*LPS*), the four rectus muscles: superior (*SR*), medial (*MR*), inferior (*IR*), lateral (*LR*), superior oblique muscle (*SO*), and inferior oblique (*IO*) muscles. (From Hayek, G., Mercier, P. H., & Fournier, H. D. [2006]. Anatomy of the orbit and its surgical approach. In: Pickard, J. D., et al. [Eds.], *Advances and technical standards in neurosurgery* [Vol. 31] [pp. 36–55]. Vienna: Springer, Figure 3.)

known as the Whitnall or Müller muscle, receiving its nerve supply from the superior cervical ganglion via the lacrimal nerve.

- The four rectus muscles form a conical space posterior to the eyeball. They arise from the common annular tendon (tendon of Zinn), which originates from the body of sphenoid, surrounding the superior, medial, and inferior edges of the optic canal and the inferomedial part of the superior orbital fissure. The common ring subsequently splits into the four rectus muscles, which continue forward for 4 cm to terminate in tendons attached to the anterior part of the sclera and control the eye movements.
- The two oblique muscles are the superior oblique and inferior oblique. The superior oblique muscle arises as a short tendon from the upper rim of the optic foramen, passing along the superomedial angle of the orbit. Then it abruptly creates a tendinous acute angle skirting over the trochlea, to continue muscular again with a lateral direction. It passes under the superior rectus muscle to end up on the superolateral side of the posterior part of the globe. The shorter and thinner inferior oblique muscle is located on the anterior edge of the floor of the orbit. It arises from the edge of the lacrimal canal, heading laterally and upward to the lower surface of the eyeball. After passing under the inferior rectus muscle, it ends up on the inferolateral side of the posterior part of the globe.

A fibrous septa system connects all these muscles, including orbital fascia or the Tenon capsule, with neurovascular content that can be considered an important accessory locomotor system contributing to the motility of eye. The role of this septa explains some motility disturbances in blow-out fractures of the orbit.

TABLE 4.2 Intraconal Space Contents

Nerves	Optic nerve (cranial nerve II)
	• Oculomotor nerve (cranial nerve III) ○ Superior division ○ Inferior division (with motor root to the ciliary ganglion)
	• Nasociliary nerve and its intraconal branches (a branch of V1) ○ Long ciliary nerves ○ Short ciliary nerves ○ Small communicating branch of the ciliary ganglion (sensory root)
	• Abducens nerve (cranial nerve VI)
	• Ciliary ganglion
Ophthalmic artery	• Intraconal branches • Central retinal artery • Short posterior ciliary arteries • Long posterior ciliary arteries • Muscular branches
	• Extraconal branches with intraconal origin ○ Posterior ethmoidal artery ○ Supraorbital artery ○ Lacrimal artery
Fat	

Intraconal Space

The intraconal space of the orbit is a musculofascial cone that contains important neurovascular structures and fat (Table 4.2). The base of intraconal space is formed by the posterior part of the globe, whereas the four rectus muscles and their fascia surround this space and converge on the common tendinous ring at the orbital apex.[11-13] The space formed externally between the extraocular muscles and the bony walls is called the extraconal space (Fig. 4.6). The superior and medial rectus muscles arise from the part of the annulus attached to the body of the sphenoid, adjacent to the optic foramen. A tendinous portion of the annulus spanning from the body of sphenoid to the greater wing gives rise to the inferior rectus. The lateral rectus muscle arises from the body of the greater wing along the lateral border of the superior orbital fissure. The Zinn ring corresponds to the bulging end of the superior orbital fissure and provides a passage for the optic nerve, superior and inferior divisions of the oculomotor nerve (cranial nerve [CN] III), the nasociliary branch of CN V1, the abducens nerve (CN VI), and the sympathetic root of the ciliary ganglion, which traverse the intraconal space. The superior ophthalmic vein can also pass through or above this opening, and the inferior ophthalmic vein may pass inside or below it. The remaining structures enter the orbital apex outside the annulus of Zinn, within the extraconal space. They include the lacrimal and frontal nerves (V1 branches), probably the superior ophthalmic vein just below them, and the trochlear nerve (IV) closely applied to the superior fibers of the annulus.[9]

Arteries of the Orbit

The ophthalmic artery (branch of internal carotid artery) provides the main arterial supply of the orbit with significant anastomoses with the maxillary and middle meningeal arteries (branches of the

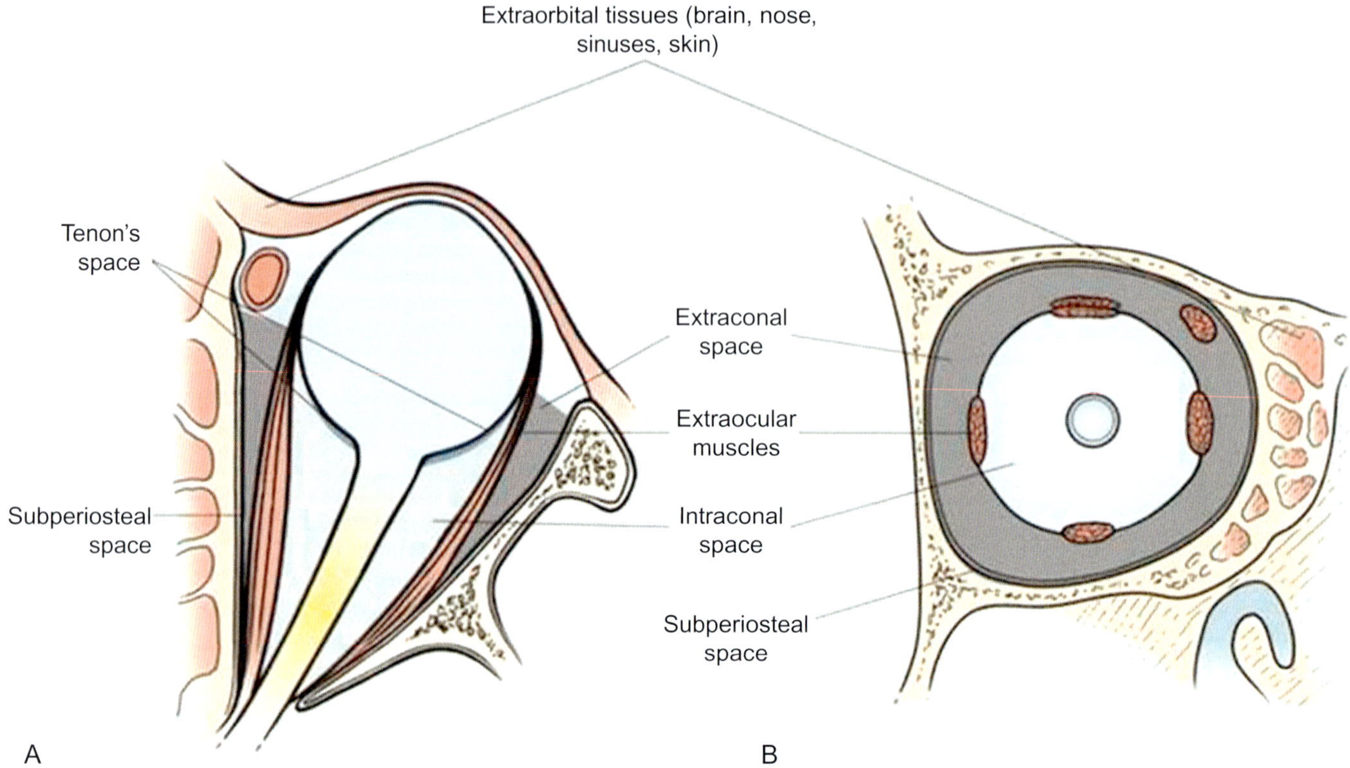

• **Fig. 4.6** The surgical spaces of the orbit. The intraconal space (central surgical space) and extraconal space (peripheral surgical space) are defined by the extraocular muscles. Subperiosteal space; Tenon space; extra-orbital space. A, Axial view. B, Coronal view. (From Nerad J. A. [2010]. *Techniques in ophthalmic plastic surgery: a personal tutorial.* Philadelphia: Elsevier, Figure 14-2.)

external carotid artery), creating further anatomic variations of the branching pattern[14] (Fig. 4.7). The ophthalmic artery stems from the internal carotid artery next to the cavernous sinus, medial to the anterior clinoid process, and then runs through the optic canal below and lateral to the optic nerve within the dural sheath to enter the orbit. It traverses the orbital cavity primarily lateral to the optic nerve and medial to the ciliary ganglion, carrying on from the lateral to medial above the optic nerve in about 80% of cases.[15] Obliquely and accompanied by the nasociliary nerve, the ophthalmic artery continues forward and toward the medial orbital wall between the superior oblique and the medial rectus muscles. It passes under the trochlea and ultimately gives off two terminal branches, the supratrochlear artery and the dorsal artery. The latter forms anastomosis with the angular artery of the nose. Collateral branches of the ophthalmic artery vary in number from 10 to 19. One of the smallest, yet present in all cases, is the central artery of the retina, which arises near the orbital apex and penetrates the optic nerve to occupy a central position at a distance of 10 to 15 mm from the posterior pole of the globe. There are 2 or 3 posterior ciliary arteries, which give rise to as many as 15 short branches, which supply the optic nerve and choroid, and to 2 long posterior ciliary arteries, which enter the sclera supplying the ciliary body and iris.

The lacrimal artery emerges above and outside the optic nerve and travels forward along the lateral rectus muscle as far as the lacrimal gland. As one of the largest branches, it gives off one or two zygomatic branches (zygomaticotemporal, zygomaticofacial anastomosis), lateral palpebral branches, and a recurrent branch that run through the superior orbital fissure to make an anastomosis with a branch of the middle meningeal artery.

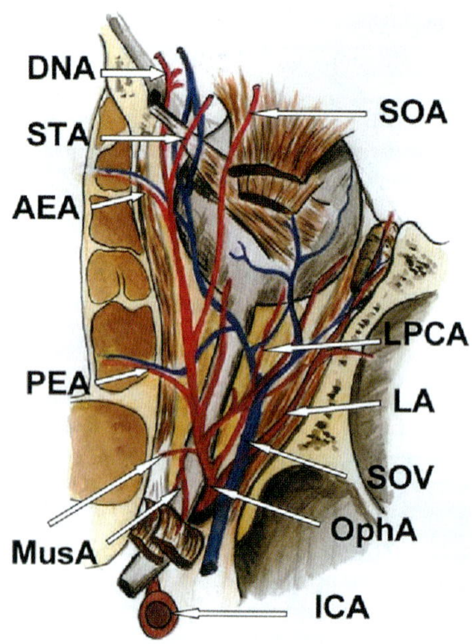

• **Fig. 4.7** Ophthalmic artery and vein of the right orbit and their branches. *AEA,* anterior ethmoidal artery; *DNA*. dorsal nasal artery; *ICA,* Internal carotid artery; *LA,* lacrimal artery; *LPCA,* long posterior ciliary artery; *MusA*. muscle artery; *OphA,* ophthalmic artery; *PEA,* posterior ethmoidal artery; *SOA,* supraorbital artery; *SOV,* superior ophthalmic vein; *STA,* supratrochlear artery. (From Hayek, G., Mercier, P. H., & Fournier, H. D. [2006]. Anatomy of the orbit and its surgical approach. In: Pickard, J. D., et al. [Eds.] *Advances and technical standards in neurosurgery* [Vol. 31] [pp. 36–55]. Vienna: Springer, Figure 4.)

The posterior ethmoidal artery arises within the intraconal space medial and above the optic nerve, and then exits between the superior oblique and the levator muscle toward the posterior ethmoid canal. The anterior ethmoidal artery starts near the anterior ethmoid canal, where it enters accompanied by the respective nerve. The numerous muscular branches supply the extraocular muscles. Within the rectus muscles they divide into two anterior ciliary arteries, except the lateral rectus, which contains only one, that pierce the globe at the tendinous insertion to join with the long posterior ciliary arteries.

The supraorbital artery travels forward in the superior orbit between the levator and the periorbita, and then leaves the cone and accompanied by the supraorbital nerve enters the supraorbital foramen. The medial palpebral arteries (superior and inferior) start below the trochlea. The supratrochlear artery and the dorsal artery exit the orbit medially as the terminal branches, accompanied by the supratrochlear nerve to supply the forehead and scalp. The infraorbital artery, a terminal branch of the maxillary artery, passes through the inferior orbital fissure and gives branches to the orbital fat and to the inferior rectus and inferior oblique muscles before entering the infraorbital canal until the infraorbital foramen. It forms anastomoses with the angular and the inferior palpebral artery.[15]

Veins of the Orbit

The orbital venous drainage to the cavernous sinus is carried out by a very dense venous network consisting of the two valveless ophthalmic veins[5] (Fig. 4.8). The larger superior ophthalmic vein originates in the superonasal quadrant of the orbit near the trochlea, formed by the angular, supraorbital, and supratrochlear veins. This vessel extends posterolaterally under the superior rectus muscle to enter the superior orbital fissure, outside the annulus of Zinn, and ultimately drains into the cavernous sinus. On its course, it receives many of collateral tributaries, including ethmoidal, muscular, ciliary, vorticose (from the choroid), lacrimal, palpebral, conjunctival, and the episcleral rami and the central vein of the retina.

The inferior ophthalmic vein is more variable and usually originates in the anterior inferomedial part of the orbit. It receives tributaries from muscular, vortex, medial, and lateral collateral veins. It courses posteriorly above the inferior rectus muscle and usually joins the superior ophthalmic vein before reaching the apex, although in some cases it terminates into the cavernous sinus as a distinct vessel. It also communicates with the pterygoid plexus via the inferior orbital fissure. The connection between the facial vein, pterygoid plexus, and cavernous sinus through the orbital venous drainage system is of paramount clinical significance, as it harbors an underlying risk of infection, spreading from the face to the intracranial contents.

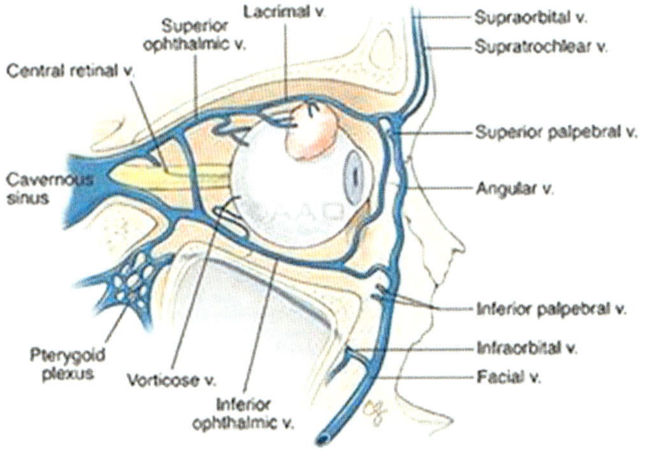

• **Fig. 4.8** Veins of the eye and of the orbit, right side; lateral view into the orbit; after removal of the lateral wall of the orbit. The superior and inferior ophthalmic veins drain the venous blood from the orbit and eye. Venous anastomoses exist to the veins of the superficial and deep facial regions (pterygoid plexus) and to the cavernous sinus. *v,* Vein. (From Paulsen, F., & Waschke, T. [2019]. *Sobotta atlas of human anatomy* [Vol. 3] [15th ed., English]. Munich: Elsevier GmbH, Figure 9.16.)

Nerves of the Orbit

The optic nerve (CN II) along with the ophthalmic artery runs through the optic canal. CNs III, IV, and VI and the ophthalmic and maxillary branch of CN V pass through the cavernous sinus, closely related to each other and to the plexus of sympathetic fibers of the internal carotid artery on their course to the orbit. Apart from the maxillary branch, all of them enter through the superior orbital fissure[5] (Table 4.3, Fig. 4.9).

The optic nerve is conventionally divided into three different parts: intraorbital, intracanicular, and intracranial. The intraorbital segment (30 mm) traverses the orbit inside fatty tissue surrounded by the extraocular muscles; its sinuous course enables the eyeball movement without neural damage. At this part the ophthalmic artery crosses over the nerve, and the ciliary ganglion juxtaposed is located medial to the lateral rectus. The intracanicular segment (5 mm) is accompanied inferiorly by the ophthalmic artery and medially by the nasociliary nerve. A very thin lamella separates this segment from the sphenoidal sinus and the posterior ethmoidal cells. The intracranial segment (10 mm) extends beyond the orbit to the optic chiasm.

The oculomotor nerve (CN III) divides the into superior and inferior branches, which enter through the medial part of the superior orbital fissure inside the annulus of Zinn and subsequently diverge away from each other. The superior division supplies the levator palpebrae superioris and superior rectus muscles, whereas the inferior division supplies the medial rectus, inferior rectus, and the inferior oblique muscle. The branch to the inferior oblique muscle travels along and crosses the inferior rectus, where it is susceptible to iatrogenic injury. In addition, after a synapse at the ciliary ganglion, a small branch carrying preganglionic parasympathetic fibers joins the short ciliary nerves that innervate the intraocular muscles.

The trochlear nerve (CN IV) passes through the superior orbital fissure medial to the frontal nerve. It runs above the muscle cone heading forward and medial to reach the superior oblique muscle. As the thinnest cranial nerve with the longest intracranial course, it is particularly vulnerable to traumatic injury causing double vision.

The abducens nerve (CN VI) enters through the medial part of the superior orbital fissure within the common tendinous ring, lateral to the oculomotor nerve branches. Then it passes along the medial surface of lateral rectus, piercing the muscle with four or five terminal branches.[5,9]

The ophthalmic division of the trigeminal nerve (CN V1) and some contribution from the maxillary division (V2) are the sensory nerves of the orbit. In the lateral wall of the cavernous sinus the ophthalmic nerve divides into the lacrimal, frontal, and nasociliary branches.[16]

TABLE 4.3 Nerves of the Orbit

Nerve	Function	Destination
Optic (cranial nerve II)	Sensory: Sight (from retinal ganglion cells)	Lateral geniculate body
Oculomotor (cranial nerve III) Superior branch Inferior branch	Motor: elevation of eyelid Adduction, depression, abduction, extorsion, elevation of the globe Parasympathetic: motor to iris sphincter and ciliary muscle	Superior: Superior palpebrae levator muscle Superior rectus muscle Inferior: Medial rectus muscle Inferior rectus muscle Inferior oblique muscle Ciliary ganglion
Trochlear (cranial nerve IV)	Motor: depression, abduction, intorsion of the globe	Superior oblique muscle
Abducens (cranial nerve VI)	Motor: abduction	Lateral rectus muscle
Ophthalmic branch (V1): Lacrimal branch Frontal branch Nasociliary branch	Sensory: fibers to skin and conjunctiva Parasympathetic: secretomotor fibers to lacrimal nerve	Eyeball Lacrimal gland Upper lid skin Conjuctiva Mucosa of the nasal cavity Skin of the nose, forehead, scalp
Maxillary branch (V2): Infraorbital nerve Zygomatic branch	Sensory: fibers to skin and conjunctiva Parasympathetic: secretomotor fibers to lacrimal nerve	Lower lid skin Conjunctiva Upper lip, cheek skin Temporal skin Lacrimal gland
Ciliary ganglion	Autonomic center: Sympathetic: fibers from carotid plexus Parasympathetic: motor to iris sphincter and ciliary muscle Sensory: nasociliary nerve and 5-6 short ciliary nerves	Iris dilator Ocular blood vessels Iris sphincter and ciliary muscle Globe

The lacrimal nerve enters the fissure outside the cone and travels along the lateral rectus muscle besides the lacrimal artery toward the lacrimal fossa. Parasympathetic secretomotor fibers coming from the pterygopalatine ganglion via the zygomaticotemporal nerve join the lacrimal nerve on the way to the lacrimal gland.

The frontal nerve passes through the tapered part of the fissure, outside the cone, between the lacrimal nerve and the trochlear nerve. It continues anteriorly between the levator muscle and the periorbita. It divides into to the smaller medial supratrochlear nerve and the large lateral supraorbital nerve. The first passes above the trochlea of the superior oblique muscle and supplies the medial upper lid, conjunctiva, and forehead, whereas the second runs through the supraorbital foramen and distributes to the brow, forehead, and scalp skin.

The nasociliary nerve enters the superior orbital fissure within the common tendinous ring. Then it crosses the optic nerve together with the ophthalmic artery and continues obliquely toward the medial wall, between the medial rectus and the superior rectus and superior oblique muscles. On its trajectory, the nasociliary nerve gives off various sensory branches, which include the following from back to front:

- The communicating branch (sensory root) of the ciliary ganglion leaves the nasociliary nerve early when entering the cone. It is composed of sensory fibers for the corneal as well as sympathetic fibers for the iris dilator, coming from the cervicotrigeminal anastomosis.
- The posterior ethmoidal nerve enters the corresponding canal and distributes to the sphenoidal sinus and posterior ethmoidal cells.
- Two or three long ciliary nerves join the short ciliary nerves (from the ciliary ganglion) containing the sympathetic fibers for the iris dilator. They perforate the sclera and terminate in the ciliary body, the iris, and the cornea.
- The anterior ethmoidal nerve crosses the corresponding canal with the same artery and then passes over the cribriform plate of the ethmoidal bone.
- The infratrochlear nerve, the lateral terminal branch, continues under the trochlea of the superior oblique muscle. It supplies the medial canthus, part of the conjunctiva and lacrimal ducts, part of the eyelid, and the root of the nose.
- The maxillary nerve (CN V2), after giving off sphenopalatine and zygomatic branches, enters through the inferior orbital fissure as the infraorbital nerve. It continues forward into the infraorbital canal, exiting the infraorbital foramen to supply the lower lid and conjunctiva, upper lip, and cheek skin. The zygomaticotemporal and zygomaticofacial branches that supply the temporal skin come from the zygomatic branch of CN V2, as it has traversed the inferior orbital fissure.[17] The lacrimal nerve also receives secretomotor fibers carried by the zygomaticotemporal branch, destined for the lacrimal gland.
- The ciliary ganglion is located close to the orbital apex between the lateral aspect of the optic nerve and the lateral rectus muscle, inside fatty tissue. It receives three roots: a sympathetic, parasympathetic, and sensory root[9] (Fig. 4.10).
- The sympathetic fibers are a branch of the carotid plexus, which enters the orbit via the common tendinous ring, destined for the iris dilator and ocular blood vessels.

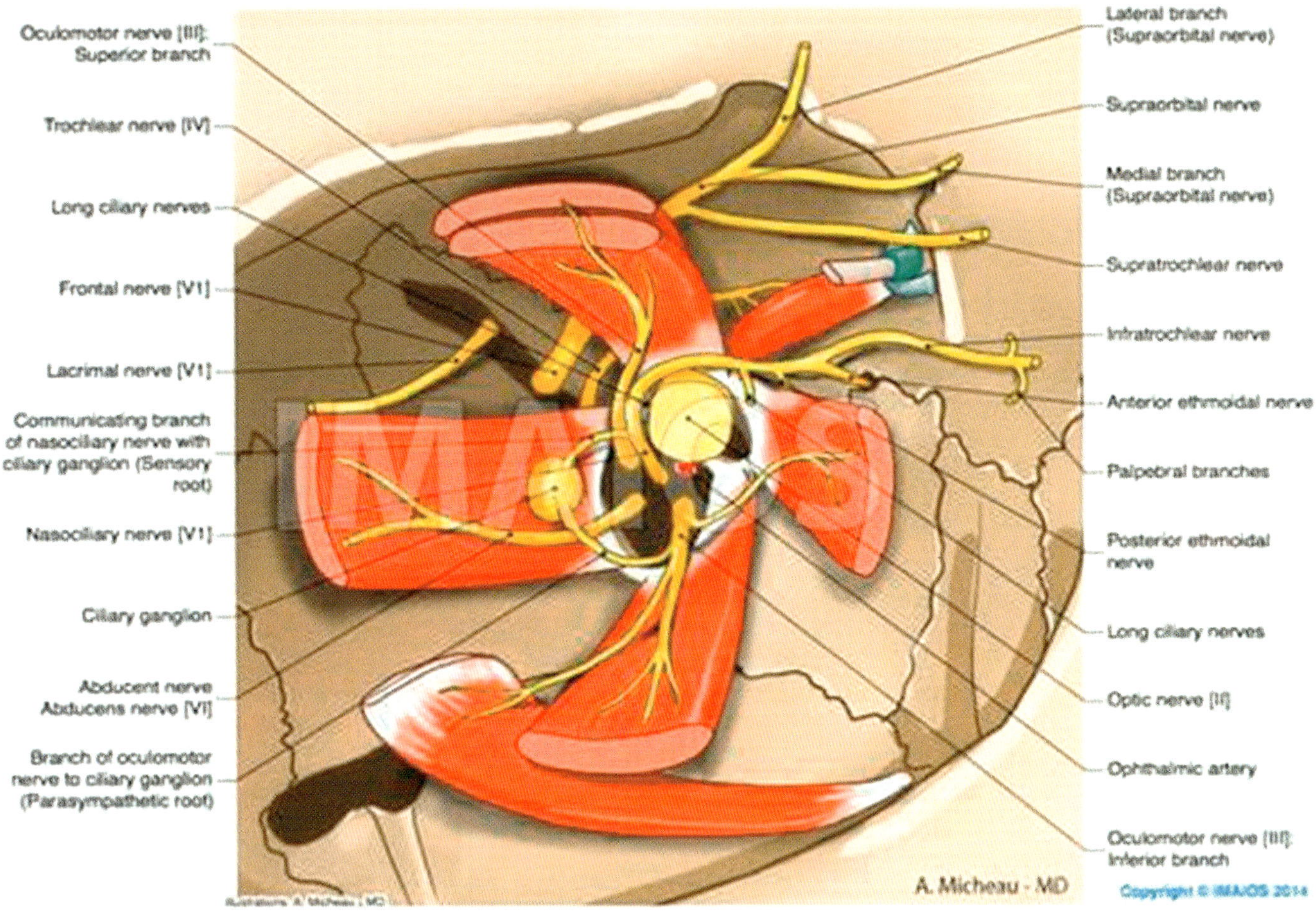

• **Fig. 4.9** Orbital nerves. Lacrimal nerve (V1); frontal nerve (V1): supraorbital branch, supratrochlear branch; trochlear nerve (IV); oculomotor nerve (III): superior branch, inferior branch. Nasociliary nerve (V1): long ciliary nerves, infratrochlear nerve, communicating branch, anterior ethmoidal nerve. Ciliary ganglion, optic nerve (II), abducens nerve (VI). (From Dutton J. J. [2011]. *Atlas of clinical and surgical orbital anatomy* [2nd ed.] [pp. 51–82]. Philadelphia: Elsevier, Figure 4-7.)

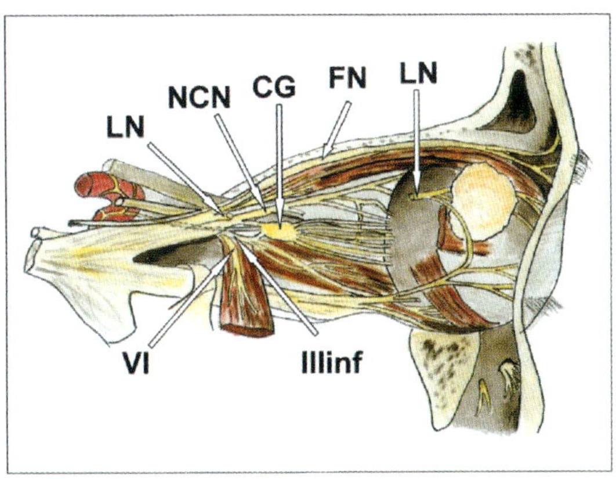

• **Fig. 4.10** Orbital nerves. Right orbit, lateral view. *CG*, ciliary ganglion; *FN*, frontal nerve; *IIIinf*, inferior division of oculomotor nerve; *LN*, Lacrimal nerve; *NCN*, nasociliary nerve; *VI*, abductor nerve. (From Hayek, G., Mercier, P. H., & Fournier, H. D. [2006]. Anatomy of the orbit and its surgical approach. In: Pickard, J. D., et al. [Eds.], *Advances and technical standards in neurosurgery* [Vol. 31] [pp. 36–55]. Vienna: Springer.)

- The motor or preganglionic parasympathetic fibers come from the inferior branch of the third cranial nerve (by the inferior oblique branch) to the iris sphincter and ciliary muscle. Only the parasympathetic fibers synapse in the ciliary ganglion.
- The sensory fibers, heading to the globe and cornea, are supplied by the nasociliary nerve. Five or six short ciliary nerves pass from the ciliary ganglion to the globe, inserting around the optic nerve.

Lacrimal System

The lacrimal system consists of the lacrimal gland and the lacrimal excretory system[18] (Fig. 4.11). The main lacrimal gland is located in the superotemporal part of orbit, contained within the periorbita. It consists of two different parts, separated by the levator muscle fascia: the upper, orbital lobe and the lower, palpebral lobe. The orbital part lies in the shallow lacrimal fossa of the zygomatic process of the frontal bone. The palpebral part extends below the levator muscle sheath in the lateral part of the upper eyelid. The lacrimal gland is composed of multiple secretory units, progressively draining into ducts that pour into the conjunctiva. The secretory system includes also numerous accessory glands, located in the middle of the lid (the Wolfring gland) or in the conjunctival fornix (the Krause gland).[7] The lacrimal artery and ophthalmic vein are responsible for the blood supply and drainage of the gland, respectively.

The lacrimal apparatus is supplied by a sympathetic root of the carotid plexus and parasympathetic secretomotor fibers of the facial nerve. Sensory innervation is via the lacrimal nerve of ophthalmic branch of CN V. The lacrimal excretory system begins at the

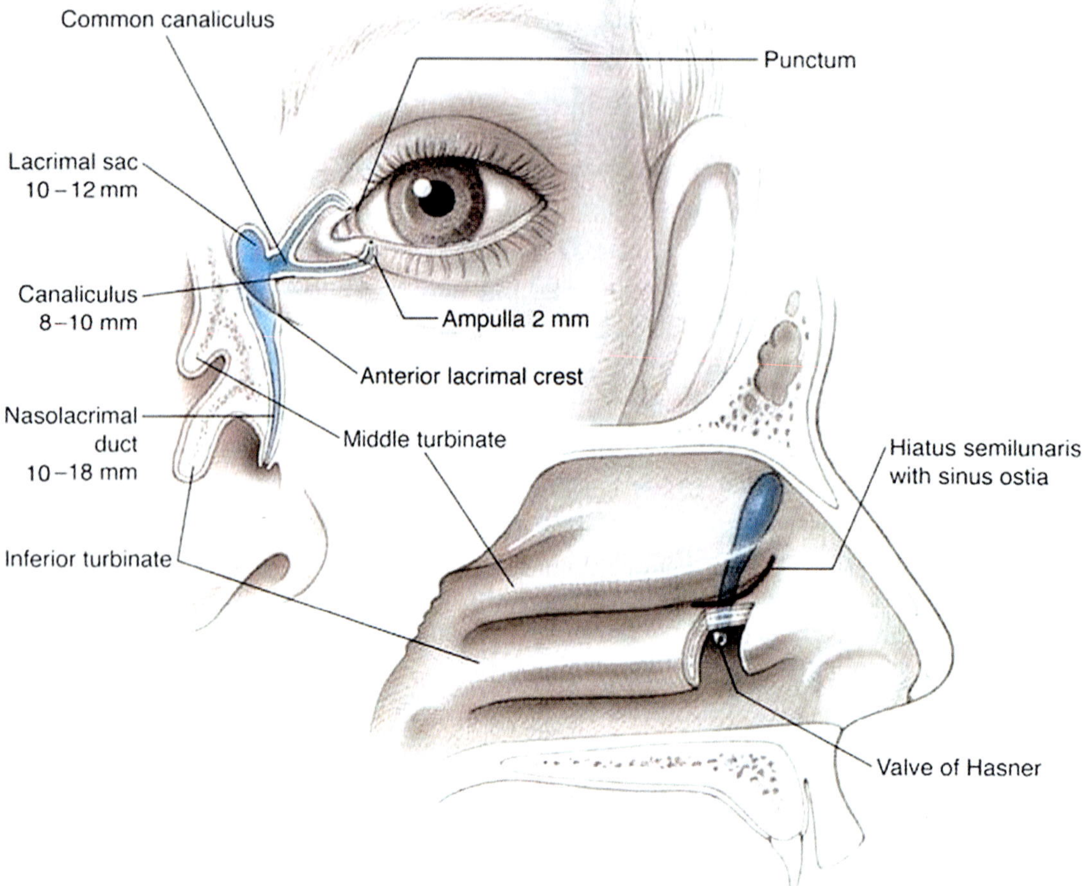

• **Fig. 4.11** Anatomy of the lacrimal apparatus. Lacrimal gland and conjunctival sac. Lacrimal punctum-Ampulla-Lacrimal canaliculus. Lacrimal sac. Nasolacrimal duct. (From Holland, E. J., Mannis, M. J., & Lee, W. B. [2013]. *Ocular surface disease: cornea, conjunctiva and tear Film*. Philadelphia: Elsevier, Figure 2.6.)

punctum in the medial end of each eyelid and then widens into ampulla and drains into the canaliculus. The superior and inferior canaliculi ultimately unite into a common canaliculus, which terminates at the lacrimal sac with the Rosenmüller valve. The lacrimal sac resides in the lacrimal fossa, confined by the anterior lacrimal crest of frontal process of maxilla and by the posterior lacrimal crest of the lacrimal bone itself. The sac concealed by the periorbita, forming the lacrimal fascia, opens below and continues with the nasolacrimal duct. The Hasner valve is found at the lower end of the duct at the level of the inferior nasal meatus.

References

1. Rootman, J., Stewart, B., & Goldberg, R. A. (1995). Orbital anatomy. In *Orbital surgery: A conceptual approach* (pp. 79–146). Philadelphia: Lippincott-Raven.
2. Romanes, G. J. (1964). *Cunningham's textbook of anatomy* (10th ed.). London: Oxford University Press.
3. Rontal, E., Rontal, M., & Guilford, F. T. (1979). Surgical anatomy of the orbit. *Annals of Otolology, Rhinolology & Laryngology*, *88*(3 Pt1), 382–386.
4. Doxanas, M. T., & Anderson, R. L. (1984). *Clinical orbital anatomy.* Baltimore: Williams & Wilkins.
5. Hayek, G., Mercier, P. H., & Fournier, H. D. (2006). Anatomy of the orbit and its surgical approach. In: Pickard, J. D., et al. (Eds.), *Advances and technical standards in neurosurgery* (Vol. 31) (pp. 36–55). Vienna: Springer.
6. Shi, X., Han, H., Zhao, J., & Zhou, C. (2007). Microsurgical anatomy of the superior orbital fissure. *Clinical Anatomy (New York, N.Y.)*, *20*(4), 362–366.
7. Koorneef, L. (1979). Orbital septa: Anatomy and function. *Ophthalmology*, *86*, 876–885.
8. Thiagarajan, B. (2013). Anatomy of orbit: Ptolaryngologist's perspective. *ENT Scholar*, 1–15. Available at: https://www.researchgate.net/publication/235418410. Accessed February 9, 2013.
9. Rene, C. (2006). Update on orbital anatomy. *Eye*, *20*(10), 1119–1129.
10. Turvey, T. A., & Golden, B. A. (2012). Orbital anatomy for the surgeon. *Oral and Maxillofacial Surgery Clinics of North America*, *24*(4), 525–536.
11. Ochs, M. W., & Buckley, M. J. (1993). Anatomy of the orbit. *Oral and Maxillofacial Surgery Clinics of North America*, *5*, 419–429.
12. Kainz, J., & Stammberger, H. (1992). Danger areas of the posterior rhinobasis: An endoscopic and anatomical-surgical study. *Acta Oto-Laryngologica*, *112*, 852–861.
13. Raza, S. M., Quiñones-Hinojosa, A., & Subramanian, P. S. (2012). Multimodal treatment of orbital tumors. In A. Quiñones-Hinojosa (Ed.), *Schmidek and Sweet: Operative neurosurgical techniques* (pp. 597–602) (6th ed.). Philadelphia: Saunders.

14. Hayreh, S. S. (1964). The ophthalmic artery. III: Branches. *British Journal of Ophthalmology*, *46*(4), 212–247.
15. Hayreh, S. S., & Dass, R. (1962). The ophthalmic artery. II: Intra-orbital course. *British Journal of Ophthalmology*, *46*(3), 165–185.
16. Moore, K. L., Dalley, A. F., Agur, A. M. R., & Dalley, A. F. (2014). *Clinically oriented anatomy* (7th ed.). Baltimore: Lippincott Williams & Wilkins.
17. Ference, E. H., Smith, S. S., Conley, D., & Chandra, R. K. (2015). Surgical anatomy and variations of the infraorbital nerve. *Laryngoscope*, *125*(6), 1296–1300.
18. Tasman, W., & Jaeger, E. A. (2007). Embryology and anatomy of the orbit and lacrimal system. In *Duane's ophthalmology*. Baltimore: Lippincott Williams & Wilkins.

5

Surgical Anatomy of the Nose, Septum, and Sinuses

EDWARD C. KUAN, MD, MBA AND JAMES N. PALMER, MD

The nasal cavity and paranasal sinuses are intimately associated with the orbit, and as such frequently serve as an appropriate surgical corridor for endoscopic access to orbital pathology. For instance, the lamina papyracea, or the medial wall of the orbit, serves as the lateral boundary of a complete ethmoid sinus dissection, and inadvertent orbital entry is possible during routine endoscopic sinus surgery. A high nasal septal deviation may challenge the orbital surgeon during endoscopic orbital decompression or dacryocystorhinostomy. Finally, the superolateral wall of the sphenoid sinus or, in some cases, a posterolateral ethmoid air cell is indented by the optic canal, and recognition of these anatomic variants is important to avoid optic nerve injury. Thus a thorough understanding of the surgical anatomy of the nose, septum, and paranasal sinuses is critical for ensuring optimal outcomes in endoscopic orbital surgery.

Surgical Anatomy and Principles Relevant to the Orbital Surgeon

Nares

The orbital surgeon's corridor begins at the nares (nostrils), or the entry point into the nasal cavity. The most anterior aspect of the nares, termed the *nasal vestibule*, is circumferentially lined by skin. The keratinized squamous epithelial lining abruptly transitions to respiratory mucosa (ciliated pseudostratified columnar epithelium) at the limen nasi, or mucocutaneous junction. From this point posteriorly, the entire nasal cavity, including within the paranasal sinuses, is lined by respiratory mucosa.

Airflow into the nasal passages is regulated at two levels of potential resistance. The external nasal valve is at the level of the nasal vestibule and is bordered by the columella medially, including the caudal nasal septum and medial crura, the nasal sill inferiorly, and the alar cartilage superolaterally. This area is also especially important for endoscopic surgeons, as effective use of the endoscope requires the ability to provide enough distraction and stability against the edges of the nares for maneuvering instruments. More posteriorly, the internal nasal valve, which is the major resistor of airflow and is located at the level of the limen nasi, is bounded by the upper lateral cartilage superiorly, the nasal septum medially, and the anterior head of the inferior turbinate laterally. Recognizing these potential areas for narrowing of the nasal passages, and the potential need to surgically address these areas before orbital surgery, is crucial.

Nasal Septum

The nasal septum divides the left and right nasal cavities (Fig. 5.1). It is lined by mucoperichondrium anteriorly (covering the quadrangular cartilage) and mucoperiosteum posteriorly (covering the bony septum), and superiorly becomes continuous with the cribriform plate mucosa, and inferiorly with the nasal floor mucosa. In the absence of trauma or surgical manipulation, the posterior aspect of the quadrangular cartilage articulates neatly with the bony septum at the bony-cartilaginous junction. The bony septum consists of the perpendicular plate of the ethmoid bone superiorly, extending to the cribriform plate, and the vomer inferiorly, which borders the choana. The most inferior aspect of the nasal septum is the bony maxillary crest, which consists of the maxillary bone anteriorly and the palatine bone posteriorly.

The septum has a notably rich vascular supply and is the most common site of epistaxis (nosebleeds), accounting for more than 90% of cases (Fig. 5.2). Specifically, the Kiesselbach plexus is a rich arcade of terminal arterial anastomoses located at the anterior septal mucosa bilaterally; it receives tributaries from the sphenopalatine artery, anterior ethmoidal artery, greater palatine artery, and superior labial artery.

Just anterior to the middle turbinates, the bilateral nasal septum may form a symmetrically protuberant zone known as the septal swell bodies. This is a specialized area of the nasal septum containing a higher proportion of venous sinusoids and may impede the surgeon from posterior surgical access.[1] However, topical decongestion generally allows for vasoconstriction and transient shrinkage of the swell bodies, thereby permitting maneuverability around them.

In general, no septum is naturally straight, and there is always some degree of curvature or the presence of cartilaginous or bony spurs (Fig. 5.3). Despite the presence of septal deviations, many patients do not experience clinically significant nasal obstruction in the absence of mucosal edema or inflammation, or a history of nasal trauma. In fact, many septal deviations are high and do not obstruct the nasal airway, which is lower down along the nasal floor. However, high septal deviations pose a unique problem for the endoscopic orbital surgeon, as they may preclude surgical access to the sinuses and thus limit the corridor to the orbit (Fig. 5.4).

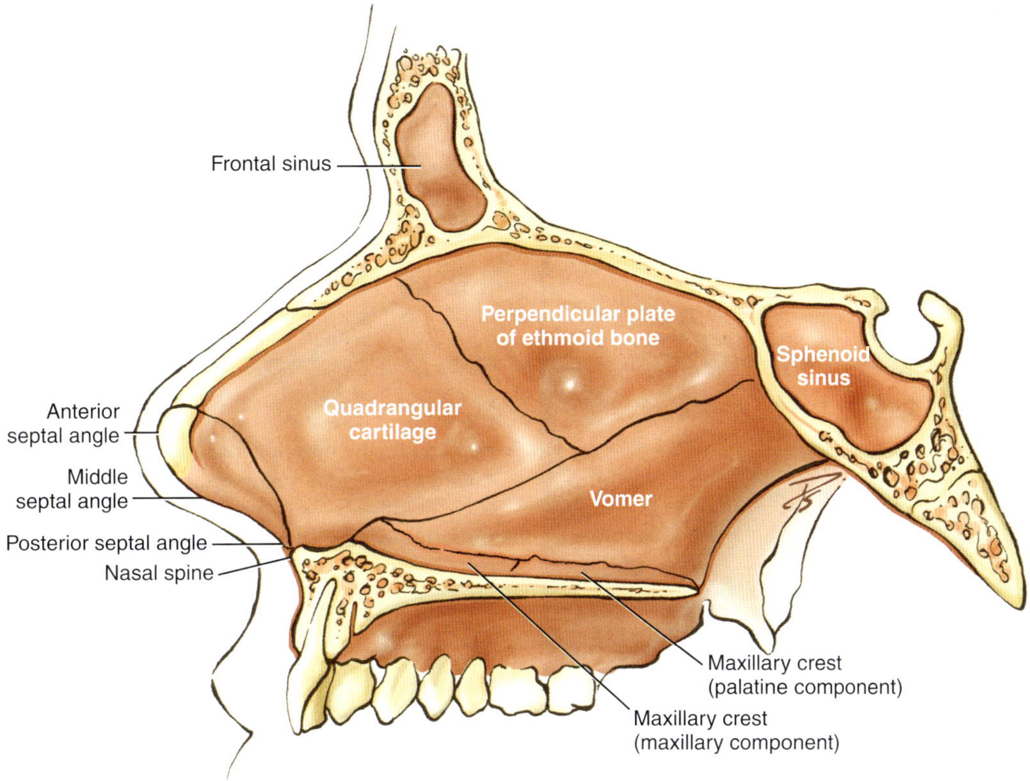

• **Fig. 5.1** Anatomy of the nasal septum. (From Chiu, A. G., Palmer, J. N., & Adappa, N. D. (Eds.). (2019). *Atlas of endoscopic sinus and skull base surgery* (2nd ed., Figure 1.1). Philadelphia: Elsevier.)

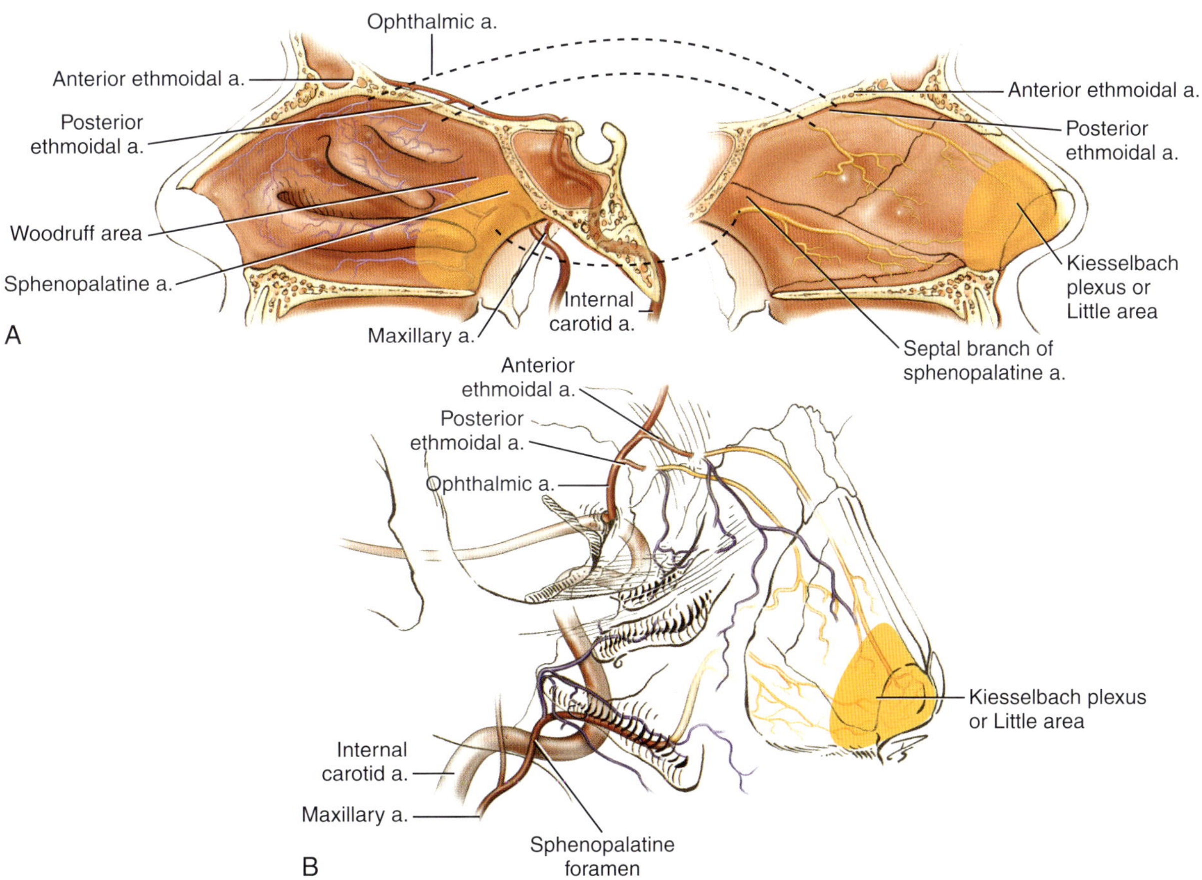

• **Fig. 5.2** Vascular supply of the nasal cavity. A, The lateral nasal wall and nasal septum are supplied by the various tributaries of the internal and external carotid arteries (B). *a,* Artery. (From Chiu, A. G., Palmer, J. N., & Adappa, N. D. (Eds.). (2019). *Atlas of endoscopic sinus and skull base surgery* (2nd ed., Figure 3.1). Philadelphia: Elsevier.)

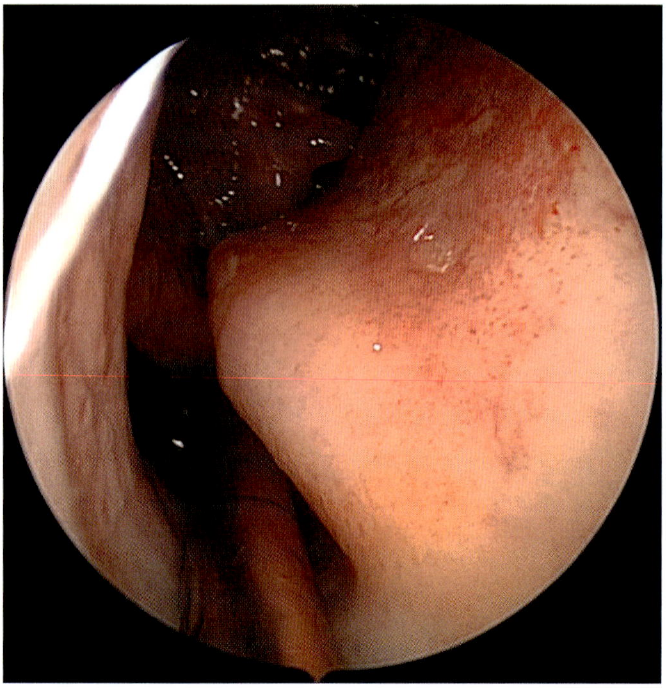

• **Fig. 5.3** Right anterior septal spur causing nasal obstruction. The inferior turbinate can be seen laterally, with nasal polyps more posteriorly emanating from the middle meatus.

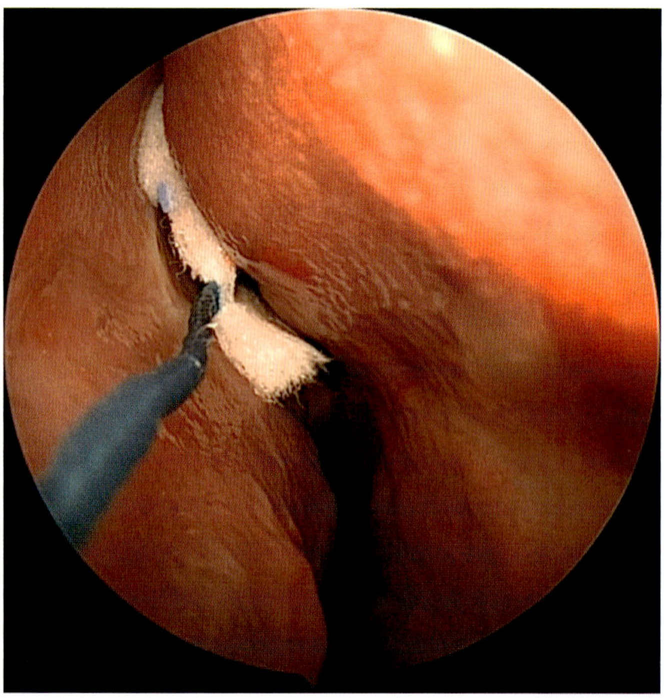

• **Fig. 5.4** High right septal deviation. These deviations, though often not causing symptomatic nasal obstruction, pose a unique challenge to the endoscopic endonasal surgeon owing to lack of access to the middle meatus. A cotton pledget sits between the lateral nasal wall and the deviated part of the septum.

Septoplasty to correct the deviated nasal septum may be approached through a standard incision (hemitransfixion, along the caudal edge of the caudal septum, or Killian, more posteriorly, along the mucocutaneous junction) or a directed "spurectomy" (incision made right anterior to the area of deviation). Care must be taken to preserve a 1- to 1.5-cm L-shaped dorsal and caudal strut of cartilage anteriorly to preserve nasal tip support. Elevation of a submucoperichondrial flap, followed by incision of the quadrangular cartilage and elevation of a contralateral flap, allows for adequate exposure of the deviated bone and cartilage, which may then be removed. Superior dissection during septoplasty must be avoided, as cerebrospinal fluid leak, though rare, is possible.

Inferior Turbinate

The bilateral inferior turbinates are located along the inferior half of the lateral nasal wall and through the entire length of the nasal passage. These paired structures increase the overall surface area of the nasal mucosa and aid in humidification of inhaled air. The submucosa of the inferior turbinate is rich in venous supply and undergoes regular congestion and decongestion approximately every 90 minutes as part of the nasal physiologic cycle. For this reason, the inferior turbinates are very sensitive to inflammatory changes of the nasal mucosa (e.g., allergic, vasomotor), and commonly serve as an area of nasal obstruction. Similarly, they are very sensitive to decongestants (e.g., oxymetazoline, phenylephrine, epinephrine, cocaine), and tend to shrink in girth with topical application. The major blood supply of the inferior turbinate arises from branches of the sphenopalatine artery, which enters the turbinate from posteriorly.

A simple and high-yield procedure at the outset of any endonasal orbital surgery involves manipulating the inferior turbinates to create room in the nasal cavity for surgical dissection. Inferior turbinate infracture and outfracture is accomplished using a Freer elevator (Skylar Surgical Instruments, West Chester, PA), where it is first placed within the inferior meatus against the lateral edge of the anterior head of the inferior turbinate and fractured medially (should result in a palpable and/or audible "crack"), and is then followed with a lateral fracture against the medial surface of the turbinate head (Fig. 5.5). This is carried along the entire length of the inferior turbinate and serves to create a working channel for instrument maneuvering, dissection, and creating of drip spaces. By performing both infracture and outfracture, a complete fracture through the inferior turbinate bone is created, which allows long-term remodeling of the nasal airway.

Middle Turbinate

The middle turbinate consists of three components (Fig. 5.6). The first component is the most readily visible when inspecting the nasal cavity, and appears as a vertical and sagittally oriented structure attached to the skull base superiorly. The septum is medial to the middle turbinate, and the space between the vertical component of the middle turbinate and the lateral nasal wall is termed the *middle meatus*. The middle meatus is the "gateway" to endoscopic orbital surgery, as full exposure of the lamina papyracea can be accomplished only through complete dissection of structures beyond the middle meatus. The second component of the middle turbinate, also known as the basal lamella, is coronally oriented and attached to the lamina papyracea. This important landmark separates the anterior and posterior ethmoid air cells. The third component is horizontal and posteroinferior, and attaches to the perpendicular plate of the palatine bone just medial to the sphenopalatine foramen. Like the inferior turbinate, the dominant blood supply of the middle turbinate comes from branches of the sphenopalatine artery, which enter the turbinate through the horizontal component from posteriorly.

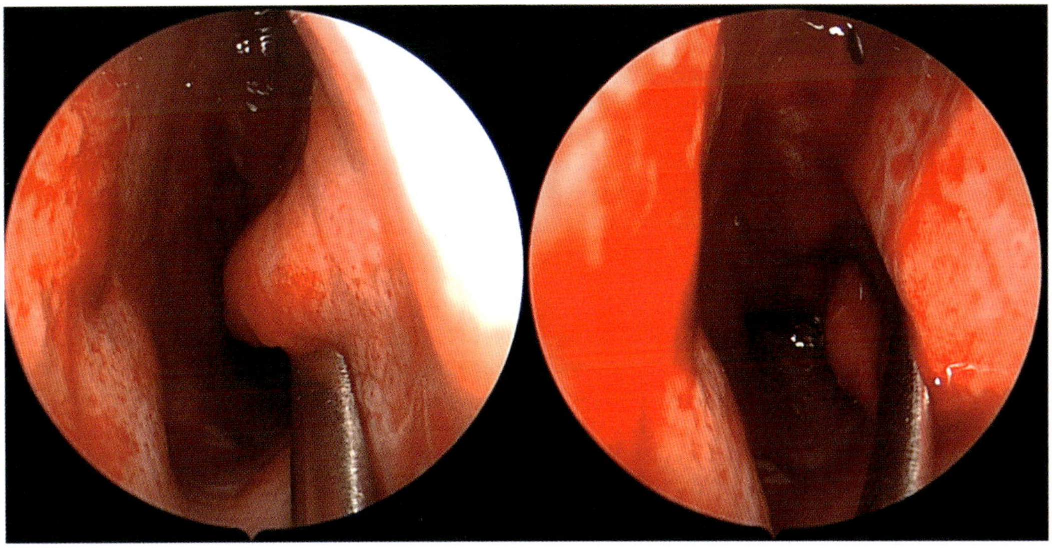

• **Fig. 5.5** Infracture (medial, *left*) and outfracture (lateral, *right*) of the inferior turbinate using a Freer elevator. This provides additional room for the surgical corridor.

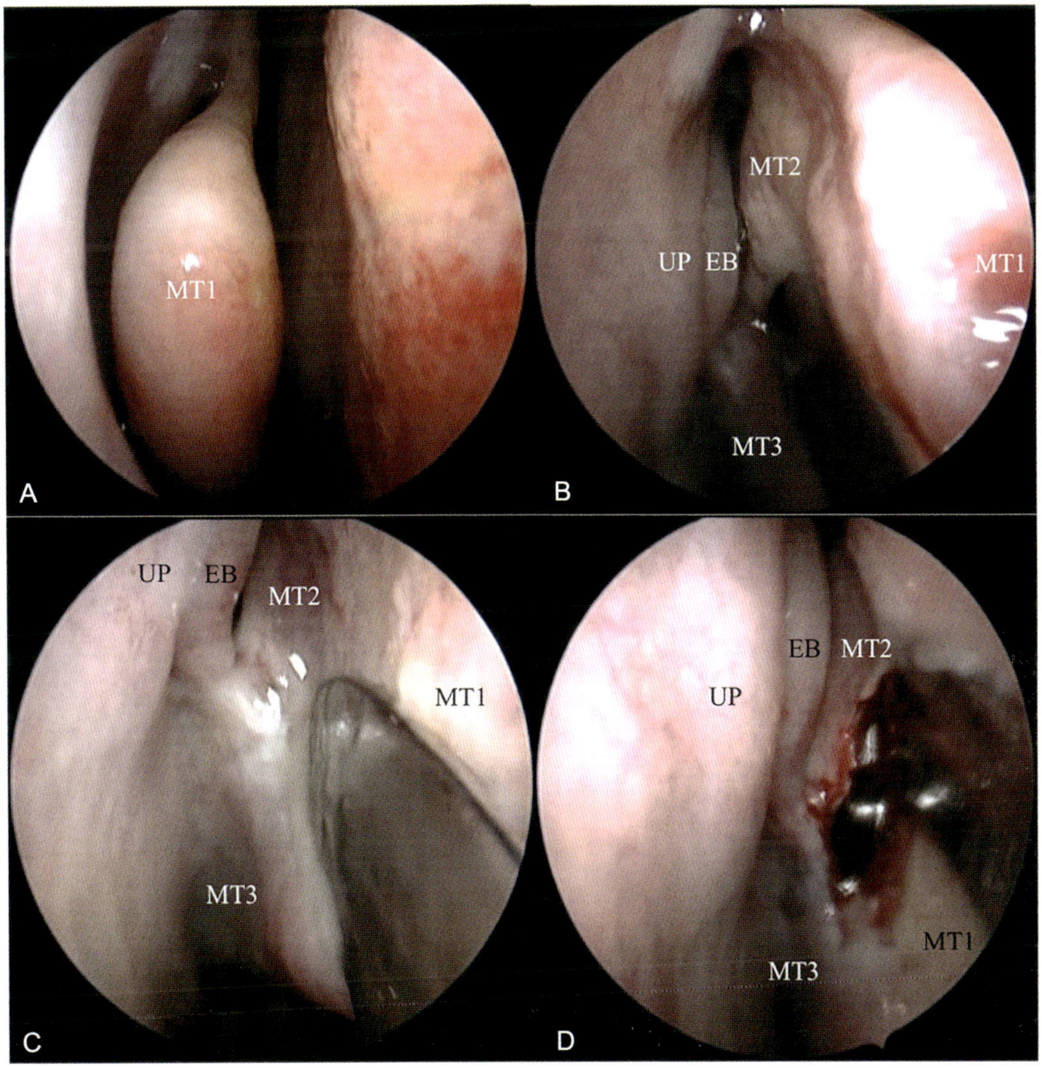

• **Fig. 5.6** Parts of the middle turbinate. A, The vertical/sagittal part (*MT1*) is the most apparent in nasal endoscopy. B, Distraction of the vertical part reveals the basal lamella (*MT2*) and horizontal part (*MT3*) within the middle meatus. C, Further medial distraction reveals the three sequential lamella to remove in endoscopic sinus surgery: the uncinate process (*UP*), ethmoid bulla (*EB*), and basal lamella. D, Here, a relaxing incision is made in the basal lamella to keep the vertical part of the middle turbinate from lateralizing during sinus surgery.

There are several nuances related to surgery of the middle turbinates. The first and third components of the middle turbinate are responsible for maintaining its structure and stability within the nasal cavity, and thus preservation of the middle turbinate requires that both components remain naturally attached. Care must be taken when dissecting the vertical component of the middle turbinate superiorly, as dissection too high may lead to a cerebrospinal fluid leak along the ethmoid skull base. For most purposes, dissection should remain lateral to the vertical component of the middle turbinate, as the cribriform plate is medial to it, and inadvertent skull base entry may arise if dissection proceeds superiorly.

In prior years, middle turbinate resection was potentially thought of as a cause of "empty nose syndrome" and thus was not generally performed. Other advocates of middle turbinate preservation state that it is a helpful landmark should patients require revision surgery. However, the middle turbinate is frequently diseased, osteitic, or undergoes polypoid degeneration, and resecting the vertical part of it may decrease disease burden (Fig. 5.7). Furthermore, resection of the middle turbinate provides more room medially in the nasal cavity to accommodate two-surgeon, four-handed dissection, which is helpful for manipulation of orbital tumors. Recently studies have demonstrated that middle turbinate resection is not associated with an increased risk of empty nose syndrome,[2] does not increase the risk of postoperatively bleeding (provided the stump containing the blood supply is cauterized),[3] does not have an adverse effect on olfaction,[4] and, when diseased, may actually improve symptom scores.[5]

Maxillary Sinus

The maxillary sinus is the largest of the paranasal sinuses. When visualizing the middle meatus, the maxillary sinus is generally not readily visible given its lateral location. Instead, the uncinate process and the ethmoid bulla, as coronally oriented structures, are apparent (Fig. 5.8). The two-dimensional slitlike space between the uncinate process and the ethmoid bulla is termed the semilunar hiatus and represents the anatomic correlate of the ostiomeatal complex. More laterally, the semilunar hiatus opens into the ethmoid infundibulum, which is a three-dimensional space containing the outflow tracts of the maxillary, anterior ethmoid, and, sometimes, the frontal sinus.

The superior attachment of the uncinate process serves a clinically significant role, as it determines the trajectory of the frontal sinus outflow tract (Fig. 5.9). In most cases, the uncinate process attaches to the lamina papyracea, and the frontal sinus drains medially and directly into the middle meatus, bypassing the ethmoid infundibulum. However, the uncinate process may also attach to the skull base or middle turbinate, in which case the frontal sinus shares a common drainage pathway with the maxillary and anterior ethmoid sinuses. Understanding these anatomic variants is also important for the first step of frontal recess dissection, which consists of removing the superior uncinate process.

The natural ostium of the maxillary sinus is located anterosuperiorly just lateral to the uncinate process and posterior to the lacrimal bone. Mucociliary clearance proceeds uniformly toward this ostium, and thus it is important to connect any surgical antrostomies to the natural ostium to prevent a recirculation phenomenon, where mucus continues to run between the natural ostium and the surgical antrostomy, thereby leading to increased mucus production, facial pressure, and a potentially increased risk of sinus infections.

The roof of the maxillary sinus is an important fixed anatomic landmark. First, it defines the inferior floor of the orbit, which is important for orientation when performing any form of orbital surgery. Second, the maxillary sinus roof approximates the same level of the sphenoid ostium, far below the skull base, and can be used to guide entry through the basal lamella and identification of the natural sphenoid ostium (Fig. 5.10).[6]

Ethmoid Sinus

The ethmoid sinus is often the most complex of the sinuses, with highly variable anatomy and intimate relationships to the orbit and skull base. The first ethmoid cell encountered is the ethmoid bulla, which is located posterior to the semilunar hiatus and anterior to the basal lamella. It is a rounded structure that is attached laterally to the lamina papyracea. For this reason, meticulous dissection of the bulla is an extremely reliable way to identify the plane of orbital axis early.

Posterior to this, the coronally oriented basal lamella, or the second part of the middle turbinate, serves as the division point between the anterior and posterior ethmoid cells. A good rule of thumb when dissecting the basal lamella is to enter it low and medially, approximately at the level just above the horizontal (third part) attachment of the middle turbinate. This location is always below the level of the skull base and would be unlikely to skew

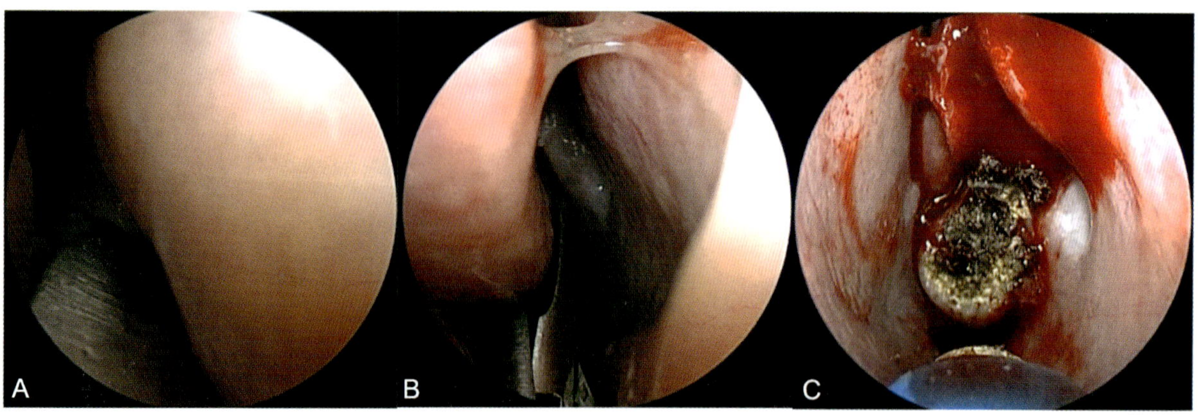

• **Fig. 5.7** Steps of middle turbinate resection. A, First, endoscopic scissors are used to transect the vertical attachment below the axilla, with care not to torque along the skull base. B, A second cut is made along the horizontal part of the middle turbinate and the entire turbinate removed using grasping forceps. C, The posterior stump, which contains the blood supply of the turbinate, is then meticulously cauterized.

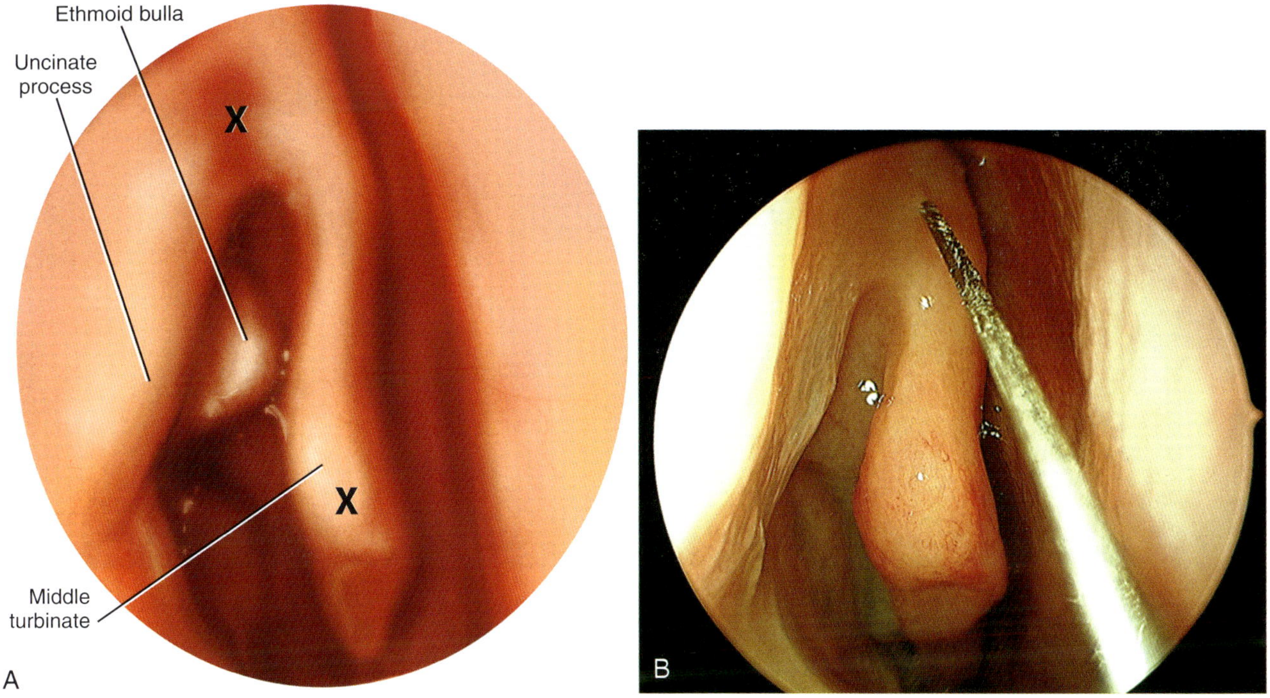

• **Fig. 5.8** When viewed with the endoscope, the uncinate process and ethmoid bulla are both coronally oriented (A). The *X* marks where infiltration of local anesthetic and decongestant is helpful for hemostasis during surgery, and as demonstrated in vivo (B). (From Chiu, A. G., Palmer, J. N., & Adappa, N. D. (Eds.). (2019). *Atlas of endoscopic sinus and skull base surgery* (2nd ed., Figure 6.8). Philadelphia: Elsevier.)

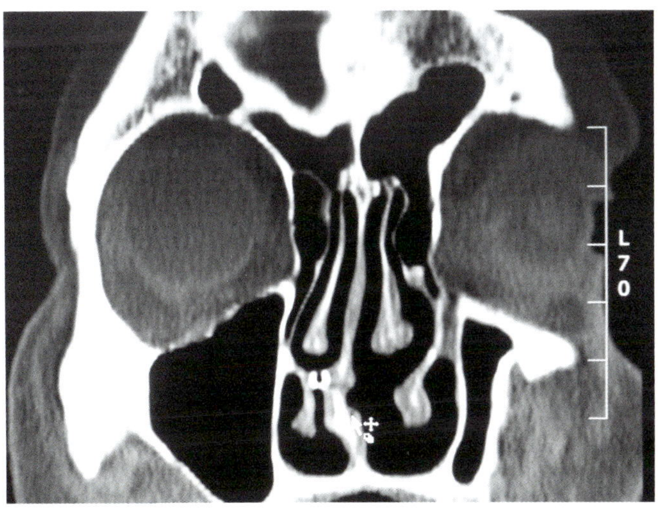

• **Fig. 5.9** Coronal CT sinus view demonstrating different superior attachments of the uncinate process. On the left, the superior uncinate attaches to the middle turbinate. On the right, it attaches to the lamina papyracea.

dissection superiorly, especially when the ethmoid sinuses are small relative to the maxillary sinus height.[7]

The first structure encountered posterior to the basal lamella is the superior turbinate, which is a vertical structure positioned medially, just lateral to the nasal septum. Removal of the inferior one-third to one-half of this structure leads to the natural ostium of the sphenoid sinus, which also approximates the level of the roof of the maxillary sinus.[6]

Lateral to the superior turbinate, the remainder of the posterior ethmoid air cells are highly variable in nature, and display highly complex relationships to the orbit and skull base. It is helpful to identify the anterior face of the sphenoid sinus and follow this up superiorly to the low point of the skull base, and then work from posterior to anterior while using an angled through-cutting forceps to palpate behind partitions, and only transecting them if there is a ledge.

Another helpful landmark to the medial orbital wall is the orbitoethmoidal plate, which is an obliquely oriented posterior ethmoid partition located laterally posterior to the basal lamella, and which is also attached to the lamina papyracea laterally. It also serves as a guide to the retromaxillary cell area, where there are posterior ethmoid cells inferomedial to the medial orbital wall that are commonly missed during the dissection.[8]

To completely skeletonize the lamina papyracea for orbital dissection, an angled endoscope (e.g., 30 or 45 degrees) is invaluable in visualizing the residual bony partitions. The globe push test, where gentle pressure is placed against the eye externally, can often be translated to movement of the medial orbital wall, suggesting that the surgeon is in the correct location.

Sphenoid Sinus

The sphenoid sinus houses the optic canal superolaterally and the carotid artery inferolaterally. Adequate exposure of the optic canal is critical for optic nerve decompression. In these cases, complete removal of the anterior face of the sphenoid sinus to the skull base superiorly and the lamina papyracea medially should be performed. An important anatomic variant is the Onodi cell, where a posterolateral ethmoid cell may aerate into the superolateral area typically occupied by the sphenoid sinus (Fig. 5.11). In these cases, the optic canal would actually be located within the Onodi cell itself as opposed to the sphenoid sinus.

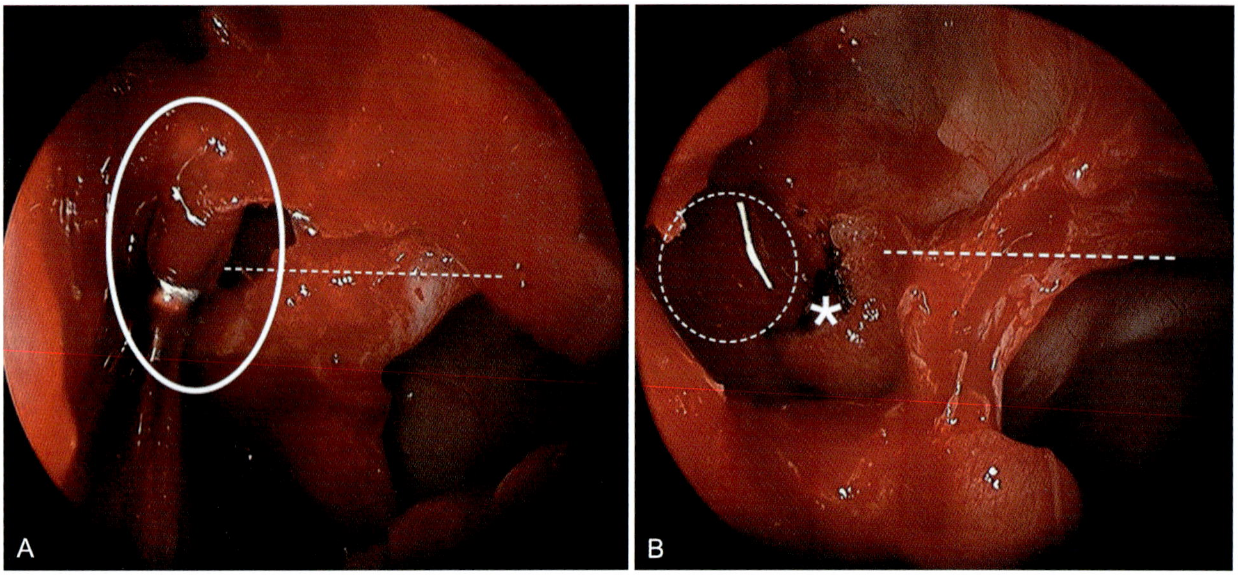

• **Fig. 5.10** The roof of the maxillary sinus, or the floor of the orbit, serves as a reliable landmark for safe entry through the basal lamella (*left*) and identification of the sphenoid ostium (*asterisk, right*). (From Chiu, A. G., Palmer, J. N., & Adappa, N. D. (Eds.). (2019). *Atlas of endoscopic sinus and skull base surgery* (2nd ed., Figures 7.11 and 7.13). Philadelphia: Elsevier.)

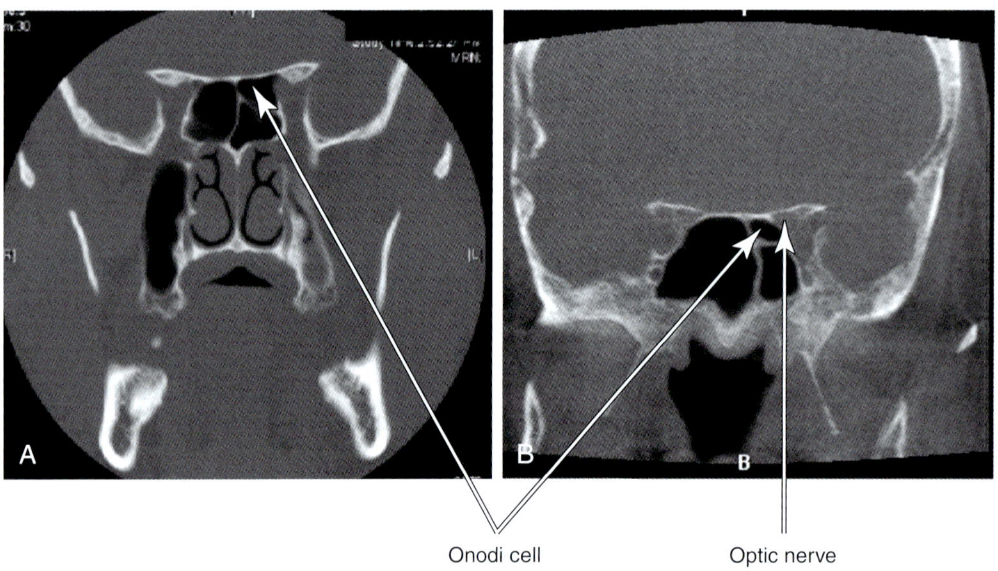

• **Fig. 5.11** Coronal computed tomography sinus scan at the level of the sphenoid sinus indicating left Onodi cell (A) and proximity to optic nerve (B). (From Chiu, A. G., Palmer, J. N., & Adappa, N. D. (Eds.). (2019). *Atlas of endoscopic sinus and skull base surgery* (2nd ed., Figure 8.3). Philadelphia: Elsevier.)

Frontal Sinus

Dissection of the frontal sinus generally takes place with an angled endoscope (e.g., 30, 45, or 70 degrees). As skull base dissection proceeds from posterior to anterior, the frontal recess is encountered and is located between the agger nasi (the most anteriorly positioned anterior ethmoid cells) anteriorly, middle turbinate medially, and lamina papyracea laterally. Identifying the frontal sinus has two important roles. First, it allows for visualization of the posterior table of the frontal sinus, which is a helpful landmark for the skull base more superiorly. Second, in cases of orbital decompression, iatrogenic obstruction of the frontal sinus may occur, thereby potentially leading to mucocele formation. It is easier to dissect the frontal sinus before opening the periorbita to avoid the need to work around the orbital contents.

Just posterior to the frontal recess, the anterior ethmoidal artery travels from posterolaterally to anteromedially between the orbit and the nasal cavity. This structure is identifiable on a coronal computed tomography (CT) scan as a "nipple" arising between the superior oblique and medial rectus muscles (Fig. 5.12). Although this structure is frequently situated within the skull base, in approximately 20% of cases it may be present within a mesentery and is at risk of injury.[9] Transection of the artery medially tends to be

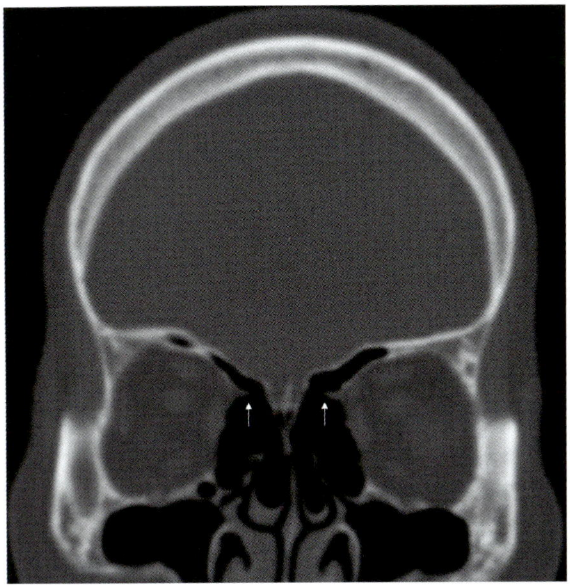

• **Fig. 5.12** *White arrows* indicate the anterior ethmoidal arteries bilaterally in this coronal CT sinus scan, also termed the "nipple" sign.

inconsequential and could be readily controlled with bipolar electrocautery. However, transection more laterally risks retraction of the arterial stump into the orbit, which may lead to a retrobulbar hematoma and thus risk vision loss. In this rare scenario, the surgeon should be prepared to perform a lateral canthotomy and cantholysis, as well as a medial orbital decompression.

Evaluation

Nasal Endoscopy

Currently the gold standard for evaluation of nasal anatomy and mucosal health is nasal endoscopy, which can often be performed in the office. The authors favor a 30-degree angled endoscope, which offers the ability to look at superior and lateral structures in addition to those straight ahead. Before performing endoscopy, topical anesthesia and decongestant spray using a mixture of lidocaine and oxymetazoline are extremely helpful to improve the examination and aid in patient comfort.

The procedure should examine the nasal septum, inferior turbinate, middle turbinate, middle meatus (uncinate process, ethmoid bulla, basal lamella), superior turbinate, sphenoethmoidal recess, olfactory cleft, eustachian tube, and nasopharynx. The presence of any polyps, masses, or purulent discharge should be noted. Both sides are examined and anatomic findings documented.

Imaging

Computed Tomography

CT scanning of the nasal cavity and paranasal sinuses is another essential tool for evaluating the sinonasal tract. A noncontrast, thin axial cut (1 mm) protocol is most useful, and the most commonly used view is the coronal sections. Aside from the anatomic considerations discussed above, CT can determine the degree of mucosal inflammation, the presence of mucus or fungal debris, osteitic changes and osteoneogenesis, and any dehiscences within the orbital wall and skull base. Furthermore, preoperative CT scanning is often used for image guidance during surgery, especially in revision cases.

Magnetic Resonance Imaging

Magnetic resonance imaging plays a less pronounced role in sinonasal surgery, although the ability to provide high-resolution assessment of soft-tissue structures (e.g., muscle, fat, nerves) makes it a helpful adjunct in orbital surgery.

Conclusion

Successful navigation through the sinonasal corridor is the first step to successful endoscopic orbital surgery. The orbital surgeon should be familiar with the surgical anatomy and various approaches of the sinonasal tract. Maximizing exposure while minimizing sinonasal morbidity is of key importance.

References

1. Costa, D. J., Sanford, T., Janney, C., Cooper, M., & Sindwani, R. (2010). Radiographic and anatomic characterization of the nasal septal swell body. *Archives of Otolaryngology–Head Neck Surgery, 136*(11), 20101107–1110.
2. Tan, N. C., Goggin, R., Psaltis, A. J., & Wormald, P. J. (2018). Partial resection of the middle turbinate during endoscopic sinus surgery for chronic rhinosinusitis does not lead to an increased risk of empty nose syndrome: A cohort study of a tertiary practice. *International Forum of Allergy & Rhinology. 8*(8). https://doi.org/10.1002/alr.22127.
3. Miller, A. J., Bobian, M., Peterson, E., & Deeb, R. (2016). Bleeding risk associated with resection of the middle turbinate during functional endoscopic sinus surgery. *American Journal of Rhinology & Allergy, 30*(2), 140–142.
4. Choby, G. W., Hobson, C. E., Lee, S., & Wang, E. W. (2014). Clinical effects of middle turbinate resection after endoscopic sinus surgery: A systematic review. *American Journal of Rhinology & Allergy, 28*(6), 502–507.
5. Scangas, G. A., Remenschneider, A. K., Bleier, B. S., Holbrook, E. H., Gray, S. T., & Metson, R. B. (2017). Does the timing of middle turbinate resection influence quality-of-life outcomes for patients with chronic rhinosinusitis? *Otolaryngology–Head Neck Surgery, 157*(5), 874–879.
6. Harvey, R. J., Shelton, W., Timperley, D., Byrd, K., Buchmann, L., Gallagher, R. M., et al. (2010). Using fixed anatomical landmarks in endoscopic skull base surgery. *Am J Rhinol Allergy, 24*(4), 301–305.
7. Ramakrishnan, V. R., Suh, J. D., & Kennedy, D. W. (2011). Ethmoid skull-base height: A clinically relevant method of evaluation. *Int Forum Allergy Rhinol, 1*(5), 396–400.
8. Kuan, E. C., Mallen-St Clair, J., Frederick, J. W., Tajudeen, B. A., Wang, M. B., Harvey, R. J., et al. (2016). Significance of undissected retromaxillary air cells as a risk factor for revision endoscopic sinus surgery. *American Journal of Rhinology & Allergy, 30*(6), 448–452.
9. Poteet, P. S., Cox, M. D., Wang, R. A., Fitzgerald, R. T., & Kanaan, A. (2017). Analysis of the relationship between the location of the anterior ethmoid artery and keros classification. *Otolaryngology–Head Neck Surgery, 157*(2), 320–324.

6

Rhinologic Evaluation in Orbital and Lacrimal Disease

PETER VALENTIN TOMAZIC, MD, PhD, NORA DEWART, BSc(Hon), AND IAN J. WITTERICK, MD, MSc, FRCSC

Sinonasal Examination

Examination and palpation of the external nose shows deformities and crepitation and confirms soft-tissue or firm masses. Transillumination of the frontal and maxillary sinuses is an unreliable maneuver. Anterior rhinoscopy can assess the anterior septum and inferior turbinates but rarely provides the entire picture. Tests of olfaction, nasal airflow, or mucociliary flow are rarely indicated in orbital or lacrimal disease. The most important rhinologic examination technique is performed via endoscopy. Endoscopic examination reveals the full range of pathology within the nasal cavity and provides a strong indication of problems within the sinuses as they may relate to the orbit.

Rigid nasal telescopes provide an excellent view of the nasal structures but, depending on the size of the scope, may be difficult to maneuver into certain areas such as the sphenoethmoidal recess. Angled scopes (e.g., 30 degrees, 45 degrees) may help in visualization, or alternatively a flexible nasolaryngoscope may be used. With modern versions of the flexible scope, such as with the camera in the tip of the scope, excellent views of sinonasal anatomy and pathology can be obtained with less discomfort for the patient compared with rigid telescopes.

For endoscopic evaluation, some clinicians use no topical pretreatment. Others prefer some combination of a topical vasoconstrictor and/or local anesthetic. It is helpful to view the mucosa before decongestion to assess swelling and color. Although color and swelling per se are not specific to any disease, the presence of granular, friable mucosa should raise the suspicion of an underlying granulomatous process such as sarcoidosis or granulomatosis with polyangiitis.

After decongestion, a better assessment into the inferior meatus, middle meatus, and sphenoethmoidal recess can be obtained. A systematic approach is advisable so as not to miss anything. Classically three passes with a rigid 30-degree endoscope were described by Stammberger and Wolf, including passes along the nasal floor, middle meatus, and sphenoethmoidal recess.[1] Regardless of which approach is used, the examiner needs to carefully assess the septum, inferior meatus, middle meatus, sphenoethmoidal recess, and the area of the cribriform plate and then repeat the examination on the contralateral side. The nasopharynx, opening of the eustachian tubes, and fossa of Rosenmüller should be assessed.

The region of the middle turbinate is carefully examined identifying the agger nasi ("agger mound") at the junction of the middle turbinate anteriorly with the lateral wall of the nose. The middle turbinate is assessed for pneumatization (concha bullosa), lateralization, or paradoxical bend. In some patients, the endoscope can be passed between the middle turbinate and septum to visualize the superior turbinate, sphenoethmoidal recess, and opening of the sphenoid sinus.

The examiner is looking for changes in color, swelling, asymmetry, displacement of structures, purulence, polyps, and abnormal fluid. Sometimes palpation of the eye or any external deformity helps to show their connection to intranasal structures by movement intranasally while palpating externally. For sinonasal neoplasms, sensation of branches of the trigeminal nerve should be assessed and extraocular motion and pupillary reflexes should be assessed. The dentition and palate should be assessed for loosening of teeth and abnormal swelling or fullness. The face and neck should be assessed for lymphadenopathy in suspected neoplasia.

The quality and quantity of mucus should be considered. Unilateral watery discharge should raise suspicion of a cerebrospinal fluid leak. Thick tenacious secretions may be associated with an underlying mucociliary problem such as primary ciliary dyskinesia. Discoloration may indicate infection and/or a cellular infiltrate. Thick inspissated secretions may point to allergic fungal rhinosinusitis.

Polypoid changes are commonly seen in the nasal cavity, most often affecting the area of the middle meatus. Typical nasal polyposis is a bilateral disease except in the case of an antrochoanal polyp. The degree of polyposis on both sides is often asymmetric and the polyps are described as smooth, glistening with a "peeled grape" appearance. The size of the polyps can be documented by a variety of grading scales. Unilateral masses of any kind should raise the possibility of a neoplastic process and be considered for biopsy. It is important to consider imaging before any biopsy of a unilateral nasal mass to rule out a connection between the dura and brain, especially in children.

Lacrimal Disease

Anatomy

The anatomy of the lacrimal system is important in understanding rhinologic evaluation. The lacrimal canaliculi and sac lie between the deep and superficial fibers of the orbicularis muscle. The anterior and superficial fibers of the pretarsal orbicularis insert along the anterior lacrimal crest on the frontal process of the maxillary bone and onto the frontal bone. Aberration or loss of structural integrity in any of these structures (e.g., lid laxity, ectropion, or ectropion) can result in symptomatic epiphora.

The lacrimal fossa is made up of the frontal process of the maxillary bone anteriorly and the lacrimal bone posteriorly, forming the anterior and posterior lacrimal crests, respectively. The lacrimal fossa contains the lacrimal sac and occasionally the proximal portion of the nasolacrimal duct. The approximate dimensions of the sac are 14 to 16 mm vertically, 4 to 8 mm anteroposteriorly, and 3 to 5 mm in width.[2] Approximately one-third of the lacrimal sac lies above the level of the medial canthal tendon. The amount of lacrimal sac covered by the bone varies significantly.

The lacrimal sac lies anterior to the anterior tip of the middle turbinate. It then courses posteriorly, inferiorly, and laterally to form the nasolacrimal canal, which terminates in the inferior meatus. The bones that contribute to the canal are the maxillary and lacrimal bones and, in some cases, the inferior turbinate bone. The anterior, posterior, and lateral walls of the canal are usually formed by the maxillary bone. The medial wall is composed of the lacrimal bone superiorly and an extension of the inferior turbinate inferiorly.[3] Significant variation occurs in the width, length, and angulation of the canal, which is often experienced at the time of probing of the nasolacrimal duct.

The length and extent of the nasolacrimal duct vary, ranging from 22 mm in the infant to approximately 35 mm in the adult. There are diverticula and valves in the duct, but the most critical is the valve of Hasner lying in the inferior meatus. The location and patency of this valve varies significantly. The angulation anteroposteriorly and laterally determine the actual point of exit of the duct underneath the inferior turbinate. An abnormally positioned valve of Hasner or a narrow inferior meatus for any reason may impede the flow of tears.

Rhinologic Evaluation

Because of the significant role of the lacrimal gland, the accurate assessment of lacrimal gland diseases is a matter of clinical importance. The endoscope paved the way for the advent of endoscopic transnasal dacryocystorhinostomy in the 1970s and 1980s and became an additional tool in the rhinologic evaluation for diseases of the lacrimal gland. Lacrimal diseases are assessed through inspection and palpation of the eyes, the medial canthus (specifically, the inferior and superior punctum), and the nasolacrimal sac. Inspection focuses on observing periorbital asymmetry and abnormal positioning of eyelids. Common eyelid position abnormalities include entropion and ectropion, inverted and everted eyelids, respectively. Inspection and palpation of the nasolacrimal sac can reveal signs of tumors as well as inflammation of the skin and eye, purulent discharge, or resistance. Although inspection and palpation can provide insight on lacrimal diseases, the first step in diagnosis is the standard nasal endoscopy.

Lacrimal diseases can be diagnosed through nasal endoscopy by placing focus on the maxillary line, the middle and inferior meatus, and the valve of Hasner.[4,5] The endoscope should be used after decongestion and topical anesthesia. The maxillary line is a curvilinear mucosal projection that is not well defined and is found at the middle to inferior turbinate of the nasal wall.[6] Below the inferior turbinate is the inferior meatus, which can best be reached by orienting the endoscopic toward the posterior end of the inferior turbinate and then rotating the scope along the turbinate into the meatus and following it posteriorly to anteriorly. The valve of Hasner, found within the inferior meatus,[7] can appear in a variety of forms from a true opening in the mucosa to a small indentation of the mucosa only visible on palpation of the sac.

Endoscopy allows for the detection of obstruction and swelling in the nasolacrimal system. Obstruction or swelling can indicate the presence of tumors, mucoceles, polyps, or cysts[8] (Fig. 6.1). Septal deviation, nasal polyps, and tumors should be further evaluated with a full physical examination, including inspection, palpitation, and endoscopy.[8,9] Obstruction caused by nasal pathology can also be ruled out through endoscopy. It should be noted that dacryocystoceles can sometimes be mistaken for ethmoidal mucoceles owing to their similar appearance as cystic, smooth lesions in the vicinity of the nasolacrimal duct.[10] Further, if the inferior meatus and the valve can be seen with the endoscope, tear consistency can be evaluated by gently palpating the medial canthus. Tears can be analyzed for purulence, sanguineous nature, and viscous characteristics that can indicate and help differentiate between acute infection, tumors, or chronic inflammation.[8,11] If no tears can be provoked, a stenosis in the system may be present.

To further evaluate the nasolacrimal system during endoscopy, a swab for culture, a biopsy, or simple maneuvers, such as resection of polyps or cysts, can be performed. Dacryolithiasis, a disorder involving the presence of tear stones, can be diagnosed only indirectly via concomitant infection and reduced tear flow. The stones are associated with infection, when a foreign body promotes the formation of a bacterial protein stone. The stones can also be caused by high concentrations of phosphate and calcium in the tears because of reduced tear flow.[12] The stones themselves can only be seen endoscopically during dacryocystorhinostomy. Surgical excision is often needed to remove the stones. On rare occasions, a stone can be massaged out of the nasolacrimal system and hence will remain in the inferior meatus.

A functional test to assess tear flow is the Jones dye test.[2] The Jones I test assesses tear drainage under physiologic conditions. It is performed by placing a drop of fluorescein dye into the eye, followed by endoscopy of the nose and evaluation of tear flow. If dye can be detected, it can be inferred that some flow is still occurring; conversely, if no dye is present, this suggests some obstruction in the lacrimal system. It should be noted that false-positive results may occur with this assessment. After the Jones I test, the Jones II test can be performed. The Jones II test is performed under nonphysiologic conditions. Here, a lacrimal cannula or 26-gauge needle is inserted into the inferior punctum. A 3-mL syringe is used to flush the lacrimal system with saline solution. If saline solution is noted in the nose, patency or partial obstruction may be diagnosed. Reflux of the saline solution from the superior punctum is caused by an obstruction of the sac or duct. If no saline solution is sensed, obstruction of the inferior canaliculus is present. Diaphanoscopy can be helpful to more accurately assess the region of nasolacrimal stenosis.[13] Here, a 0.5-mm light fiber is inserted in the superior canaliculus and the area is illuminated. The stenosis is located at the area where the light cannot shine through or is less intense compared with the remaining duct and/or sac.

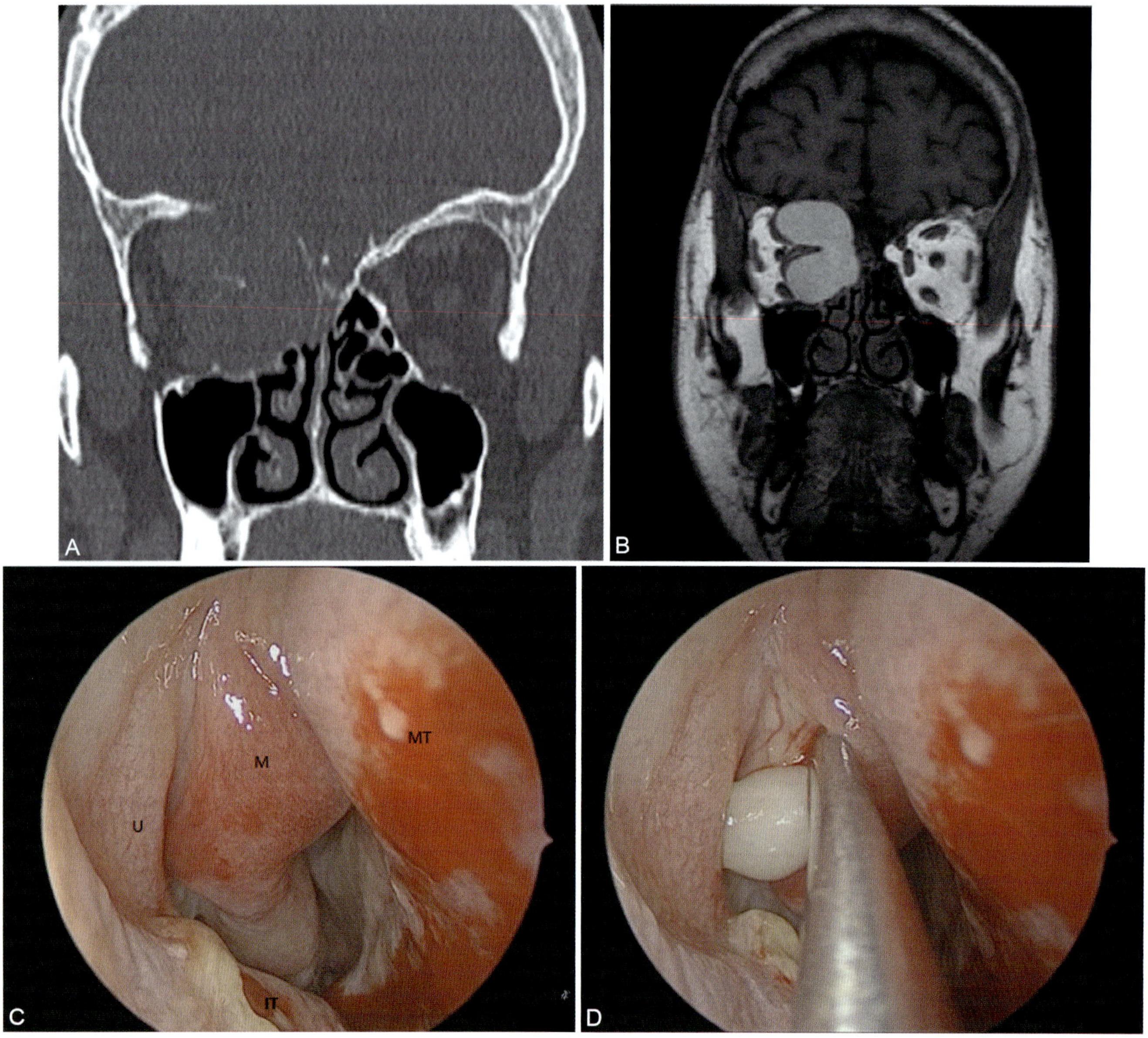

• **Fig. 6.1** Right ethmoid mucocele compressing the right orbit. A, Coronal computed tomography scan shows a large mass occupying the right ethmoid sinus and compressing the orbit with thinning of the bone over the medial orbital roof. B, Coronal T1 magnetic resonance image. C, Endoscopic view of the right middle meatus. D, Endoscopic puncture of the mucocele shows thick white discharge coming out. *IT,* inferior turbinate; *M,* mucocele; *MT,* middle turbinate; *U,* uncinate process.

Orbital Disease

The major symptom of orbital disease is exophthalmos and/or displacement of the globe with lid edema or deformity. Exophthalmos is the anterior bulging of the eye from its orbit. Exophthalmos may be caused by inflammation of the eye's membranous lining (such as with Graves disease) or from the presence of a tumor (such as with neoplastic disease). Graves disease is caused by an overproduction of thyroid hormone, which can ultimately result in the activation of inflammatory cytokines, which can alter orbital tissue response.[14] Benign nasal tumors such as inverted papilloma or osteoma, or malignant lesions such as squamous cell carcinoma, may be growing toward or into the orbit, which can also cause exophthalmos. The mass can be seen endoscopically and may be biopsied.[15] Tumors originating in the orbit can grow extraconally or intraconally. If a tumor grows medial and/or inferior to the medial rectus and inferior recuts muscle, respectively, the lamina papyracea may protrude into the middle meatus, which could be seen endoscopically. Intraconal tumors can grow eccentrically and enlarge the intraconal space and displace the muscles.[16] The vector of the mass effect would be directed outside the orbit and protrusion of the lamina papyracea would be less likely. Here CT and magnetic resonance imaging would further facilitate the diagnosis. Mucoceles may also be extending from the paranasal sinuses toward the orbit causing exophthalmos. Depending on the size and location of a mucocele, it may be seen endoscopically as a smooth cystic mass covered by normal mucosa[17] (Figs. 6.2 and 6.3). Allergic rhinitis can present as rhinoconjunctivitis with itching and redness of the eye; however, the orbit or the nasolacrimal system are usually not affected.[18]

A nasal finding potentially presenting with enophthalmos is silent sinus syndrome. Silent sinus syndrome is typically unilateral and can be identified by usually asymptomatic enophthalmos and decreased maxillary sinus space.[19] Endoscopically, atelectasis and lateralization of the uncinate process can be seen. The sinus CT scan reveals the definite diagnosis with maxillary sinus hypoplasia and opacification, lowering of the orbital floor, and lateralization of the uncinate process against the lamina papyracea.[20]

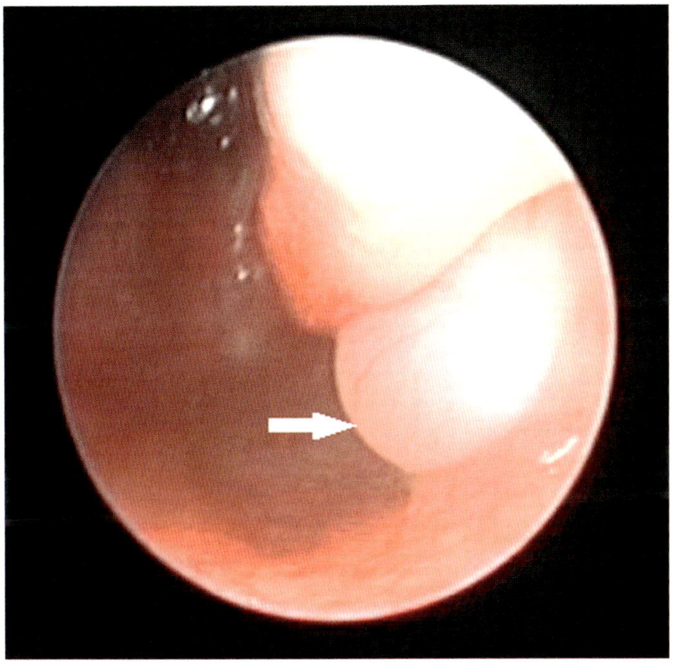

• **Fig. 6.2** Left nasolacrimal cyst (arrow) seen under the left inferior turbinate.

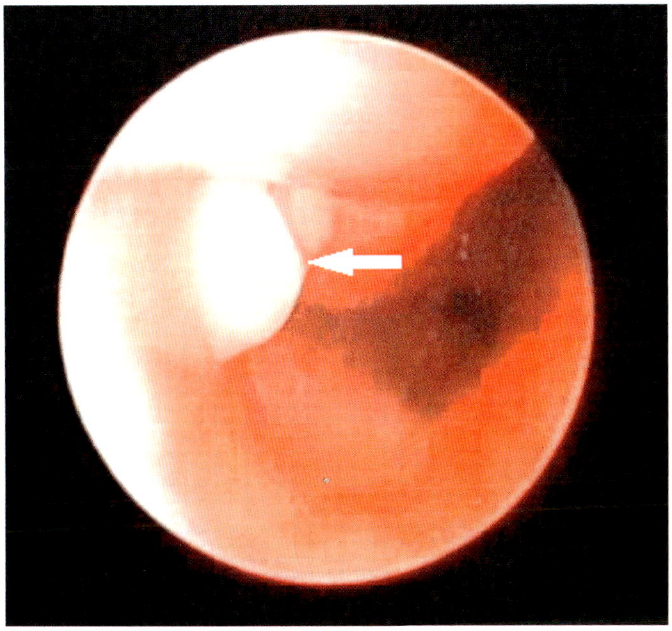

• **Fig. 6.3** Right nasolacrimal cyst (arrow) seen under the right inferior turbinate.

The most prevalent forms of orbital complications include subperiosteal or intraorbital abscess and orbital phlegmon.[21] Cavernous sinus thrombosis is a complication from nasal or maxillary infections, which as the name suggests leads to thrombosis in the cavernous sinus. Patients with cavernous sinus thrombosis may present with visual symptoms, pulsatile exophthalmos, and may rapidly become medically unstable. Additionally, on endoscopic examination pus may be encountered in the middle meatus, in which case orbital decompression may be indicated. Nasal polyps, resulting from severe chronic rhinosinusitis and sometimes caused by aspirin intolerance and high eosinophilia, may decalcify bone and exert pressure on the periorbita. The most severe form of nasal polyps in children is known as Woakes syndrome, in which there is the potential for destruction of the nasal pyramid.[22]

Summary

A variety of nasal and sinus problems affect the lacrimal system and orbit. Careful external and internal assessment of the nose and sinuses, especially with thorough endoscopy, and aided by imaging and laboratory investigation, facilitate appropriate diagnosis and management.

References

1. Stammberger, H., & Wolf, G. (1988). Headaches and sinus disease: The endoscopic approach. *Ann Otol Rhinol Laryngol Suppl*, *134*, 3–23.
2. Bailey, J. H. (1923). Surgical anatomy of the lacrimal sac. *Am J Ophthalmol*, *6*(8), 665–669.
3. Jones, L. T. (1961). An anatomical approach to problems of the eyelids and lacrimal apparatus. *Arch Ophthalmol*, *66*, 111–124.
4. Lund, V. J., Stammberger, H., Fokkens, W. J., Beale, T., Bernal-Sprekelsen, M., Eloy, P., et al. (2014). European position paper on the anatomical terminology of the internal nose and paranasal sinuses. *Rhinol Suppl*, *24*, 1–34.
5. Onerci, M. Dacryocystorhinostomy. (2002). Diagnosis and treatment of nasolacrimal canal obstructions. *Rhinology*, *40*(2), 49–65.
6. Chastain, J., Cooper, M., & Sindwani, R. (2005). The maxillary line: Anatomic characterization and clinical utility of an important surgical landmark. *Laryngoscope*, *115*(6), 990–992.
7. Cnaan, R., Moosajee, M., Heatley, C., & Olver, J. (2012). Endoscopic endonasal retrieval of a nasolacrimal duct stone via the valve of Hasner in the inferior meatus. *Ophthalmic Plast Reconstr Surg*, *28*(2), e48–e50.
8. Strong, E. B. (2013). Endoscopic dacryocystorhinostomy. *Craniomaxillofac Trauma Reconstr*, *6*(2), 67–74.
9. Taban, M., Jarullazada, I., Mancini, R., Hwang, C., & Goldberg, R. A. (2011). Facial asymmetry and nasal septal deviation in acquired nasolacrimal duct obstruction. *Orbit, 30*(5), 226–229.
10. Wong, E., Leith, N., Wilcsek, G., & Sacks, R. (2018). Endoscopic resection of a huge orbital ethmoidal mucocele masquerading as dacryocystocele. *BMJ Case Rep*. bcr-2018-226232. https://doi.org/10.1136/bcr-2018-226232.
11. Schwarcz, R. M., Coupland, S. E., & Finger, P. T. (2013). Cancer of the orbit and adnexa. *Am J Clin Oncol*, *36*(2), 197–205.
12. Mishra, K., Hu, K. Y., Kamal, S., Andron, A., Rocca Della, R. C., Ali, M. J., et al. (2017). Dacryolithiasis: A review. *Ophthalmic Plast Reconstr Surg*, *33*(2), 83–89.
13. Siegert, R. (2007). Localization of lacrimal drainage system obstruction by diaphanoscopy. *Laryngorhinootologie*, *86*(4), 252–254 (in German).

14. Gianoukakis, A., Khadavi, N., & Smith, T. (2008). Cytokines, Graves' disease, and thyroid-associated ophthalmopathy. *Thyroid, 18*(9), 953–958.
15. Lund, V. J., Stammberger, H., Nicolai, P., Castelnuovo, P., Beal, T., Beham, A., et al. (2010). European position paper on endoscopic management of tumours of the nose. Paranasal sinuses and skull base. *Rhinol Suppl, 22*, 1–143.
16. Tomazic, P. V., Stammberger, H., Habermann, W., Gerstenberger, C., Braun, H., Gellner, V., et al. (2011). Intraoperative medialization of medial rectus muscle as a new endoscopic technique for approaching intraconal lesions. *Am J Rhinol Allergy, 25*(5), 363–367.
17. Samil, K. S., Yasar, C., Ercan, A., Hanifi, B., & Hilal, K. (2015). Nasal cavity and paranasal sinus diseases affecting orbit. *J Craniofac Surg, 26*(4), e348–e351.
18. Bousquet, J., Schunemann, H. J., Samolinski, B., Demoly, P., Baena-Cagnani, C. E., Bachert, C., et al. (2012). Allergic rhinitis and its impact on asthma (ARIA): Achievements in 10 years and future needs. *J Allergy Clin Immunol, 130*(5), 1049–1062.
19. Yosuf, K., Velázquez-Villaseñor, L., & Witterick, I. (2009). Silent sinus syndrome: Case series and literature review. *J Otolaryngol Head Neck Surg, 38*(5), E110–E113.
20. Lee, D. S., Murr, A. H., Kersten, R. C., & Pletcher, S. D. (2018). Silent sinus syndrome without opacification of ipsilateral maxillary sinus. *Laryngoscope, 128*(9), 2004–2007.
21. Teinzer, F., Stammberger, H., & Tomazic, P. V. (2015). Transnasal endoscopic treatment of orbital complications of acute sinusitis: The Graz concept. *Ann Otol Rhinol Laryngol, 124*(5), 368–373.
22. Schoenenberger, U., & Tasman, A. J. (2015). Adult-onset Woakes' syndrome: Report of a rare case. *Case Rep Otolaryngol, 2015*, 857675.

7

Ophthalmologic Evaluation in Orbital and Lacrimal Disease

CATHERINE J. HWANG, MD, BRIAN H. CHON, MD, AND JULIAN D. PERRY, MD

The orbit and lacrimal system is bounded by the paranasal sinuses, eyelids, temporal region, and intracranial fossa (Figs. 7.1 and 7.2). The orbit contains all of the supporting structures of the eye and produces unique signs and symptoms depending on the location and pathology of the underlying disease. Careful evaluation of these structures and their function allows for localization and identification of many processes, and represents a key step in determining the next steps of the workup. Processes that affect the orbit and lacrimal system include vascular, inflammatory, cystic, neural, muscular, lymphoid, fibrous, and osseous diseases. In addition, infections or diseases can extend from periorbital regions or metastasize to the orbit.

History

The location, quality, and timing of symptoms, as well as modifying factors, can aid in diagnosis and management of orbital and lacrimal disease. Review of old photographs helps to document a change in appearance.

Visual symptoms should be reviewed during the workup of both orbital and lacrimal diseases. Symptoms may include blurred vision, loss of vision, double vision, and light sensitivity. Diplopia must be clarified as either monocular or binocular. Monocular diplopia does not resolve with each eye closed; it is typically due to media opacities, such as cataract or tear film irregularities. Binocular diplopia resolves with either eye closed; it is due to misalignment of the eyes and may be due to orbital disease.

Inflammatory symptoms include the four classic symptoms of tenderness or pain (dolor), swelling (tumor), warmth (calor), and redness (rubor). Infections may present with similar findings and/or mucopurulent or purulent discharge. Because the orbit represents a compartment with vast sensory innervation passing through it, pain may occur in a variety of other orbital processes, including orbital hemorrhage and malignancy.

The timing and progression of symptoms may point to particular diagnoses. Infections (dacryocystitis, orbital cellulitis, mucormycosis) and hemorrhage (orbital hemorrhage, pituitary apoplexy) typically present acutely. Inflammations (nonspecific orbital inflammation, dacryoadenitis, myositis) and some tumors such as metastases may present subacutely. A more indolent presentation may occur with benign orbital tumors, such as cavernous malformations, lymphomas, dermoid cysts, mucoceles, or neurogenic tumors.

Tearing represents the most common symptom of lacrimal disease and may result from primary or secondary tear hypersecretion or from underdrainage of tears. Epiphora specifically relates to excess tears that overflow onto the cheek, which often implies underdrainage of tears owing to lacrimal outflow obstruction or tear pumping abnormality. Hypersecretion may occur from inflammation of the ocular surface. The most common cause of surface inflammation is keratoconjunctivitis sicca, or dry eye syndrome. Dry eye syndrome is often accompanied by burning, irritation, redness, ocular ache, foreign body sensation, blurred vision, photophobia, and mattering of eyelashes; however, tearing may be the sole symptom of dry eye. Other surface inflammations that may produce tearing include blepharitis, conjunctivitis, keratitis, allergies, Stevens-Johnson syndrome, and ocular cicatricial pemphigoid. Mechanical abrasion of the ocular surface may also result in tearing. This can occur with trichiasis, eyelid malpositions such as entropion, or tumors abutting the globe. Exacerbating factors for tearing could include wind, smoke, smog, or other environmental irritants. Lacrimal sac malignancies may present with blood-tinged tears (hemolacria), epistaxis, or a mass extending superior to the medial canthal tendon in addition to tearing. Infants with tearing should be evaluated by a pediatric ophthalmologist, as the differential diagnosis includes congenital glaucoma.

Medical History, Medications, and Allergies

The medical history should be reviewed for diseases that may affect the lacrimal system and orbit, including sinusitis or rhinitis, allergies and atopy, autoimmune disorders (in particular thyroid disease, Sjögren syndrome, sarcoidosis, granulomatosis with polyangiitis, rheumatoid arthritis, and systemic lupus erythematosus), Stevens-Johnson syndrome, ocular cicatricial pemphigoid, diabetes mellitus, history of local or systemic malignancies, and periocular trauma.

The ocular history should include previous eye surgeries or interventions. For patients with tearing, a history of punctal plug placement is particularly important. Certain ocular medications can exacerbate tearing or nasolacrimal duct obstruction (NLDO), such as topical glaucoma medications (timolol, dorzolamide, pilocarpine) and antivirals (idoxuridine, trifluridine).

Prior surgical history and interventions, including past nasal, sinus, dental, lacrimal, facial and cosmetic surgeries, history of radiation treatment, or a history of skin cancer and treatments, should be elicited.

Medication history pertinent to the orbital examination includes the use of corticosteroids or other immunosuppressants,

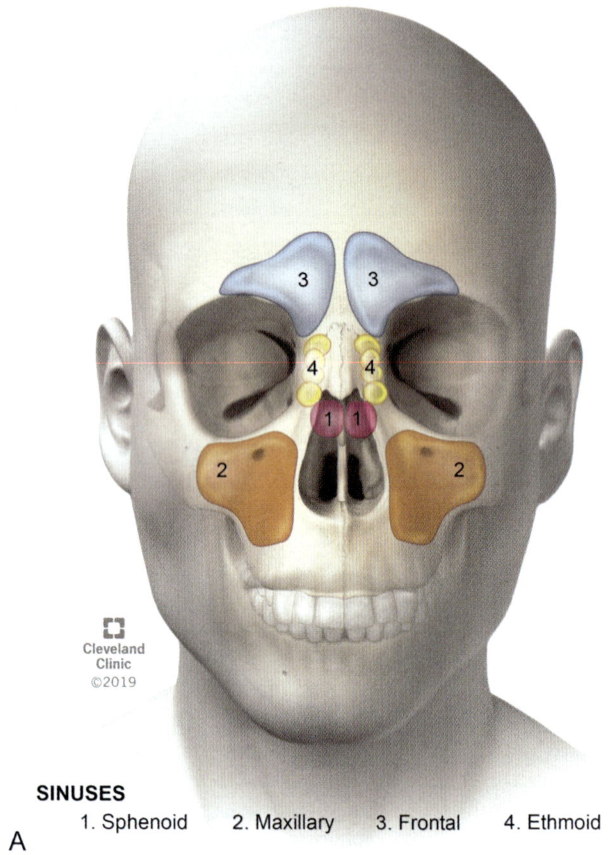

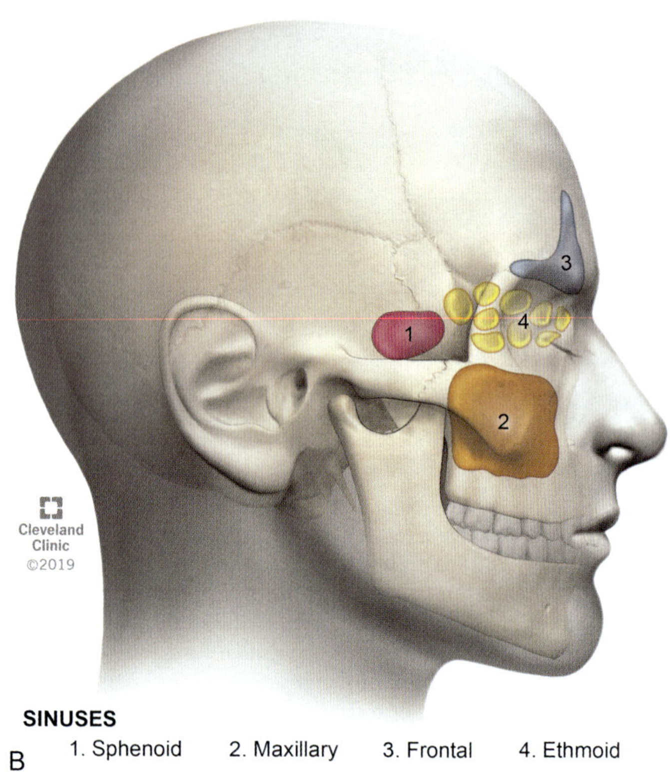

• **Fig. 7.1** (A) Paranasal sinuses, frontal view. Note the proximity of the orbit to the sinuses. (B) Paranasal sinuses, side view.

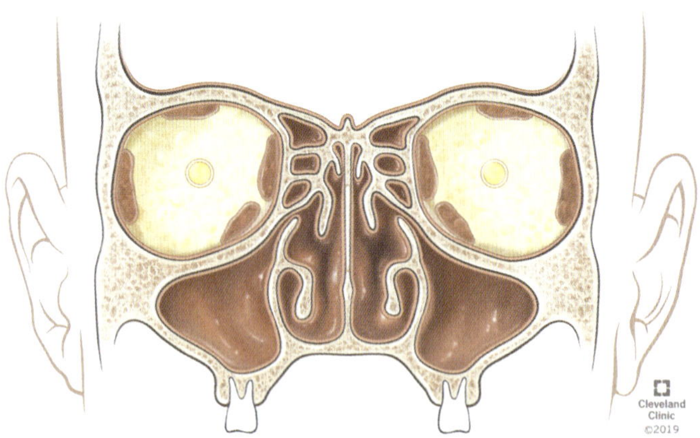

• **Fig. 7.2** Coronal view of the orbit and paranasal sinuses. The orbit is bound superiorly by the cranial fossa, medially by the ethmoid sinus and nasal cavity, and inferiorly by the maxillary sinus.

thyroid medications, and blood thinners. For the lacrimal evaluation, pertinent medications include allergy medications, radioactive iodine 131, chemotherapy (paclitaxel, docetaxel, 5-fluorouracil, and others), and topical ocular lubricants. Dry eye syndrome can be exacerbated with antihistamines, antidepressants, antihypertensives, and oral contraceptives.

Pertinent substance history includes cocaine use (nasal septum defects) and tobacco smoking history (thyroid eye disease and other inflammatory disorders, malignancy).

The family history may play a role in some orbital and lacrimal diseases, such as thyroid eye disease, nasolacrimal duct obstruction, and certain malignancies.

Ophthalmic Examination

The ophthalmic examination must evaluate the function of myriad structures within the orbit and lacrimal system, including the visual sensory system, the oculomotor system, the globe, the somatic sensory system, the periocular structures, and the lacrimal system. The examination can localize a disease process and point to the proper imaging or other evaluation techniques.

Visual Sensory System

Although it is obviously critical to determine the exact cause of vision loss, the most important aspect of vision regarding the orbit is whether vision loss is due to a problem of the eye itself, or due to compression of the optic nerve from an orbital process. Optic nerve function can affect visual acuity, but so can many other disorders that are not orbital in origin.

Optic nerve function can be further characterized by assessing visual acuity, pupillary response, visual fields, and color vision. Visual acuity should be performed one eye at a time either at near or distance, with the patient wearing glasses or contact lenses, or with a pinhole. The swinging flashlight test detects a relative afferent pupillary defect, and this test is critical to master for any surgeon operating on the orbit. In general, the pupil of each eye should constrict in a similar fashion when the light is brought in front of the eye. If the affected eye dilates when the light is brought over from the unaffected eye, this signifies optic nerve dysfunction. The dilation may be very subtle. Other tests for optic nerve function include confrontational visual field testing, which can be done with the examiner's fingers placed in peripheral quadrants while the patient gazes straight ahead. Static perimetry (e.g., Humphrey visual field analyzer [Carl Zeiss Meditec Inc., Dublin, CA]) using special devices provides a much more detailed assessment to detect smaller degrees of nerve damage and is recommended in most cases other than at the bedside and in urgent situations.

Color vision is another test of optic nerve function. Color vision is more likely to be reduced in vision loss due to optic neuropathy compared with other types of vision loss, such as media opacities, macular disease, or amblyopia.[1] This is particularly important for orbital disease. Compressive diseases may affect color vision before affecting other optic nerve function parameters. It is best tested using books with standardized Ishihara color plates (Kanehara Shuppan Co., LTD, Tokyo, Japan), but if these are unavailable, color vision can be tested by subjectively asking the patient to compare the saturation of a red object presented to each eye.

To complete the visual sensory examination, a slit-lamp examination should be performed. This biomicroscopic examination evaluates both the surface and the contents of the eye. It can detect an elevated tear meniscus in lacrimal disease, or signs of exposure keratopathy in orbital disease. Vision loss from an ocular surface issue such as exposure of the cornea must be distinguished from that caused by an optic neuropathy to guide proper treatment. Similarly, a slit-lamp examination can tease out other causes of vision loss, such as cataract, media opacities such as vitreous hemorrhage, or retinal disease. Evaluation of the optic nerve using the slit lamp and a handheld lens, or direct ophthalmoscope, can detect swelling of the optic nerve in more acute and anterior orbital cases of optic neuropathy or pallor of the optic nerve in chronic cases.

Oculomotor System

The oculomotor system should evaluate the function of the extraocular muscles. The position of the eyes can be determined by asking the patient to look at the examiner's nose while covering one eye and looking for movement of the other. Eyes that are aligned (orthophoria) will not move with this test. If, for example, the eye moves laterally to find the examiner's nose while the fellow eye is being occluded, this signifies the eye is deviated inward (esotropia). This could be due to restriction of the medial rectus muscle or to weakness of the lateral rectus muscle. Next, ductions, or examination of extraocular motility, are performed by asking the patient to move the eyes in all cardinal directions of gaze. The degree of movement in the four cardinal directions should be compared to the fellow eye. Some processes in the orbit can restrict eye movement. These include fractures entrapping a muscle or inflammatory diseases affecting extraocular muscle(s). In the example provided, a medial restriction would cause limited lateral (abduction) movement of the eye. However, limited eye movement may be due to causes other than restriction, such as cranial nerve (CN) III, IV, and VI palsy. Each nerve palsy presents with unique extraocular movement (EOM) patterns. Neuromuscular diseases, such as myasthenia gravis, may also limit eye movement. To determine whether a limited eye movement is due to a restrictive cause or other cause, forced ductions may be performed (Fig. 7.3). Classically, after numbing the ocular surface, forceps can be used to grasp the muscle insertion and move the eye in

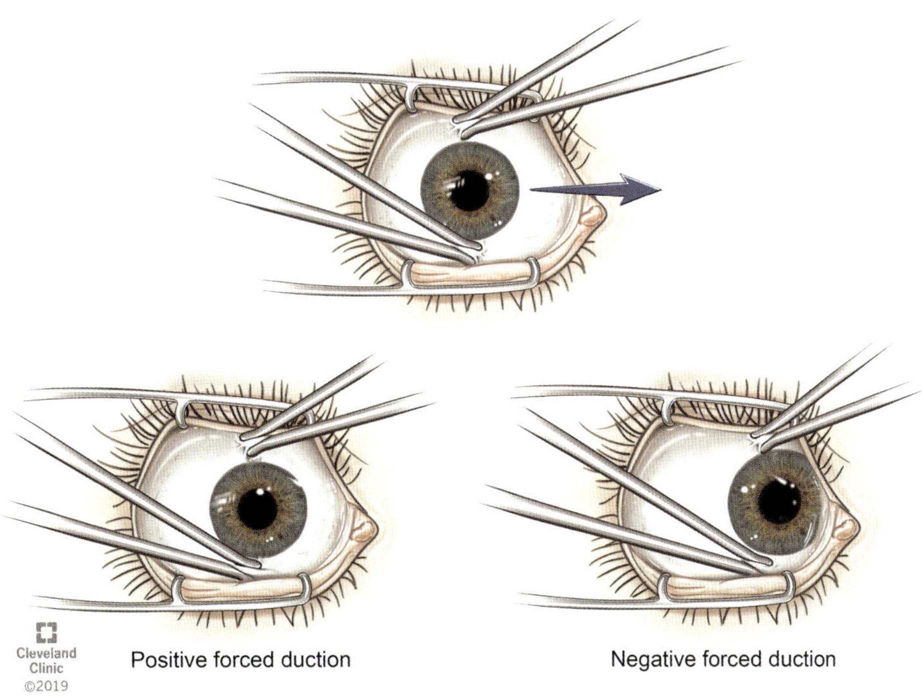

• **Fig. 7.3** Forced duction testing. After anesthetizing the eye, the conjunctiva can be grasped with two forceps. The bottom left image shows a positive forced duction test with restriction of eye movement. The bottom right image shows a negative forced duction test with a normal range of eye movement in the direction of pull.

the opposite direction to determine if the muscle is mechanically restricted. In the case of medial rectus muscle restriction, if the medial rectus insertion is grasped, the eye cannot be pushed laterally to its full extent. In the case of palsy, the eye can be moved to its full extent. Caution is recommended, however, as forced ductions can be uncomfortable and can result in oculocardiac reflex and bradycardia if there is restriction. Some examiners use a cotton-tipped applicator instead of forceps.

Globe Evaluation

The globe position should also be measured. The globe may be higher (hyperglobus) or lower (hypoglobus) than the fellow/normal eye, or it may be further forward (proptosis) or more recessed (enophthamos) than the fellow/normal eye. Hyperglobus and hypoglobus can be measured using a dedicated device, a straight ruler, or qualitatively. Proptosis/enophthalmos is typically measured with a dedicated mirrored device called an exophthalmometer. Even in skilled hands, the reading can be different between examiners, and serial measurements are best compared by repeat examinations by a single examiner.

A general sense of proptosis can be evaluated by looking at the patient from below, or the "worm's eye view" position. A difference of 2 mm between eyes is considered clinically significant, but any difference can be meaningful. The direction of globe dystopia may be related to the location of orbital disease. Typically, the globe will displace away from the mass lesion (Fig. 7.4). In axial proptosis, lesions tend to be posterior to the globe or may involve most of

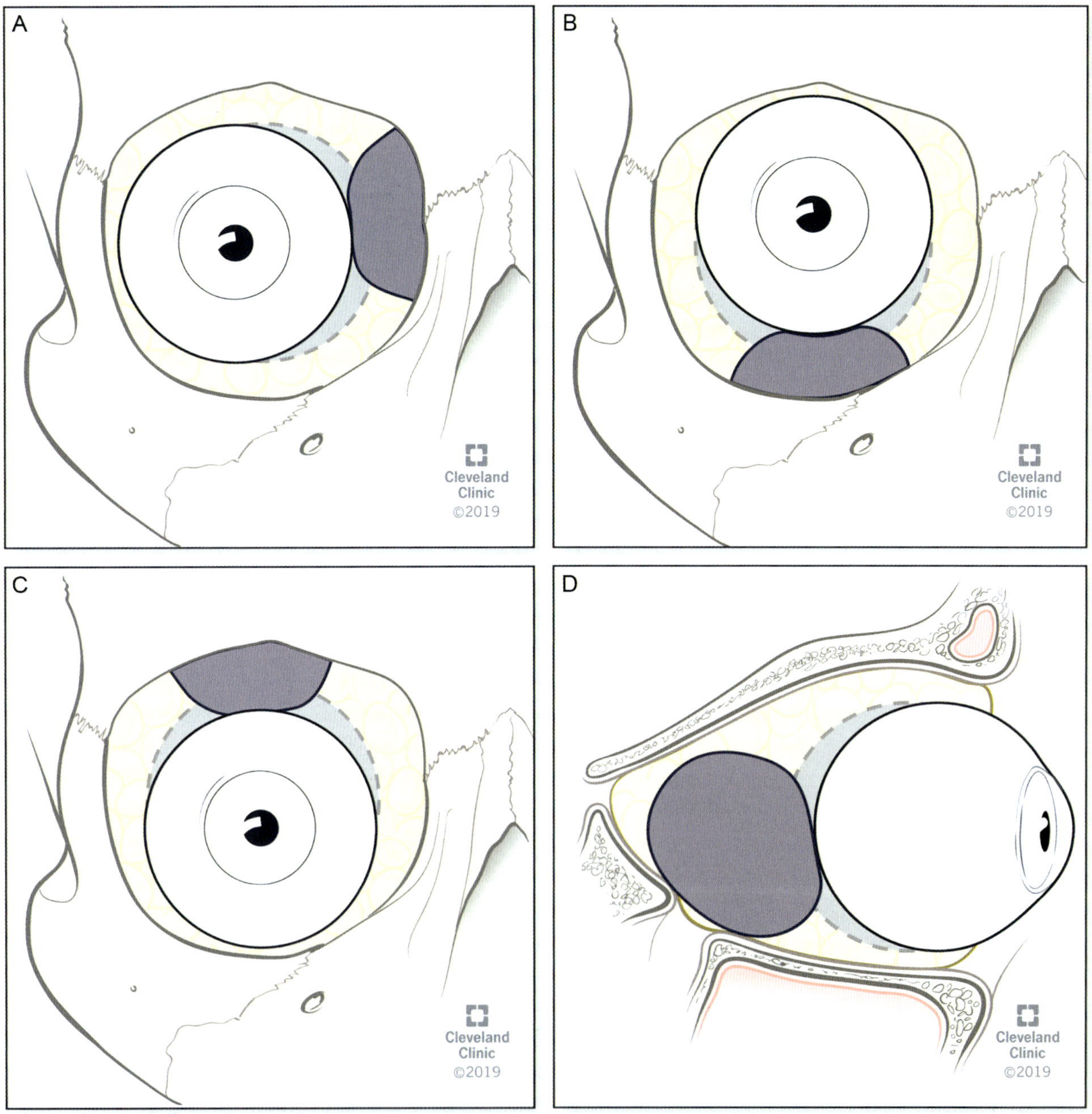

• **Fig. 7.4** Globe dystopia and proptosis. (A) A medial mass lesion is present, displacing the globe laterally. (B) An inferior lesion displaces the globe superiorly. (C) A superior lesion displaces the globe inferiorly. (D) A retroorbital lesion, causing proptosis or axial globe displacement.

the orbit. This may occur in cavernous malformation, optic nerve glioma, meningioma, diffuse nonspecific orbital inflammation, and thyroid eye disease. Superotemporal lesions, such as a lacrimal gland mass, are more likely to displace the globe inferonasally. Superonasal lesions, such as a dermoid cyst, would displace the globe inferotemporally. Thyroid eye disease, the most common cause of unilateral or bilateral proptosis in adults, tends to produce axial (anterior) proptosis.

Diseases increasing the orbital bony volume (silent sinus syndrome, fracture) or decreasing orbital soft-tissue volume (sclerosing metastatic breast cancer, granulomatosis with polyangiitis) may reduce globe projection, producing enophthalmos, or produce movement of the globe in the direction of the orbital process.

Because the globe resides within the orbital compartment, intraocular pressure (IOP) may provide a general sense of orbital pressure. A normal intraocular pressure is 10 to 21 mm Hg and is typically measured with either Goldmann applanation at the slit lamp or a handheld tonometer (Tono-Pen, Reichert, Buffalo, NY). The experienced practitioner can use digital palpation to compare the pressure on each side and provide a general estimate of eye and orbital pressure. Similarly, the technique of digital retropulsion of the globe can be used to determine a rough estimate of orbital compliance. In addition to palpating/retropulsing the globe, the warmth, tenderness, mobility, and pulsation of the orbit should be assessed. Pulsation increases the suspicion of a vascular lesion or pulsation from cerebrospinal fluid, such as in sphenoid wing dysplasia. Palpation of regional lymph nodes should also be performed.

Periocular Examination

The somatic sensory system of the eyelids extending from the orbit should be evaluated. The supraorbital branch of the trigeminal nerve (CN V1) traverses along the roof of the orbit to exit at the supraorbital notch/foramen to supply sensation to the forehead (Fig. 7.5). The infraorbital nerve (CN V2) passes just beneath the very thin bone of the orbital floor to exit approximately 1 cm beneath the rim. Trigeminal sensation should be tested with a tissue or touch and asking the patient to compare the sensation of each side. The tissue can be twisted and gently placed on the cornea to check corneal sensation (CN V1). This is an important test in any patient with lagophthalmos or facial nerve paresis.

The only motor system of the eyelid that extends from the orbit consists of the eyelid retractor muscles: the levator palpebrae superioris of the upper eyelid and the eyelid retractors of the lower eyelid. These muscles affect the height of the eyelid, and mainly the upper eyelid becomes manifest in disease states. Inflammatory diseases such as thyroid eye disease may cause retraction of the upper eyelid, whereas ptosis of the upper eyelid may occur from mechanical or neurologic causes from orbital disease. The height of the eyelid is characterized by the marginal reflex distance-1 (MRD-1). This is the distance from the upper eyelid margin to the pupillary light reflex in primary gaze. Levator function represents the amount in milimeters of excursion of the upper eyelid when the eye moves from downgaze to upgaze. It characterizes the strength of the levator muscle. The normal marginal reflex distance-1 (MRD-1) is 3 to 5 mm and normal levator function is 12 to 15 mm.

The motor system controlling eyelid height is balanced by the eyelid protractor muscles, which are controlled by the facial nerve, entering the eyelids mostly laterally, but some fibers enter the upper eyelid medially as well. The protractors are not primarily affected in orbital disease, but they play an integral role in the lacrimal secretory and excretory functions.

The normal eyelid is apposed to the globe along its entire length. Eyelid laxity can be assessed in three directions. Medial

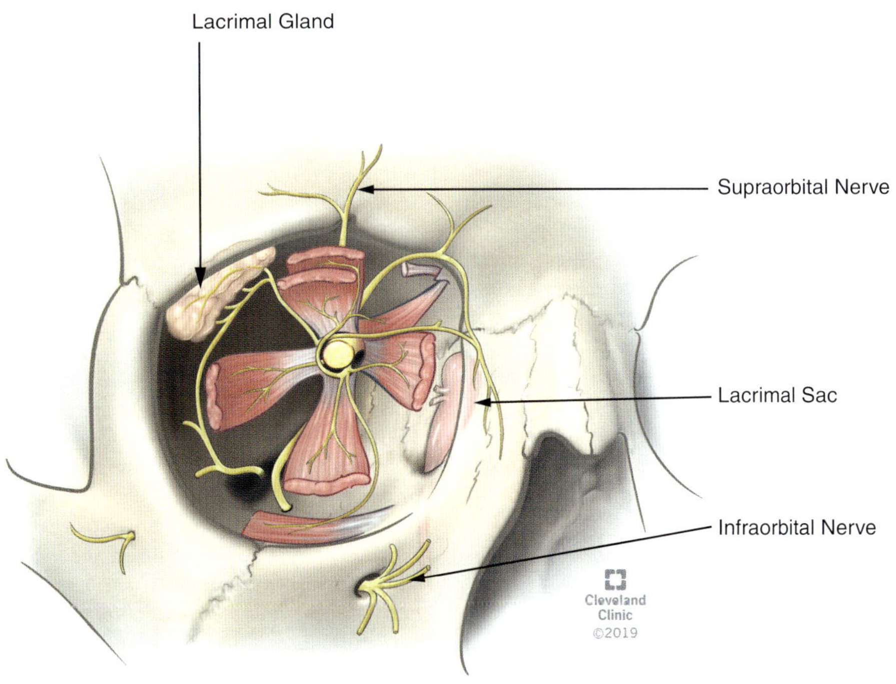

• **Fig. 7.5** Soft-tissue contents of the orbit. The lacrimal gland is located in the superotemporal orbit, whereas the lacrimal sac is positioned in the inferomedial orbit. Note the position of the supraorbital nerve (cranial nerve V1) and the infraorbital nerve (cranial nerve V2).

eyelid laxity can be tested by stretching the eyelid laterally and determining the extent of lateral displacement of the punctum, which generally should not exceed 2 mm. Mild laxity is present if the punctum reaches the medial limbus, and severe laxity is present if the punctum reaches the central pupil.[2] Similarly, lateral eyelid laxity can be tested by stretching the eyelid medially. To test generalized laxity of the eyelid, the eyelid is distracted from the globe by pinching it and stretching it away from the globe. The central eyelid should not extend more than 6 mm from the surface of the globe. The snap-back test can also be performed: After distraction of the eyelid from the globe surface, the eyelid should return spontaneously and immediately to appose the globe without the need for eyelid blinking. Eyelid laxity is seen if the eyelid returns to normal position only after several seconds or after blinking.

Eyelid laxity may occur with age but may also occur with facial nerve paresis. Other signs of facial nerve paresis include incomplete blinking of the eyelid (lagophthalmos). Pretarsal orbicularis oculi muscle weakness may be detected if the upper eyelid herniates over the lower eyelid margin on forced contraction of the eyelids.

The eyelid margin should be examined. An abnormal eyelid margin may be turned inward toward the globe (entropion) or turned away from the globe (ectropion). Trichiasis indicates aberrant eyelashes that misdirected (turned inward or touching the globe) or with an abnormal origin.

Lacrimal Examination

The lacrimal system begins with the lacrimal secretory system, consisting of the lacrimal gland and the conjunctival goblet cells (see Fig. 7.5). Upper eyelid eversion can evaluate the posterior aspect of the eyelid and the upper conjunctival fornix. The orbital lobe of the lacrimal gland can often be visualized within the upper fornix and can be visualized with eyelid eversion. Cysts and other abnormalities of the lacrimal gland can be directly visualized here. Signs of mass lesions, such as lymphoma, lacrimal gland tumors, or inflammatory disease, may become evident with this maneuver. The conjunctival goblet cells, responsible for basal tear secretion, are prominent in the conjunctival fornices.

The lacrimal excretory system begins with the puncta. Both upper and lower punctum should be assessed. The normal position of the punctum is facing toward the globe and tear lake. Punctal eversion can be noted in cases of eyelid laxity. The punctum should appear patent to the naked eye. Causes of punctal occlusion include congenital agenesis, ocular surface inflammation, or iatrogenic causes (e.g., punctal plugs or cautery). The punctum should be evaluated for erythema and discharge. As discussed previously, normal orbicularis function is essential for a normal blink reflex and a functioning tear drainage system. Signs of poor orbicularis function include poor lid apposition to the globe, weakened forced lid closure, lagophthalmos, and ectropion.

The remainder of the lacrimal system cannot be directly visualized without the use of dacryoendoscopy, an uncommonly used procedure. Thus, the function of this system relies on testing in the office.

Tear meniscus height can give an estimate of tear volume, which is a balance of tear secretion and excretion. Increased tear meniscus height indicates either hypersecretion or hypoexcretion of tears. Tear secretion may be assessed with Schirmer testing. In the basic secretion test, a drop of anesthetic is placed in the eye, the excess fluid is blotted, and a test strip is placed in the inferotemporal fornix. A normal result is more than 15 mm of wetting on the test strip over 5 minutes. Similarly, a Schirmer test can be performed in a similar fashion but without topical anesthetic to test for both basal and reflex tearing.

The fluorescein dye disappearance test is one method to evaluate tear drainage. A drop of fluorescein is placed into both fornices. The tear film is reevaluated after 5 minutes, with the degree of drainage of fluorescein evaluated. The test is easier to interpret in asymmetric dye disappearance, although grading scales have been made.[3]

The lacrimal system can be evaluated with probing and irrigation (Fig. 7.6). The punctum may be anesthetized with topical anesthetic drops or 4% lidocaine on a pledglet before testing for patient comfort. If needed, the punctum can be enlarged with a punctal dilator. A lacrimal cannula, typically on a 1- or 3-mL syringe prefilled with sterile saline solution, is inserted into the punctum and advanced. It is important to respect the anatomy during this test; the initial vertical portion of canaliculus is only for 2 mm, then horizontal for 8 to 10 mm. The eyelid should be placed on lateral stretch to prevent kinking and a false sense of a soft stop. Both the degree of canalicular stenosis and the location of the stenosis along the canaliculus can be evaluated during probing. The lacrimal system can then be irrigated. A normal lacrimal system is present if the saline solution is felt in the nasopharynx, without reflux through the opposite punctum. If some saline solution is felt in the nasopharynx with reflux through the opposite punctum, a partial NLDO is present. If no saline solution is felt in the nasopharynx with reflux through the opposite punctum, then a complete NLDO is present. If the saline solution refluxes through the same punctum, then a complete canalicular obstruction is present.

Jones testing is completed by the Jones I and Jones II tests. In the Jones I test, a drop of fluorescein is placed in each eye. After 5 minutes, a cotton-tipped applicator is placed into the inferior meatus. If fluorescein is seen on the cotton tip, the test is normal. If not, the Jones II test is performed. In the Jones II test, the eye is washed of residual fluorescein. The lacrimal system is irrigated with saline solution. Again, a cotton-tipped applicator is placed in the inferior meatus. If dye is detected, this suggests partial NLDO. If no fluorescein is detected, this indicates that the fluorescein never entered the lacrimal sac, either from a tear pump deficiency, punctal stenosis, or canalicular stenosis.[4]

Other Tests

Computed tomography and magnetic resonance imaging are useful and often used adjunctive tests for orbital and lacrimal disease. This topic is covered in Chapter 9. Beyond computed tomography and magnetic resonance imaging, dacryocystography (DCG) and lacrimal scintigraphy (LS) are two other imaging tests that may provide additional information in the evaluation of the lacrimal system; however, these tests are less commonly used. In DCG, contrast dye is injected into one or both lacrimal systems and a series of radiographs are taken. In lacrimal scintigraphy, a radionuclide, typically technetium 99m pertechnetate, is placed in the fornices. The lacrimal system is imaged with a gamma camera. These images can show the entire lacrimal system. LS has shown greater

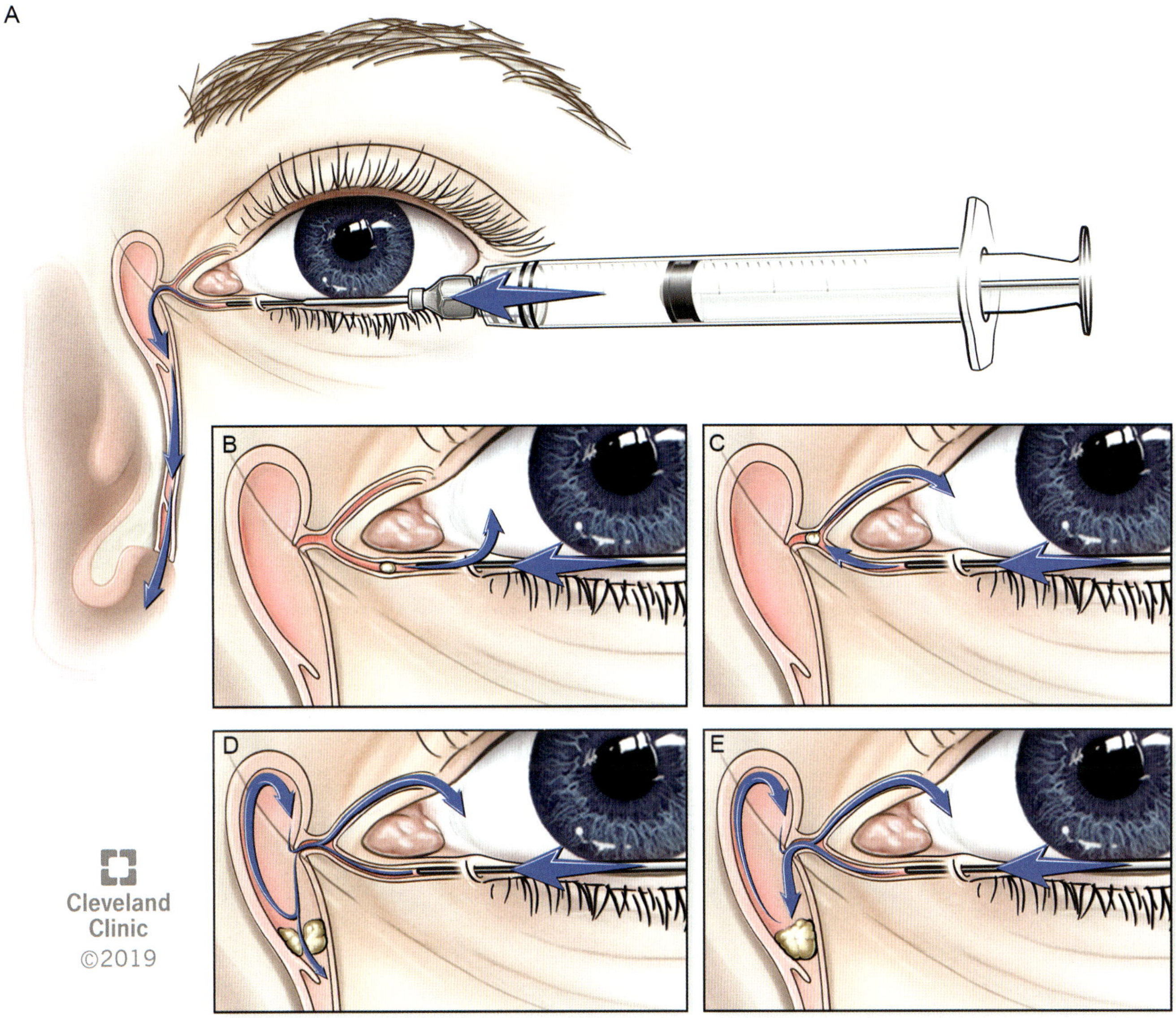

• **Fig. 7.6** Lacrimal irrigation. (A) Normal irrigation. Irrigated fluid flows into the nose/inferior meatus without regurgitation or resistance. (B) Canalicular obstruction. Fluid regurgitation through the same punctum as the irrigating cannula. (C) Common canaliculus obstruction. Fluid flowing up to the obstruction, but regurgitation through opposite punctum. (D) Partial nasolacrimal duct obstruction. Fluid partially flowing into nose/inferior meatus, but with regurgitation through the same or opposite punctum. (E) Complete nasolacrimal duct obstruction. Fluid does not flow into the nose/inferior meatus. Regurgitation through the same or opposite punctum.

agreement than DCG with clinical examination, possibly because the method of LS is more physiologic.[5] When used, dacryocystography and/or scintigraphy may help with evaluating the site of lacrimal obstruction.[6]

Summary

When evaluating patients with orbital or lacrimal disease, a thorough history and ophthalmic examination can help guide differential diagnoses and direct further studies such as imaging. The key components of an orbital examination include testing of the visual sensory system, including optic nerve function, extraocular motility, and globe position. For patients presenting with lacrimal system dysfunction, eyelid examination to evaluate the tear pump mechanism, slit-lamp examination to check for ocular surface disease, and lacrimal irrigation are integral.

References

1. Almog, Y., & Nemet, A. (2010). The correlation between visual acuity and color vision as an indicator of the cause of visual loss. *American Journal of Ophthalmology*, *149*(6), 1000–1004.
2. Olver, J. M., Sathia, P. J., & Wright, M. (2001). Lower eyelid medial canthal tendon laxity grading: An interobserver study of normal subjects. *Ophthalmology*, *108*(2), 2321–2325.

3. MacEwen, C. J., & Young, J. D. (1991). The fluorescein disappearance test (FDT): An evaluation of its use in infants. *Journal of Pediatric Ophthalmology & Strabismus*, *28*(6), 302–305.
4. Freitag, S. K., & Lefebvre, D. R. (2018). *Diagnostic techniques to evaluate obstructive or reflexive epiphora. AAO: Oculofacial Plastic Surgery Education Center.* Availabe at San Francisco, CA: American Academy of Ophthalmology: Oculofacial Plastic Surgery Education Center. (2018). https://www.aao.org/oculoplastics-center/diagnostic-techniques-to-evaluate-obstructive-refl.
5. Peter, N. M., & Pearson, A. R. (2009). Comparison of dacryocystography and lacrimal scintigraphy in the investigation of epiphora in patients with patent but nonfunctioning lacrimal systems. *Ophthalmic Plastic and Reconstructive Surgery*, *25*(3), 201–205.
6. Nagi, K. S., & Meyer, D. R. (2010). Utilization patterns for diagnostic imaging in the evaluation of epiphora due to lacrimal obstruction: A national survey. *Ophthalmic Plastic and Reconstrive Surgery*, *26*(3), 168–171.

8

Neuro-Ophthalmologic Evaluation and Testing

LISA D. LYSTAD, MD

The impact of intraorbital, intracranial, and sinus lesions on visual function and eye movement can be difficult to quantify. Imaging yields information on lesion location and possible etiology. The role of the neuro-ophthalmologist is to provide quantifiable measurements of the damage caused by disease processes in the orbit, skull base, and sinuses. This quantification allows for more concise decision making regarding lesion progression, surgical timing, and potential lesion recurrence. Functional changes may precede obvious structural progression on imaging studies. The neuro-ophthalmologist also aids in managing temporary or permanent patient issues such as diplopia and vision loss. Diagnostic tools for monitoring vision and ocular motility are reviewed, followed by use of these techniques in case presentations.

Techniques for Assessing Visual Function

The hallmarks of optic nerve dysfunction include afferent pupillary defect, color vision deficits or dyschromatopsia, and visual field loss. Afferent pupillary defect is evaluated using the standard swinging flashlight test. It is usually graded on a subjective 0 to +4 scale or by a logMAR scale (0.3 to 1.8) as measured with photo gray filters.

Color vision is assessed using Ishihara or AOH-R-R (Hardy, Rand, and Rittler) color plates or the D-15 disks. The most common test is done with the Ishihara booklet; testing is performed on each eye separately. A quick in-office test for dyschromatopsia is subjective red desaturation using any bright red object. The patient is shown the object with one eye at a time. He or she is asked whether the color red is the same or different in each eye and which eye looks the most "true red." Optic nerve dysfunction may produce a darker red, more orange, or more pink appearance. Color vision testing is not dependent on visual acuity except in cases of severe vision loss or macular degeneration.

Visual Field Testing and Automated Perimetry

Automated perimetry provides the best technology for monitoring visual field changes. Humphrey (Zeiss, Oberkochen, Germany) and Octopus (Haag-Streit USA, Mason, OH) visual field machines both give quantitative measures of peripheral vision valuable for monitoring change over time. A 24-2 visual field, measuring 24 degrees from fixation, is the standard for ophthalmic disease. I prefer to use a 30-2 test. Testing 30 degrees from fixation can allow for earlier detection of compressive optic neuropathy. This test checks for 30 degrees on all sides from fixation, providing an additional 6 degrees of periphery (Fig. 8.1).

When evaluating the visual field the physiologic blind spot is located on the temporal side of the field from the patient perspective. The right eye blind spot is on the right of the field. The left eye blind spot is on the left (Fig. 8.2).

Proptosis

Proptosis is measured using an exophthalmometer. This device takes a millimeter measurement of the distance between the anterior cornea and the temporal orbital rim for each eye. For an individual patient the measurement base is the distance between the two temporal orbital rim margins. Thus a consistent measurement of proptosis or enophthalmos over time can be tracked for an individual. There is a wide range of normal readings between individuals owing to structural differences in skull morphology and orbital fat content. The measure is independent of ptosis or eyelid retraction, which can give the illusion of proptosis. Exophalmometer readings are particularly useful to monitor changes from thyroid eye disease or orbital mass. Enophthalmos can be indicative of orbital floor fracture or a cicatrizing lesion such as metastatic breast cancer. The data are expressed as "x" millimeters right eye, "y" millimeters left eye, with a base of "z" millimeters.

Ocular Motility and Prism

Ocular motility testing yields information on the range of motion of individual eye muscles as well as binocular eye alignment. Quantifying ocular motility deficits is performed using prism bars or loose prisms. The pattern of deviation is useful in suggesting whether a deficit is due to cranial nerve or ocular muscle damage. Prism measurements allow tracking of deterioration or improvement in ocular motility deficits over time. Prisms can provide a means to at least partially rid a patient of diplopia. The goal in their use is single vision looking straight ahead with a reasonable range of fusion with eye movement. This allows better daily function and the potential for an ability to drive. It prevents the loss of peripheral vision caused by patching one eye.

(Text continues on p. 57)

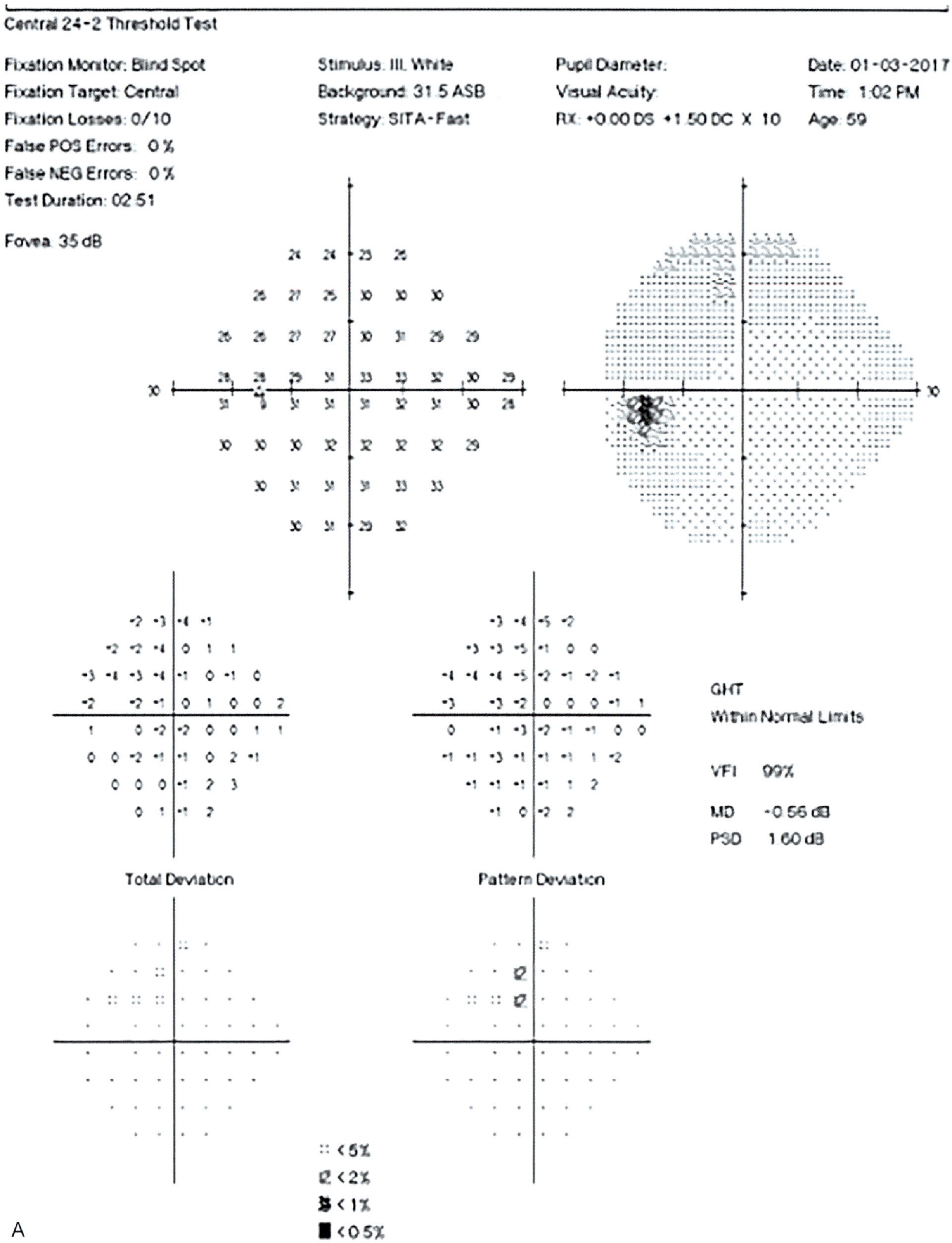

A

• **Fig. 8.1** A, Humphrey 24-2 Visual field program measures 24 degrees from fixation except at the extreme nasal field which extends two points out to 30 degrees.

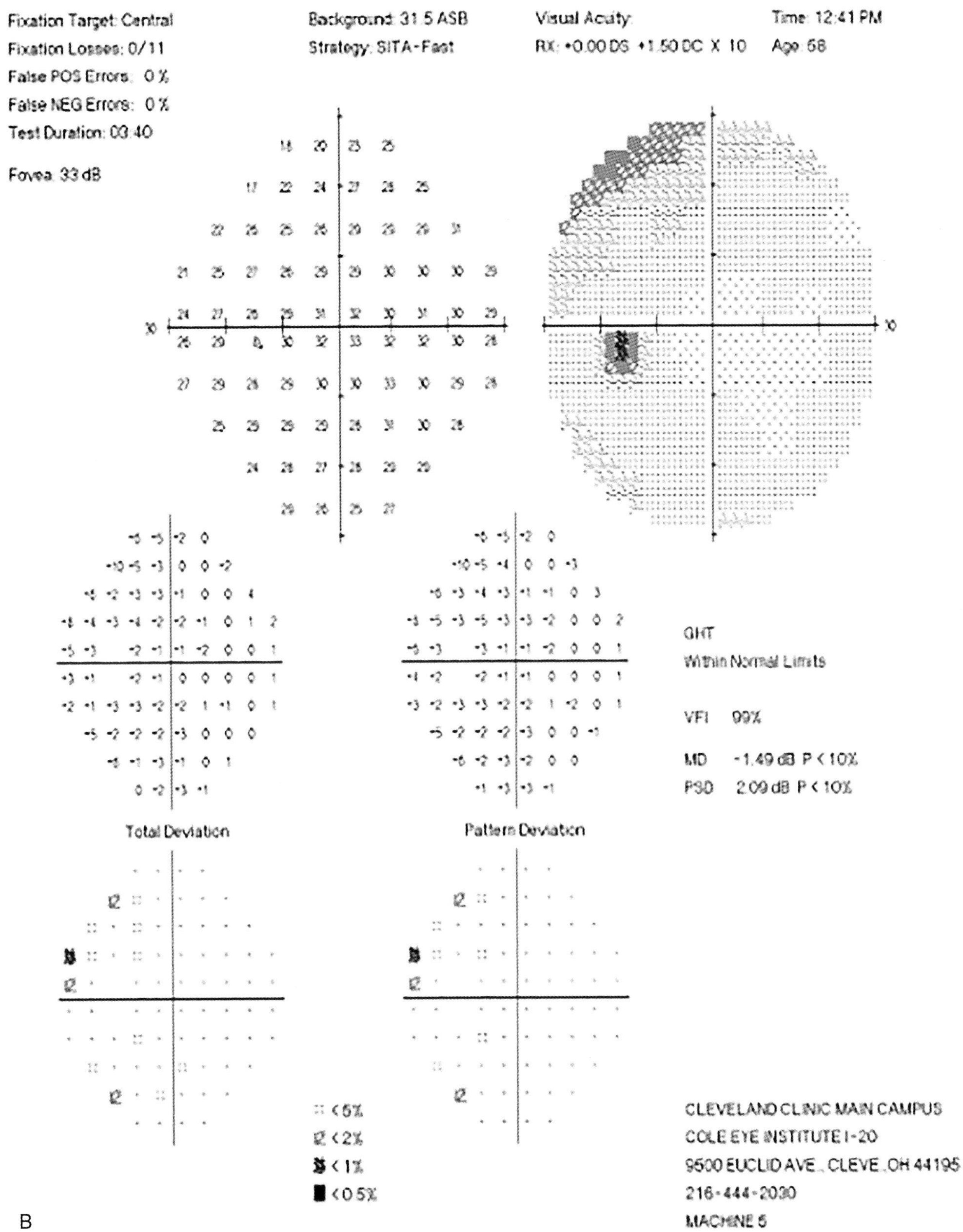

B

• **Fig. 8.1, cont'd** B, Left eye 30-degree visual field of same patient 3 weeks later reveals early superior temporal constriction. This represents early superior temporal constriction of the field from a pituitary lesion which was missed using the 24 degree field testing. *ASB,* apostilbs; *DC X,* diopters of cylinder correction at a given number of degrees; *DS,* diopter sphere; *GHT,* Glaucoma Hemifield Test; *MD,* the difference between the patient's test results and a normal age matched control; *NEG,* negative; *POS,* positive; *PSD,* pattern standard deviation; *RX,* prescription; *SITA,* Swedish Interactive Thresholding Algorithm; *VFI,* Visual Field Index.

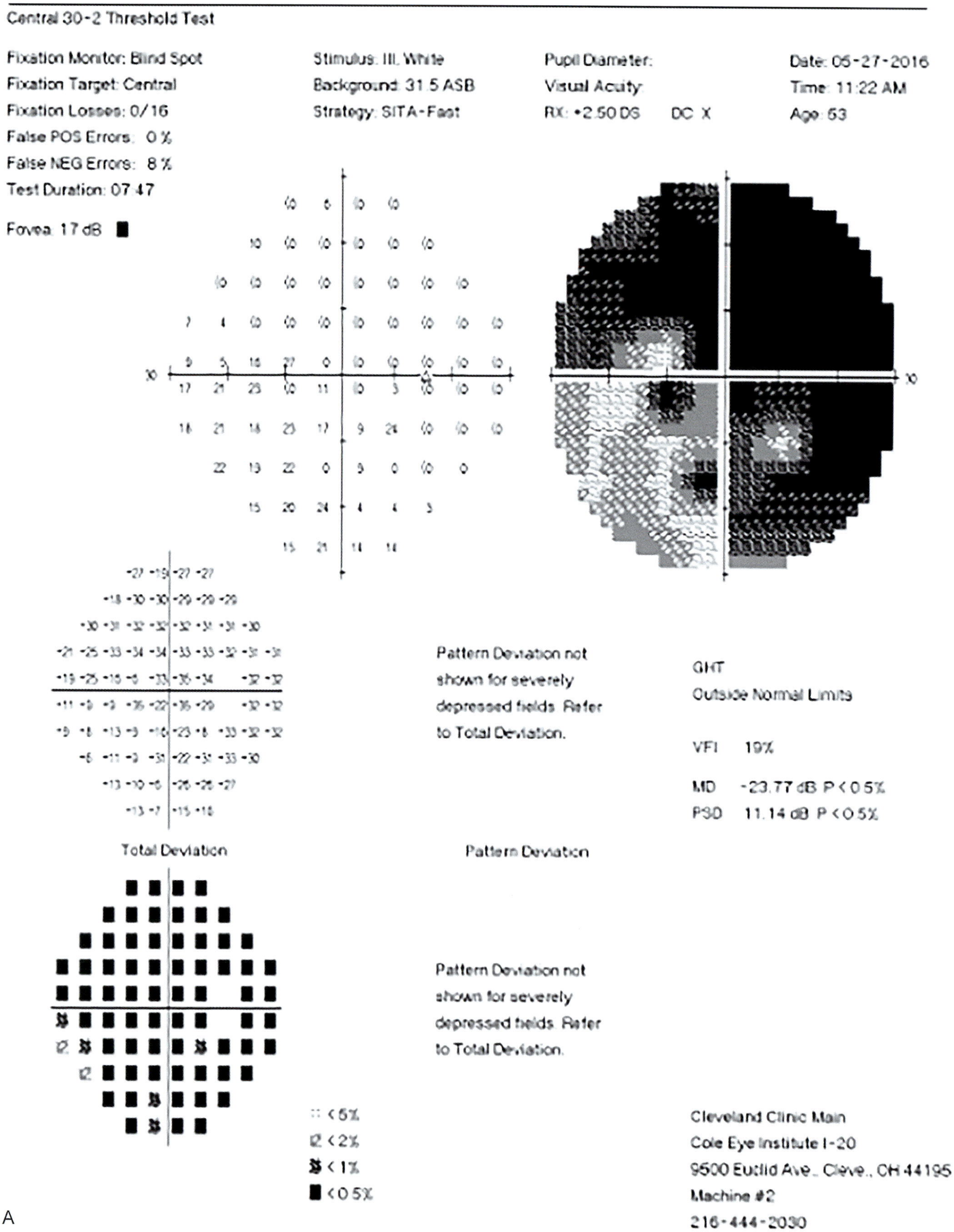

A

• **Fig. 8.2** A, Visual acuity is 20/60 in the right eye despite the severe visual field constriction. Vision is 20/20 in the left eye. There is a right afferent pupillary defect. Ocular coherence tomography (OCT) shows nerve fiber layer thinning.

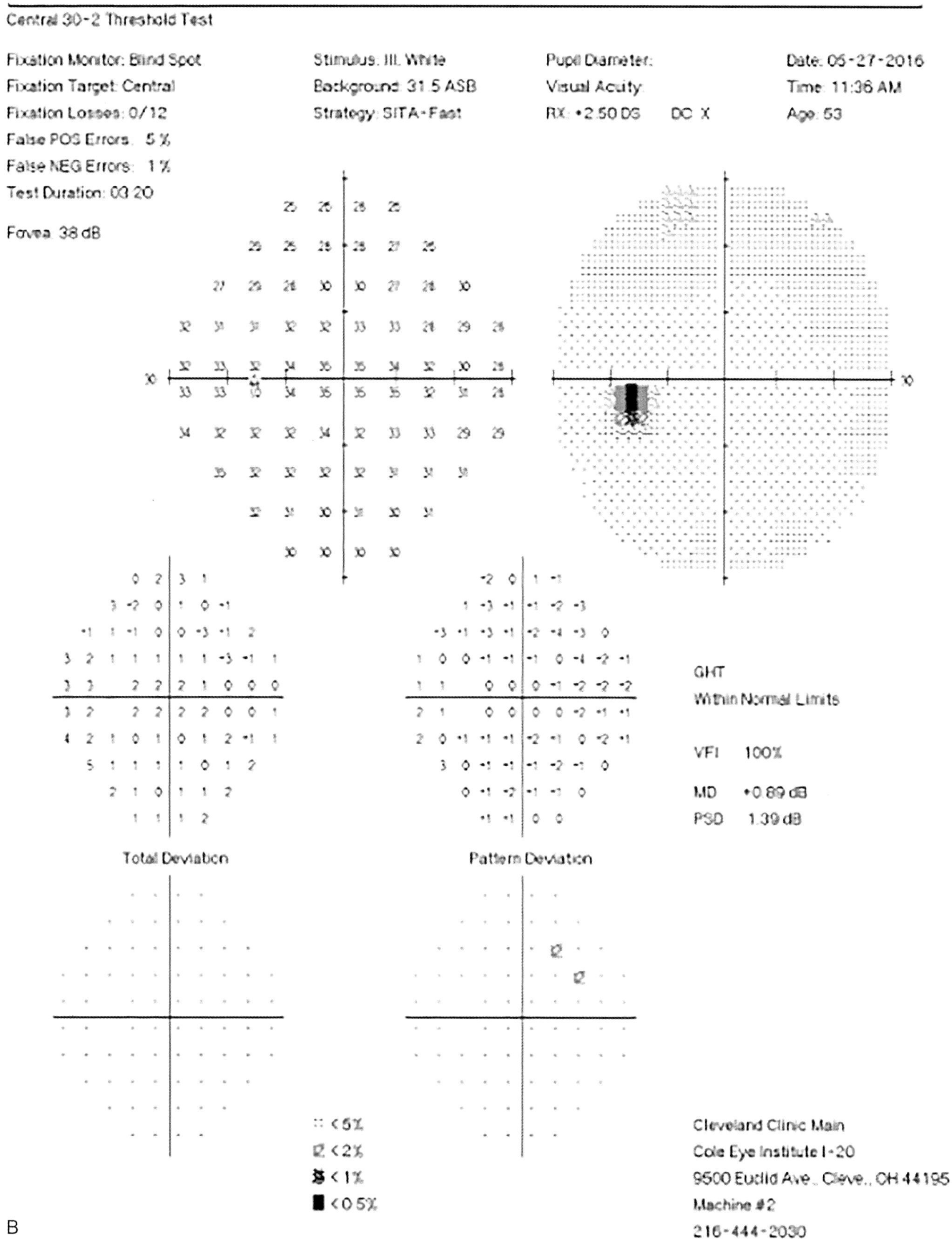

B

• **Fig. 8.2, cont'd** B, At presentation normal visual field in the left eye.

Continued

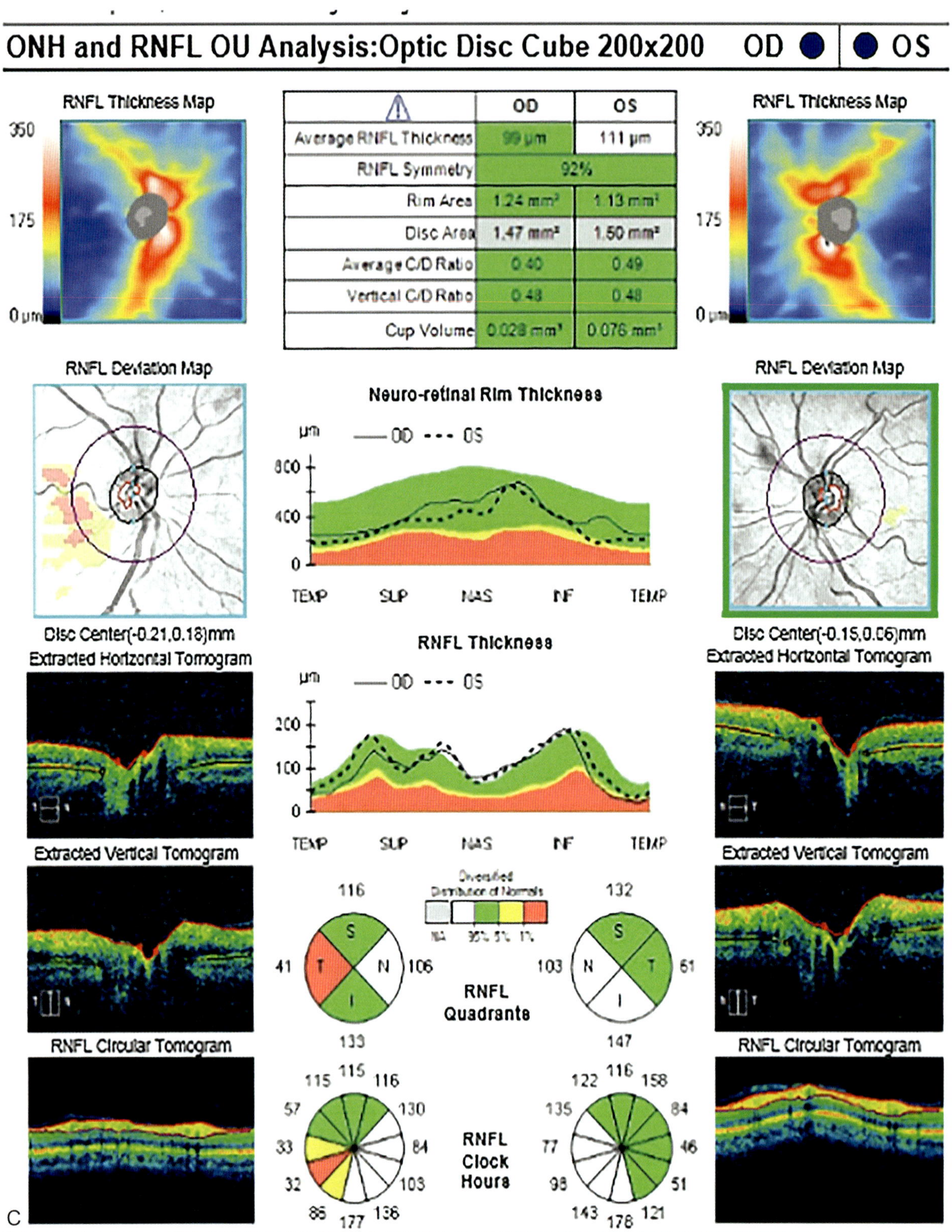

• **Fig. 8.2, cont'd** C, OCT optic nerve shows early thining in the nerve fiber layer of the right eye in the papillomacular bundle. Left eye OCT results is normal, which suggests good potential for visual improvement given the magnitude of the visual field defect.

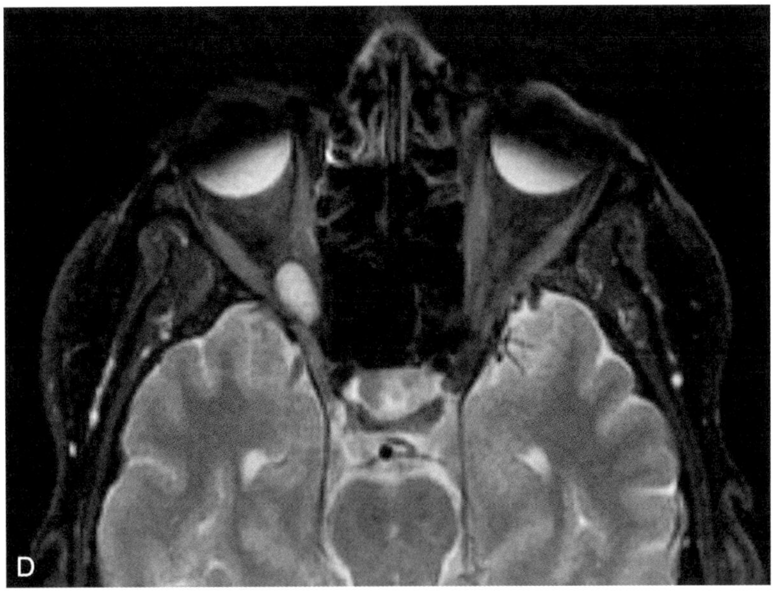

• **Fig. 8.2, cont'd** D, Magnetic resonance imaging of the orbit. T1-weighted post-gadolinium image shows a solitary well-circumscribed enhancing mass at the orbital apex with mild displacement of optic nerve.

Continued

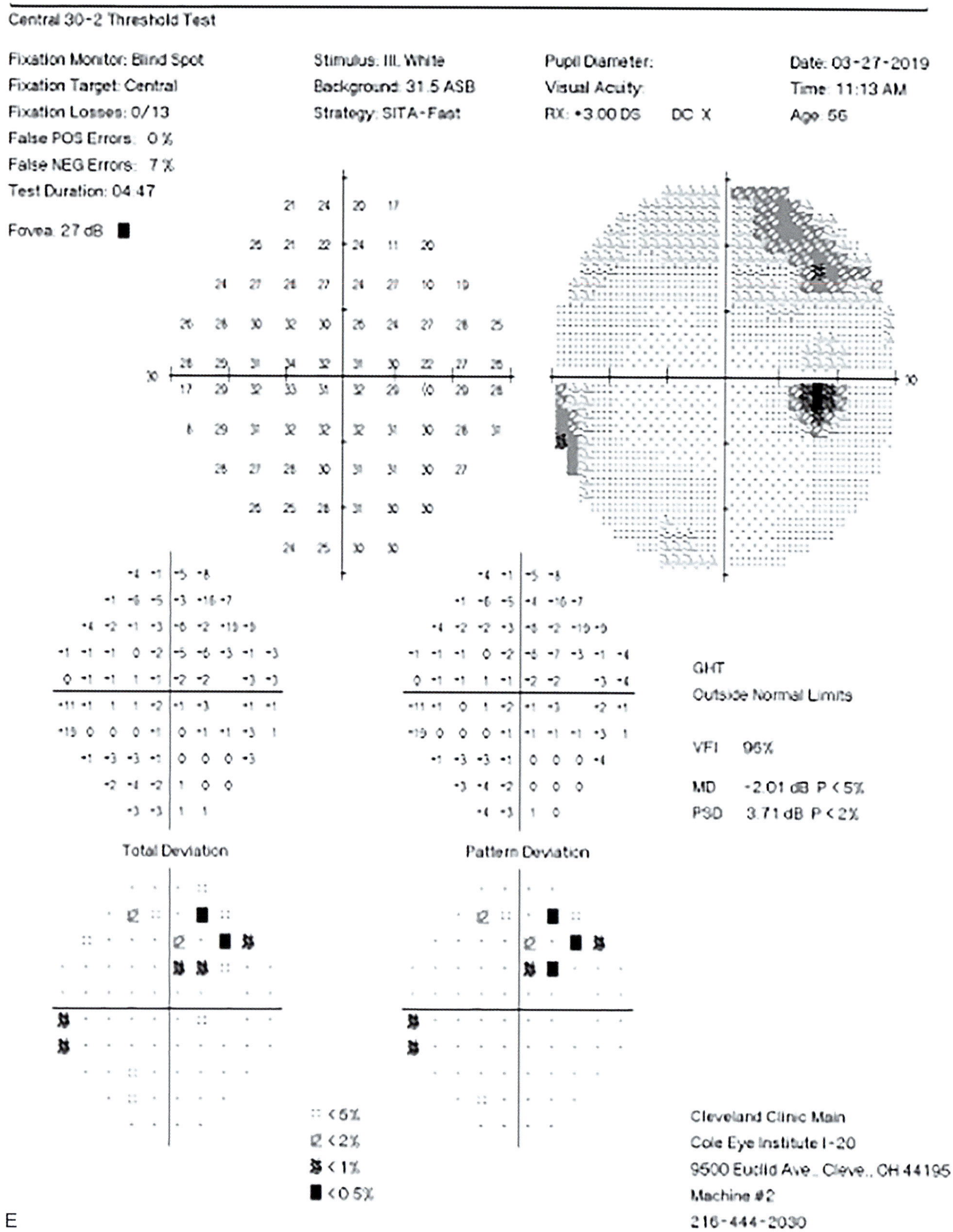

• **Fig. 8.2, cont'd** E, Postoperative improvement in the visual field in the right eye 2 months after surgical excision of the intraorbital cavernous hemangioma. Vision improved to 20/20. There was mild diplopia after surgery that resolved spontaneously.

Fresnel prisms are a means of temporarily allowing visual fusion in patients with diplopia. These are ridged sheets of clear plastic that can be placed on the back of a glasses lens using tap water. They bend light to allow centration of an image on the fovea and compensate for ocular misalignment. Easy to replace when adjusting for changes in the double vision, Fresnel prisms do not damage the glasses lens. They are particularly useful when an improvement in the magnitude of diplopia is expected and much less expensive than prism ground into glasses.

Ocular Coherence Tomography

Ocular coherence tomography (OCT) is a transpupillary means of evaluating the retinal layers in the macula and surrounding the optic nerve. It uses low-coherence light in the near-infrared spectrum to provide two- and three-dimensional images of tissue. Cross-sectional data provide a method for assessing retinal nerve fiber and ganglion cell layer thickness with a resolution of microns. When evaluating a compressive lesion of the optic nerve, OCT provides an assessment of retrograde neuronal damage in the nerve and retinal ganglion cell layer. Changes in OCT precede the development of optic atrophy. If a lesion, such as a meningioma or pituitary adenoma, is long-standing, OCT demonstrates nerve and ganglion cell layer defects that correlate with visual field loss. This information can be used to make a prediction of potential for improvement in visual function following surgical intervention (Figs. 8.2C and 8.5C).

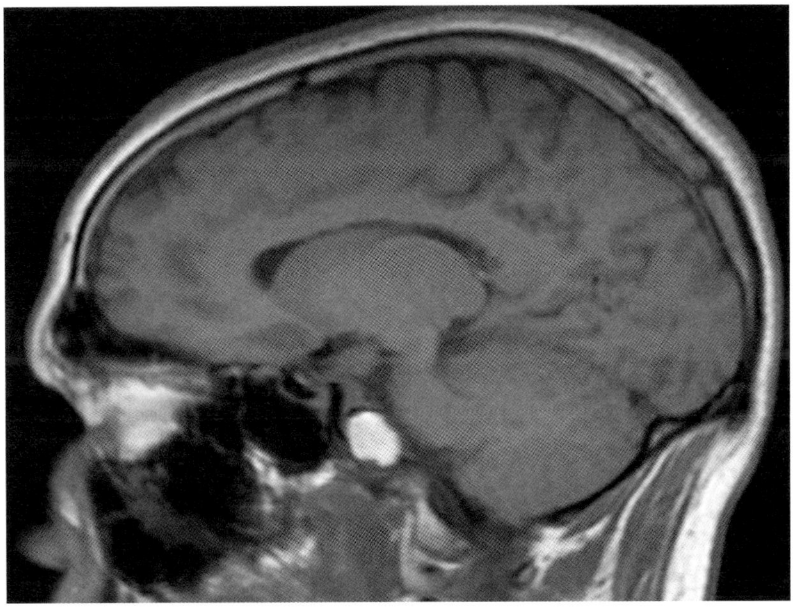

Fig. 8.3 A patient presented with a left abducens nerve palsy causing esotropia and double vision. Imaging showed a cholesterol granuloma at the petrous apex displacing the left sixth cranial nerve. Diplopia improved immediately after surgery and resolved completely within 2 weeks.

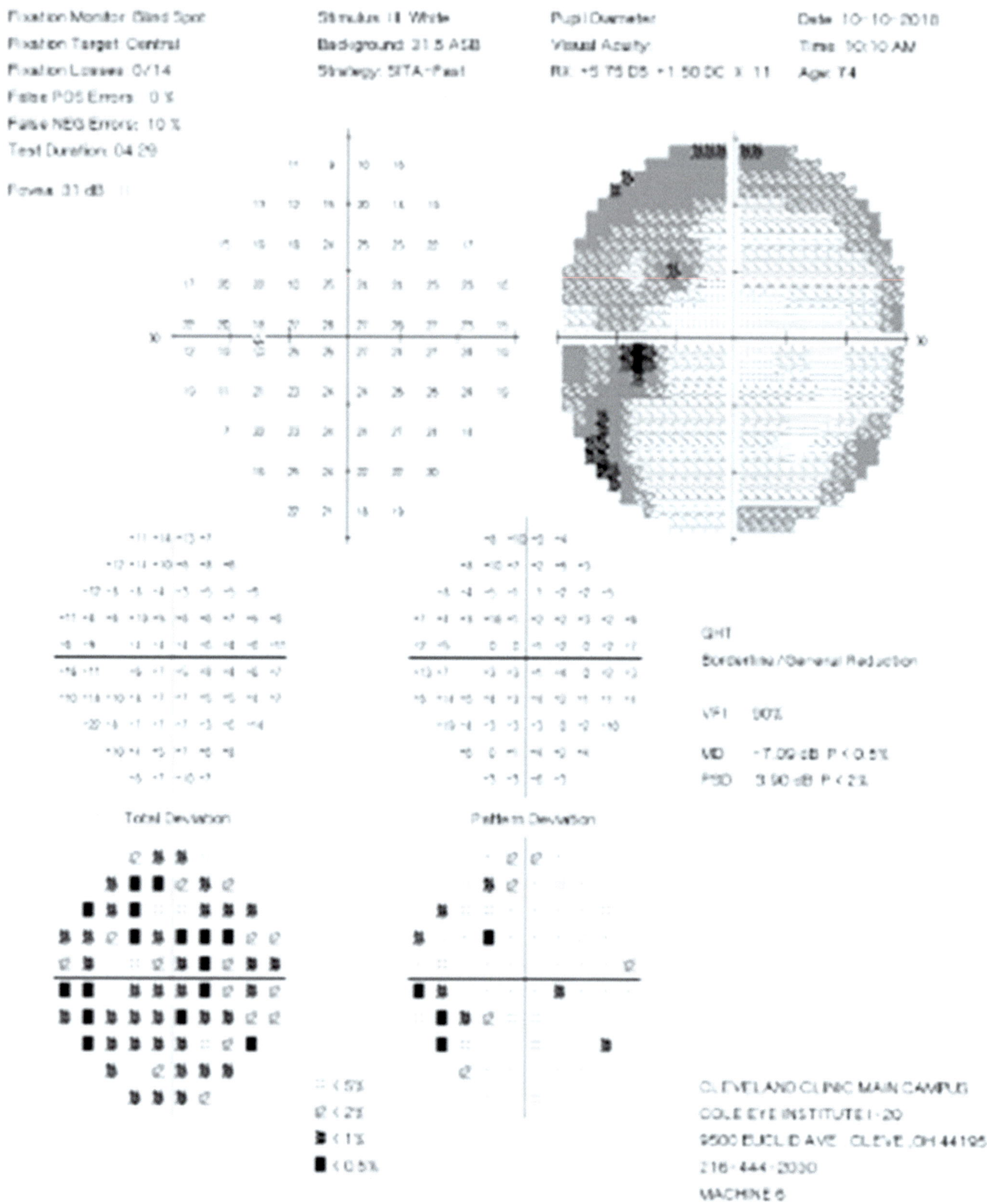

• **Fig. 8.4** A, Diffuse visual field depression in both eyes owing to compression of optic nerves from thyroid ophthalmopathy. Visual acuity was 20/20 and there was mild red color desaturation in both eyes. No afferent pupillary defect is present owing to bilateral disease. The patient began taking prednisone 60 mg daily and was scheduled for urgent bilateral orbital decompression.

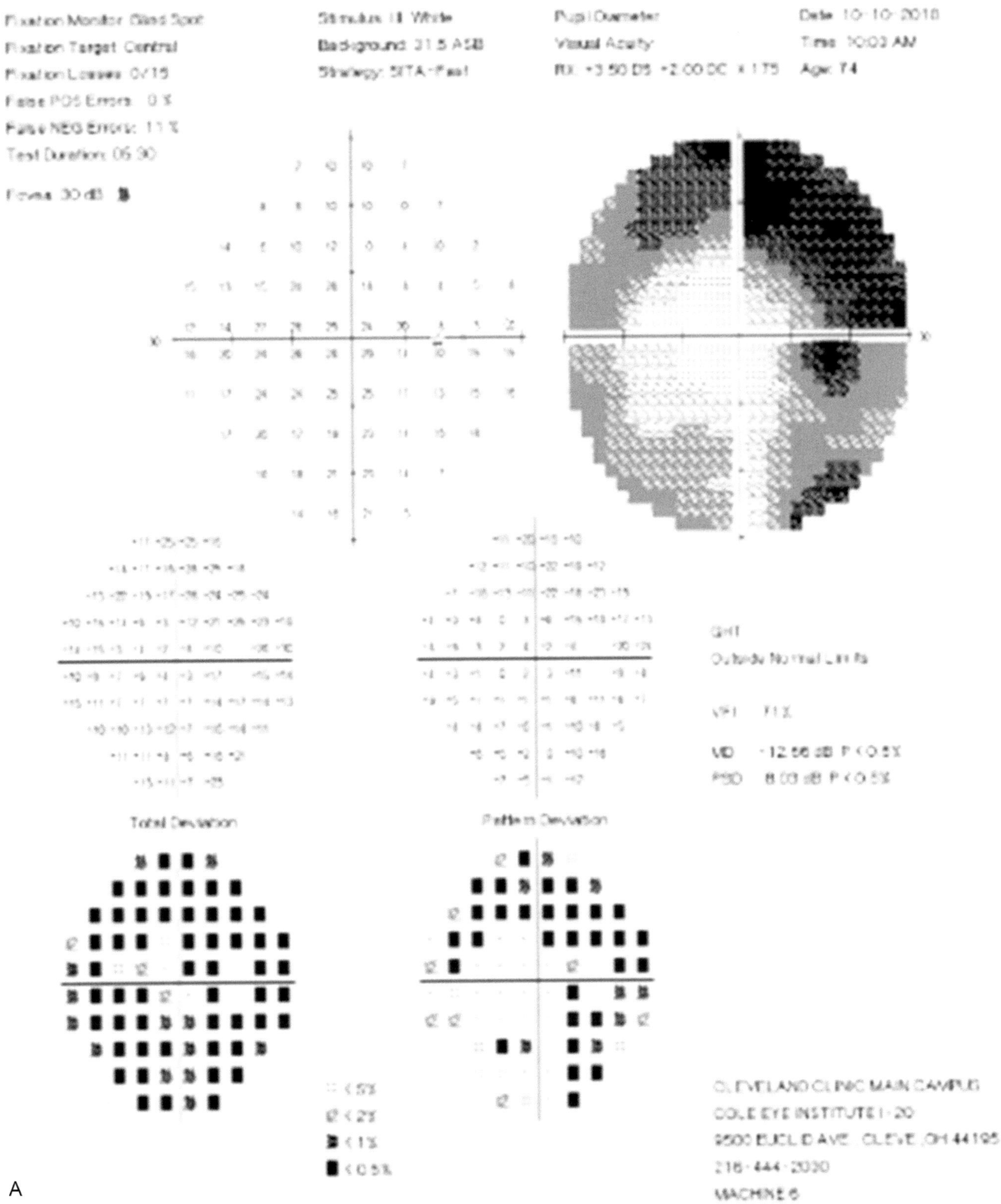

• **Fig. 8.4, cont'd**

Continued

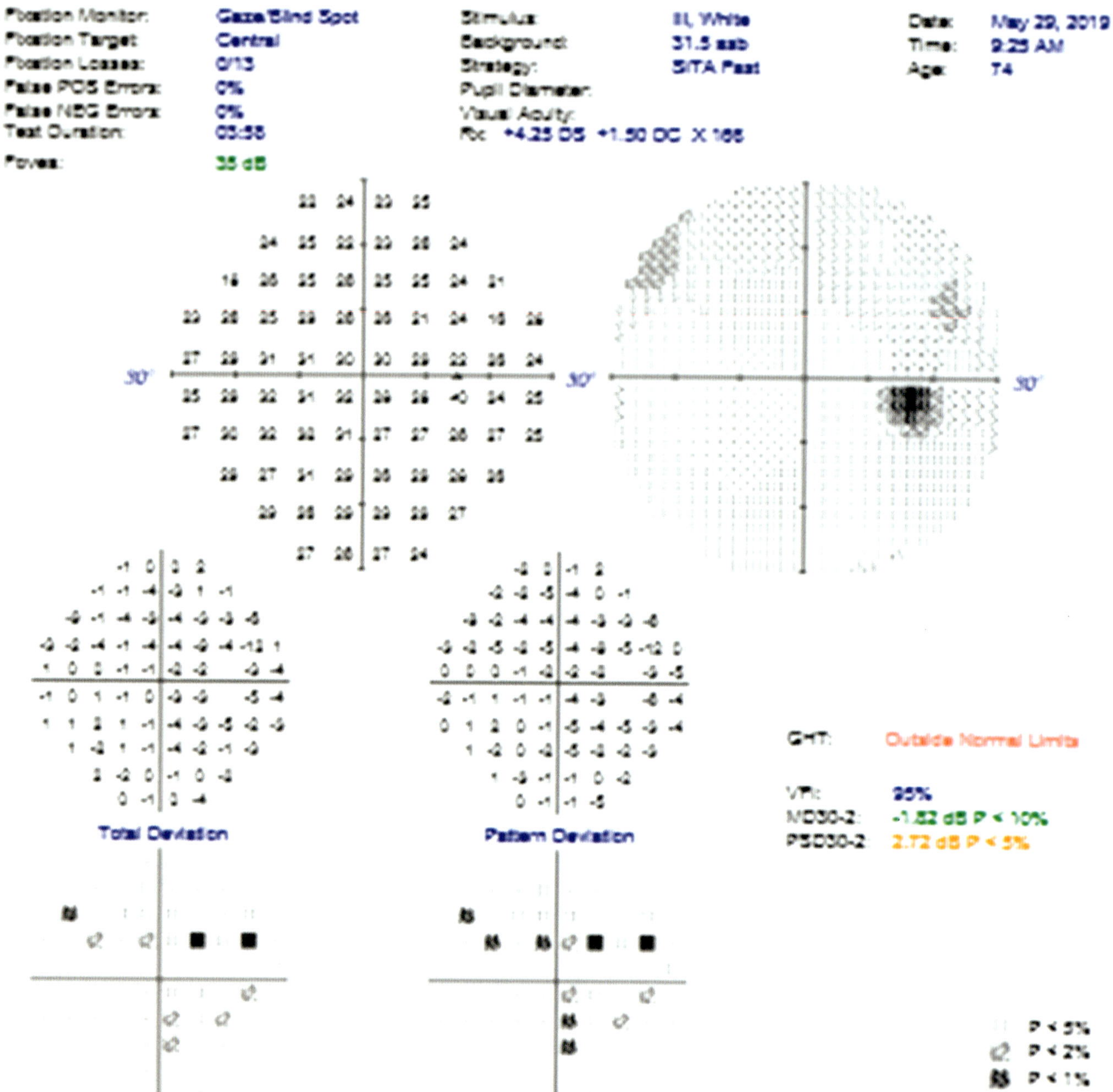

B

• **Fig. 8.4, cont'd** B and C, After orbital decompression for compressive optic neuropathy from thyroid disease, the visual field defects resolved in both eyes. Color desaturation resolved completely. Prednisone treatment was discontinued.

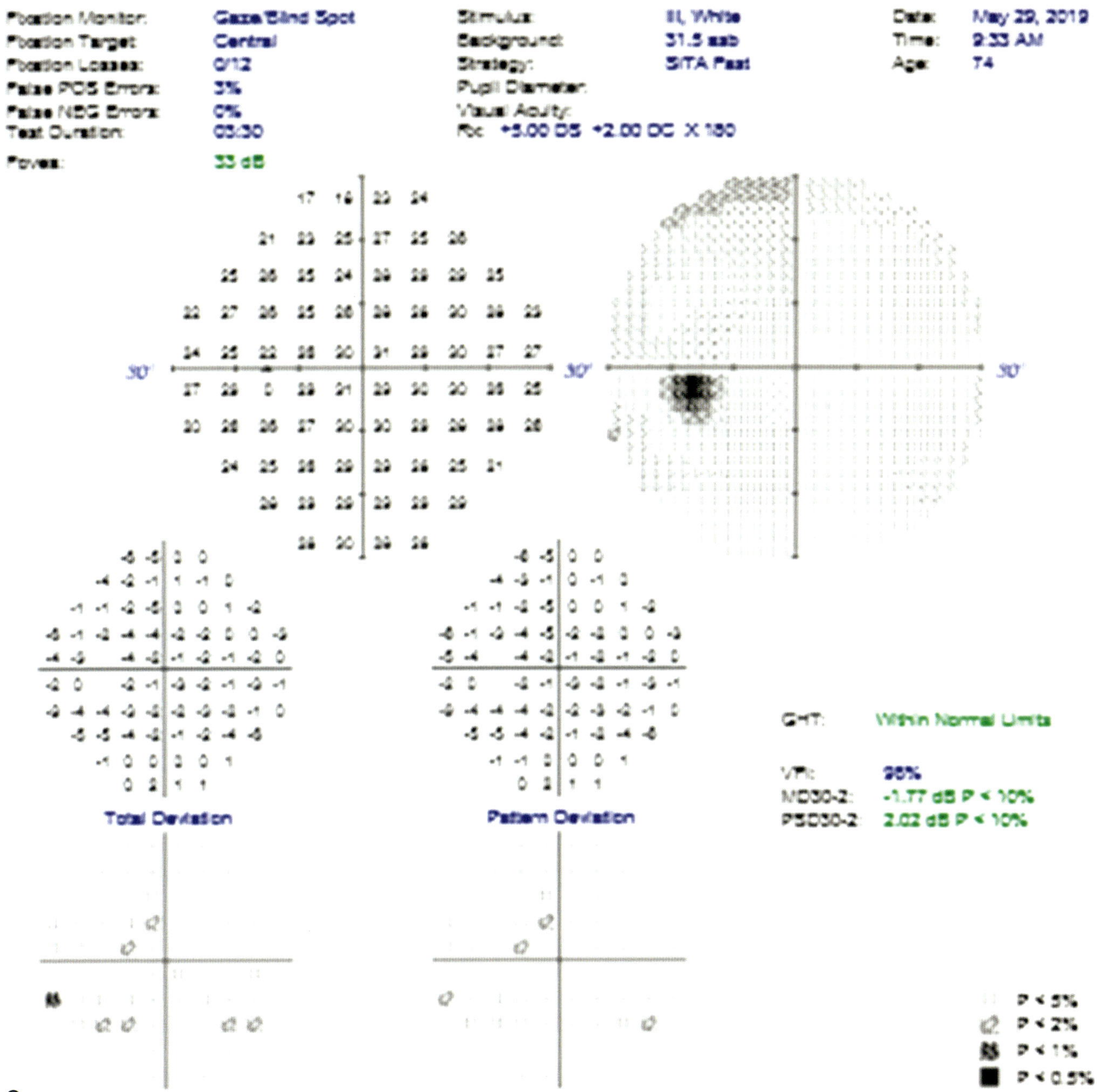

C

• **Fig. 8.4, cont'd**

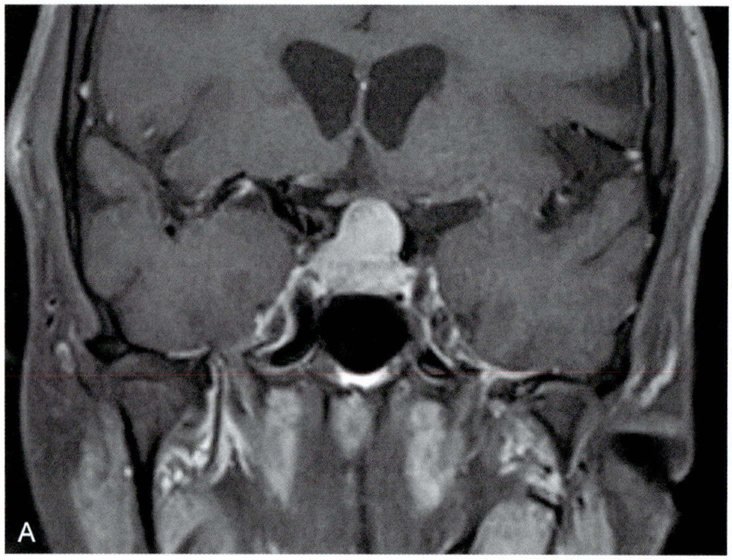

• **Fig. 8.5** A, Pituitary macroadenoma with chiasmal compression.

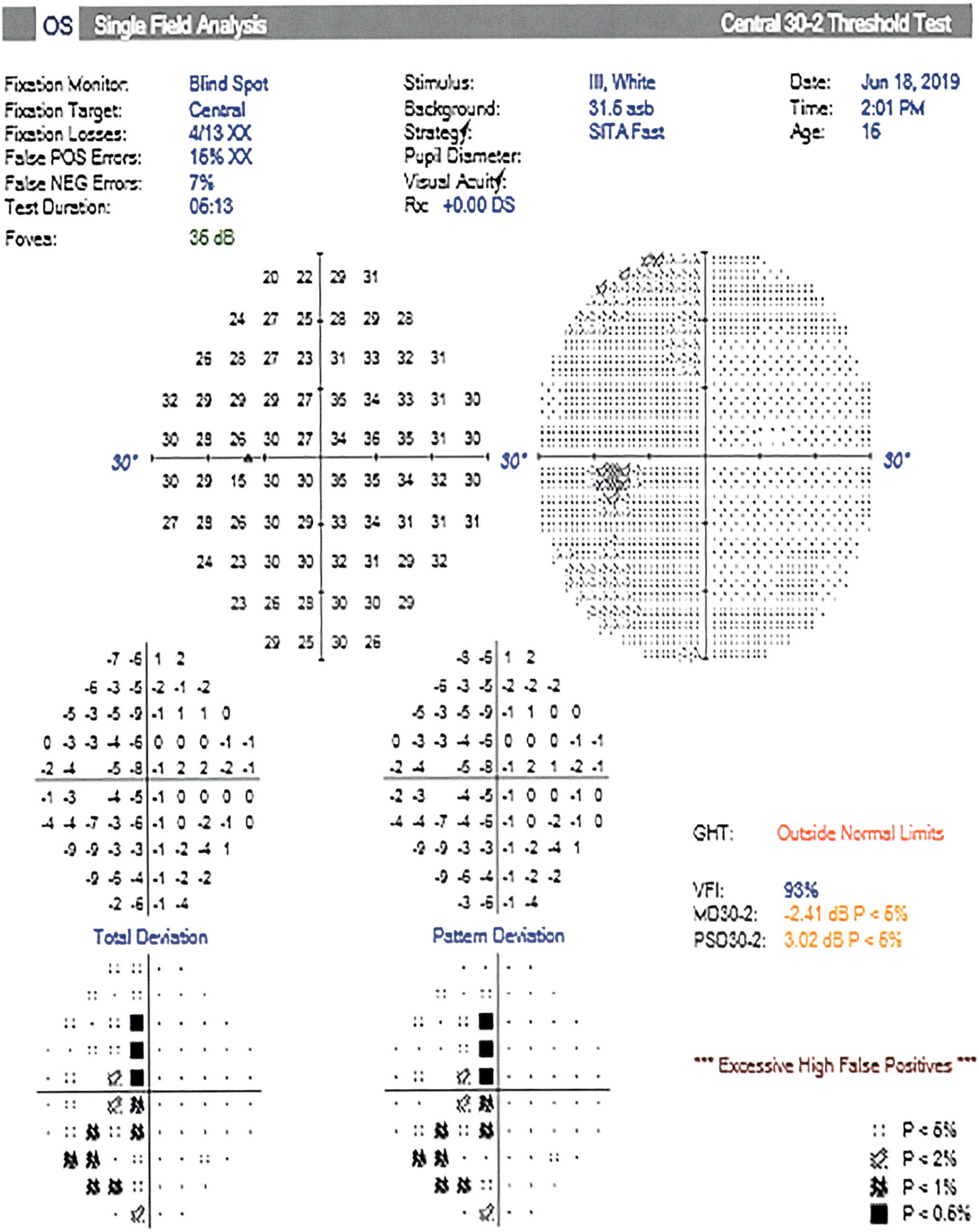

• **Fig. 8.5, cont'd** B, Early bitemporal visual field constriction in both eyes.

Continued

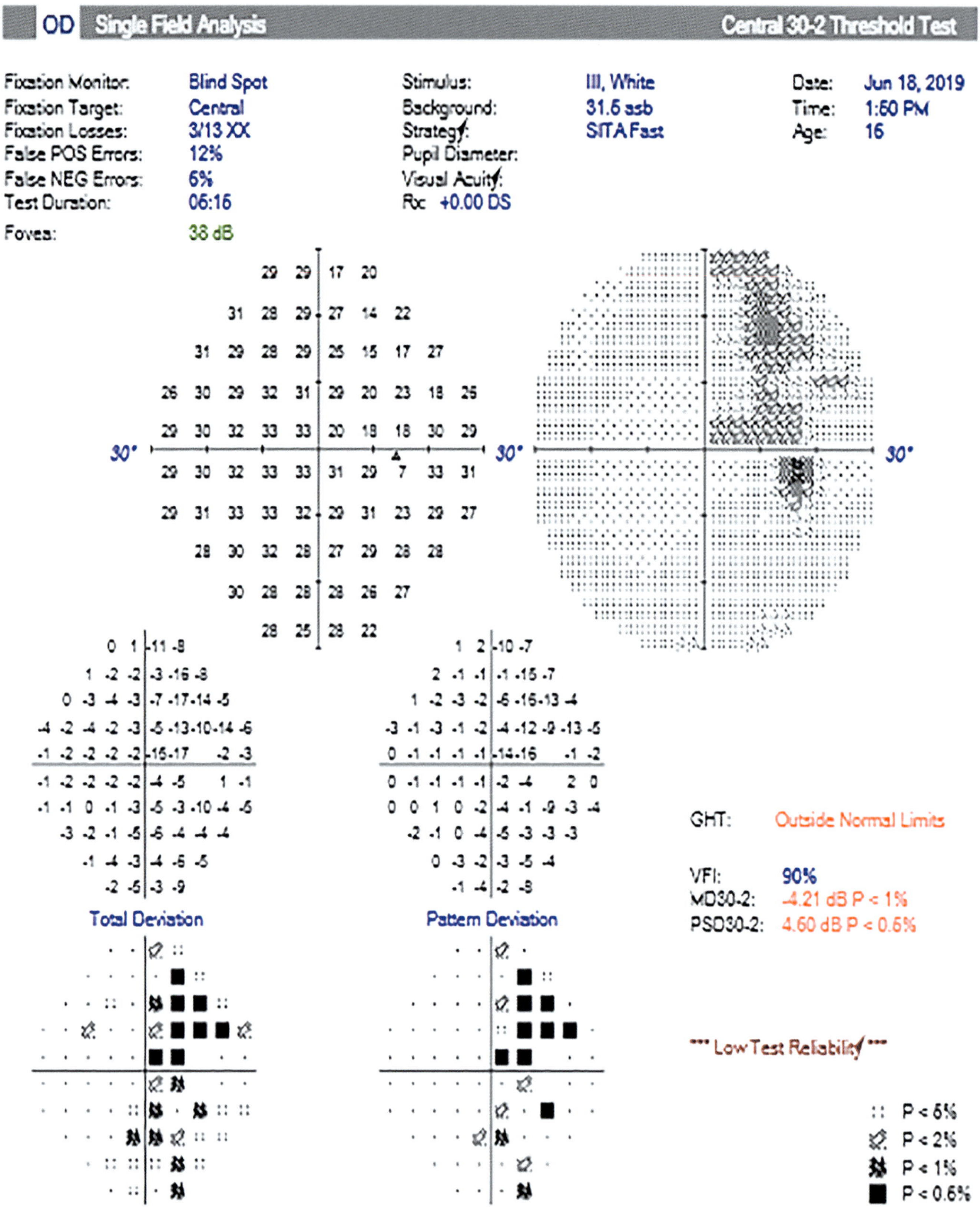

B

• **Fig. 8.5, cont'd**

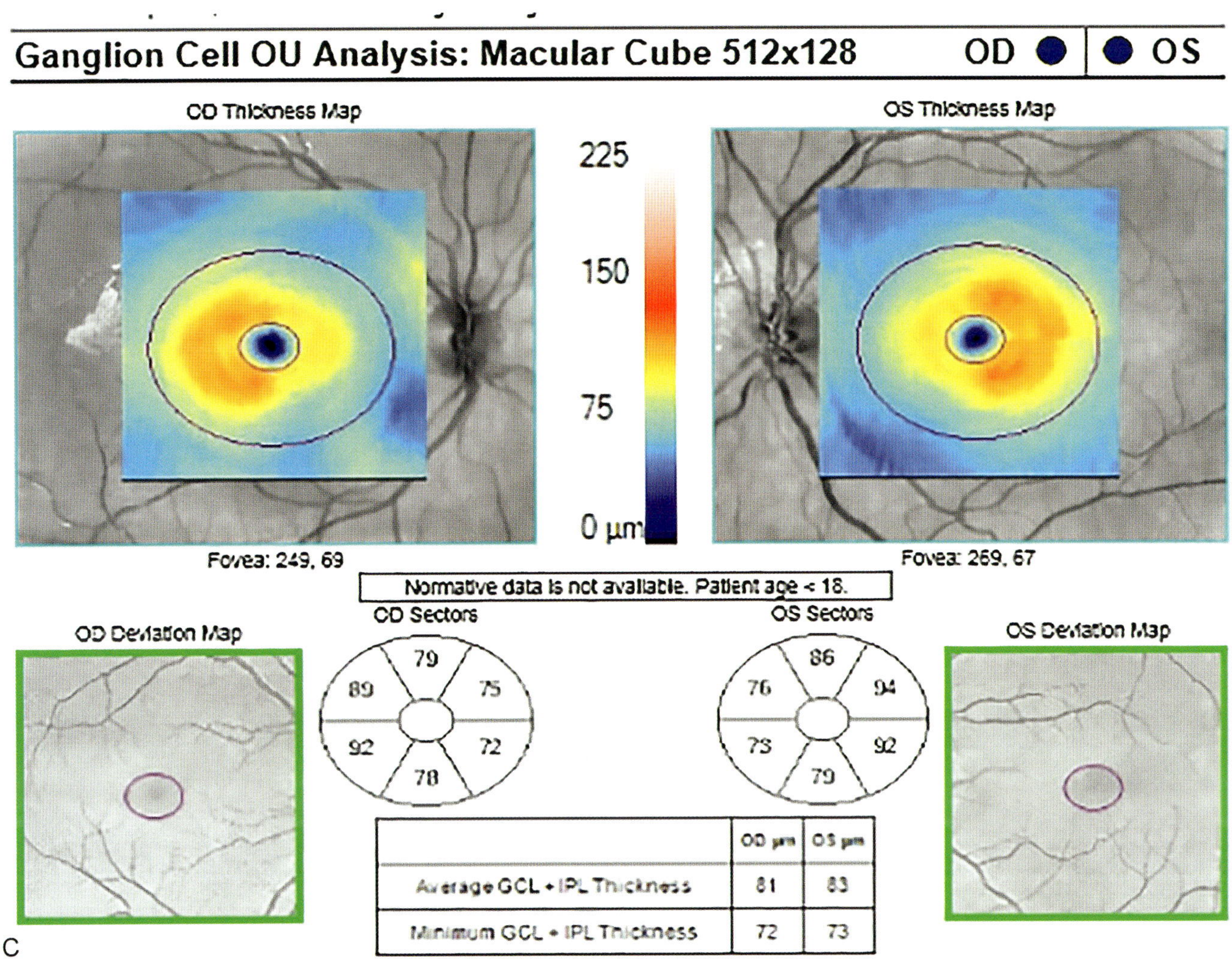

C

• **Fig. 8.5, cont'd** C, The upper two images show the Ganglion cell layer plot in the macula. The large circle delineates the area studied. Within the circle there is an area of decreased brightness in the nasal macula. This implies prolonged chiasmal compression with retrograde and transynaptic nerve damage in the retina. It makes improvement in the bitemporal field defects less likely post operatively. *ASB,* apostilbs; *DC X*, diopters cyl; *DS,* diopter sphere; *GHT,* Glaucoma Hemifield Test; *OD*, right eye; *OS*, left eye; *MD30-2*, Mean Deviation of 30-2 program (30-2 is the type of visual field program that was used); *MD*, the difference between the patient's test results and a normal age matched control; *PSD30-2*, Pattern Standard Deviation. This is the result when the MD is corrected for cataract, decreased visual acuity or diffuse depression of the Visual field. It reveals focal areas of abnormal visual field; *GCL*, Ganglion Cell Layer of the retina, *IPL*, Inner Plexiform Layer of the retina *NEG;* negative; *POS,* positive; *PSD,* pattern standard deviation; *Rx,* prescription; *SITA,* Swedish Interactive Thresholding Algorithm; *VFI,* Visual Field Index.

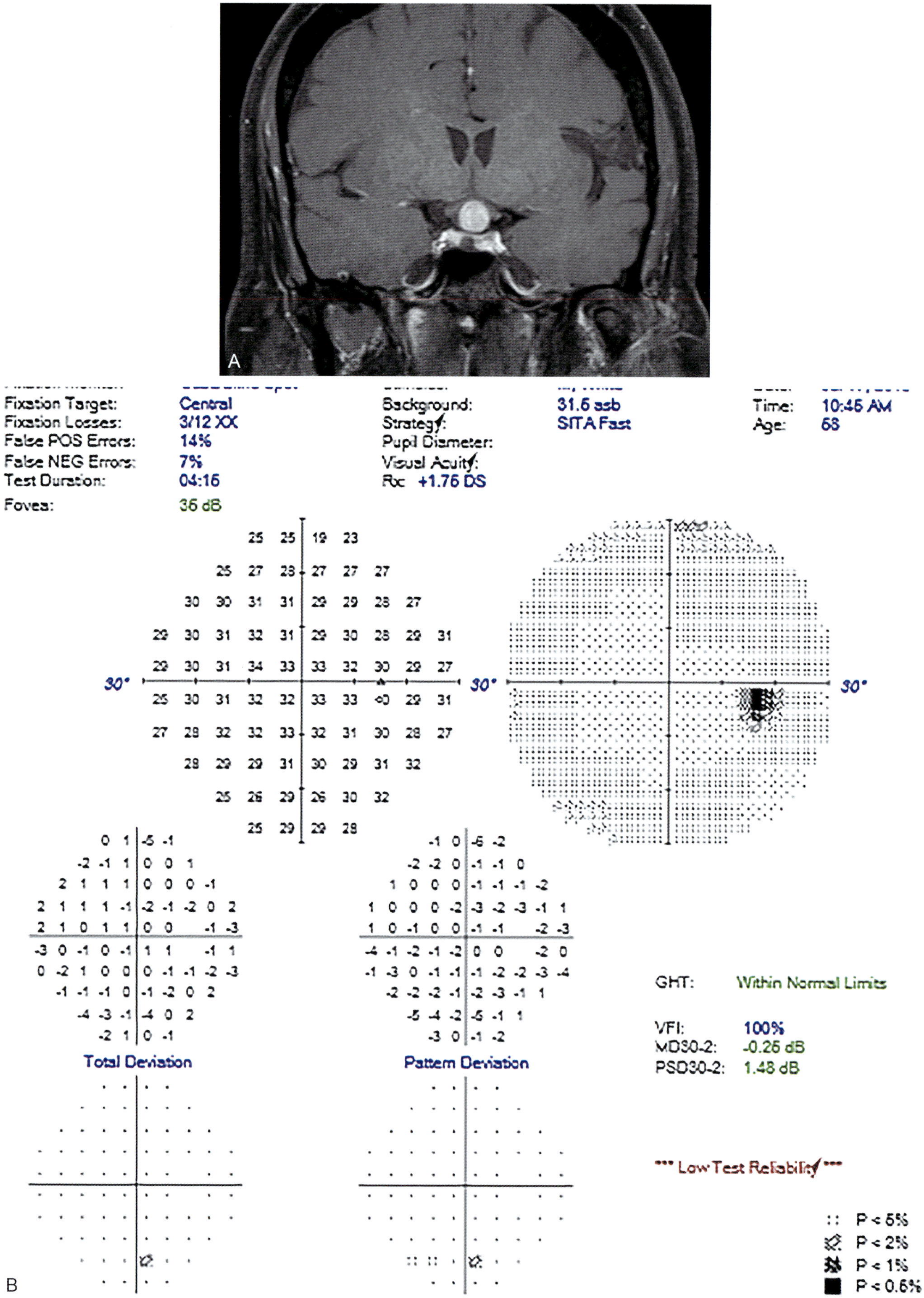

• **Fig. 8.6** A, Pituitary macroadenoma with chiasmal compression monitored for 5 years without surgery. B, Right eye visual field.

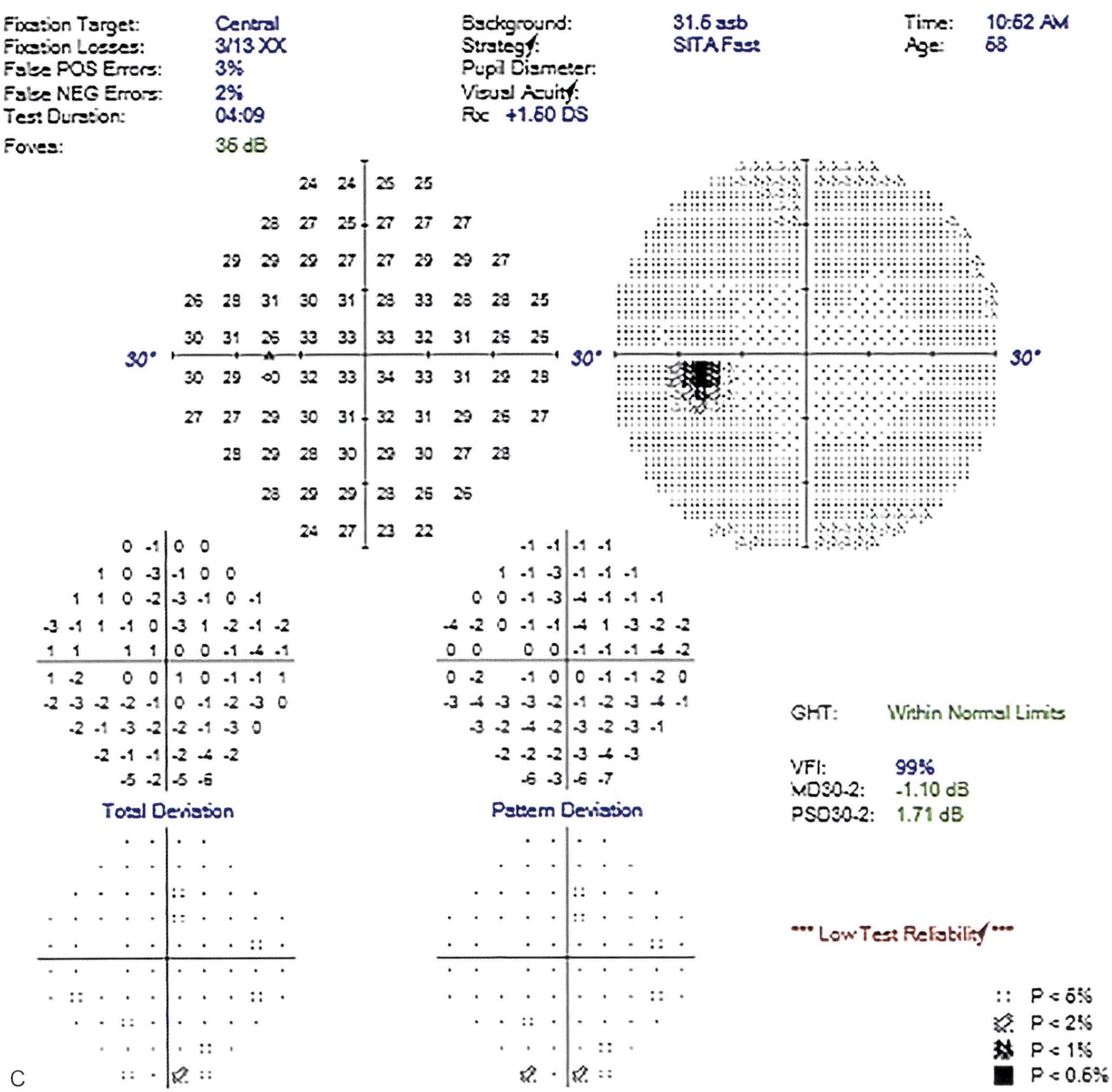

C

• **Fig. 8.6, cont'd** C, The visual fields in both eyes have remained full and normal despite elevation of the chiasm for more than 5 years. *ASB,* apostilbs; *DC X,* diopters of cylinder correction at a given number of degrees; *DS,* diopter sphere; *GHT,* Glaucoma Hemifield Test; *MD,* mean deviation; *MD30-2,* Mean Deviation of 30-2 program (30-2 is the type of visual field program that was used) *NEG;* negative; *POS,* positive; *PSD,* pattern standard deviation; *PSD30-2,* Pattern Standard Deviation. This is the result when the MD is corrected for cataract, decreased visual acuity or diffuse depression of the Visual field. *RX,* prescription; *SITA,* Swedish Interactive Thresholding Algorithm; *VFI,* Visual Field Index.

9

Radiologic Evaluation of the Orbit: Computed Tomography and Magnetic Resonance Imaging

CHRISTOPHER KARAKASIS, MD AND PAUL RUGGIERI, MD

Imaging plays an important role in the evaluation of patients with suspected orbital disease. Radiography, ultrasonography, computed tomography (CT), and magnetic resonance imaging (MRI) are commonly used in clinical practice. Each modality has its advantages and disadvantages in terms of diagnostic value, accessibility, speed of acquisition, and radiation exposure. This chapter focuses on the cross-sectional modalities of CT and MRI, as these methods have evolved to occupy a central role in the assessment, preoperative planning, and intraoperative guidance of orbital pathology.

Anatomy

Osseous Anatomy

The orbital region is a complex coalescence of seven craniofacial bones—namely, the frontal, maxillary, zygomatic, sphenoid, ethmoid, lacrimal, and palatine bones, which form the conical boundaries of the orbit whose apex is directed dorsally and medially. The orbital roof is also the floor of the frontal fossa and frontal sinus and is composed of the orbital plate of the frontal bone and a portion of the lesser wing of the sphenoid bone. The orbital roof is quite thin and tends to become thinner with age.[1] The orbital apex is primarily composed of the sphenoid and ethmoid bones and the orbital process of the palatine bone. Importantly, these bones form the optic canal along the medial superior margin, with the obliquely oriented superior orbital fissure (SOF) lateral to this, and inferolaterally is the inferior orbital fissure. The medial orbital wall serves as the lateral boundary of the ethmoid sinus, slightly angles laterally and inferiorly, and is largely formed by the delicate lamina papyracea of the ethmoid bone, with a portion of the body of the sphenoid bone dorsally and the lacrimal plate of the lacrimal bone anteriorly. The orbital floor or roof of the maxillary sinus is also very thin, slopes anteriorly and inferiorly, and is formed by the orbital portion of the maxillary bone and the orbital processes of the zygomatic and palatine bones. The orbital floor contains the infraorbital canal, which follows an anteroposterior course in the floor from the inferior orbital fissure to the infraorbital foramen. The lateral wall is considerably thicker and is formed by a portion of the greater wing of the sphenoid bone and the orbital plate of the zygomatic bone.[2] The Whitnall tubercle (lateral orbital tubercle) is an important small bony protuberance along the lateral wall, caudal to the zygomaticofrontal suture and 1 cm dorsal to the orbital rim, which serves as a point of attachment for the levator aponeurosis, a suspensory ligament for the globe, and the lateral palpebral ligament.[3] The sutural distinction between these bones within the orbit is not always possible with standard CT imaging. In the mid orbit, the relatively thin caliber of the bones can result in poor visibility, which reinforces the necessity of high-resolution imaging.

The bony orbit is best evaluated with CT. The bony orbit contains several important foramina and canals, which demonstrate variability in anatomic shape but consistent relationships. The superior orbital fissure is formed by the greater and lesser sphenoid wings and the ethmoid and palatine bones, located at the orbital apex (Fig. 9.1). The superior orbital fissure transmits cranial nerves (CN) III (oculomotor), IV (trochlear), V1 (ophthalmic), and VI (abducens), in addition to vascular structures, such as the superior ophthalmic vein and branches of the meningeal and lacrimal arteries.[4] The optic foramen is the ventral termination of the optic canal, situated at the medial margin of the superior orbital fissure (Figs. 9.1 and 9.2) and transmits the optic nerve and the ophthalmic artery. The inferior orbital fissure is formed primarily by the maxillary, sphenoid, and zygomatic bones and is contiguous with the foramen rotundum and pterygopalatine fossa (Figs. 9.1 and 9.3). The inferior orbital fissure receives CN V2 (maxillary) from the foramen rotundum and transmits V2 fibers and the inferior ophthalmic vein. Along the dorsal margin of the floor, the inferior orbital fissure communicates with pterygopalatine fossa and the temporal fossa. Continuing ventrally from the inferior orbital fissure and pterygopalatine fossa, the infraorbital canal (Fig. 9.4) carries the infraorbital nerve (V2) through the orbital floor to the maxilla, terminating at the ventral margin of the maxilla as the infraorbital foramen (see Fig. 9.1). The supraorbital foramen is visualized as a small notch along the superior orbital rim (see Fig. 9.1) and contains the supraorbital nerve (V1). The nasolacrimal canal extends caudally from the lacrimal sac in the lacrimal groove of the lacrimal plate and transmits the nasolacrimal duct (Fig. 9.5), draining into the inferior meatus of the nasal cavity below the inferior turbinate.

Multiple fracture patterns involving the orbital walls are encountered in the setting of trauma, including orbital blowout

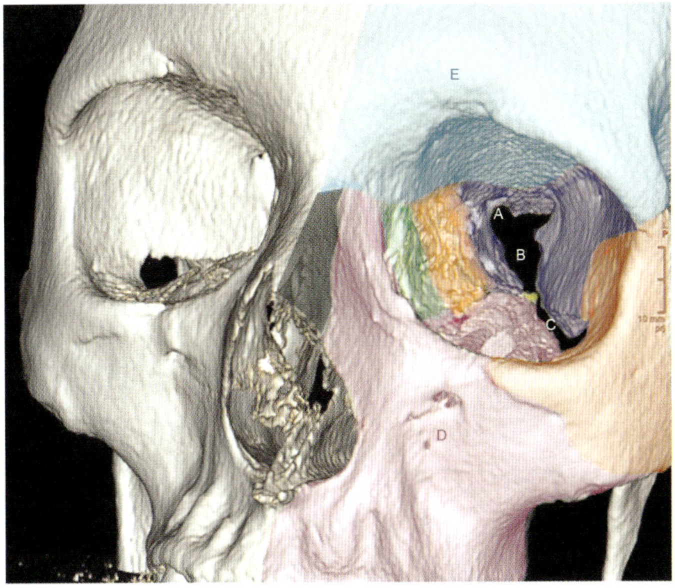

• **Fig. 9.1** Anatomy. Three-dimensional reconstruction from thin-section computed tomography orbits in slightly oblique coronal plane. *Bright blue:* Frontal bone. *Dark blue:* Sphenoid bone. *Red:* Zygomatic bone. *Purple:* Maxillary bone. *Light green:* Lacrimal bone. *Orange:* Ethmoid bone (lamina papyracea). *Yellow:* Palatine bone. *Dark green:* Nasal bone. A, Optic foramen. B, Superior orbital fissure. C, Inferior orbital fissure. D, Infraorbital foramen. E, Supraorbital foramen.

fractures, nasoorbitoethmoidal, LeFort II/III, and zygomaticomaxillary complex fractures. Potential sequelae of orbital trauma include diplopia as the result of extraocular muscle impingement or entrapment, or hypoesthesia in the maxillary sensory distribution as the result of fracture involving the infraorbital canal (Fig. 9.6). Only the resolution and contrast of CT can effectively characterize such fractures for clinical decision making. Similarly, only the bony detail of CT can distinguish bony remodeling and attenuation from frank bony destruction in the setting of infection or neoplasm within or adjacent to the bony orbit.

Soft-Tissue Anatomy

The soft-tissue structures of the orbit typically assessed on imaging consist of the globe, extraocular muscles, optic nerve, intraorbital fat, lacrimal gland, periorbita or orbital fascia, orbital septum, and neurovascular structures.

The orbital septum is an important imaging landmark, although it is not typically visible on CT and is infrequently evident on MRI. It is composed of a fibrous septum contiguous with the aponeurosis of levator palpebrae superioris, the capsulopalpebral fascia, and the tarsal plates and extends to the orbital rims to blend with the periorbita.[5] The orbital septum effectively serves as the anterior border of the orbit and plays a significant role as a barrier to intraorbital extension of infection. Thus assessment of preseptal and/or postseptal involvement is an important distinction on imaging because patients present very differently and the distinction has a considerable impact on the type and duration of therapy (Fig. 9.7).

The striated extraocular muscles involved in movement of the globe include the medial, superior, lateral and inferior rectus muscles, and the superior and inferior oblique muscles (see Fig. 9.4B). The four rectus muscles and the levator palpebrae superioris all arise from a thickened, conical tendinous ring that surrounds the optic foramen and medial aspect of the superior orbital fissure and is contiguous with the periorbita, known as the annulus of Zinn.[1] The superior oblique muscle lies in the upper medial quadrant of the orbit, arises from the sphenoid bone periosteum, passes anteriorly through a fibrocartilaginous ring (trochlea), and then courses dorsally, medially, and inferiorly, subjacent to the superior rectus, to insert onto the sclera of the dorsal superior globe. The inferior oblique arises from the orbital floor, dorsal and lateral to the lacrimal sac, and then follows a dorsal lateral superior course below the inferior rectus to insert on the dorsal lateral sclera of the globe. The levator palpebrae superioris functions to elevate the eyelid, running parallel and cephalad to the superior rectus muscle. The levator palpebrae superioris and superior rectus demonstrate variable separation on imaging and are sometimes apposed in the coronal plane. The extraocular muscles demonstrate hypointense T1 and T2 MRI signal relative to intraorbital fat, with normal mild, uniform postcontrast enhancement. The muscles normally demonstrate a tapered caliber at their ventral and dorsal tendinous margins, whereas each muscle belly has a larger, flattened ovoid configuration in the coronal plane. The extraocular muscles are surrounded by orbital fat and form the boundaries of the intraconal and extraconal spaces within the orbit (Fig. 9.8), which are useful aids to predict the nature of orbital pathology on imaging studies.

The globe is encased by the elastic tissue of the sclera from the periphery of the cornea to the optic nerve, where it is fused with its dural sheath. The choroid and retina are not typically distinguishable from the scleral margin on standard imaging. The sclera is surrounded by the capsule of Tenon, which is a fibrous sheath that envelops the Tenon (episcleral) space, inserts in the sclera anteriorly, is pierced dorsally by the optic nerve and its sheath, and separates the globe from the surrounding orbital fat. The optic nerve runs through the optic canal along with the ophthalmic artery. A dural sheath surrounds the optic nerve as it traverses the canal, after which the dura inserts to the periosteum of the bony orbit.[1] The optic nerve normally demonstrates uniform hypointense T1 and T2 signal without postcontrast enhancement. There is normal hyperintense T2 signal in the CSF space within the optic nerve sheath (Fig. 9.9) that is contiguous with the intracranial subarachnoid space. On CT, it is not typically possible to distinguish the nerve from the dural sheath and the interposed subarachnoid space; however, this is possible with MRI.

The periorbita is the periosteum of the bony orbit but is more loosely adherent to the bone than the periosteum elsewhere. The periorbita is continuous with the dura in the orbital apex and with the orbital septum anteriorly. It is not normally discernible with imaging but is important to consider in the setting of neoplasm or infection because direct involvement or extension through the periorbita is an important distinction that alters prognosis and clinical management in such settings (Fig. 9.10). Making this distinction can be difficult on imaging, but subperiosteal tissue is generally sharply defined and crescentic or lentiform in configuration confined to the extraconal space, whereas tissue extending through the periosteum is generally larger, focal, lobulated, or irregular and ill defined.

The lacrimal gland is a compound tuboloacinar gland located in the lacrimal recess in the ventral superolateral orbit, contained within periorbita and supported inferiorly by the Whitnall capsule. Frequently overlooked on imaging, assessment of the lacrimal gland is important as it may be involved with infection, primary neoplasm (such as adenoid cystic, adenocarcinoma, squamous cell or mucoepidermoid carcinoma), lymphoma, pseudotumor, and granulomatous disease among other etiologies. The lacrimal gland normally demonstrates hyperintense T2 signal, isointense T1

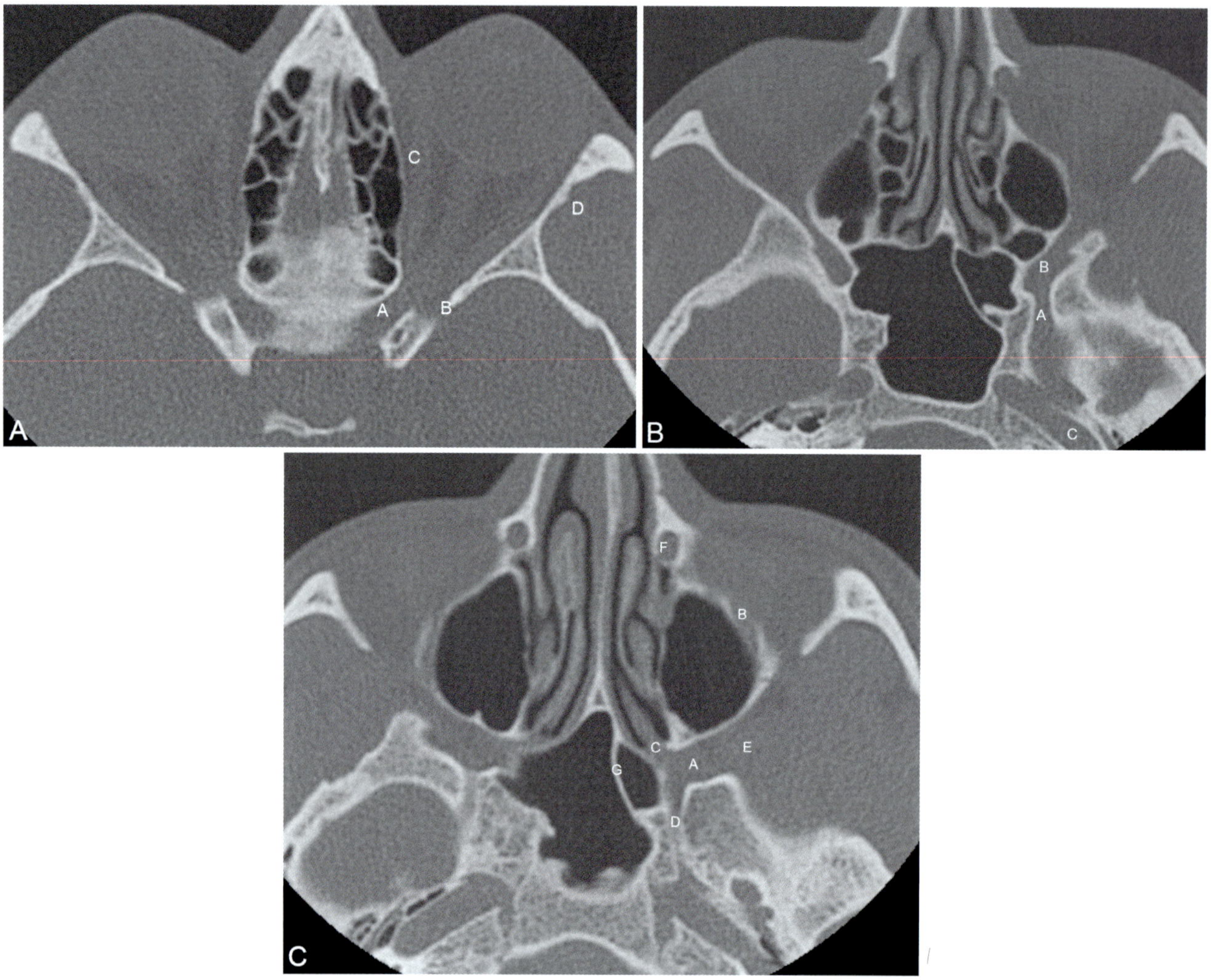

• **Fig. 9.2** Anatomy. *a,* Axial computed tomography (CT) at the level of the superior orbits demonstrates the axial relationship of the optic canal and superior orbital fissure. A, Optic canal. B, Superior orbital fissure. C, Medial orbital wall formed by lamina papyracea of ethmoid bone. D, Lateral orbital wall formed by zygomatic bone. *b,* Axial CT at the inferior orbit demonstrates the axial relationship of the foramen rotundum and inferior orbital fissure. A, Foramen rotundum. B, Inferior orbital fissure. C, Foramen lacerum with internal carotid artery. *c,* Axial CT just inferior to part *b)* demonstrates the axial relationships of the pterygopalatine fossa. A. Pterygopalatine fossa. B. Inferior orbital canal. C, Sphenopalatine foramen. D, Vidian canal. E, Pterygomaxillary fissure. F, Nasolacrimal duct. G, Sphenoid sinuses.

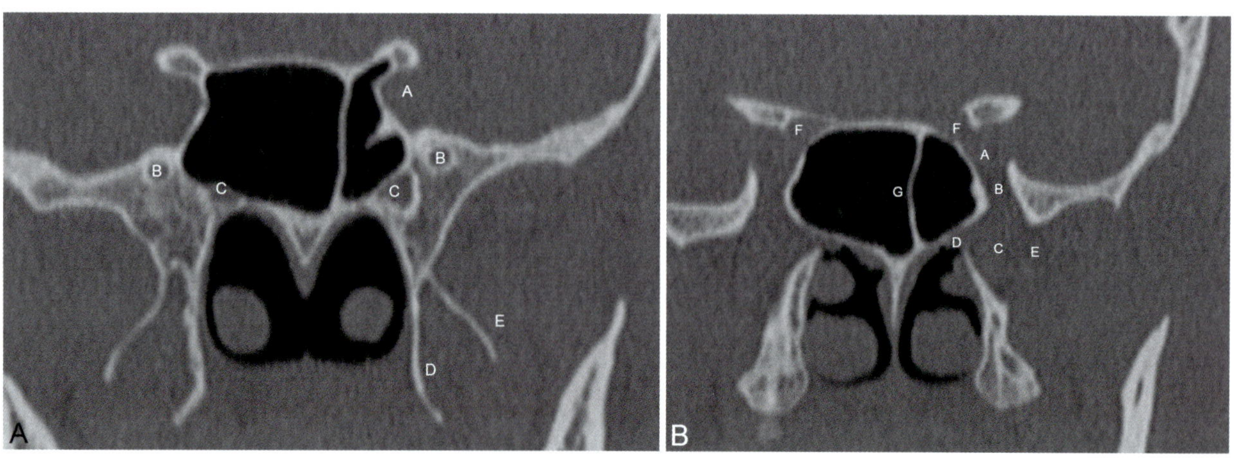

• **Fig. 9.3** Anatomy. *a,* Coronal computed tomography (CT) dorsal to the orbit demonstrates the relationship of greater sphenoid wing foramina. A, Superior orbital fissure. B, Foramen rotundum. C, Vidian canal. D, Medial pterygoid process. E, Lateral pterygoid process. *b,* Coronal CT just ventral to part *(a)* demonstrates the relationships of the pterygopalatine fossa. A, Superior orbital fissure. B, Inferior orbital fissure. C, Pterygopalatine fossa. D, Sphenopalatine foramen. E, Pterygomaxillary fissure. F, Optic canal G, Sphenoid sinuses.

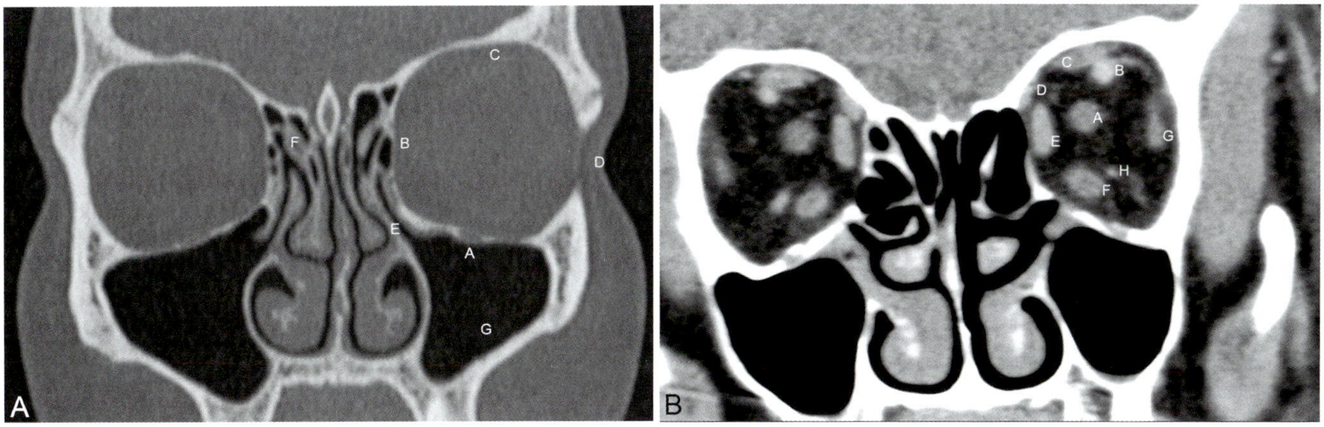

• **Fig. 9.4** Anatomy. *a,* Coronal computed tomography (CT) at the level of the mid orbits demonstrates the relationship of the orbit to the sinonasal cavity. A, Infraorbital canal along the orbital floor. B, Lamina payracea. C, Orbital roof formed by frontal bone. D, Lateral orbital wall. E, Uncinate process along the medial margin of maxillary ostium. F, Ethmoid air cells. G, Maxillary antrum. *b,* Coronal CT with contrast in soft-tissue windows. A, Optic nerve and sheath complex. B, Superior ophthalmic vein. C, Superior rectus and levator palpebrae superioris. D, Superior oblique. E, Medial rectus. F, Inferior rectus. G, Lateral rectus. H, Inferior ophthalmic vein.

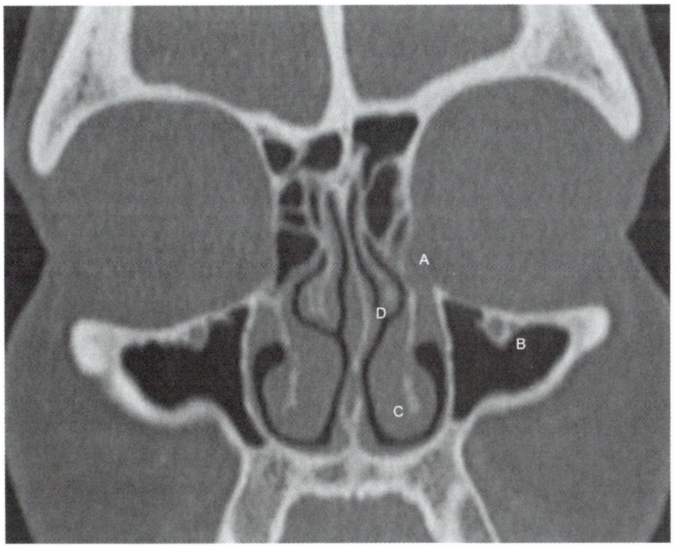

• **Fig. 9.5** Anatomy. Coronal computed tomography at the level of the ventral orbit. A, Nasolacrimal canal. B, Infraorbital canal along the orbital floor. C, Inferior turbinate. D, Middle meatus along inferior margin of middle turbinate.

signal, and uniform postcontrast enhancement (Fig. 9.11). Keys to pathology include atypical signal intensity characteristics, restricted diffusion, and irregular enhancement or enlargement, noting that pathology may be bilateral.

The orbits contain many vascular structures, the most important of which are the ophthalmic arteries, which arise directly from the internal carotid arteries and traverse the optic canals along with the optic nerves, providing the main arterial supply to the globe. The extraocular muscles are supplied by muscular branches of the ophthalmic artery as well as the lacrimal and infraorbital arteries. The superior ophthalmic veins (SOVs) are readily visualized on imaging and follow a circuitous course: initially along a posterolateral course medial to the superior rectus muscle, then the veins pass caudal to the superior rectus but superior and lateral to the nerve sheath, and then posteriorly and medially to the superior orbital fissure to the cavernous sinus but lateral to the superior rectus. The SOVs should be assessed on imaging for enlargement and/or thrombosis, which can portend cavernous sinus thrombosis or cavernous-carotid fistula (Fig. 9.12). The inferior ophthalmic veins are considerably smaller and arise inferiorly and laterally, course dorsally along the inferior rectus muscle, and drain into the pterygoid plexus through the inferior orbital fissure but also communicate with the SOVs.

Imaging Considerations

The American College of Radiology (ACR) Appropriateness Criteria provide a valuable resource for the assessment of imaging protocols as they pertain to clinical presentation,[6] providing information regarding the diagnostic value for the different modalities along with expected radiation dose. These criteria are becoming interlinked with reimbursement for imaging; thus it would seem essential that all providers in the clinical and imaging settings become familiar with the contents.

Computed Tomography

A central tenet to imaging with ionizing radiation (i.e., CT scans, radiographs) is the as low as reasonably achievable principle, which states that radiation doses should be as low as reasonably achievable. Prudence is recommended, particularly in the setting of younger populations who have more long-term risk for stochastic events. Cumulative dosimetry is recorded with more frequency across institutions and is undergoing continued investigation.

The primary question in the setting of CT orbital imaging is the indication for the examination—that is, trauma, foreign body, infiltrative/destructive osseous process, presurgical evaluation of bony anatomy, or postoperative assessment of a reconstruction procedure. Noncontrast CT is typically adequate in the setting of trauma for fracture, foreign body, or soft-tissue injury, including lens dislocation or globe rupture. CT of the brain is the initial examination of choice for acute vision loss, such as homonymous hemianopsia, to assess for stroke. CT of the brain is also the gold standard for initial assessment of the presence of acute intracranial hemorrhage.

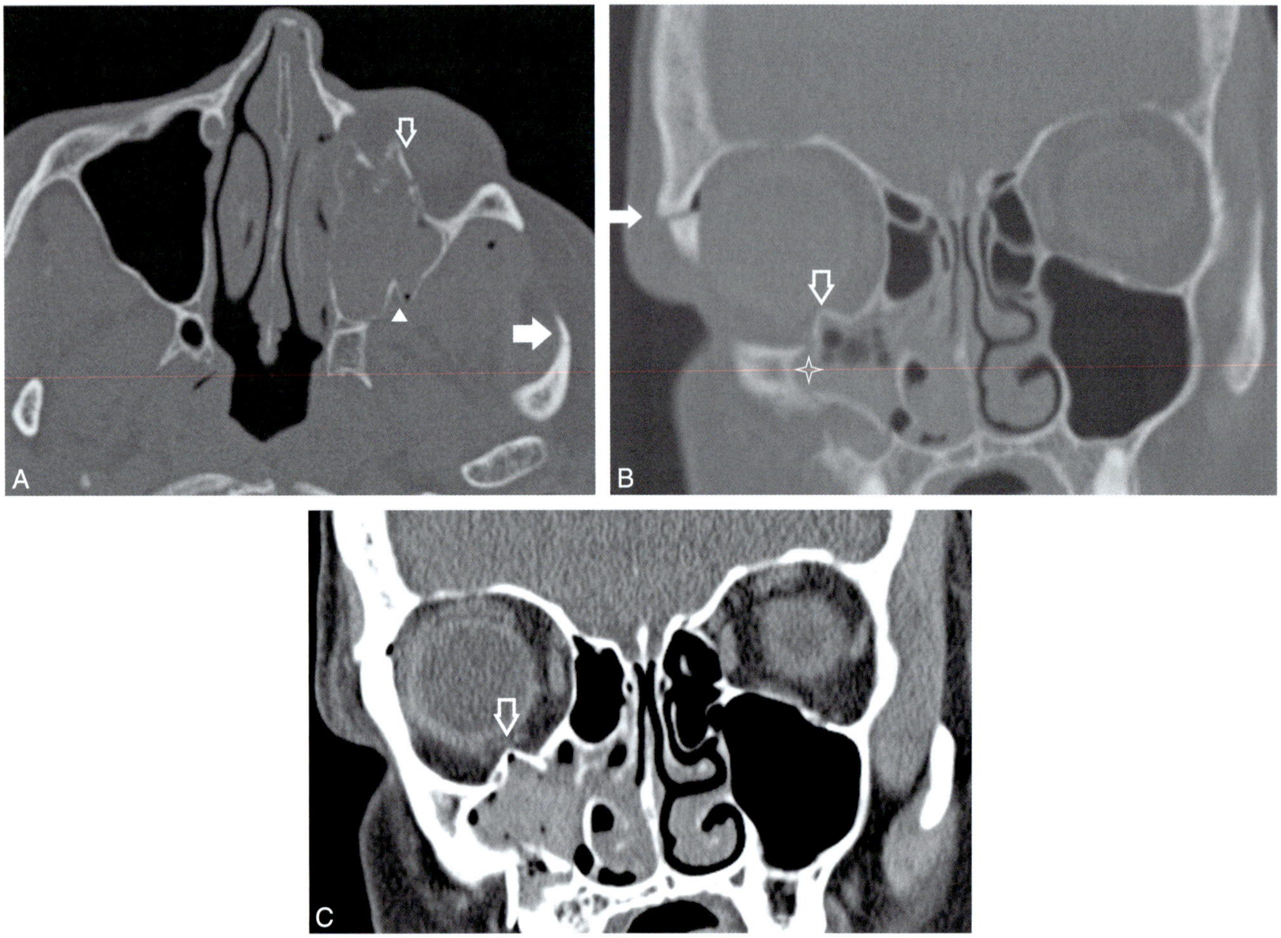

• **Fig. 9.6** Orbital Trauma With Zygomaticomaxillary Complex Fracture. *a,* Axial CT with bone windows at the level of the orbital floor demonstrates fractures of the right zygomatic arch (*solid white arrow*), posterior maxillary wall (*arrowhead*), and anterior maxillary wall (*open arrow*). *b,* Coronal computed tomography with bone windows at the level of the ventral orbit demonstrates fracture of the right lateral orbital rim (*solid white arrow*), fracture of the infraorbital canal (*star*), and orbital floor with displaced fragments. *c,* Impingement upon the inferior rectus muscle (*open arrow* in parts *b* and c). This highlights the importance of viewing the orbits in both bone and soft-tissue windows.

In general, intravenous contrast is indicated in evaluation of neoplastic, infectious, inflammatory, and vascular pathologies. Iodinated CT contrast is accompanied by the risk of nephrotoxicity and allergic reaction, which must be weighed against the added benefit of contrast imaging. Allergy premedication protocols exist and although they are institution specific, generally consist of steroid administration at 6-hour intervals at 13, 6, and 1 hour before injection along with antihistamine administration 1 hour before injection of the contrast. CT with or without contrast may be appropriate for surgical planning depending on the nature of the underlying orbital pathology. Conversely, in most settings CT with and without contrast adds little diagnostic information while doubling the radiation dose to the patient. Dual-energy CT is an emerging technology helpful in the assessment of hyperdense lesions on postcontrast imaging (i.e., orbital mass vs. hematoma), because dual-energy CT has the capability to isolate and subtract the energy peak for iodine, thus allowing for virtual noncontrast images to confirm whether the lesion truly enhances. When available, this approach typically uses slightly less radiation dose than two separate scans without and with contrast.

In pregnant patients CT is not optimal; however, it may be obtained with consent of the patient if there is sufficient clinical indication. Although the long-term risk to the fetus is very low, no data exist to precisely quantify the risk and, as such, this must be weighed against the clinical benefits of imaging.

Also note that in patients with retinoblastoma inherited mutation, CT imaging should be avoided because a greater risk of malignancy in the contralateral orbit from ionizing radiation.[7]

Magnetic Resonance Imaging

MRI is not generally indicated in the setting of acute orbital trauma owing to its reduced sensitivity for the assessment of osseous structures and increased time of acquisition. MRI is predisposed to motion artifact in unstable or uncooperative patients. The indication for contrast administration in MRI in many ways parallels the role in CT imaging. However, magnetic resonance orbital imaging without and with contrast is almost always indicated in the setting of evaluation for neoplastic, infectious, inflammatory, vascular, granulomatous, or autoimmune etiologies.

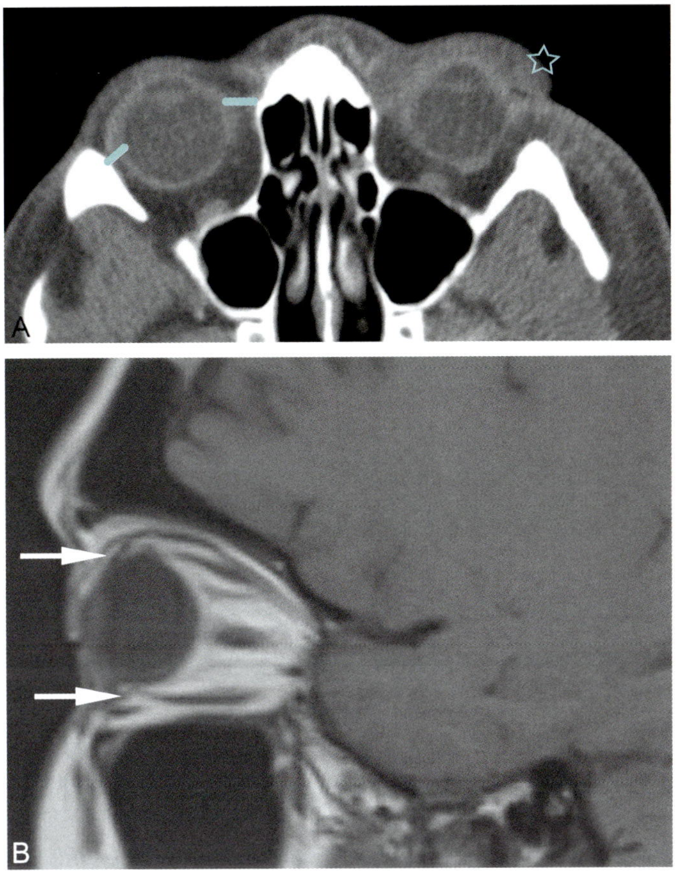

• **Fig. 9.7** A, Periorbital cellulitis. Axial postcontrast computed tomography of the orbits demonstrates left periorbital cellulitis (*star*) without evidence of postseptal extension. The right orbit is normal, with *blue lines* delineating the expected anatomic location of the orbital septum. B, Anatomy. Sagittal noncontrast T1-weighted image of the orbits in a different patient demonstrates the orbital septum above and below the globe (*white arrows*).

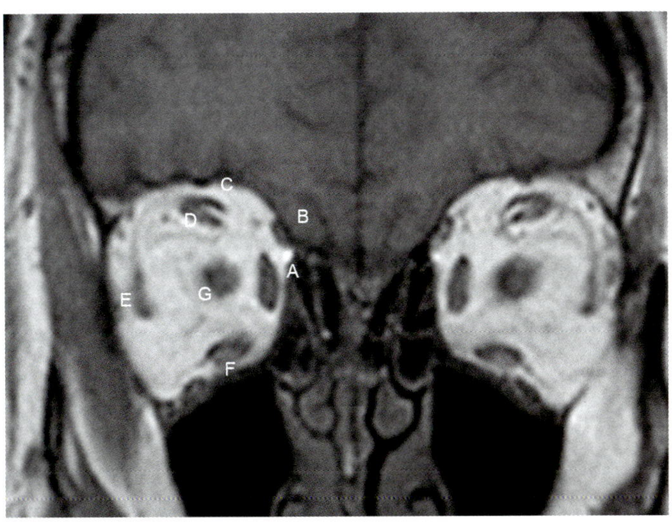

• **Fig. 9.8** Anatomy. Coronal noncontrast T1-weighted image of the mid orbit demonstrates intraorbital structures. A, Medial rectus. B, Superior oblique. C, Levator palpebrae superioris. D, Superior rectus. E: Lateral rectus. F: Inferior rectus. G: Optic nerve. The space contained within the boundary of the extraocular muscles is termed the intraconal space.

In the case of MRI, it is important to assess the intrinsic signal intensity characteristics on the unenhanced T1 images to determine if there is truly enhancement with intravenous contrast. For example, subacute blood is normally high in signal on T1 without contrast and might be misinterpreted as enhancing without the precontrast images for comparison. Depending on the clinical indication, the addition of diffusion-weighted imaging (DWI) or fluid-attenuated inversion recovery sequences of the whole brain may be of value, particularly in the setting of suspected infarct or demyelination. DWI may also be useful for evaluation of aggressive or densely cellular (e.g., lymphoma) orbital masses.

Although gadolinium-based agents do not result in nephrotoxicity, the primary concern is nephrogenic systemic fibrosis, the risk of which can be significantly mitigated by avoiding contrast administration in patients with severe renal dysfunction (glomerular filtration rate <30 mL/min) and by using macrocyclic agents. There is growing evidence of gadolinium retention in body tissues including the brain.[8,9] At this time, no evidence exists that gadolinium retention results in patient harm. Current U.S. Food and Drug Administration guidelines do not restrict gadolinium administration on this basis; however, study is ongoing.

Patients who are requested to undergo MRI must also be thoroughly screened for safety, including for the presence of ferromagnetic foreign bodies, particularly within tissues sensitive to the potential effect of motion/dislodgment or electromagnetic heating. Radiographs may be ordered to rule out orbital metallic foreign body if there is compatible clinical history upon screening. Implantable devices need to be disclosed and evaluated before imaging and generally are categorized as MRI safe, conditional, or unsafe. The radiology department will assess these concerns before imaging approval and protocoling. MRI-safe devices may be scanned using field strengths within which the device has been tested; MRI conditional refers to an item that poses no known hazard within a specifically defined MRI environment. MRI-unsafe devices should not be scanned. MRI is considered safe in the setting of pregnancy, although administration of gadolinium contrast is currently not advised as there are insufficient data to judge the safety of retained gadolinium in the fetus.

Patients should be asked to close their eyes during scanning to reduce ocular motion. Iron oxide from tattoos or cosmetic products in the eyelid region can result in susceptibility artifact, but this is generally insignificant unless the structural lesion of concern is very superficial.

Protocols

Computed Tomography of the Orbits

A typical orbital CT protocol uses thin-section axial imaging of approximately 2-mm slice thickness and high in-plane resolution with reconstructions in the coronal and sagittal planes. The inclusion of soft-tissue and bone kernel reconstructions from the raw data is important as the former highlights soft-tissue contrast and the latter fine bony detail. The typical field of view is approximately 20 cm, with slices extending from the frontal sinuses to the maxilla to include the orbits and paranasal sinuses (Table 9.1). These imaging parameters remain constant regardless of whether the study is performed with or without contrast. In an adult, a reasonable radiation dose would be expected to be on the order of 200 to 300 mGy*cm in terms of dose-length product, noting that this

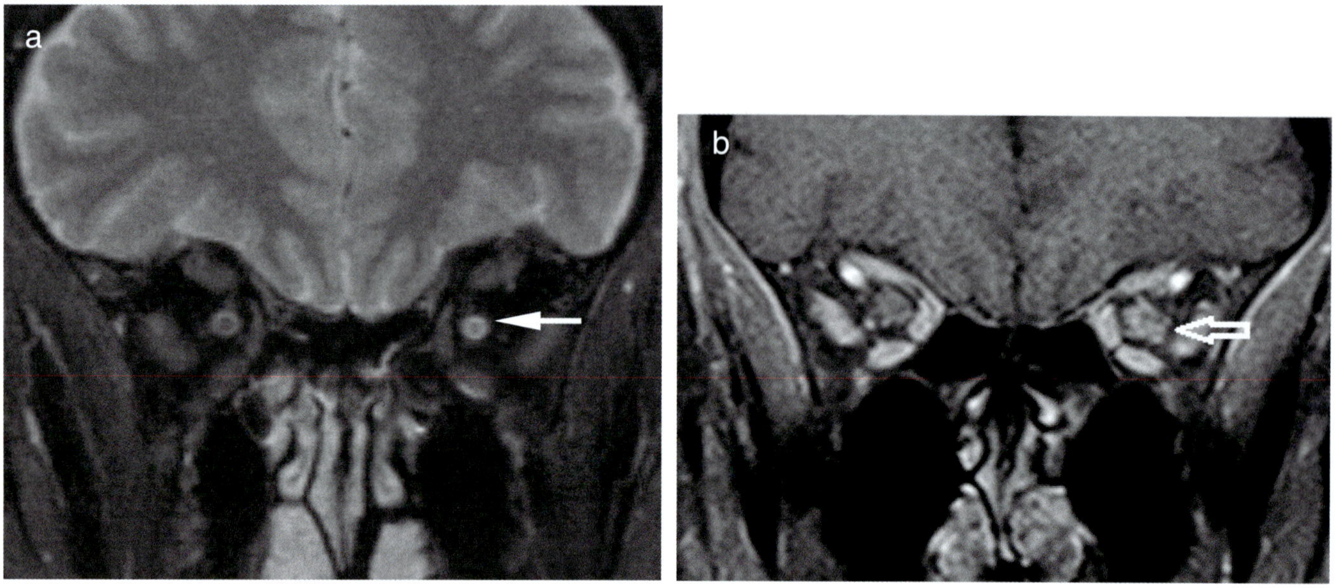

• **Fig. 9.9** Optic neuritis. *a,* Coronal T2 fat-saturated image through the orbits demonstrates abnormal hyperintense T2 signal in the left optic nerve (*arrow*), indicating sequela of prior optic neuritis or injury. There is normal hyperintense signal in the optic nerve sheaths surrounding the optic nerves bilaterally. *b,* T1 coronal fat-saturated postcontrast image demonstrates contrast enhancement of the left optic nerve (*thick open arrow*) nerve indicating active inflammation.

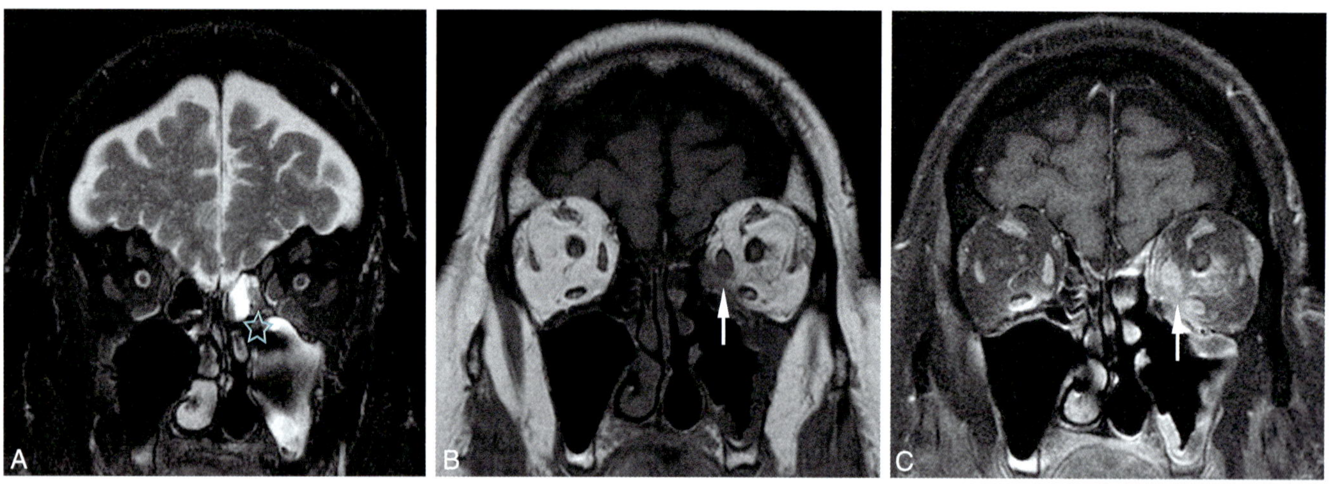

• **Fig. 9.10** Sinusitis With Extension Through Periorbita. *a,* Coronal T2 fat-saturated image through the orbits demonstrates abnormal hyperintense T2 signal in the ethmoid and maxillary sinuses (*blue star*) indicating sinus disease. *b,* Noncontrast T1-weighted coronal image demonstrates stranding in the extraconal fat (*white arrow*). *c,* Postcontrast T1 fat-saturated image demonstrates enhancement of the intracornal and extraconal fat (*arrow*), as well as the extraocular muscles, better delineating the extent of orbital infection/inflammation. No rim-enhancing abscess is present.

number should be considerably lower in a child. Dose reduction techniques should be used whenever feasible to minimize radiation exposure to the lens.

Magnetic Resonance Imaging of the Orbits

A typical MRI examination of the orbits uses multiple pulse sequences with an approximate field of view of 16 × 16 cm. Sequences should be used in a protocol that maximizes diagnostic utility and minimizes time, with attention to patient comfort/cooperation as well as departmental efficiency. Multiple trade-offs become evident; however, the prime consideration in designing MRI protocols is the diagnostic needs of the patient.

Although it increases acquisition time, high-resolution imaging is necessary; a reasonable protocol includes 3-mm thick two-dimensional (2D) slices with 0 to 10% interslice spacing for spin echo sequences or 1- to 2-mm contiguous slices in a turbo-spin echo or three-dimensional (3D) gradient echo acquisition (Table 9.2). The latter affords planar reconstructions when

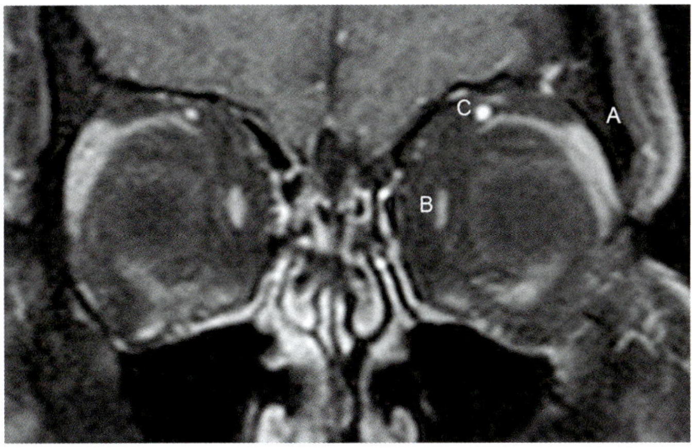

• **Fig. 9.11** Anatomy. Coronal T1 postcontrast fat-saturated image through the mid orbits demonstrates structures with normal enhancement. A, Lacrimal gland. B, Extraocular muscles. C, Superior ophthalmic vein.

TABLE 9.1 Computed Tomography Protocol[a]

Number of Detectors	Variable (Range 8-256)
Kilovolt peak (peak voltage)	100 kV (range 100-120)
Current (mA)	Automatic (maximum limit 300 mA)
Slice thickness	2 mm (range 1.25-3 mm)
Scan field of view	20 cm (range 20-25)
Display field of view	15 cm (range of 12.5 to 15)
Pitch	1
Rotation time	1 second
Dose-length product	200 mGy*cm (range 120-300)

[a]The table shows an example of a typical computed tomography orbits protocol. Note that the protocol details would be unchanged with or without intravenous iodinated contrast, and reconstruction in soft tissue or bone kernel may be performed from either.

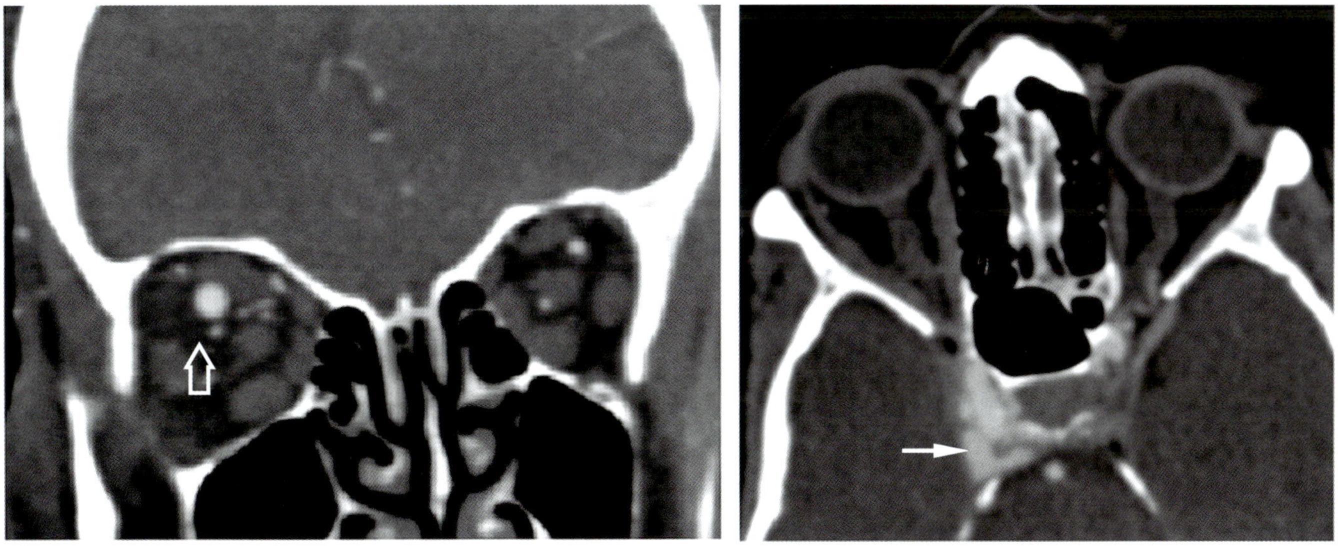

• **Fig. 9.12** Cavernous-Carotid Fistula. *a,* Coronal computed tomography (CT) angiogram through the orbits demonstrates marked enlargement of the right superior ophthalmic vein (*open arrow*). *b,* Intracranial CT angiogram demonstrates early filling of the right cavernous sinus (*solid arrow*), confirming cavernous carotid fistula. There is also engorgement within the right orbit with proptosis.

acquired with isotropic (equal dimensions of imaging voxels in all three planes) or near isotropic resolution. Although 3D acquisitions afford advantages in resolution, artifact from globe or gross patient motion is considerably worse than in 2D acquisitions, and image contrast is altered relative to conventional spin echo sequences. The use of a higher signal-to-noise ratio of 3-Tesla imaging allows for higher in-plane and through-plane resolution to identify subtle pathology, whereas 1.5-Tesla imaging is less prone to susceptibility from air in the paranasal sinuses. Surface coil imaging can significantly enhance the signal-to-noise ratio but is generally indicated only if the concern is diagnostic and limited to the orbits because there is considerable signal drop-off dorsal to the orbits with such coils. For surgical planning, uniform volume coils (e.g., head coils) are considered preferable because of their greater uniformity of signal and contrast across the entire volume.

Essential MR imaging concepts include a carefully selected combination of pulse sequences and imaging planes to effectively characterize the nature and distribution of pathologic tissues in the orbits relative to adjacent normal tissue. A typical protocol consists of T1 precontrast axial and coronal imaging, T1 postcontrast fat-saturated axial and coronal imaging, T2 fat-saturated sequences, and DWI. Standard T1 imaging generally consists of 2D spin echo or fast-spin echo sequences.

TABLE 9.2 Example of Magnetic Resonance Orbits Protocol at 1.5 Tesla[a]

Sequence	Slice Thickness (mm)	Slice Gap (mm)	Repetition Time (ms)	Echo Time (ms)	No. of Excititations/ Averages	Matrix	Field of View (cm)	Bandwidth	Inversion Time (ms)	Flip Angle (degrees)
Noncontrast T1 coronal spin echo	3	0.3	500	11	2	256 × 154	15 × 20	190	N/A	90
Noncontrast T1 axial spin echo	3	0.3	600	11	3	256 v 320	21 × 21	190	N/A	90
Postcontrast T1 coronal spin echo FS	3	0.3	500	11	2	256 × 192	20 × 20	190	N/A	90
Postcontrast T1 axial spin echo FS	3	0.3	500	11	3	256 × 156	170 × 210	130	N/A	90
T1 axial gradient echo Postcontrast volumetric	1	0	9	2.4	1	256 × 256	25.6 × 25.6	230	N/A	8
Diffusion weighted	5	2	4200	TE1 66, TE2 114	1	150 × 150	23 × 23	695	N/A	180

[a]The device used is the Siemens Magnetom Aera (Siemens, Munich Germany). Note that additional brain sequences (axial FLAIR, sagittal T1) may be added before contrast administration for diagnostic evaluation of the brain and orbital pathways.

FS, fat-saturated; *FLAIR*, fluid-attenuated inversion recovery; *N/A*, not applicable.

Three-dimensional volumetric gradient echo sequences obtain isotropic voxels (typically on the order of 1 mm^3) that allow for high-resolution imaging and reconstructions in any plane. However, gradient echo sequences are more prone to susceptibility artifact and magnetic field inhomogeneity/nonlinearity at the level of the skull base because of the air/soft-tissue or bone/soft-tissue interfaces in this region. Presurgical planning is enhanced by fusion of the isotropic, short echo time 3D MRI sequences with high-resolution, isotropic CT images to compensate for the nonlinearity of MRI at the skull base, thereby allowing more accurate and concomitant assessment of osseous and soft-tissue structures for intraoperative guidance (Fig. 9.13).

Non–fat-saturated T1 sequences preserve the intrinsic hyperintensity of fat. This accentuates pathology, such as masses and inflammation, by taking advantage of the intrinsically hypointense stranding or confluent signal of inflammatory or neoplastic processes relative to the normally T1-hyperintense signal of fat in the orbit and other fat-containing structures, such as the adjacent pterygopalatine fossa or skull base. Suppression of fat is useful as an adjunct to confirm the presence of fat within a lesion, such as a lipoma, dermoid cyst, or teratoma. Fat-saturated imaging is most useful after intravenous contrast as the T1 shortening effect of gadolinium results in hyperintense signal in structures that take up gadolinium, such as masses and their infiltrative margins, inflammation, and perineural disease, whereas the suppression of underlying intrinsic fat signal improves conspicuity of the enhancement that would otherwise be indiscernible from the bright fat.

Fat-saturated imaging can be obtained using several methods, as discussed by Delfaut et al.,[10] the most common of which include frequency-selective saturation, inversion recovery, opposed-phase imaging, and the Dixon technique. Frequency-selective saturation is highly susceptible to inhomogeneities in the magnetic field as might be introduced by air or metal/soft-tissue interfaces such as the paranasal sinuses, metal in the face or scalp from prior trauma, surgery, or braces. These situations may result in a lack of fat suppression in and around the orbit, signal loss, geometric distortion, as well as the inadvertent suppression of water signal. These susceptibility effects are worse at higher MRI field strengths (3 Tesla vs. 1.5 Tesla); however, there is lower quality of frequency-selective fat suppression at lower field strengths. In addition, imaging time is increased by fat-saturated imaging. These factors highlight some of the many trade-offs necessary to consider in protocol design.

Fat-saturated T2-weighted coronal and/or axial sequences are essential for complete evaluation of tissues because the combination of T1 and T2 imaging helps to characterize the pathologic tissues. Because the commonly used fast-spin echo T2-weighted sequences also cause fat to be bright and most pathologic tissue is T2 hyperintense, the fat suppression makes the pathology more obvious on imaging. In the setting of susceptibility artifact, short-tau inversion recovery sequence is an alternative as it has less susceptibility effect. Note that its mechanism of suppression of substances with short T1 relaxation times is noteworthy in the sense that it is not uniquely selective for fat and can also inadvertently suppress gadolinium enhancement. Heavily T2-weighted

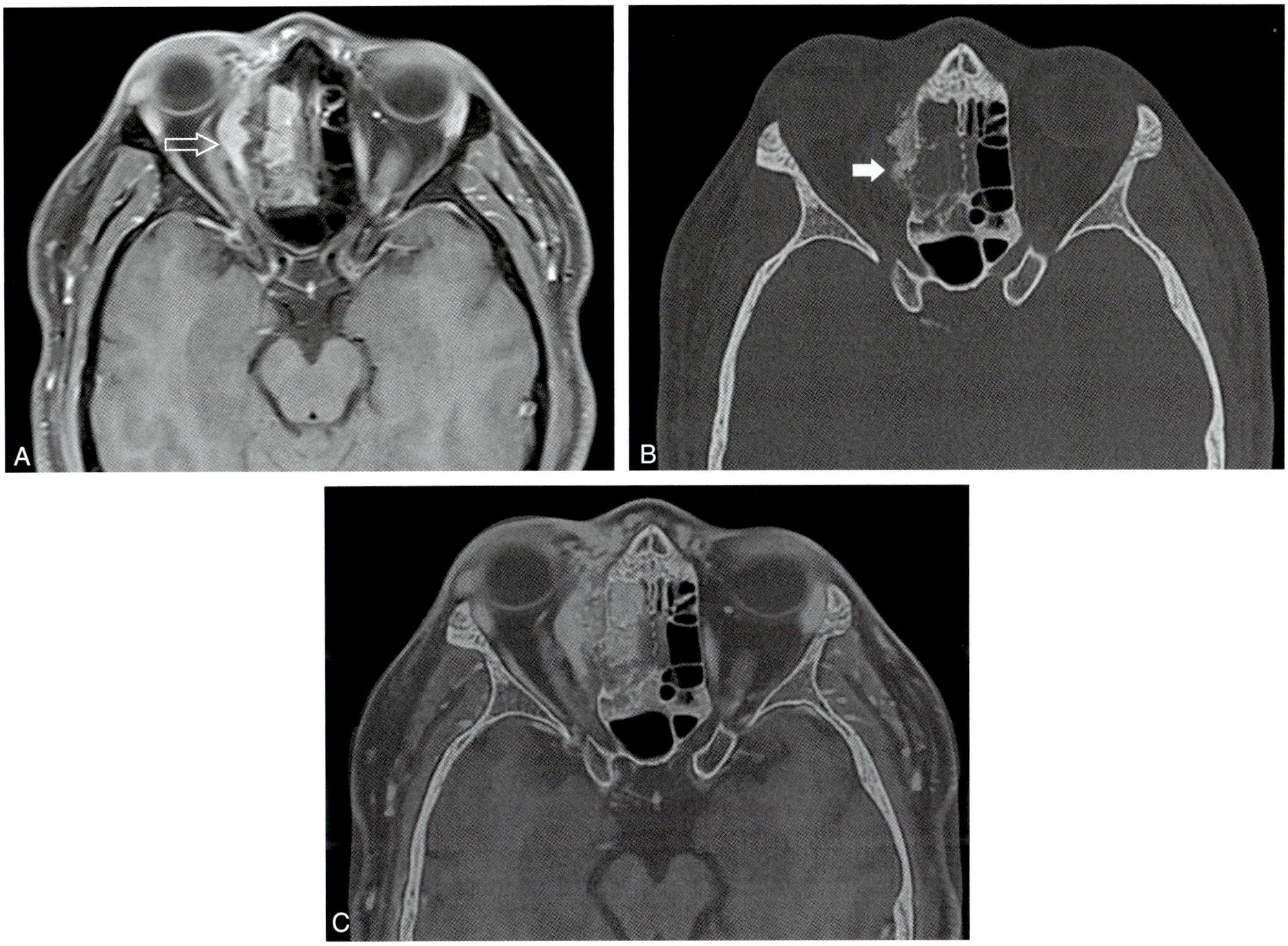

• **Fig. 9.13** Fused Computed Tomography/Magnetic Resonance Imaging for Presurgical Planning. Patient With NUT Midline Carcinoma. *a,* Axial postcontrast magnetic resonance imaging (MRI) with T1 fat-saturated gradient echo technique with isotropic voxels demonstrates an enhancing mass centered in the right ethmoid extending to the medial right orbit with mass effect and proptosis (*open arrow*). *b,* Axial high-resolution computed tomography (CT) through the orbits demonstrates osseous permeation and periosteal reaction (*closed arrow*). *c,* Fused MRI/CT offers excellent delineation of the mass soft-tissue components and osseous involvement relative to the underlying anatomy.

3D gradient echo with steady-state free procession sequences offer isotropic voxels and high-resolution imaging (<1-mm voxels) and marked contrast distinction between T2 hyperintense cerebrospinal fluid and other structures. These sequences are most useful as high-resolution cisternograms in the evaluation of retroorbital/suprasellar lesions to visualize fine structures such as the CNs, although the sequences are prone to susceptibility and inhomogeneity artifact at the skull base, which limits their utility within the orbit.

DWI is most useful in the setting of stroke to demonstrate infarction, playing a role in the setting of visual field defects owing to infarcts in the occipital lobe or along the optic tracts or radiations, as well as of the CNs III, IV, and VI nuclei in the brainstem. Assessment of the apparent diffusion coefficient (ADC) map is paramount, as true restricted diffusion appears hyperintense on the DWI image with corresponding dark signal on the ADC map, whereas hyperintense signal on ADC indicates a T2 shine-through effect. DWI has additional benefit in demonstrating lesions with tightly packed cells, such as epidermoid cyst or abscess, or high nuclear-to-cytoplasmic ratio as in malignant tumors (Fig. 9.14). Standard echo planar DWI may be limited by susceptibility effects (metal, bone, air interfaces), which may be improved but not eliminated through the use of multishot echoplanar techniques. DWI is frequently added to the orbital protocol in the precontrast portion as the time impact is low and the diagnostic value can be high in certain cases.

Conclusion

Orbital imaging, particularly cross-sectional imaging, is a key component of the diagnostic evaluation of orbital pathology, frequently complementing diagnostic findings obtained during clinical examination, as well as bringing new data to light that may be otherwise undetectable. A collaborative role between the clinical and radiology services best serves the patient with the advent of personalized care with customizable imaging protocols and advanced imaging techniques.

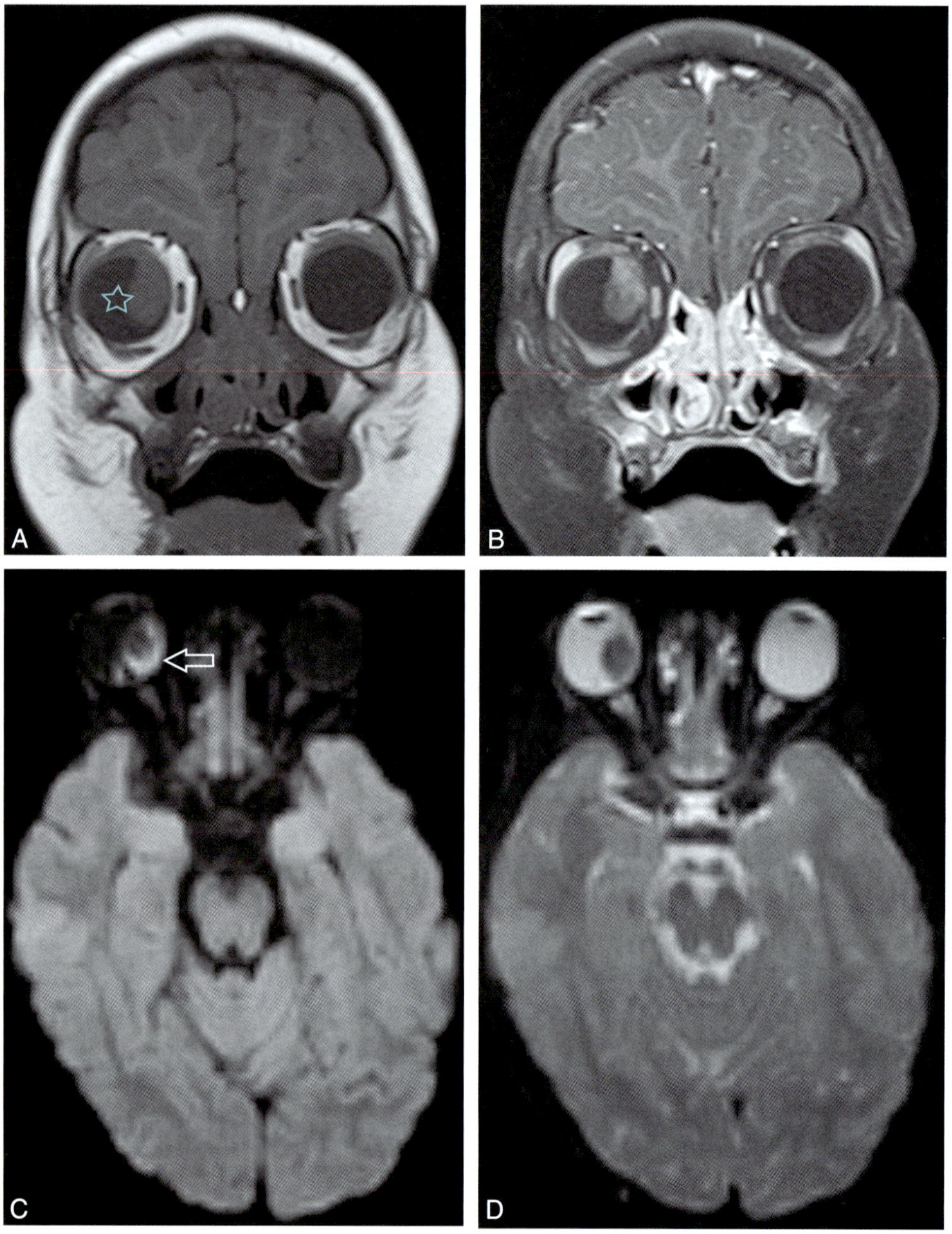

• **Fig. 9.14** Retinoblastoma. *a,* Coronal T1 non–fat-saturated image through the orbits demonstrates a right ocular mass (*blue star*). *b,* Axial T1 fat-saturated postcontrast image demonstrates enhancement of the lesion. *c,* Axial diffusion-weighted imaging demonstrates hyperintense signal. *d,* Corresponding hypointense signal on apparent diffusion coefficient within the mass, indicating true restricted diffusion from a highly cellular malignant lesion.

References

1. Turvey, T. A., & Golden, B. A. (2012). Orbital anatomy for the surgeon. *Oral and Maxillofacial Surgery Clinics of North America*, (*4*), 525–536.
2. Moore, K. L., & Agur, A. M. R. (2007). *Essential clinical anatomy.* Baltimore, MD: Lippincott Williams & Wilkins.
3. Som, P. M., & Curtin, H. D. (2003). *Head and neck imaging.* St. Louis, MO: Mosby.
4. Aviv, R. I., & Casselman, J. (2005). Orbital imaging: Part 1. Normal anatomy. *Clinical Radiology*, *60*, 279–287.
5. Grech, R., Cornish, K. S., Galvin, P. L., et al. (2014). Imaging of adult ocular and orbital pathology—a pictorial review. *Journal of Radiology Case Reports*, (*2*), 1–29.
6. American College of Radiology. ACR Appropriateness Criteria: Orbits, vision and visual loss. Available at https://acsearch.acr.org/docs/69486/Narrative. Accessed September 16, 2018.
7. De Graaf, P., Goricke, S., Rodjan, F., et al. (2012). Guidelines for imaging retinoblastoma: Imaging principles and MRI standardization. *Pediatric Radiology*, (*1*), 2–14.
8. Radbruch, A., Weberling, L. D., Kieslich, P. J., et al. (2015). Gadolinium retention in the dentate nucleus and globus pallidus is dependent on the class of contrast agent. *Radiology*, *275*, 783–791.
9. Kanal, E., & Tweedle, M. F. (2015). Residual or retained gadolinium: Practical implication for radiologists and our patients. *Radiology*, *275*, 630–634.
10. Delfaut, E. M., Beltran, J., Johnson, G., Rousseau, J., Marchandise, X., & Cotton, A. (1999). Fat suppression in MR imaging: Techniques and pitfalls. *Radiographics*, *19*, 373–382.

10 Optimizing Visualization and Localization During Endoscopic Orbital Surgery

PETER VALENTIN TOMAZIC, MD, PhD AND HEINZ STAMMBERGER, MD†

Surgical Technique

The endoscopic transnasal approach to the orbit usually starts with complete sphenoethmoidectomy and wide opening of the maxillary ostium to oversee the orbital floor. Then the papyraceus lamina is identified and resected, and the periobit is opened to gain access to the intraorbital space. To facilitate identification of the lamina, the periorbit, or the tumor at a later stage, a simple trick is to exert gentle pressure to the eyeball to push and medialize the orbital wall or content. An alternative to that approach was proposed by Shah et al.[1] to avoid moving one hand of the surgeon out of the field or require an assistant to push the globe. With this technique a blunt instrument is used to apply pressure to the expected location of the papyraceus lamina. If the lamina has been adequately exposed, the whole lamina will be seen moving. If residual ethmoid lamellae are attached, no movement or partial movement can be seen. Theses first steps can easily be accomplished with 0-degree endoscopes. When intraorbital pathology is addressed, angulated scopes (e.g., 30-degree or 45-degree) may help to increase visualization of the surgical field because the optical angle becomes wider the more lateral one dissects. Sometimes a partial septectomy or a septal window is helpful to approach the orbit from both nasal cavities and through both nostrils, especially in a four-handed technique.[2] With the advent of three-dimensional (3D) endoscopy, spatial orientation may be enhanced, especially when targeting the orbital apex and skull base.[3] In particular, the approach to the intraconal space harbors two major sources of difficulties for visualization and localization of pathology: the protruding orbital fat and the extraocular muscles.[2] Contrary to orbital decompression, when protrusion of orbital fat and decrease of intraorbital pressure is desired, here it hampers the view and working space if intraorbital lesions, predominantly tumors, are addressed.[4] Because of the mass effect of the tumor, intraorbital pressure is elevated, promoting the protrusion of fat after incision of the periorbit. However, it is advised not to remove the fat to maintain normal eyeball movement and ocular muscle function and to avoid enophthalmos postoperatively.[5] Therefore incision through the periorbit should be limited before the ethmoidectomy has been completed to avoid obstruction of the surgical field. The fat should be dissected bluntly with standard instruments such as elevators or dissectors until the tumor capsule is identified. It is also helpful to use cottonoids or cotton-tipped applicators to gently dissect the connective tissue and spread the fat out of the way. Here, tactile feedback is very important, and advanced endoscopic techniques such as 3D endoscopy may not be as helpful as in fixed structures such as the skull base, because the fat is constantly manipulated and changes its orientation in space. Moreover, the endoscope lens could be obstructed more easily when closer to the fat and intraorbital space, which would additionally be of disadvantage for the 3D effect. In general—as in all endoscopic approaches—a clear field and endoscope lens is of utmost importance. Classically antifog solutions of different preparations and patties or small beakers are used to keep the lens clean. Automated self-cleaning devices for the scopes are beneficial to avoid frequent egress of the endoscope for extra nasal cleaning. Here the endoscope is put into an extra shaft that is linked to an irrigation device and pump and can be flushed on demand by operating a foot petal.[6] The only disadvantage may be that the endoscope's working diameter is increased owing to the extra shaft, which could hamper movement of instruments in narrow spaces and corridors (e.g.. if the nostrils are tight).

Handling of Bleeding During Surgery to Improve Visualisation

If bleeding occurs during the dissection, it can usually be handled with swabs soaked in adrenaline 1:1.000. When using adrenaline, however, vasospasms to the centralis retinae and ciliares posteriores arteries may occur. Distinct arterial bleeders may be cauterized with bipolar devices if properly identified. When the superior/medial compartment needs to be addressed, the ethmoidal arteries may be in the surgical field. In particular, the anterior ethmoidal artery can be identified on computed tomography by looking for a pyramidal notch at the papyraceus lamina between the superior oblique and medial rectus muscles. This notch marks the exit of the artery from the orbit. If it is likely to be crossed during the intraorbital approach, it can be dissected and ligated easiest by bipolar

†Deceased.

cautery forceps. Care is needed to cauterize the entire intranasal length of the artery and dissect it in the middle to avoid retraction and intraorbital bleeding. If the notch cannot be seen on CT, the artery runs in the skull base. If it needs to be crossed to gain access superiorly, the skull base must be thinned out carefully with a diamond burr to expose the artery and cauterize it thereafter. The same can be done for the posterior ethmoidal artery, especially for posterior lesions close to or in the orbital apex.[7] However, extensive cauterization of the orbital fat should be avoided for the same reason as not resecting it. Furthermore, the nerves and muscles can be endangered by excessive cautery. Other hemostatic agents such as Oxicell (Apex Energetics, Irvine, CA), TachoSil Fibrin Sealant Patch (Johnson & Johnson Ethicon, Bridgewater, NJ), or Floseal (Baxter International, Deerfield, IL) may be applied. Oxicell and TachoSil are helpful after surgery to avoid minor oozing; however, intraoperative use of Floseal is suitable because it can be easily suctioned away once the bleeding stops and would not obstruct the view or access. Oxicell also expands and hardens when soaked with blood; thus it should not be left/put intraorbitally but may be placed over the orbital fat or remaining periorbit. Fibrin glue—particularly, autologous fibrin glue—can be sprayed into the cavity to prevent oozing and to seal the orbit. However, postoperative infection of the orbit is very rare and orbital reconstruction is rarely necessary.[8,9]

Adjuncts for Intraorbital Tumor Dissection

Once the tumor is identified, extracapsular dissection may be facilitated by enlarging the incision of the periorbit. The tumor itself can be cauterized to reduce its volume and facilitate dissection and removal. An alternative to cautery may be cryoassisted tumor ablation as described by Campbell et al. and Castelnuovo et al.[10,11] Here, once the lesion is exposed medial and inferior, a cryoprobe (modified ophthalmic standard cryoprobe) is placed in contact with the capsule of the tumor and activated, which creates temporary adhesion owing to the so-called Joule-Thompson effect. Once the probe is activated, freezing temperatures are reached at its tip and the tissue becomes frozen white, which proofs the adherence of the tumor and its capsule to the probe. Care is needed to avoid freezing of surrounding structures. When adhesion of the lesion is achieved, it can be manipulated by gentle torsional traction to separate it from surrounding connective tissue. This process can be repeated to achieve extracapsular dissection, and the lesion can subsequently be pulled out of the orbit, which makes further dissection and visualization easier.

For intraconal tumors, another obstacle toward the anticipated lesion is the medial rectus muscle.[12] Damage to it may lead to severe diplopia, and restoring the muscle after iatrogenic dissection is challenging, if not impossible.[13]

Dealing With Extraconal Muscles

A simple technique to avoid damage to the muscle and keeping it out of the visual field is a temporary medialization through sutures or slings. Here the muscle is identified before entering the intraconal space, and a suture or vessel loop is placed around the muscle. Thereafter it can be gently pulled out of the field and be positioned as desired (Fig. 10.1). Monofilic, larger-diameter sutures (e.g., 2-0) should be used to decrease trauma to the muscle tissue and its delicate capsule. After completion of the surgery, the suture is removed.[2,14] In addition, a trocar can be inserted via the canine fossa to provide a third corridor for instruments or scopes and thus gain space and better angulation intranasally (Fig. 10.2).

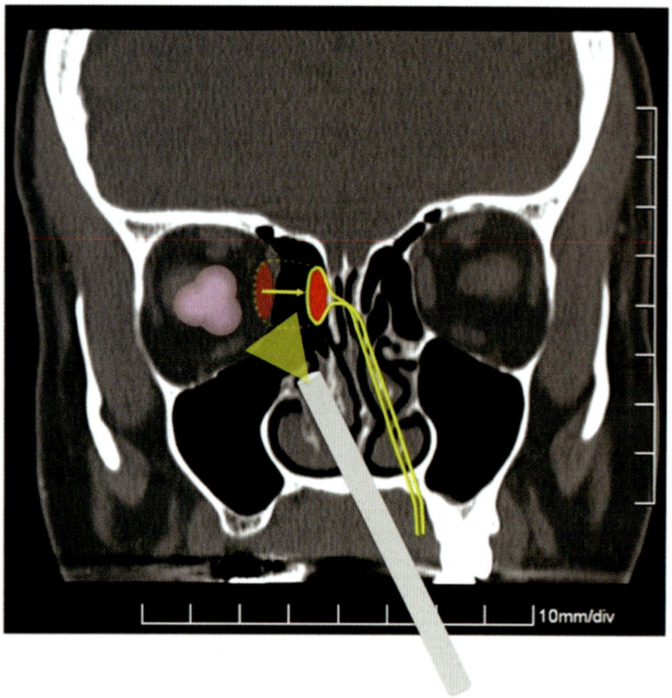

• **Fig. 10.1** Schematic display of the medialization technique with the medial rectus muscle secured by a suture and gently pulled medially to expose the tumor.

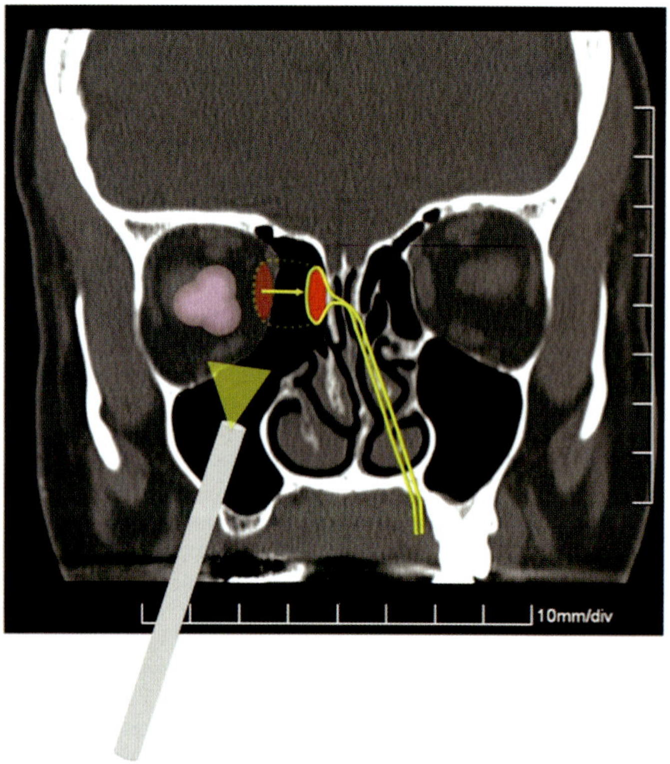

• **Fig. 10.2** Schematic display of the medialization technique with a trocar in the maxillary sinus to gain an additional port for access.

Identification of the pathology is easiest when either the tumor is large and/or the amount of intraorbital fat is limited. To assist in orienting inside the orbit and identifying tumors or foreign bodies, computer-assisted navigation, especially a CT/magnetic resonance imaging (MRI) fusion technique, can be helpful as in standard functional endoscopic sinus surgery procedures.[5,15–17] In the majority of cases electromagnetic navigational devices are used. Their major advantage lies in a variety of malleable instruments from suction to dissectors without the need of reregistration. This facilitates the work at a high angulation as required inside the orbit. Moreover, the small size of the instruments favors the four-handed work intranasally compared with the optical devices. Novel software adjuncts to navigation devices can mark critical structures preoperatively on CT and/or MRI datasets. This can be used either to avoid damaging tissue like the optic nerve or to mark out the tumor location so that acoustic and optical feedback is given to the surgeon if the lesion is approached. This can be helpful in small tumors or if massive orbital fat hampers the dissection, orientation, and visualization. Because this information is entered preoperatively on the respective datasets, which are not updated unless intraoperative CT or MRI is available, the surgeon must be aware that the location of the tumor may have changed as the result of manipulation, such as incision of the periorbit or dissection of the orbital fat.

Recently Castelnuovo et al.[18] reported a "push-pull" technique to remove an intraorbital venous malformation located superomedially in the orbit. With this technique the external approach improves visualization of the lesion by pushing it down via a superior eyelid approach while removing it endoscopically. In addition to the endoscopic approach, external approaches and combined approaches to the orbit are well described.[19]

References

1. Shah, R. R., Thomas, W. W., Kuan, E. C., & Kennedy, D. W. (2018). The lamina push test: An alternative to the globe push test for identifying the medial orbit during endoscopic sinus surgery. *International Forum of Allergy & Rhinology*, *8*, 1073–1075.
2. Tomazic, P. V., Stammberger, H., Habermann, W., Gerstenberger, C., Braun, H., Gellner, V., et al. (2011). Intraoperative medialization of medial rectus muscle as a new endoscopic technique for approaching intraconal lesions. *American Journal of Rhinology & Allergy*, *25*, 363–367.
3. Roth, J., Fraser, J. F., Singh, A., Bernardo, A., Anand, V. K., & Schwartz, T. H. (2011). Surgical approaches to the orbital apex: Comparison of endoscopic endonasal and transcranial approaches using a novel 3D endoscope. *Orbit*, *30*, 43–48.
4. Castelnuovo, P., Turri-Zanoni, M., Battaglia, P., Locatelli, D., & Dallan, I. (2015). Endoscopic endonasal management of orbital pathologies. *Neurosurgery Clinics of North America*, *26*, 463–472.
5. Castelnuovo, P., Dallan, I., Locatelli, D., Battaglia, P., Farneti, P., Tomazic, P. V., et al. (2012). Endoscopic transnasal intraorbital surgery: Our experience with 16 cases. *European Archives of Oto-Rhino-Laryngology*, *269*, 1929–1935.
6. Sindwani, R. (2017). Technological advances in sinus and skull base surgery. *Otolaryngology Clinics of North America*, *50*, xix–xx. https://doi.org/10.1016/j.otc.2017.03.002.
7. Felippu, A., Mora, R., & Guastini, L. (2011). Endoscopic transnasal cauterization of the anterior ethmoidal artery. *Acta Oto-Laryngologica*, *131*, 1074–1078.
8. Tomazic, P. V., Edlinger, S., Gellner, V., Koele, W., Gerstenberger, C., Braun, H., et al. (2015). Vivostat: An autologous fibrin sealant as useful adjunct in endoscopic transnasal CSF-leak repair. *European Archives of Oto-Rhino-Laryngology*, *272*, 1423–1427.
9. Barham, H. P., Sacks, R., & Harvey, R. J. (2016). Hemostatic materials and devices. *Otolaryngologic Clinics of North America*, *49*, 577–584.
10. Campbell, P. G., Yadla, S., Rosen, M., Bilyk, J. R., Murchison, A. P., & Evans, J. J. (2011). Endoscopic transnasal cryo-assisted removal of an orbital cavernous hemangioma: A technical note. *Minimally Invasive Neurosurgery*, *54*, 41–43.
11. Castelnuovo, P., Arosio, A. D., Leone, F., Ravasio, A., Azzolini, C., De Maria, F., et al. (2019). Endoscopic transnasal cryo-assisted removal of orbital cavernous hemangiomas: Case report and technical hints. *World Neurosurgery*, *126*, 66–71.
12. Lenzi, R., Bleier, B. S., Felisati, G., & Muscatello, L. (2016). Purely endoscopic trans-nasal management of orbital intraconal cavernous haemangiomas: A systematic review of the literature. *European Archives of Oto-Rhino-Laryngology*, *273*, 2319–2322.
13. Thacker, N. M., Velez, F. G., Demer, J. L., Wang, M. B., & Rosenbaum, A. L. (2005). Extraocular muscle damage associated with endoscopic sinus surgery: An ophthalmology perspective. *American Journal of Rhinology*, *19*, 400–405.
14. McKinney, K. A., Snyderman, C. H., Carrau, R. L., Germanwala, A. V., Prevedello, D. M., Stefko, S. T., et al. (2010). Seeing the light: Endoscopic endonasal intraconal orbital tumor surgery. *Otolaryngology–Head and Neck Surgery*, *143*, 699–701.
15. Łysoń, T., Sieskiewicz, A., Rogowski, M., & Mariak, Z. (2013). Transnasal endoscopic removal of intraorbital wooden foreign body. *Journal of Neurological Surgery Part A. Central European Neurosurgery*, *74*(Suppl 1), e100–e103.
16. Tomazic, P. V., Stammberger, H., Habermann, W., Gerstenberger, C., Braun, H., Gellner, V., et al. (2011). Intraoperative medialization of medial rectus muscle as a new endoscopic technique for approaching intraconal lesions. *American Journal of Rhinology & Allergy*, *25*, 363–367.
17. Kent, J. S., Allen, L. H., & Rotenberg, B. W. (2010). Image-guided transnasal endoscopic techniques in the management of orbital disease. *Orbit*, *29*, 328–333.
18. Castelnuovo, P., Fiacchini, G., Fiorini, F. R., & Dallan, I. (2018). "Push-pull technique" for the management of a selected superomedial intraorbital lesion. *Surgery Journal (New York, NY)*, *4*, e105–e109.
19. Paluzzi, A., Gardner, P. A., Fernandez-Miranda, J. C., Tormenti, M. J., Stefko, S. T., Snyderman, C. H., et al. (2015). "Round-the-clock" surgical access to the orbit. *Journal of Neurological Surgery Part B, Skull Base*, *76*, 12–24.

PART 3

Nasolacrimal Duct Obstruction and Endoscopic-DCR

11

Evaluation and Management of Congenital Nasolacrimal Duct Obstruction

KAPIL MISHRA, MD AND COURTNEY LYNN KRAUS, MD

Congenital nasolacrimal duct obstruction (NLDO) is a blockage of the lacrimal drainage system and the most common cause of persistent tearing and ocular discharge in infants and young children.[1–4] The anatomic site of obstruction is an imperforate membrane at the valve of Hasner located at the distal end of the nasolacrimal duct. The obstruction can be unilateral or bilateral, and signs usually consist of epiphora, discharge, and an increased tear lake. Although most cases resolve spontaneously by age 6 months, several effective treatment options exist for persistent cases. Because of the high rate of resolution, conservative measures are preferred before considering surgical treatment. Recent studies assist the clinician in selection and timing of treatment. Endoscopy has become an important diagnostic and therapeutic tool in patients with anomalous anatomy and surgical failures.

Epidemiology and Risk Factors

Epidemiology

NLDO is diagnosed in up to 6% of newborns,[5,6] although evidence of impaired lacrimal drainage reportedly exists in up to 20% of infants during the first year of life.[3] Signs of NLDO occur early, with one study reporting 95% of children with NLDO were symptomatic in the first month of life.[3] There is an age-dependent decrease in the rate of spontaneous resolution, with 90% of cases resolving spontaneously by 6 months of age. For cases persisting to 6 to 10 months, about 66% demonstrate resolution. NLDO beyond 1 year is less likely to resolve spontaneously.[3]

Most patients have unilateral NLDO, although about 31% have bilateral disease. Unilateral obstructions appear to resolve slightly earlier than bilateral obstructions. One study found that in infants with NLDO, 38% affected the right eye and 32% affected the left eye.[7] Males and females are equally affected. However, males have symptom resolution slightly earlier than females, which has been hypothesized to be secondary to an anatomically larger nasolacrimal fossa.[7]

Risk Factors

Prematurity may be a risk factor for the development of NLDO, and some degree of blockage has been observed in 16% of premature infants.[8] Bilateral obstruction has been observed in extremely premature children, with the percentage affected inversely correlated with gestational age. Patients with midface anomalies also have higher rates of NLDO. One study found NLDO to be present in almost 22% of patients with Down syndrome.[9] Patients with Down syndrome were found to have distal sites of obstruction, in addition to higher rates of canalicular atresia and stenosis.[10] Children with mandibulofacial dysostosis are also at increased risk of NLDO, and high rates of punctal atresia have been found in this patient population.[11]

Pathophysiology

The nasolacrimal system begins development at gestational day 32.[12] Initially the ectoderm thickens within the nasooptic fissure. This thickened ectoderm resides between the nasal and maxillary processes and eventually becomes more well differentiated. As it extends, an upper branch forms the canaliculi and a lower forms the nasolacrimal duct. Canalization is already occurring in the 60-day embryo. The interface between the distal end of the nasolacrimal duct and the mucus membrane of the inferior meatus, known as the valve of Hasner, is the last point in the ductal system to become patent (Fig. 11.1).[13]

Perhaps not coincidentally, the valve of Hasner is the most common site of obstruction.[14] An assessment of stillborn infants found that 73.3% did not have a patent nasolacrimal passage to the nose.[12] More complicated sites of obstruction include diffuse stenosis of the nasolacrimal duct, intranasal mucoceles/dacryocystoceles, and proximal outflow dysgenesis occurring concurrently with distal obstruction.

Diagnosis

Symptoms of NLDO are often observed within the first weeks of life.[14] The three hallmark signs are epiphora, mucoid discharge, and increased tear lake. Each may present in varying degrees. One study showed that 95% of patients had an increased tear lake, 80% had epiphora, and 68% had mucoid discharge,[15] whereas another study found tearing was the main presenting symptom in 93.4%.[16] Lack of irritation or photophobia is an important consideration when differentiating from other causes of tearing and discharge.

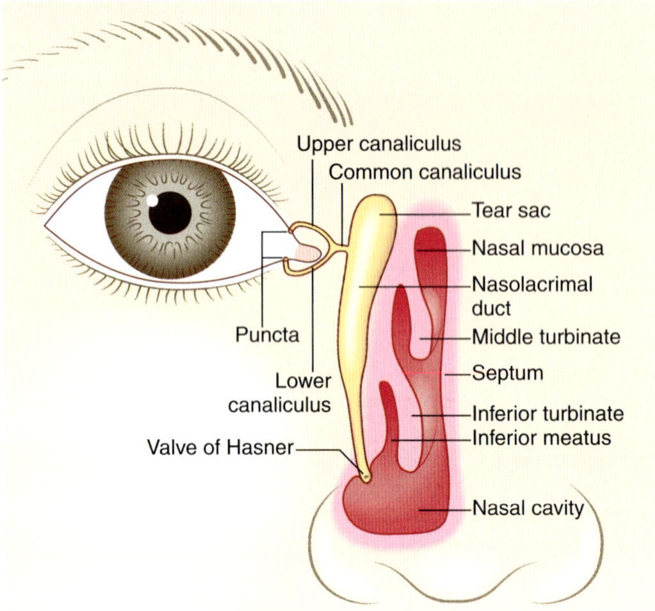

• **Fig. 11.1** Lacrimal drainage system.

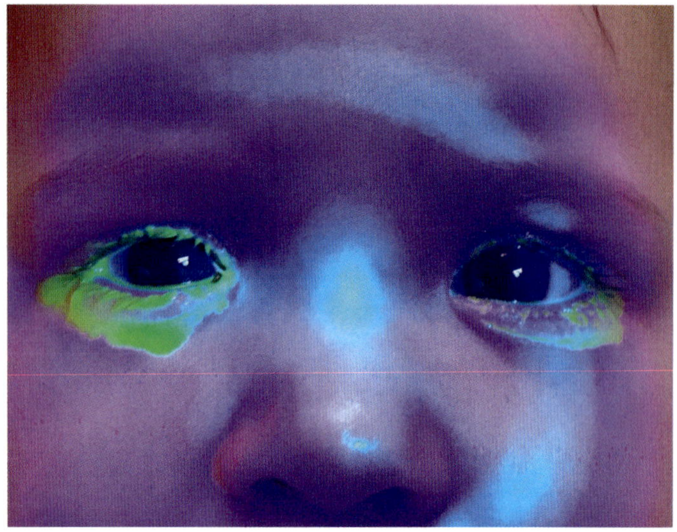

• **Fig. 11.2** Increased tear lake and tear overflow of the right eye highlighted using cobalt blue light and fluorescein dye.

Differential Diagnosis

When a child presents with epiphora, whether it is due to tear overproduction or outflow obstruction must be explored. Causes of tear overproduction include ocular irritation from causes such as foreign body, corneal abrasion, or infection. Tearing when sucking or chewing may suggest a rare congenital cranial dysinnervation disorder caused by aberrant facial salivary fibers innervating the lacrimal gland.[17]

It is critical that congenital glaucoma be ruled out, as it can present with epiphora. However, glaucoma uniquely is accompanied by blepharospasm and photophobia. Signs include corneal haze/opacification and eye enlargement (buphthalmus). Ruling out congenital glaucoma requires a full ophthalmologic examination, including intraocular pressure measurement, assessment of corneal diameter and haze, inspection of the optic nerve, and cycloplegic refraction.

Although an imperforate valve of Hasner is the most common cause of tear outflow obstruction, other anatomic anomalies present in the same manner. Congenital canalicular atresia is an uncommon cause of NLDO that may be identified during NLDO surgery.[18] Another condition is a lacrimal fistula that may be internal, from nasal mucosa to lacrimal sac or external, connecting the skin to the common canaliculus or lacrimal sac.[19] Lacrimal fistulas have been estimated to occur in 1 in 2000 births.[20] The location is characteristically inferonasal to the medial canthus. Although they are usually asymptomatic, some patients have clear mucoid discharge at the fistula's ostium.

Another important phenomenon to rule out is a congenital dacryocystocele, which presents around the time of birth as a blue- or pink-colored mass just inferior to the medial canthus. This mass represents a dilated lacrimal sac, which is thought to arise secondary to simultaneous proximal and distal obstruction of the lacrimal system.[21] The proximal obstruction acts as a one-way valve leading to accumulation of mucus, tears, and cellular debris. Secondary infection causing dacryocystitis is common and warrants intravenous antibiotics and procedural intervention. Dacryocystocele with significant nasal extension is an uncommon but important cause of respiratory distress in infants, who are obligate nasal breathers.[22]

Testing

In an infant presenting with epiphora, a fluorescein dye disappearance test can be used to evaluate for obstruction. A drop of fluorescein is instilled in the eye and the tear film is observed after 5 minutes using cobalt blue light (Fig. 11.2). Persistence of significant dye or asymmetric clearance between the eyes suggests an outflow obstruction. One prospective study showed this test to be 90% sensitive and 100% specific in aiding in the diagnosis of NLDO.[23] Contrast dacryocystography and dacryoscintigraphy have been described in the literature as possible diagnostic tools but are rarely performed in clinical practice. Computed tomography and magnetic resonance imaging may have a role in evaluating congenital craniofacial deformities and concomitant nasal or sinus disease.[24]

Management

Conservative Management

Because of the high rate of spontaneous resolution of NLDO, initial treatment usually involves conservative, nonsurgical measures. For patients older than 1 year who have a lower likelihood of spontaneous resolution, several studies have generated treatment algorithms.

Lacrimal massage has long been advocated as a first-line treatment option for NLDO. Crigler first described his technique for massaging the lacrimal sac in 1923.[25] The technique involved placing one finger over the common canaliculus to prevent upward flow and simultaneously stroking downward along the lacrimal sac with the intent to increase hydrostatic pressure to break the membrane at the valve of Hasner. This particular technique, called the Crigler massage, has been shown to have higher success rates than simple massage or no massage.[4,26–29]

Antibiotic drops can be prescribed concurrently with lacrimal massage, although their efficacy has been debated. Investigation into the bacterial flora of the lacrimal system has suggested no difference for patients with and without NLDO.[30] Other studies have suggested trends: *Streptococcus pneumoniae* was the most common gram-positive and *Haemophilus influenza* the most common gram-negative bacteria.[31–33] The organisms in these studies were susceptible to ofloxacin.

Procedural Management

Optimal duration of conservative management has been debated extensively, in part because conflicting reports exist on the rate of spontaneous resolution with age. Some studies seem to suggest high rates of resolution with conservative management even after the age of 1 year.[28,34] As part of the Pediatric Eye Disease Investigator Group (PEDIG) studies, researchers found that 66% of patients between 6 and less than 10 months had resolution of symptoms with 6 months of conservative treatment alone.[35] These findings were mirrored by another study with a similar age group.[36] If surgery was attempted in patients older than 1 year, some studies did not find an age-related decline in surgical success.[37,38] However, other reports suggested a delay in surgical treatment led to poorer outcomes.[5,16,39,40]

Because of the differing reports in the literature, there is no consensus on optimal management after 6 months of age. The physician must take into account symptom severity, caregiver concerns, and feasibility of surgery when deciding on further treatment options. Deferring invasive techniques until after 12 months of age spares a portion of patients from procedural intervention. However, there are advantages to escalating care after 6 months of age. In younger patients probing can usually be performed in an office setting with topical anesthetic, whereas older patients need to undergo general anesthesia in a surgical facility. Immediate office-probing ($562) appear to be more cost-effective than observing for 6 months followed by facility-probing ($701) for those children without spontaneous resolution. This, combined with 3 fewer months of symptoms, argues for early probing. However, a very strong argument against early probing is that two of every three infants have spontaneous resolution.[41]

Probing the Nasolacrimal Duct

If conservative management fails, probing is the next possible intervention. The procedure involves dilation of the punctum followed by insertion of a Bowman probe. The probe is gently advanced along the canaliculus while exerting lateral traction on the lid until a "hard stop" at the nasal bone is felt. The probe is then rotated 90 degrees to align with the nasolacrimal duct and is advanced. If a distal membrane at the valve of Hasner is present, a "pop" can be felt as the probe penetrates it. Correct passage into the nasal cavity and patency can be confirmed in several ways: introducing a second Bowman probe in the nostril to allow metal-metal contact of the two probes, injecting fluorescein into the punctum and aspirating from the nose, or endoscopy-assisted visualization (Fig. 11.3).[42]

Endoscopy has become a valuable tool in confirming patency of the nasolacrimal drainage pathway, particularly in cases of abnormal anatomy or dacryocystoceles. Patients with dacryocystoceles have a high likelihood of a nasolacrimal duct cyst at the valve of Hasner,[43] and endoscopy aids in direct visualization and tissue removal. Endoscopic-assisted probing may facilitate improved outcomes in older patients or in those for whom prior probing has failed.[44,45]

Overall, 80% of patients have resolution of symptoms with a single probing.[46] In a prospective, nonrandomized study, PEDIG found probing successful in 78% of eyes overall, 78% success for patients 6 to 12 months of age, 79% for those 1 to 2 years, 79% for those 2 to 3 years, and 56% for patients 3 to 4 years.[15] This age-related decline has been replicated by other studies, with lower success rates postulated to be secondary to diffuse stenosis in the setting of chronic obstruction.[47,48]

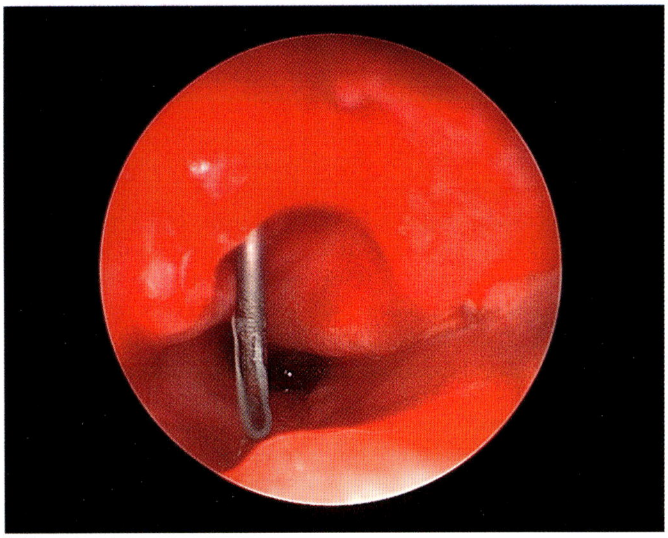

• **Fig. 11.3** Endoscopic image of metal Bowman probe exiting the nasolacrimal duct immediately below the inferior meatus.

Balloon Dilation

An alternative to simple probing is balloon catheter dilation, a technique introduced in the 1990s that uses a semi-flexible wire probe with an inflatable balloon tip (Fig. 11.4).[49] Manufacturer protocol advises passing the balloon catheter through the nasolacrimal duct system into the nasal cavity and confirming its position by touching the catheter with a second probe or by direct visualization. The balloon is then inflated for 90 seconds, deflated, inflated again for 60 seconds, deflated, then withdrawn 5 mm, and finally inflated/deflated again for 90 and 60 seconds before withdrawing. Retrospective case series found high success rates with balloon dilation and in the PEDIG prospective study, 82% of patients were successfully treated.[50] Balloon dilation is a reasonable option as a primary procedure, but the higher cost of the procedure compared with simple probing should be considered.

Silicone Intubation

Placement of a temporary silicone tube after probing to maintain patency was first introduced in the 1960s and remains a common

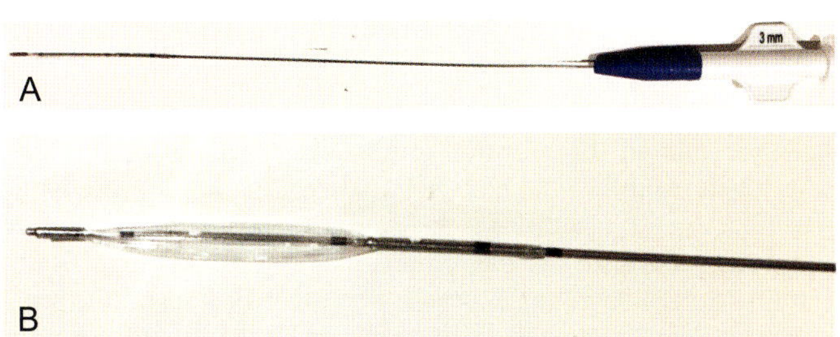

• **Fig. 11.4** A, Uninflated LacriCath probe (Quest Medical, Secaucus, NJ). B, Inflated balloon catheter.

treatment for all causes of NLDO.[51] The procedure traditionally involved bicanalicular stenting (e.g., Crawford and Ritleng stents). However, this technique requires an additional trip to the operating room and general anesthesia for stent removal, and therefore is a less ideal primary procedure for congenital NLDO. It is best suited for complex cases, failed prior probings, or in older patients.

Monocanalicular stents (e.g., Monoka stent, FCI Ophthalmics, Pembroke, MA) are advantageous in eliminating the need for another exposure to general anesthesia as removal can be done in an office setting. Both monocanalicular and bicanalicular tubes can be secured in the nose with a nasal mucosal suture or simple tying. Success rates of stenting as a primary procedure range from 79% to 96%.[52–55] PEDIG performed a prospective study and found success in 90% of cases; monocanalicular stents were used in the majority of cases.[56] A meta-analysis that included studies comparing monocanalicular to bicanalicular stents found no difference in success or dislocation rate.[57] A randomized controlled trial suggested similar rates of success between probing only and silicone intubation in simple NLDO; however, bicanalicular silicone intubation appeared to confer a significant advantage in cases of complex NLDO.[58]

Complications

Across all techniques, postprocedural complications are uncommon and can be managed conservatively. In simple probing, studies have indicated low rates of minor bleeding from the punctum, resulting in blood-tinged tears or mild epistaxis.[15] A large series of office-based nasolacrimal duct probing reported no complications.[59] Probing can create a false passage into the nose, resulting in incomplete obstruction resolution. Balloon dilation is also well tolerated, with no complications reported in a large PEDIG study.[50]

The most common complication of nasolacrimal silicone intubation is tube migration and the subsequent need for removal. One series found early tube removal (defined as less than 2 months) in 41% of eyes.[56] Far less common complications include corneal abrasion, pyogenic granuloma formation, canalicular slitting, and cellulitis.[53]

Follow-up

Treatment success is defined as the absence of signs of obstruction several weeks after the procedure. Symptom resolution is apparent within the first few days and can be identified by the caregiver. Therefore the first postoperative visit can take place 4 to 6 weeks after surgery, by which time treatment failure is obvious.

Several options exist if the primary procedure fails to resolve the obstruction. If probing were chosen as the primary procedure, the surgeon may elect to repeat probing with or without endoscopy, balloon dilation, or silicone intubation. In their prospective study, PEDIG reported a 56% success rate with repeat probing, echoing previous retrospective studies.[60–62] When assessing the efficacy of balloon dilation or silicone intubation after failed probing, researchers found 77% and 84% success rates, respectively.[63] The difference in success rates was not statistically significant, making either procedure a viable secondary option. Endoscopic visualization in recalcitrant cases serves a valuable diagnostic purpose, especially if aberrant anatomy is suspected. If secondary treatment also does not lead to resolution, more invasive surgical procedures such as dacryocystorhinostomy or conjunctivodacryocystorhinostomy may be considered depending on the anatomy.

Even after NLDO resolution, patients require ongoing comprehensive eye examinations to monitor for amblyopia. In pediatric patients presenting with NLDO, 22% had amblyogenic risk factors such as refractive error or strabismus.[64] Patients with unilateral NLDO have a higher risk of anisometropia, specifically higher hyperopia on the obstructed side, a risk factor for amblyopia.[65,66]

Conclusion

Observation with or without massage is the preferred first-line treatment option. Continued observation or procedural therapies are reasonable strategies for persistent cases. Although balloon dilation or silicone intubation have high success rates even in cases of prior failed probing, there is support for endoscopy-assisted probing for better visualization, particularly in older children or in those with abnormal nasal anatomy.

References

1. Ffooks, O. (1962). Dacryocystitis in infancy. *British Journal of Ophthalmology, 46*(7), 422–434. https://doi.org/10.1136/bjo.46.7.422.
2. Örge, F. H., & Boente, C. S. (2014). The lacrimal system. *Pediatric Clinics of North America, 61*(3), 529–539. https://doi.org/10.1016/j.pcl.2014.03.002.
3. Mac Ewen, C. J., & Young, J. D. H. (1991). Epiphora during the first year of life. *Eye (London), 5*(Pt5), 536–600. https://doi.org/10.1038/eye.1991.103.
4. Petersen, R. A., & Robb, R. M. (1978). The natural course of congenital obstruction of the nasolacrimal duct. *Journal of Pediatric Ophthalmology and Strabismus, 15*(4), 246–250.
5. Paul, T. O., & Shepherd, R. (1994). Congenital nasolacrimal duct obstruction: Natural history and the timing of optimal intervention. *Journal of Pediatric Ophthalmology and Strabismus, 31*(6), 362–367.
6. Guerry, D., & Kendig, E. L. (1948). Congenital impatency of the nasolacrimal duct. *Archives of Ophthalmology (Chicago), 39*(2), 193–204. http://www.ncbi.nlm.nih.gov/pubmed/18868825 Accessed September 3, 2018.
7. Sathiamoorthi, S., Frank, R. D., & Mohney, B. G. (2019). Incidence and clinical characteristics of congenital nasolacrimal duct obstruction. *British Journal of Ophthalmology, 103*(4), 526–529.
8. Lorena, S. H. T., Silva, J. A. F., & Scarpi, M. J. (2013). Congenital nasolacrimal duct obstruction in premature children. *Journal of Pediatric Ophthalmology & Strabismus, 50*(4), 239–244. https://doi.org/10.3928/01913913-20130423-01.
9. Berk, A. T., Saatci, A. O., Erçal, M. D., Tunç, M., & Ergin, M. (1996). Ocular findings in 55 patients with Down's syndrome. *Ophthalmic Genet.* https://doi.org/10.3109/13816819609057864.
10. Coats, D. K., Brady McCreery, K. M., Plager, D. A., Bohra, L., Kim, D. S., & Paysse, E. A. (2003). Nasolacrimal outflow drainage anomalies in Down's syndrome. *Ophthalmology.* https://doi.org/10.1016/S0161-6420(03)00410-X.
11. Bartley, G. B. (1990). Lacrimal drainage anomalies in mandibulofacial dysostosis. *Am J Ophthalmol.* https://doi.org/10.1016/S0002-9394(14)70688-9.
12. CASSADY, J. V. (1952). Developmental anatomy of nasolacrimal duct. *AMA Arch Ophthalmol, 47*(2), 141–158. http://www.ncbi.nlm.nih.gov/pubmed/14894015. Accessed August 19, 2018.
13. Sevel, D. (1981). Development and congenital abnormalities of the nasolacrimal apparatus. *J Pediatr Ophthalmol Strabismus.*
14. Kapadia, M. K., Freitag, S. K., & Woog, J. J. (2006). Evaluation and management of congenital nasolacrimal duct obstruction. *Otolaryngol Clin North Am.* https://doi.org/10.1016/j.otc.2006.08.004.
15. Repka, M. X., Chandler, D. L., Beck, R. W., et al. (2008). Primary treatment of nasolacrimal duct obstruction with probing in children

younger than 4 years. *Ophthalmology*. https://doi.org/10.1016/j.ophtha.2007.07.030.
16. Kashkouli, M. B., Beigi, B., Parvaresh, M. M., Kassaee, A., & Tabatabaee, Z. (2003). Late and very late initial probing for congenital nasolacrimal duct obstruction: What is the cause of failure? *Br J Ophthalmol*. https://doi.org/10.1136/bjo.87.9.1151.
17. Gutowski, N. J., & Chilton, J. K. (2015). The congenital cranial dysinnervation disorders. *Archives of Disease in Childhood, 100*(7), 678–681. https://doi.org/10.1136/archdischild-2014-307035.
18. Soliman, M., & Lueder, G. T. (2015). Initial management of congenital canalicular atresia. *J AAPOS*. https://doi.org/10.1016/j.jaapos.2015.02.009.
19. Birchansky, L. D., Nerad, J. A., Kersten, R. C., & Kulwin, D. R. (1990). Management of congenital lacrimal sac fistula. *Archives of Ophthalmology (Chicago, Ill, 1960), 108*(3), 388–390. (1990). http://www.ncbi.nlm.nih.gov/pubmed/2310340. Accessed August 19, 2018.
20. François, J., & Bacskulin, J. (1969). External congenital fistulae of the lacrimal sac. *Ophthalmologica, 159*(4), 249–261. https://doi.org/10.1159/000305922.
21. Mansour, A. M., Cheng, K. P., Mumma, J. V., et al. (1991). Congenital dacryocele: A collaborative review. *Ophthalmology*. https://doi.org/10.1016/S0161-6420(91)32063-3.
22. Hepler, K. M., Woodson, G. E., & Kearns, D. B. (1995). Respiratory distress in the neonate: Sequela of a congenital dacryocystocele. *Archives of Otolaryngology–Head Neck Surgery, 121*(12), 1423–1425. http://www.ncbi.nlm.nih.gov/pubmed/1757852. Accessed August 19, 2018.
23. MacEwen, C. J., & Young, J. D. (1991). The fluorescein disappearance test (FDT): An evaluation of its use in infants. *Journal of Pediatric Ophthalmology & Strabismus, 28*(6), 302–305. http://www.ncbi.nlm.nih.gov/pubmed/9373120. Accessed September 3, 2018.
24. Guzek, J. P., Ching, A. S., Hoang, T. A., Dure-Smith, P., Llaurado, J. G., Yau, D. C., et al. (1994). Clinical and radiologic lacrimal testing in patients with epiphora. *Ophthalmology, 104*(11), 1875–1881. http://www.ncbi.nlm.nih.gov/pubmed/7488375. Accessed August 19, 2018.
25. Crigler, L. W. (1923). The treatment of congenital dacryocystitis. *J Am Med Assoc*. https://doi.org/10.1001/jama.1923.02650010027009.
26. Kushner, B. J. (1982). Congenital nasolacrimal system obstruction. (1982). *Archives of Ophthalmology (Chicago, IL, 1960), 100*(4), 597–600. http://www.ncbi.nlm.nih.gov/pubmed/6896140. Accessed August 19, 2018.
27. Nelson, L. B., Calhoun, J. H., & Menduke, H. (1985). Medical management of congenital nasolacrimal duct obstruction. *Pediatrics, 76*(2), 172–175. http://www.ncbi.nlm.nih.gov/pubmed/4022689. Accessed August 19, 2018.
28. Nucci, P., Capoferri, C., Alfarano, R., & Brancato, R. (1989). Conservative management of congenital nasolacrimal duct obstruction. *Journal of Pediatric Ophthalmology & Strabismus, 26*(1), 39–43. http://www.ncbi.nlm.nih.gov/pubmed/2915312. Accessed August 19, 2018.
29. Karti, O., Karahan, E., Acan, D., & Kusbeci, T. (2016). The natural process of congenital nasolacrimal duct obstruction and effect of lacrimal sac massage. *International Ophthalmology, 36*(6), 845–849. https://doi.org/10.1007/s10792-016-0208-5.
30. CJ, M., Phillips, M. G., & Young, J. D. (1994). Value of bacterial culturing in the course of congenital nasolacrimal duct (NLD) obstruction. *J Pediatr Ophthalmol Strabismus*.
31. Usha, K., Smitha, S., Shah, N., Lalitha, P., & Kelkar, R. (2006). Spectrum and the susceptibilities of microbial isolates in cases of congenital nasolacrimal duct obstruction. *J AAPOS*. https://doi.org/10.1016/j.jaapos.2006.04.009.
32. Kuchar, A., Lukas, J., & Steinkogler, F. J. (2000). Bacteriology and antibiotic therapy in congenital nasolacrimal duct obstruction. *Acta Ophthalmol Scand*. https://doi.org/10.1034/j.1600-0420.2000.078006694.x.
33. Bareja, U., & Ghose, S. (1990). Clinicobacteriological correlates of congenital dacryocystitis. *Indian Journal of Ophthalmology, 38*(2), 66–69 http://www.ncbi.nlm.nih.gov/pubmed/2387604. Accessed August 19, 2018.
34. Young, J. D., MacEwen, C. J., & Ogston, S. A. (1996). Congenital nasolacrimal duct obstruction in the second year of life: A multicentre trial of management. *Eye (London, England), 10*(4), 485–491. https://doi.org/10.1038/eye.1996.107.
35. Pediatric Eye Disease Investigator Group (2012). Resolution of congenital nasolacrimal duct obstruction with nonsurgical management. *Archives of Ophthalmology (Chicago, IL, 1960), 130*(6), 730–734. https://doi.org/10.1001/archophthalmol.2012.454.
36. Paul, T. O. (1985). Medical management of congenital nasolacrimal duct obstruction. *Journal of Pediatric Ophthalmology & Strabismus, 22*(2), 68–70. http://www.ncbi.nlm.nih.gov/pubmed/3989643. Accessed August 19, 2018.
37. Robb, R. M. (1998). Success rates of nasolacrimal duct probing at time intervals after 1 year of age. *Ophthalmology*. https://doi.org/10.1016/S0161-6420(98)97038-5.
38. Kushner, B. J. (1998). The management of nasolacrimal duct obstruction in children between 18 months and 4 years old. *J AAPOS*.
39. Katowitz, J. A., & Welsh, M. G. (1987). Timing of initial probing and irrigation in congenital nasolacrimal duct obstruction. *Ophthalmology*. https://doi.org/10.1016/S0161-6420(87)33392-5.
40. Kashkouli, M. B., Kassaee, A., & Tabatabaee, Z. (2002). Initial nasolacrimal duct probing in children under age 5: Cure rate and factors affecting success. *J AAPOS*. https://doi.org/10.1067/mpa.2002.129041.
41. Pediatric Eye Disease Investigator Group. (2012). A randomized trial comparing the cost-effectiveness of 2 approaches for treating unilateral nasolacrimal duct obstruction. *Archives of Ophthalmology, 130* (12), 1525–1533. https://doi.org/10.1001/archophthalmol.2012.2853.
42. Avram, E. (2018). Insights in the treatment of congenital nasolacrimal duct obstruction. *Rom J Ophthalmol, 61*(2), 101–106. http://www.ncbi.nlm.nih.gov/pubmed/29450381. Accessed August 19.
43. Lueder, G. T. (2012). The association of neonatal dacryocystoceles and infantile dacryocystitis with nasolacrimal duct cysts (an American Ophthalmological Society thesis). *Trans Am Ophthalmol Soc, 110*, 74–93. http://www.ncbi.nlm.nih.gov/pubmed/23818736. Accessed September 6, 2018.
44. Wallace, E. J., Cox, A., White, P., & MacEwen, C. J. (2006). Endoscopic-assisted probing for congenital nasolacrimal duct obstruction. *Eye, 20*(9), 998–1003. https://doi.org/10.1038/sj.eye.6702049.
45. Lueder, G. T. (2004). Endoscopic treatment of intranasal abnormalities associated with nasolacrimal duct obstruction. *Journal of the American Association for Pediatric Ophthalmology and Strabismus, 8*(2), 128–132. https://doi.org/10.1016/S1091853103003100.
46. Schnall, B. M. (2013). Pediatric nasolacrimal duct obstruction. *Curr Opin Ophthalmol*. https://doi.org/10.1097/ICU.0b013e3283642e94.
47. Arora, S., Koushan, K., & Harvey, J. T. (2012). Success rates of primary probing for congenital nasolacrimal obstruction in children. *Journal of the American Association for Pediatric Ophthalmology and Strabismus, 16*(2), 173–176. https://doi.org/10.1016/j.jaapos.2011.12.151.
48. Perveen, S., Sufi, A. R., Rashid, S., & Khan, A. (2014). Success rate of probing for congenital nasolacrimal duct obstruction at various ages. *Journal of Ophthalmic and Vision Research, 9*(1), 60–69. http://www.ncbi.nlm.nih.gov/pubmed/24982734. Accessed September 6, 2018.
49. Becker, B. B., Berry, F. D., & Koller, H. (1996). Balloon catheter dilatation for treatment of congenital nasolacrimal duct obstruction. *American Journal of Ophthalmology, 121*(3), 304–309. http://www.ncbi.nlm.nih.gov/pubmed/8597274. Accessed September 6, 2018.
50. Repka, M. X., Melia, B. M., Beck, R. W., et al. (2008). Primary treatment of nasolacrimal duct obstruction with balloon catheter dilation in children younger than 4 years of age. *J AAPOS*. https://doi.org/10.1016/j.jaapos.2008.07.001.
51. Keith, C. G. (1968). Intubation of the lacrimal passages. *American Journal of Ophthalmology, 65*(1), 70–74. http://www.ncbi.nlm.nih.gov/pubmed/5635571. Accessed September 6, 2018.
52. Lim, C. S., Martin, F., Beckenham, T., & Cumming, R. G. (2004). Nasolacrimal duct obstruction in children: Outcome of intubation. *Journal of the American Association for Pediatric Ophthalmology and Strabismus, 8*(5), 466–472. https://doi.org/10.1016/S1091853104001594.

53. Kaufman, L. M., & Guay-Bhatia, L. A. (1998). Monocanalicular intubation with Monoka tubes for the treatment of congenital nasolacrimal duct obstruction. *Ophthalmology*. https://doi.org/10.1016/S0161-6420(98)93445-5.
54. Engel, J. M., Hichie-Schmidt, C., Khammar, A., Ostfeld, B. M., Vyas, A., & Ticho, B. H. (2007). Monocanalicular silastic intubation for the initial correction of congenital nasolacrimal duct obstruction. *Journal of the American Association for Pediatric Ophthalmology and Strabismus*, *11*(2), 183–186. https://doi.org/10.1016/j.jaapos.2006.09.009.
55. Tao, S., Meyer, D. R., Simon, J. W., & Zobal-Ratner, J. (2002). Success of balloon catheter dilatation as a primary or secondary procedure for congenital nasolacrimal duct obstruction. *Ophthalmology*, *109*(11), 2108–2111. https://doi.org/10.1016/S0161-6420(02)01216-2.
56. Pediatric Eye Disease Investigator Group. (2008). Primary treatment of nasolacrimal duct obstruction with nasolacrimal duct intubation in children younger than 4 years of age. *Journal of the American Association for Pediatric Ophthalmology and Strabismus*, *12*(5), 445–450. https://doi.org/10.1016/j.jaapos.2008.03.005.
57. Lin, A. E., Chang, Y.-C., Lin, M.-Y., Tam, K.-W., & Shen, Y.-D. (2016). Comparison of treatment for congenital nasolacrimal duct obstruction: A systematic review and meta-analysis. *Canadian Journal of Ophthalmology/Journal Canadien d. Ophtalmologie*, *51*(1), 34–40. https://doi.org/10.1016/j.jcjo.2015.10.002.
58. Al-Faky, Y. H., Mousa, A., Kalantan, H., Al-Otaibi, A., Alodan, H., & Alsuhaibani, A. H. (2015). A prospective, randomised comparison of probing versus bicanalicular silastic intubation for congenital nasolacrimal duct obstruction. *British Journal of Ophthalmology*, *99*(2), 246–250. https://doi.org/10.1136/bjophthalmol-2014-305376.
59. Miller, A. M., Chandler, D. L., Repka, M. X., Hoover, D. L., Lee, K. A., Melia, M., et al. (2014). Office probing for treatment of nasolacrimal duct obstruction in infants. *Journal of the American Association for Pediatric Ophthalmology and Strabismus*, *18*(1), 26–30. https://doi.org/10.1016/j.jaapos.2013.10.016.
60. Pediatric Eye Disease Investigator Group. (2009). Repeat probing for treatment of persistent nasolacrimal duct obstruction. *Journal of the American Association for Pediatric Ophthalmology and Strabismus*, *13*(3), 306–307. https://doi.org/10.1016/j.jaapos.2009.02.008.
61. Stager, D., Baker, J. D., Frey, T., Weakley, D. R., & Birch, E. E. (1992). Office probing of congenital nasolacrimal duct obstruction. *Ophthalmic Surgery*, *23*(7), 482–484. http://www.ncbi.nlm.nih.gov/pubmed/1407947. Accessed September 11, 2018.
62. Katowitz, J. A., & Welsh, M. G. (1987). Timing of initial probing and irrigation in congenital nasolacrimal duct obstruction. *Ophthalmology*, *94*(6), 698–705. http://www.ncbi.nlm.nih.gov/pubmed/3627719. Accessed September 11, 2018.
63. Repka, M. X., Chandler, D. L., Holmes, J. M., Hoover, D. L., Morse, C. L., Schloff, S., et al. (2009). Balloon catheter dilation and nasolacrimal duct intubation for treatment of nasolacrimal duct obstruction after failed probing. *Archives of Ophthalmology*, *127*(5), 633–639. https://doi.org/10.1001/archophthalmol.2009.66.
64. Matta, N. S., Singman, E. L., & Silbert, D. I. (2010). Prevalence of amblyopia risk factors in congenital nasolacrimal duct obstruction. *Journal of the American Association for Pediatric Ophthalmology and Strabismus*, *14*(5), 386–388. https://doi.org/10.1016/j.jaapos.2010.06.012.
65. Matta, N. S., & Silbert, D. I. (2011). High prealence of amblyopia risk factors in preverbal children with nasolacrimal duct obstruction. *Journal of the American Association for Pediatric Ophthalmology and Strabismus*, *15*(4), 350–352. https://doi.org/10.1016/j.jaapos.2011.05.007.
66. Saleem, A., Siddiqui, S., Wakeel, U., & Asif, M. (2018). Anisometropia and refractive status in children with unilateral congenital nasolacrimal duct obstruction. *Taiwan Journal of Ophthalmology*, *8*(1), 31. https://doi.org/10.4103/tjo.tjo_77_17.

12

Evaluation and Management of Acquired Nasolacrimal Duct Obstruction

LIOR OR, MD, INBAL GAZIT, MD, AND MORRIS E. HARTSTEIN, MD, FACS

In the evaluation of patients with acquired tearing, the first step is to assess whether epiphora (tearing caused by insufficient drainage) or lacrimation (hypersecretion of tears) is the cause of tearing. Systematic examination helps isolate the cause of acquired tearing and distinguish patients with obstruction of the lacrimal drainage system from those with secondary hypersecretion.

This chapter discuss the symptoms, clinical characteristics, causes, and management options of acquired nasolacrimal duct obstruction (NLDO).

Etiology

NLDO is the most common cause of persistent epiphora. Acquired NLDO can be classified in to two categories[1]: primary acquired nasolacrimal duct obstruction (PANDO) and secondary acquired nasolacrimal duct obstruction (SANDO).

Primary Acquired Nasolacrimal Duct Obstruction

PANDO most frequently affects middle-aged adults and more women than men. In studies on the osseous nasolacrimal canal, it been observed that women have significantly narrower dimensions in the lower nasolacrimal fossa and middle nasolacrimal duct (NLD), as well as changes in the anteroposterior dimensions of the bony nasolacrimal canal.[1] These changes coincide with osteoporotic changes throughout the body and may explain the higher incidence of PANDO in women. Menstrual and hormonal fluctuations and a heightened immune status have also been suggested as factors that may contribute to the disease process in lacrimal obstruction. These may explain the prevalence of NLDO in middle-aged and elderly women. Hormonal changes that bring about a generalized de-epithelialization in the body may cause the same within the lacrimal sac and duct. An already narrow lacrimal fossa in women may predispose them to obstruction by sloughed-off debris.[1]

Secondary Acquired Nasolacrimal Duct Obstruction

SANDO may result from several causes, including infection, inflammation, neoplastic, trauma, and mechanical. Bacteria, viruses, fungi, and parasites have been implicated as underlying causes of infectious lacrimal drainage obstruction. SANDO has no sexual or age predilection.[2–5]

Bacterial infection can be caused by different bacteria, such as *Staphylococcus aureus, Actinomyces, Pseudomonas, Propionibacterium, Fusobacterium, Bacteroides, Mycobacterium, Chlamydia, Nocardia, Aeromonas, Enterobacter, and Treponema pallidum.*[5] Viral causes of lacrimal obstruction most commonly are seen with herpetic infection. Obstruction is due to the damage to the elastic tissue of the substantia propria as well as to the canalicular elastic tissue and/or the adherence of the inflammatory membranes to the raw epithelial surface of the canaliculus.[5,6]

Fungi may obstruct lacrimal passages by forming a stone (dacryolith) or cast. This mechanical obstruction has been associated with *Aspergillus, Candida, Pityrosporum,* and *Trichophyton.*[6]

Parasitic obstruction is unusual but is reported in patients infected with *Ascaris lumbricoides,* which enters the lacrimal system retrograde through the valve of Hasner.[6]

Inflammation may be endogenous or exogenous in origin. Wegener granulomatosis and sarcoidosis are two examples of conditions that lead to obstruction caused by progressive inflammation within the nasal and lacrimal sac mucosa. Other endogenously arising inflammations associated with lacrimal obstruction are cicatricial pemphigoid, sinus histiocytosis, Kawasaki disease, and scleroderma.[7]

Neoplasms may cause lacrimal obstruction by primary growth, secondary spread, or metastatic spread. Primary tumors of the lacrimal drainage system are relatively uncommon but may arise in the puncta, canaliculi, lacrimal sac, or NLD. Secondary spread from nearby tissues is more common than primary tumors. This most commonly involves eyelid cancers (e.g., basal cell carcinoma, squamous cell carcinoma), although spread from the maxillary antrum and the nasopharynx also have been reported. Studies have documented lacrimal obstruction from oncocytoma and cylindroma from direct extension. Metastatic spread, an exceedingly rare phenomenon, has been reported with primary sites from the breast and prostate.[8,9]

Trauma may be iatrogenic in the case of scarring of the lacrimal passages after overly aggressive lacrimal probing. Iatrogenic causes of NLDO also may follow orbital decompression surgery, paranasal, nasal, and craniofacial procedures. Non-iatrogenic traumatic causes are either blunt or sharp and most commonly involve the canaliculus, lacrimal sac, and NLD. Posttraumatic dacryostenosis was found to have a frequent association with delayed treatment of facial fracture repair or bone loss in the lacrimal district.[10,11]

Exogenous causes may also result in inflammatory obstruction of the lacrimal drainage system. Eye drops, radiation, systemic chemotherapy (e.g., docetaxel anhydrous [Taxotere], Sanofi-Ventis), and bone marrow transplantation are all causes of treatment-related inflammatory obstruction.[12]

Mechanical lacrimal drainage obstruction may be due to intraluminal foreign bodies, such as dacryoliths or casts. These may be caused by infection (e.g., *Actinomyces, Candida*) as well as long-term administration of topical medications. Mechanical obstruction also may be caused by external compression from rhinoliths, nasal foreign bodies, or mucoceles. Dentigerous cyst in the maxillary sinus has been reported to have caused NLDO.[2]

Evaluation

Evaluation should include a detailed general medical history, ocular history, and exact description of the symptoms.[13] The clinical picture of patients with acquired NLDO may include epiphora, mucoid punctal discharge with pressure on the lacrimal sac, or dacryocystitis. Painful swelling of the medial canthus is sometimes present, and in cases of nasal, sinus, or lacrimal sac tumor, bloody tears and epistaxis.

Past medical history may include inflammatory disease such as Wegener granulomatosis, sarcoidosis, ocular cicatricial pemphigoid, Kawasaki disease, scleroderma, neoplastic disease and its treatment, such as lymphoma, previous radiation treatment to the medial canthal area, systemic chemotherapy with fluorouracil, parasitic infection, facial trauma, and previous nasal or sinus surgery.

Ocular history may include dacryocystitis, recurrent conjunctivitis or ocular pemphigus, previous eye surgery (dacryocystorhinostomy [DCR] or eyelid surgery), glaucoma, and the use of antiglaucoma medications, or other topical medications.[13]

Examination begins with evaluation of the eyelid position and blink function. The lower lid should be well opposed to the globe with good snap back tone (Fig. 12.1). Punctal patency and position relative to the tear lake are assessed. Punctal discharge may indicate canaliculitis (Fig. 12.2).

The lacrimal sac fossa is palpated to evaluate tenderness, to determine whether a mass is present, and to elicit reflux from the puncta. A tender lacrimal sac may be indicative of dacryocystitis (Fig. 12.3). Firm canthal masses, bloody reflux from the punctum, and hypervascularity are suggestive of neoplasm. Reflux from the punctum suggests an obstruction in the lacrimal system. A significantly distended sac may not regurgitate with pressure owing to the functional valve of Rosenmüller.[6]

Slit-lamp examination is performed to detect the presence of eyelid, conjunctival, or corneal inflammation that may be associated with hypersecretion, as well as to detect secondary infection.

When evaluating the tear meniscus, the size of the lacrimal lake, the presence of precipitated proteins, and stringy mucus may indicate an abnormal tear film. This in turn may cause reflex tearing.[6]

Tear breakup time can be observed after fluorescein has been placed in the conjunctival cul-de-sac. The patient is asked to open the eyes and refrain from blinking. The ophthalmologist then examines the tear film using a broad beam of the slit lamp. The time before breakup should be at least 10 seconds.[6] A more rapid tear film breakup time may indicate poor function of the mucin or meibomian layer despite an apparently sufficient amount of tears.

The mucin layer of the tear film helps spread the other layers evenly over the corneal surface. The oily layer of the tear film, secreted from the meibomian glands, helps prevent tear evaporation. Topical rose bengal and lissamine green staining can be used to evaluate corneal and conjunctival epithelium. These detect subtle ocular surface abnormalities by staining devitalized conjunctival and corneal epithelium. Fluorescein staining indicates more severe tear film malfunction with epithelial loss.[6]

When evaluating basal tear secretion, topical anesthetic is applied and the inferior cul-de-sac is dried. A Schirmer strip is bent at the notch and placed with the short end resting on the conjunctiva and the fold crease on the eyelid margin at the lateral one-third of the lower eyelid. The strip is left in place for 5 minutes and the amount of wetting is recorded. The normal amount is approximately 10 to 15 mm. Rapid saturation of the filter strip signifies hypersecretion. However, excess secretion may occur in response to irritation from the measuring strips themselves. Serial testing should be performed to confirm this assumption. Two classic but less often performed tests are the Schirmer I and Schirmer II tests. The Schirmer I test allows the physician to evaluate both basic and reflex tearing. The Schirmer II test is used to distinguish between fatigue block (when reflex secretion is suppressed because of chronic irritation) and a lack of function of the reflex secretors circumstances.[14]

Nasal examination may uncover an unsuspected cause of the epiphora, such as an intranasal tumor, turbinate impaction, or chronic allergic rhinitis. These conditions may occlude the nasal end of the NLD.

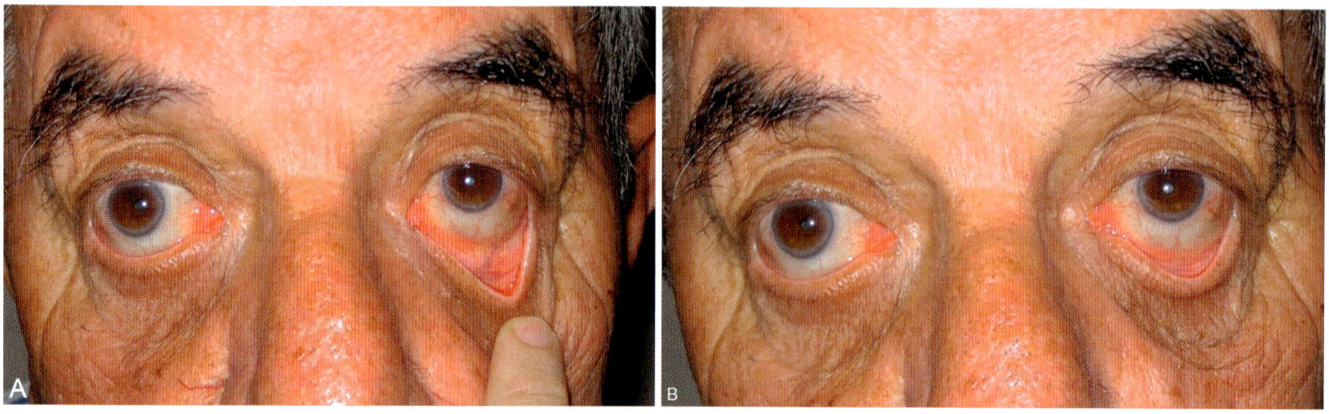

• **Fig. 12.1** (A) Snap Back Test. After distracting the lid, it does not snaps back to hug the globe before the next blink. (B) Poor snap back tone.

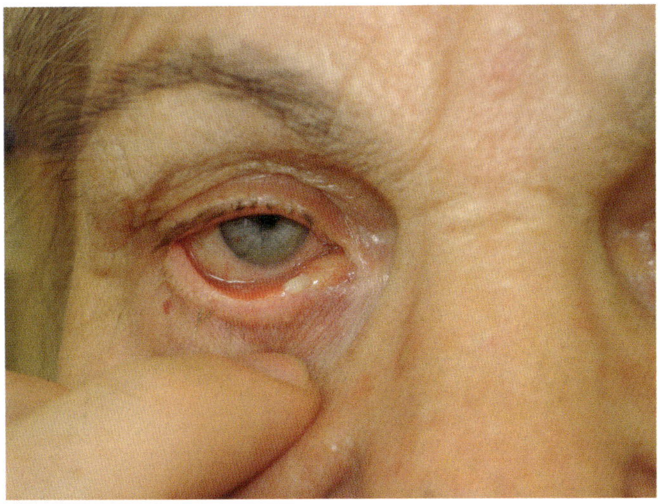

• **Fig. 12.2** Mucopurulent discharge from the punctum indicating canaliculitis. There is no swelling over the lacrimal sac, and the lacrimal system would be patent to irrigation.

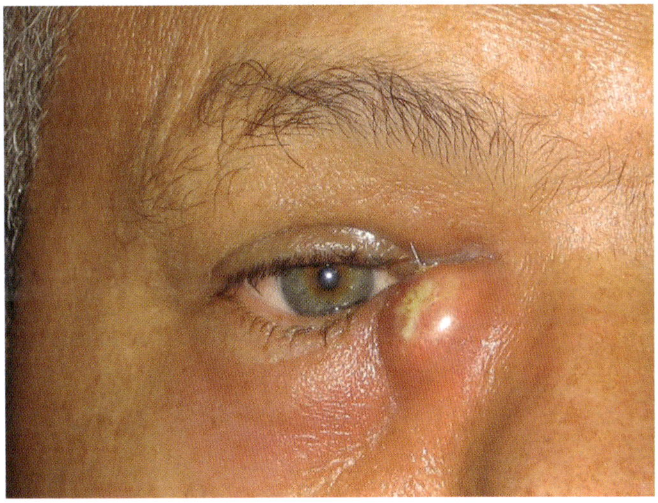

• **Fig. 12.3** Acute dacryocystitis.

Diagnostic Tests

The dye disappearance test (DDT) is a noninvasive, rapid, and convenient test that is useful for assessing PANDO, functional NLDO, congenital NLDO, and canalicular laceration.[15] The examiner instills fluorescein into the conjunctival fornix of each eye (using a drop of sterile 2% solution fluorescein solution of a moistened fluorescein strip) and then observes the tear film with the cobalt blue filter of the slit lamp. Persistence of significant dye and asymmetric clearance of the dye from the tear meniscus over a 5-minute period indicate a possible obstruction. The DDT has great value in ruling out conditions if the result is negative; if the DDT results are normal, severe lacrimal drainage dysfunction is highly unlikely. However, it does not rule out other causes of tearing, such as allergy, dacryolith, or intranasal obstruction.

The Jones I and Jones II tests have historically been used in the evaluation of epiphora and are now rarely used in clinical practice The Jones I test investigates lacrimal outflow under normal physiologic conditions, and the Jones II test determines the presence or absence of fluorescein in the irrigating saline solution fluid retrieved from the nose after irrigation in nonphysiologic conditions.[15]

The lacrimal drainage system irrigation is performed to evaluate obstruction of lacrimal drainage system occlusion and the level of obstruction. It is usually performed immediately after the DDT. Using topical anesthesia, the lower eyelid punctum is dilated (Fig. 12.4) and the irrigating cannula is placed in the canalicular system. To prevent canalicular kinking and difficulty in advancing the irrigating cannula, the clinician maintains lateral traction of the lower eyelid. Canalicular stenosis or occlusion should be noted, and if suspected should be confirmed by subsequent diagnostic probing. Once the irrigating cannula has been advanced into the horizontal canaliculus, clear saline solution is injected. Careful observation and interpretation determine the area of obstruction without additional testing. Total canalicular obstruction is suggested when it is difficult to advance the irrigating cannula and impossible to irrigate fluid. Complete blockage of the common canaliculus is suggested when irrigation passes successfully but refluxes through the upper canalicular system and no distension of the lacrimal sac is noted.

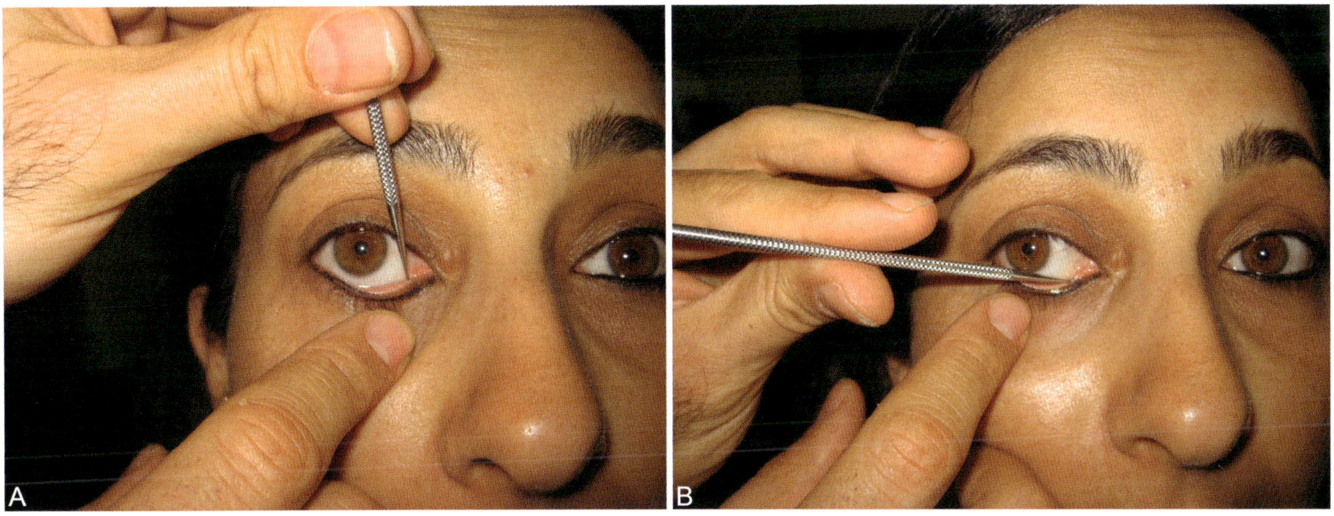

• **Fig. 12.4** (A) The punctum dilator is first inserted perpendicular to the punctum, and (B) is then advanced toward the lacrimal sac while applying counter traction on the lid.

If mucoid material or fluorescein refluxes through the opposite punctum and the lacrimal sac becomes distended, the diagnosis is complete NLDO. If saline solution irrigation is not associated with canalicular reflux or fluid passing down the NLD, the lacrimal sac will become distended, causing patient discomfort. This result confirms a complete NLDO with a functional valve of Rosenmüller, preventing reflux through the canalicular system. In partial NLD stenosis, combination of simultaneous saline reflux through the opposite canaliculus and saline irrigation through the NLD into the nose are present.[6]

Imaging

Dacryocystography allows visualization of anatomic details of the lacrimal drainage system using contrast material and imaging with x-ray or computed tomography (Fig. 12.5). It is more accurate when digital subtraction of the bone is added. Visual localization of the site of obstruction may help determine the surgical plan, especially when the patient is symptomatic but the lacrimal system is patent after syringing.[16]

Dacryoscintigraphy is used to detect functional lacrimal duct obstruction when the system appears patent but there is no drainage. The test is performed by using radionucleotide drops to follow tear flow using a scintigram (Fig. 12.6). It is a more sensitive and less invasive method, especially for incomplete blocks of the upper drainage system or functional obstructions. In these cases, silicone intubation may facilitate tear drainage. Dacryoscintigraphy, however, does not provide as much detailed anatomic imaging as contrast dacryocystography.[16]

Computed tomography scanning is useful if traumatic or mechanical causes of obstruction are suspected, in particular bony abnormalities such as fracture, and for preoperative surgical planning (Fig. 12.7). Many surgeons request a preoperative computed tomography scan for a patient undergoing endoscopic DCR.

Gadolinium-enhanced magnetic resonance dacryocystography has very high sensitivity, particularly for the detection of soft-tissue

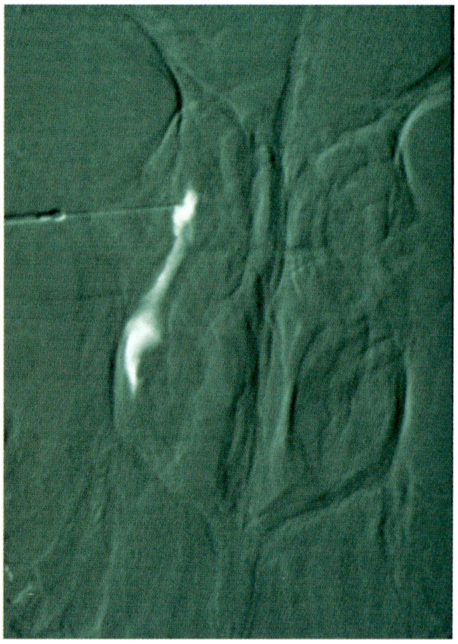

• Fig. 12.5 Digital subtraction dacryocystography demonstrating patent lacrimal system on the right.

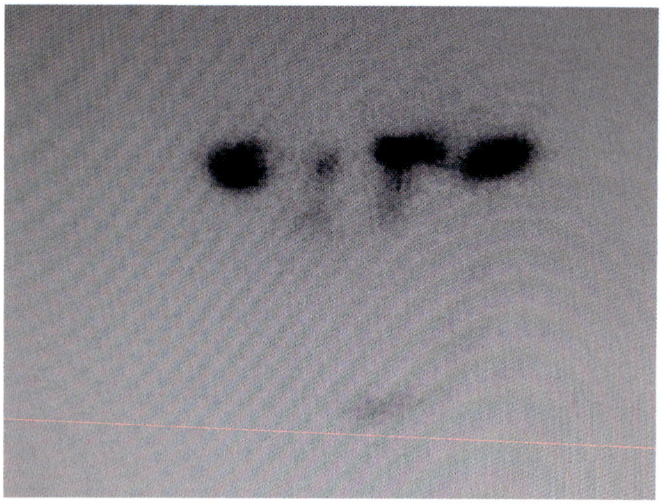

• Fig. 12.6 Early dacryoscintigraphy demonstrating normal flow on the left and obstruction on the right at the sac/duct junction.

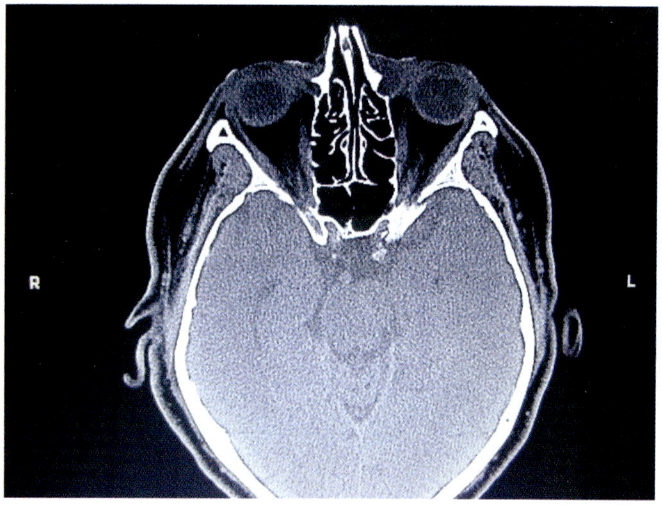

• Fig. 12.7 Axial computed tomography scan demonstrating left dacryocystitis with enlarged lacrimal sac.

masses or malignancies that may play a role in patients with an obstruction. The high cost of the examination may make it less available.

Nasal endoscopy is used for direct visualization of the nasal passages. It is especially useful before internal (endonasal) DCR and for postoperative evaluation after DCR. Nasal endoscopy can alert the surgeon preoperatively as to whether the septum is deviated toward the side of the lacrimal obstruction and to the presence of polyps or scar tissue in the nose.[17]

Management

Acquired NLDO is primary treated surgically. DCR is the procedure of choice for most patients with acquired NLDO. Surgical indications include recurrent dacryocystitis, chronic mucoid reflux, painful distention of the lacrimal sac, and bothersome epiphora. For patients with dacryocystitis, active infection should be treated, if possible, before DCR is performed. Although there are many minor variations in surgical technique, all share the feature of creating an anastomosis between the lacrimal sac and the nasal cavity through a bony ostium, with or without placing a silicone tube through this anastomosis to maintain patency. A patent punctum and canaliculus are required for this procedure.[18,19]

External DCR had been the gold standard of lacrimal bypass surgeries for many years. The procedure creates a communication between the lacrimal sac and nasal cavity through a large osteotomy, bypassing the obstructed NLD.

Advantages of the external approach include excellent success rates, reported to be up to 90% to 95%, and direct visualization of lacrimal sac abnormalities, such as lacrimal stones, foreign bodies, or tumors. In external DCR, direct suturing of the nasolacrimal sac and lateral nasal mucosal flaps allow for optimal apposition and primary intention healing of the flaps. Disadvantages of external DCR include potential for visible scar caused by the skin incision and possible longer healing time compared with the internal approach.[20–22]

Internal (endonasal) DCR involves the creation of a large ostium with or without the endoscope, and with or without construction of nasal and lacrimal sac mucosal flaps. Advantages of the internal approach include lack of a skin incision and possible scar, faster recovery, shorter operative time, less bleeding, and preservation of lacrimal pump. Disadvantages include expensive equipment and a learning curve. When endonasal DCR was first performed, success rates were less than those in external DCR. However, in recent years, endonasal success rates have approached or surpassed those of external DCR.[21,22]

When selecting a surgical technique, the surgeon should remember that second attempts after failed DCR—regardless of which approach was used—have a higher failure rate. Therefore patients should be informed that if an internal DCR fails, the likelihood of a successful external DCR is somewhat decreased.

Conjunctivodacryocystorhinostomy (CDCR) is used in cases of canalicular obstruction, using a Pyrex glass STOPLOSS™ Jones tube (FCI ophthalmics, MA, USA) and creating a bypass of the entire lacrimal system. CDCR can be performed as an external procedure through a medial canthal incision and positioning of the Jones tube at the region of the caruncle, or as endoscopic-assisted technique. The disadvantages of CDCR are the need for tube irrigation periodically, the possibility of tube migration, malposition, or infection and reflux from the nose into the eye.[23]

Some studies have recommended lacrimal surgery using antimetabolites such as mitomycin C to increase efficacy and reduce the rate of restenosis. Thus it is mainly used for revision DCR.[24,25]

References

1. Groessl, S. A., Sires, B. S., & Lemke, B. N. (1997). An anatomical basis for primary acquired nasolacrimal duct obstruction. *Archives of Ophthalmology*, *115*(1), 71–74.
2. Bartley, G. B. (1992). Acquired lacrimal drainage obstruction: An etiologic classification system, case reports, and a review of the literature. Part 1. *Ophthalmic Plastic and Reconstructive Surgery*, *8*(4), 237–242.
3. Bartley, G. B. (1992). Acquired lacrimal drainage obstruction: An etiologic classification system, case reports, and a review of the literature. Part 2. *Ophthalmic and Plastic and Reconstructive Surgery*, *8* (4). 243–29.
4. Bartley, G. B. (1993). Acquired lacrimal drainage obstruction: An etiologic classification system, case reports, and a review of the literature. Part 3. *Ophthalmic and Plastic and Reconstructive Surgery*, *9*(1), 11–26.
5. Pujari, A., & Ali, M. J. (2018). Infections of the lacrimal drainage system. In *Principles and practice of lacrimal surgery* (pp 179–188). Singapore: Springer
6. American Academy of Ophthalmology (2007-2008). Orbit, eyelids and lacrimal system (pp. 259–264). American Academy of Opthalmology: Basic and Clinical Science Course. San Francisco.
7. Ghanem, R. C., Chang, N., Aoki, L., Santo, R. M., & Matayoshi, S. (2004). Vasculitis of the lacrimal sac wall in Wegener granulomatosis. *Ophthalmic and Plastic and Reconstructive Surgery*, *20*, 254–257.
8. Berry-Brincat, A., Tomlins, P., Hall, A., Quinlan, M., & Cheung, D. (2008). Primary extrasac orbital lymphoma presenting as nasolacrimal obstruction. *Orbit*, *27*(3), 175–177.
9. Tanweer, F., Mahkamova, K., & Harkness, P. (2013). Nasolacrimal duct tumours in the era of endoscopic dacryocystorhinostomy: Literature review. *Journal of Laryngology and Otology*, *127*(7), 670–675.
10. Ali, M. J., Gupta, H., Honavar, S. G., & Naik, M. N. (2012). Acquired nasolacrimal duct obstructions secondary to naso-orbito-ethmoidal fractures: Patterns and outcomes. *Ophthalmic Plastic and Reconstructive Surgery*, *28*, 242–245.
11. Becelli, R., Renzi, G., Mannino, G., Cerulli, G., & Iannetti, G. (2004). Posttraumatic obstruction of lacrimal pathways: A retrospective analysis of 58 consecutive naso-orbitoethmoid fractures. *Journal of Craniofacial Surgery*, *15*(1), 29–33.
12. Kashkonli, M. B., Rezaee, R., Nilforonshan, N., Salimi, S., Foroutan, A., & Naseripour, M. (2008). Topical antiglaucoma medications and lacrimal drainage system obstruction. *Ophthalmic and Plastic Reconstructive Surgery*, *24*(3), 175–176.
13. Sibley, D., Norris, J. H., & Malhotra, R. (2013). Management and outcomes of patients with epiphora referred to a specialist ophthalmic plastic unit. *Clinical and Experimental Ophthalmology*, *41*, 231–238.
14. Kashkouli, M. B., Pakdel, F., Amani, A., Asefi, M., Aghai, G. H., & Falavarjani, K. G. (2010). A modified Schirmer test in dry eye and normal subjects: Open versus closed eye and 1-minute versus 5-minute tests. *Cornea*, *29*(4), 384–387.
15. Wright, M. M., Bersani, T. A., Frueh, B. R., & Musch, D. C. (1989). Efficacy of the primary dye test. *Ophthalmology*, *96*(4), 481–483.
16. Guzek, J. P., Ching, A. S., Hoang, T. A., Dure-Smith, P., Llaurado, J. G., & Yau, J. G. (1997). Clinical and radiologic lacrimal testing in patients with epiphora. *Ophthalmology*, *104*(11), 1875–1881.
17. Ali, M. J., & Naik, M. N. (2015). Image-guided dacryolocalization (IGDL) in traumatic secondary acquired lacrimal drainage obstructions (SALDO). *Ophthalmic and Plastic Reconstructive Surgery*, *31*, 406–409.
18. Anila, M., & Sulejman, Z. (2016). Nasolacrimal duct obstruction in adults. *International Journal of Science and Reseach*, *5*(1), 1327–1329. https://doi.org/10.21275/v5i1.nov152967.
19. Linberg, J. V., & McCormick, S. A. (1986). Primary acquired nasolacrimal duct obstruction: A clinicopathologic report and biopsy technique. *Ophthalmology*, *93*(8), 1055–1062.
20. Dolman, P. J. (2003). Comparison of external dacryocystorhinostomy with non-laser endonasal dacryocystorhinostomy. *Ophthalmology*, *110*(1), 78–84.
21. Huang, J., Malek, J., Chin, D., Snidvongs, K., Wilcsek, G., Tumuluri, K., et al. (2014). Systematic review and meta-analysis on outcomes for endoscopic versus external dacryocystorhinostomy. *Orbit*, *33*(2), 81–90.
22. Marcet, M. M., Kuk, A. K., & Phelps, P. O. (2014). Evidence-based review of surgical practices in endoscopic endonasal dacryocystorhinostomy for primary acquired nasolacrimal duct obstruction and other new indications. *Current Opinion in Ophthalmology*, *25*(5), 443–448.
23. Paul, L., Pinto, I., & Vicente, J. M. (2003). Treatment of complete obstruction of the nasolacrimal system by temporary placement of nasolacrimal polyurethane stents: Preliminary results. *Clinical Radiology*, *58*(11), 876–882.
24. Ali, M. J., Psaltis, A. J., & Wormald, P. J. (2014). Long-term outcomes in revision powered endoscopic dacryocystorhinostomy. *International Forum of Allergy & Rhinology*, *4*, 1016–1019.
25. Akcay, E., Yuksel, N., & Ozen, U. (2016). Revision external dacryocystorhinostomy results after a failed dacryocystorhinostomy surgery. *Ophthalmol and Therapy*, *5*, 75–80.

13

Endoscopic Dacrocystorhinostomy

JESSICA W. GRAYSON, MD, RICHARD J. HARVEY, MD, PhD, AND RAYMOND SACKS, MD

Endoscopic Dacryocystorhinostomy

Nasolacrimal duct dysfunction, whether by lacrimal pump failure or nasolacrimal obstruction, prevents the flow of tears through the lacrimal system, resulting in epiphora. Dacryocystorhinostomy (DCR) is a commonly performed procedure for cases of nasolacrimal duct dysfunction. The endoscopic approach offers a different view from the originally described endonasal approach in 1893 by Caldwell.[1] After the advent of endoscopes, the endoscopic DCR was described, allowing for better visualization of the endonasal lacrimal anatomy.[2] In 2003, Tsirbas and Wormald[3] described use of mucosal flaps for improved apposition of the lacrimal sac to the nasal mucosa. In this chapter, we discuss our endoscopic approach to DCR in the setting of nasolacrimal duct obstruction (NLDO).

Workup

NLDO can occur for many different reasons and can be divided into primary and secondary obstruction. Primary obstruction occurs as the result of inflammation and fibrosis of unknown causes, whereas secondary obstruction occurs as the result of inflammation, infection, neoplasm, or mechanical obstruction. Regardless of etiology, such patients often present with epiphora.[4] However, the diagnosis can be complicated by the possibility of hyperlacrimation, which is due to an excretory issue in the lacrimal gland instead of an obstruction, as in epiphora. To delineate the difference between these two etiologies, a full history and physical examination, including medication lists, previous operations of the lacrimal system or sinuses (including lacrimal probing), previous injuries or trauma to the face, bloody tears, initial presentation of excessive tearing, and natural history of the complaint should be obtained.

Primary hyperlacrimation is uncommon but can be due to stimulation of the lacrimal gland in lacrimal gland neoplasia or from the use of parasympathetic medications (i.e., pilocarpine). Irritation to the ocular surface can also cause a reflex as the result of stimulation of the trigeminal nerve (e.g., trichiasis, distichiasis, episcleritis, conjunctivitis, iritis, orbital chemosis). In situations of previous facial nerve dysfunction (trauma, Bell palsy, and so on), there is potential for inappropriate reinnervation of the lacrimal gland with nerve fibers originally destined for the salivary gland, leading to gustatory tearing. The treatment of these conditions is not further discussed in this chapter.

Epiphora has many potential causes; therefore a thorough history and physical examination are pertinent. The following text lists subsites of obstruction and their associated causes:

- *Punctal stenosis (complete/partial),* which can be caused by malposition or scarring
  - Congenital stenosis, occlusion, infection/radiation, pemphigoid, tumors, and so on
- Common canalicular stenosis
  - Congenital absence, canaliculitis, tumor compression or infiltration, trauma, after radiation
- Lacrimal sac stenosis
  - Sac inflammation, prelacrimal fibrosis, dacryolithiasis, primary lacrimal sac neoplasia, adnexal tumor compression
- Nasolacrimal duct
  - NLDO, delayed opening of the Hassner valve, craniofacial abnormalities, agenesis, tumor, trauma, severe septal deformity
- Eyelid malposition
  - Ectropion
    - The punctum should not be visible when the patient is recumbent.
    - Snap-back and pinch test can be used for diagnosis.
    - Entropion
- Pump dysfunction
  - Laxity of the lower eyelid or dysfunction of the orbicularis oculi

Imaging

Imaging is not required in the standard evaluation of epiphora, but in situations when the clinical picture is unclear, they can be used as adjuncts for diagnosis.

Computed Tomography

Computed tomography (CT) can be helpful to determine if there is concomitant sinus disease, as this can be managed at the time of the DCR. CT can also be useful if there is concern for neoplasia arising within the sinus cavity or the nasolacrimal system. However, CT is not required preoperatively in standard cases and in our practice, we only use these in the previously listed situations.

Contrast Dacryocystography

Dacryocystography is used to assess the anatomic features of the lacrimal system and can be combined with plain radiograph or CT. Dacryocystography requires the lacrimal sac to be injected with radiopaque material with follow-up imaging completed at 5 and 30 minutes. This can be used to identify possible locations of anatomic obstruction, including the presence of dacryoliths or diverticuli.[5] However, this is not commonly applied clinically by our team.

Dacryoscintigraphy

Dacryoscintigraphy evaluates physiologic tear drainage; therefore radioactive tracer is administered into the fornix of the conjunctiva. The patient then undergoes a series of sequential images with normal blink responses. These sequential images are captured over a range of up to 10 to 15 minutes, as normal tear transport is variable.[6] This nuclear medicine study can be used to further investigate causes of epiphora in situations of a negative result for the dye disappearance test (DDT). However, our team uses the Jones I and II tests in our clinic instead of the DDT.

Endoscopy Evaluation

All patients undergo a rigid nasal endoscopy as part of the investigation of epiphora. This is used to evaluate for concomitant sinus disease or other pathologies warranting further surgery at the time of the dacryocystorhinostomy (e.g., anatomic abnormality, neoplasia, access for DCR).

Dye Disappearance Test

Sterile 2% fluorescein or a fluorescein strip is instilled into the conjunctival fornix and clearance of the fluorescein is evaluated after 5 minutes. Both eyes should be evaluated with a slit lamp for information regarding tear film as well as puntum assessment. A positive test result is one in which the dye disappears from the conjunctiva. This test result can be weakly positive (i.e., some dye disappearance), which indicates a potential stenosis or pump failure. The DDT can be done in both eyes simultaneously and used for comparison, particularly in cases of unilateral epiphora. This test can be particularly helpful in children, as they are unlikely to tolerate sac washout testing (Jones II) without sedation.

Jones Tests

The Jones I test, also known as the primary dye test, evaluates the flow of the lacrimal system under physiologic conditions. A Jones I test is performed exactly the same as a DDT: 2% fluorescein is instilled in the conjunctival fornix, except endoscopy is used to confirm outflow. Using rigid endoscopy, the inferior meatus and the Hassner valve are then observed for flow of fluorescein through the lacrimal system at 5 minutes. If the result of this test is positive, indicating flow through the system, then no further testing is required. If this test result is negative, then progression to the Jones II test is completed.

In the Jones II test, a 27-gauge syringe with saline solution is placed through the inferior canaliculus for sac washout. At this time, probing is also undertaken with the syringe. If there is flow in the sac washout test, then this is considered a positive test result and the pathology is lacrimal pump dysfunction. Lacrimal pump dysfunction is less likely to have a successful outcome after surgery.[7] Other options may need to be considered as an adjunct to DCR pending the causation of lacrimal pump dysfunction (ectropion, orbicularis dysfunction, and so on). If there is partial regurgitation during the sac washout test, then there is a stenosis of the nasolacrimal duct that is being overcome by the forced manual washout. If there is total regurgitation of the sac washout, then it is important to note the results of the probing completed with the washout syringe. If a hard stop is present (indicating that the probe has gone to the medial orbital wall), then the stenosis is in the nasolacrimal duct. However, if a soft stop is present, this is indicative of scarring in the common canaliculus or obstruction of the tested canaliculus (Fig. 13.1).

Indications

1. Benign stricture
2. Distal common canalicular stenosis
3. Common canalicular stenosis
4. Pump dysfunction
5. Dacrolith/lithiasis
6. Primary neoplasia/exposure of sac for tumor excision
7. Trauma from previous surgery

Operative Setup

Instrumentation

1. 0-degree and 30-degree endoscope
2. Scalpel with a No. 15 blade
3. 2-mm up-biting Kerrison rongeur
4. DCR spear knife/60-degree 2.5-mm W, bevel down Beaver tympanoplasty blade (Beaver-Visitec International, part 377200, Waltham, MA)/2.4-mm slit-angled Mani Ophthalmic Knife, part MSL24 ((Mani, Tochigi, Japan)
5. Bellucci micro ear scissors (Integra LifeSciences, Cincinnati, OH)
6. Punctum dilators
7. Bowman lacrimal probes (sizes 00 and 000, Integra LifeSciences)
8. DCR sickle knife
9. Lusk pediatric through-biting forceps (Integra LifeSciences)
10. Powered diamond drill (2.5-mm 20;degree Medtronic DCR Bur, part 1882569HS, Medtronic, Fridley, MN)
11. Crawford/Infant Bika Silastic tubes (FCI Ophthalmics Paris, France)

Surgical Procedure

Step 1. Create a posteriorly based mucosal flap to expose the lacrimal bone and frontal process of the maxilla (Fig. 13.2A).
- Incise 10 mm superiorly to the axilla of the middle turbinate. The incision should be extended anteriorly 10 mm onto the frontal process of the maxilla.
- Make a vertical incision along the frontal process of the maxilla and carry this inferiorly to the area above the insertion of the inferior turbinate.
- Turn the blade horizontally and proceed from the uncinate insertion to the vertical incision.

Step 2. Raise the mucosal flap (Fig. 13.2B).
- Elevate the flap with a cottle dissector. It is important to stay directly on the bone to avoid losing the surgical plane as you transition from the hard bone of the frontal process to the soft lacrimal bone.

Step 3. Remove the overlying bone.
- Using a round knife to flake off the lacrimal bone over the anteroinferior portion of the lacrimal sac.

Step 4: Use a Kerrison to remove the hard bone of the frontal process of the maxilla overlying the anterior-inferior aspect of the lacrimal sac (Fig. 13.2C).
- Switch to a powered drill with the DCR burr when the Kerrison is no longer able to grasp the frontal process of the maxilla. Ensure complete removal of the bone to the superior incision.

Step 5. Expose the agger nasi cell (Fig.13.2D).
- This will allow for apposition of the mucosa of the lacrimal sac to the agger nasi cell mucosa.

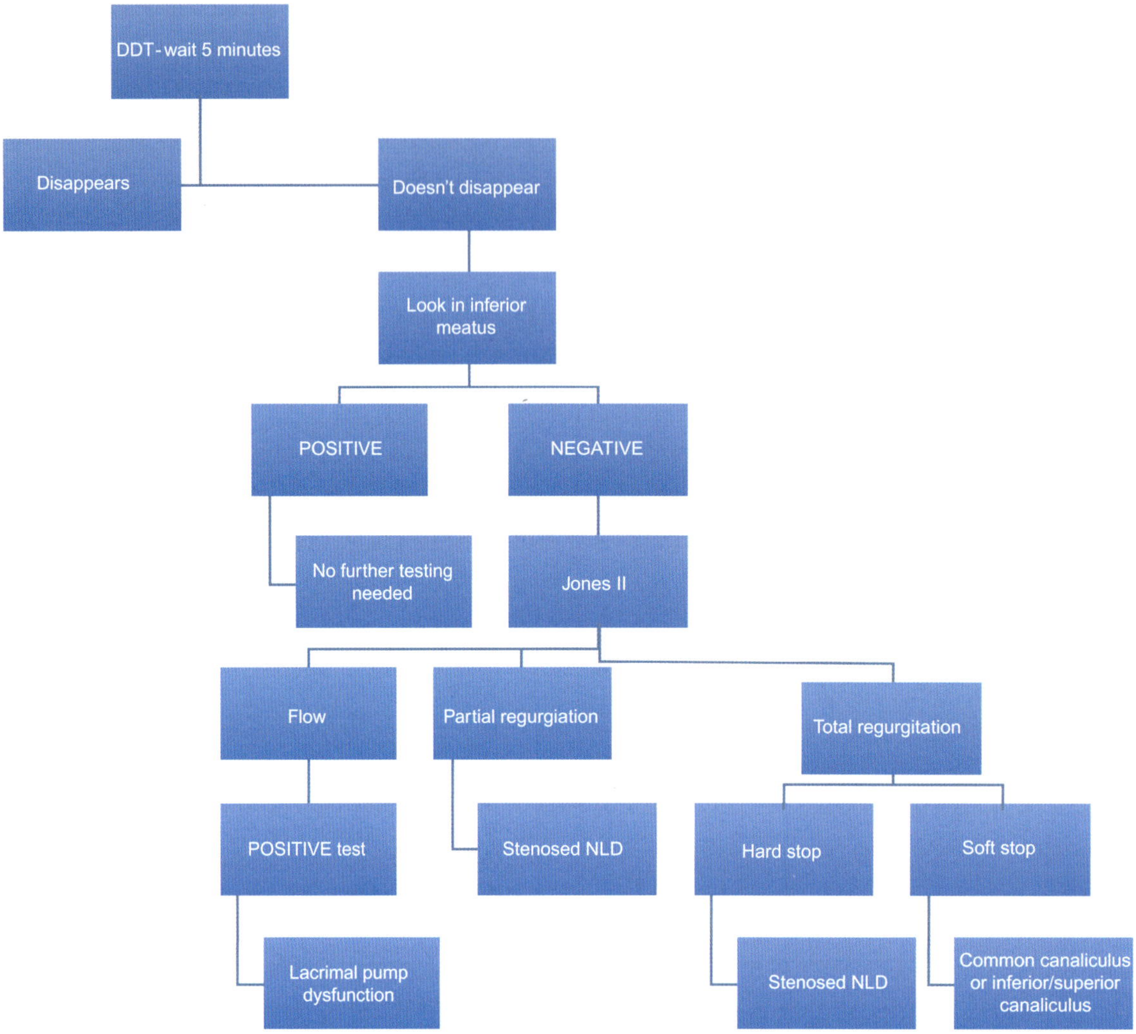

• **Fig. 13.1** Interpretation of Jones testing. DDT, dye disappearance test; *NLD,* nasolacrimal duct.

Step 6. Marsupialize the lacrimal sac.

Cannulate the lower canaliculus with a lacrimal probe. Tent the lacrimal sac and ensure visibility of the probe to prevent injury to the common canaliculus (Fig. 13.2E). Use the DCR spear knife, Beaver blade (Beaver-Visitec), or ophthalmic knife to incise the lacrimal sac posteriorly to provide the largest anterior flap possible (Fig. 13.2F).

Using the Bellucci scissors (Integra LifeSciences), create releasing incisions in the upper and lower posterior flap (Fig. 13.3A); use the sickle knife to create similar incisions in the anterior flap (Fig. 13.3B).

Once the sac is completely marsupialized, it should lie flat on the lateral nasal wall.

Step 7. Trim the mucosal flap to appose the lacrimal sac mucosa (Fig. 13.3C, D)

Trim the mucosal flap to a superior and inferior limb and place these in the corresponding borders of the marsupialized sac.

Ensure that the agger nasi cell is open and the mucosa is in apposition with the posterior superior portion of the lacrimal sac.

Step 8. Pass Crawford/Infant Bika silastic tubes (Fig. 13.3E, F)

Pass the silastic lacrimal tubes into the nasal cavity via the inferior and superior puncta. Slide a piece of Gelfoam (Pfizer, Groton, NY) on the Crawford tubes to hold the flaps in place. Secure the tubes with either a clip or tying the two ends together.

Postoperative Care and Considerations

Dressings and Stents

The use of postoperative stents is a topic of debate, with two randomized controlled trials and one meta-analysis indicating no difference in outcome between procedures with stents and no stents,[8–10] whereas another retrospective study indicates that patients with stents fare worse.[11] However, our team finds them useful and important for postoperative management. Crawford stents are used to facilitate stenting of the common canaliculus; stenosis of this area can be associated with epiphora postoperatively, particularly in cases of prolonged dacryocystitis. Other stents can be used (i.e., O'Donoghue) at the discretion of the surgeon. In the case of common canalicular obstructions, Lester Jones glass tubes are used. The Crawford stents are also used to hold the Gelfoam or Nasopore (Stryker, Groningen, Netherlands) in place, which is providing support to the mucosal flaps. The final function of stent placement is to promote tear drainage through the canalicular system via capillary action

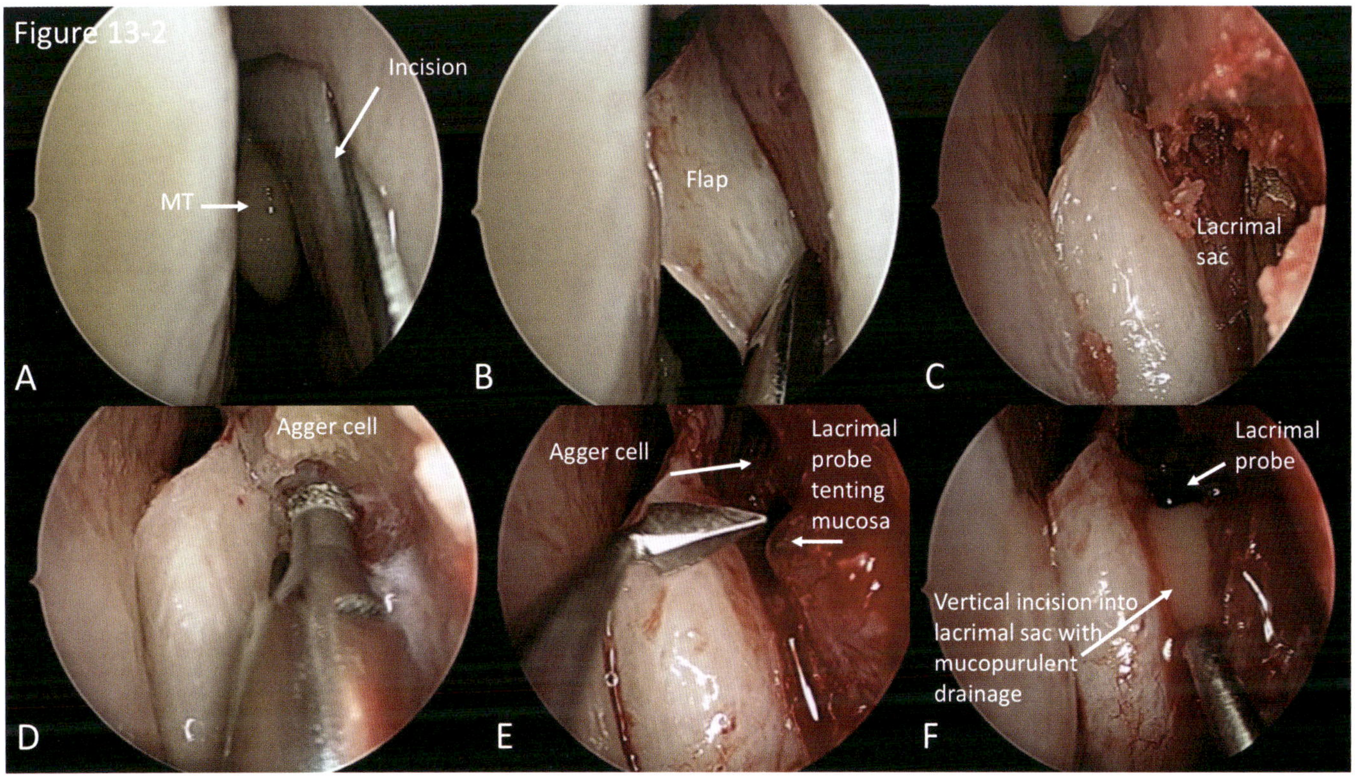

• **Fig. 13.2** Endoscopic View. A, Incision used to create posteriorly based mucosal flap to expose the lacrimal bone and frontal process of maxilla. B, Elevation of mucosal flap. C, Exposed lacrimal sac. D, Opening of agger nasi cell. E, Tenting of the medial sac wall to prevent common canalicular injury during incision. F, Vertical incision made with a dacryocystorhinostomy spear knife. *MT,* Middle turbinate.

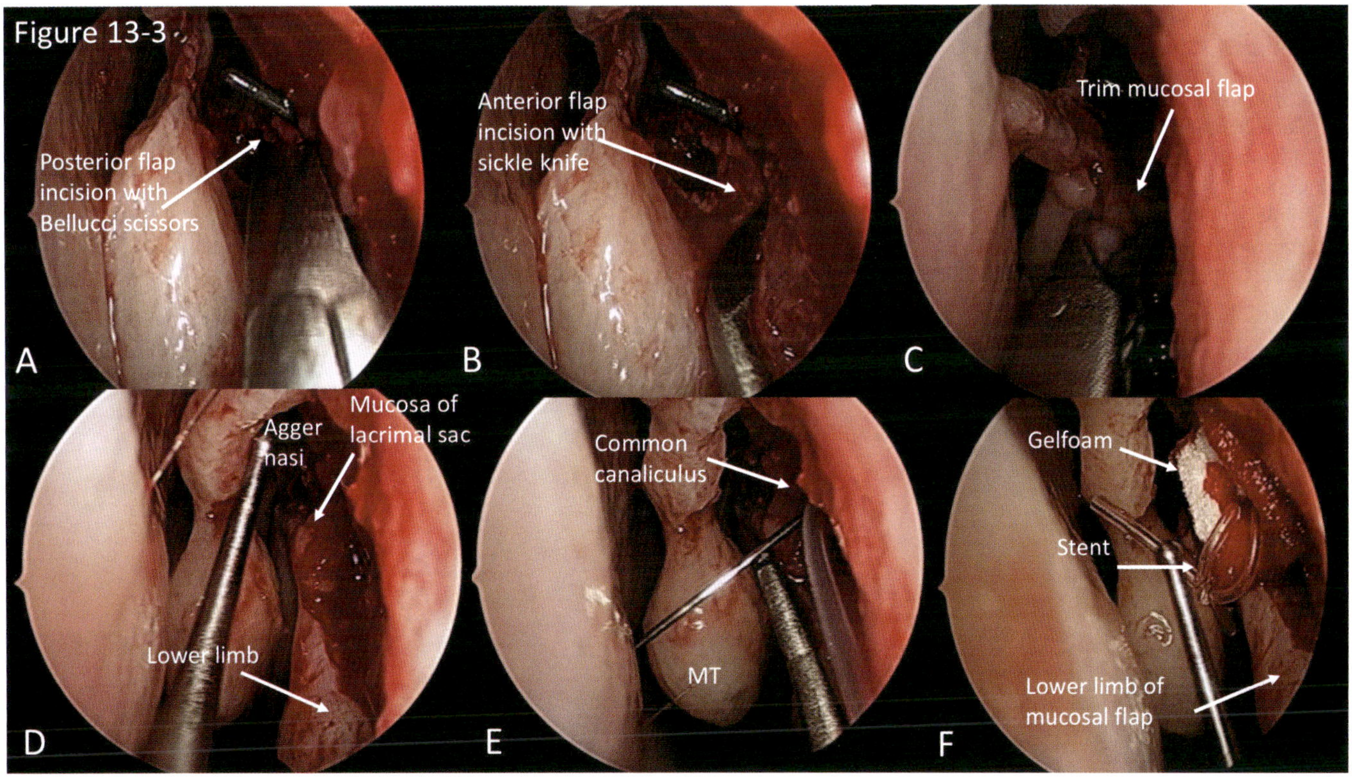

• **Fig. 13.3** Endoscopic View. A, Posterior releasing incisions made with Bellucci scissors. B, Anterior releasing incisions made with dacryocystorhinostomy knife. C, Trimming of the mucosal flap. D, Mucosal flap apposition. E, Passing of Crawford stent through the common canaliculus. F, Placement of Gelfoam up the silastic splints. Mucosal flaps in place.

along the tubes. In the event of inferior or superior canaliculus obstruction, if a probe is easily passed through obstruction, then the canaliculus will be reconstituted. However, if a probe is unable to be passed, then a monocanalicular stent will be used postoperatively.

Antibiotics and Rinses

Patients are discharged home with a 1-week supply of oral antibiotics, a 1-week supply of eye drops (chloramphenicol and dexamethasone), and saline solution irrigations to begin on postoperative day 0.

Follow-up

Patients are evaluated at the first postoperative visit at 2 weeks for removal of crusting. Crawford stents are not removed for 4 to 6 weeks. At this time, patients undergo the Valsalva bubble test. A drop of saline solution is placed in the medial canthal region and the patient is asked to use the Valsalva maneuver. In a patent DCR, bubbles are present in the saline solution.[12] If there is question of DCR patency, repeat DDT can also be completed.

Risks and Benefits

- Pain
- Bleeding
- Scarring/need for repeat surgery
- Orbital hematoma
- Resolution of epiphora

Sacks' Six Causes of Failure

1. Incorrect diagnosis
   Incorrect interpretation of Jones I and II tests
2. Inadequate bone removal
   Failure to place common canaliculus as direct opening to the lateral nasal wall
3. Bony fragments
   Prevent with meticulous surgery and clearance
4. Poor mucosal apposition
   Mucosal flaps
5. False passage
6. Sump Syndrome

References

1. Caldwell, G. (1893). Two new operations for obstruction of the nasal duct. *New York Medical Journal, 57*, 581–582.
2. Gonnering, R., Lyon, D., & Fisher, J. (1991). Endoscopic laser assisted lacrimal surgery. *American Journal of Ophthalmology, 108*, 1172–1186.
3. Tsirbas, A., & Wormald, P. (2003). Mechanical endonasal dacryocystorhinostomy with mucosal flaps. *British Journal of Ophthalmology, 87*, 4–347.
4. Linberg, J., & McCormick, S. (1986). Primary acquired nasolacrimal duct obstruction. A clinicopathologic report and biopsy technique. *Ophthalmology, 93*, 1055–1063.
5. Knisely, A., Harvey, R., & Sacks, R. (2015). Long-term outcomes in endoscopic dacryocystorhinostomy. *Current Opinion in Otolaryngology & Head and Neck Surgery, 23*, 53–58.
6. Detorakis, E. T., Zissimopoulos, A., Ioannakis, K., & Kozobolis, V. P. (2014). Lacrimal outflow mechanisms and the role of scintigraphy: Current trends. *World Journal of Nuclear Medicine, 13*, 16–21.
7. Chin, D., Harvey, R., Wilcsek, G., & Sacks, R. (2012). Can lacrimal sac washout predict outcomes of endoscopic DCR? *Otolaryngology–Head and Neck. Surgery, 147*(2), 242–243.
8. Chong, K., Lai, F., Ho, M., Luk, A., Wong, B., & Young, A. (2013). Randomized trial on silicone intubation in endoscopic mechanical dacryocystorhinostomy (SEND) for primary nasolacrimal duct obstruction. *Ophthalmology, 120*(*10*), 2139–2145.
9. Smirnov, G., Tuomilehto, H., Terasvirta, M., Nuutinen, J., & Seppa, J. (2008). Silicone tubing is not necessary after primary endoscopic dacryocystorhinostomy: A prospective randomized study. *American Journal of Rhinology, 22*(2), 214–217.
10. Feng, Y., Cai, J., Zhang, J., & Han, X. (2011). A meta-analysis of primary dacryocystorhinostomy with and without silicone intubation. *Canadian Journal of Ophthalmology, 46*, 521–527.
11. Mohamad, S., Khan, I., Shakeel, M., & Nadapalan, V. (2013). Long-term results of endonasal dacryocystorhinostomy with and without stenting. *Annals of the Royal College of Surgeons of England, 95*, 196–199.
12. Mulligan, N., Ross, C., Francis, I., & Moshegov, C. (1994). The Valsalva DCR bubble test: A new method of assessing lacrimal patency after DCR surgery. *Ophthalmic Plastic and Reconstructive Surgery, 10*(2), 121–123.

14

Endonasal Dacryocystorhinostomy With Mucosal Flaps

ERICH VYSKOCIL, MD AND PETER J. WORMALD, MD, FAHMS, FRACS, FRCS(Ed), FCS(SA), MBChB

Diseases within the tear duct system can interfere with tear drainage and result in epiphora. Poor drainage with secretion retention may result in inflammation and infection. In the majority of cases, epiphora is attributed to an outflow obstruction of the nasolacrimal duct. To date, the exact etiology is not completely understood, but inflammatory alterations with stenosis at the junction between the lacrimal sac and nasolacrimal duct represent the predominant cause of acquired nasolacrimal duct obstruction. Iatrogenic damage may also result in postoperative epiphora.[1]

As conservative care is usually ineffective, surgical procedures are the treatment of choice for distal lacrimal system pathology. Topographically there is a close proximity of the lacrimal sac and nasolacrimal duct to the nasal cavity and the paranasal sinuses, so that localized pathologic changes can also influence the tear drainage (Box 14.1).

The history of surgical interventions of the lacrimal system dates back to antiquity.[2] Modern surgical techniques were developed more than 100 years ago with the description of external dacryocystorhinostomy (DCR) by the Italian rhinologist A. Toti in 1904[3] and Caldwell's proposal of endonasal DCR.[4] Since then both methods have been competitively applied and further modified. Which method results in better outcomes is controversially discussed in the current literature.[5,6] External DCR is a well-established procedure performed since the early 20th century with stable outcomes between 90% and 95% in the best hands.[7] After Caldwell's first description of endoscopic DCR, surgeons discovered this technique again about three decades ago. Despite significant technical progress, these early attempts to perform endoscopic DCR were not as successful as the external approach, with success ranging from 55% to 90%.[8,9]

• BOX 14.1 Causes of Tear Duct Stenosis or Occlusions

- Chronic polypous rhinosinusitis
- Chronic dacryocystitis
- Dacryolithiasis by infections (e.g., *Chlamydia, herpes, Actinomycetes*)
- Systemic vascular diseases (e.g., Wegener disease, sarcoidosis)
- Trauma (midfacial fracture, injury of the tear drainage pathway as the result of surgical interventions; e.g., osteotomy in rhinoplasty or maxillary sinus surgery)
- Tumors in the area of the tear ducts, the nasal cavity, or the paranasal sinuses

Various studies showed that the main reason for unsuccessful surgery is creating an opening in the lacrimal duct that is too small. Recent publications have shown that only a significant endoscopic resection of the lacrimal bone and the frontal process of maxilla with exposure of the entire lacrimal sac guarantees success rates equivalent to external approaches.[10–15] In contrast, laser DCR allows creation of only a small ostia and has significantly lower success rates.[16] A crucial factor contributing to success has been the understanding of the endoscopic anatomy of the lacrimal sac. Initially it was assumed that the sac extends only slightly beyond the level of the axilla of the middle turbinate (Fig. 14.1). However, imaging procedures revealed that it extends significantly above the insertion of the middle turbinate (about 8 mm above the axilla).[12] Various clinical and cadaveric studies further elucidated intranasal anatomy of the lacrimal sac in relation to other structures on the lateral nasal wall, which led to safer and more effective surgical techniques.[17] The accurate definition of the exact intranasal position of the lacrimal sac was an essential step toward successful endoscopic DCR. The second important factor was wide marsupialization of the completely exposed sac with approximation of the lacrimal and nasal mucosa that allowed the sac to heal without granulation tissue and subsequent scarring. As a result, a novel powered endoscopic DCR approach was developed.[11,18–21]

Preoperative Assessment

Endoscopic DCR directly communicates the lacrimal sac with the nasal cavity. Evaluation of the exact site of tear flow impairment is crucial to guarantee successful outcome of DCR, as proximal lacrimal blockage needs to be separately addressed.[22] A stenosis, obstruction, or aplasia of the canaliculus or an occlusion of the lacrimal punctum is a more complex problem to solve and identifying this before surgery allows the patient to understand the likely success rate of the surgery and will change the surgical procedure performed. Therefore evaluation of the site of obstruction is very important before surgery. It is important to assess both the lacrimal system and the nasal cavity. Nasal endoscopy can identify inflammatory or infectious diseases, tumors, foreign body, or scarring or abnormality of the inferior turbinate. It can also identify the need to perform a septoplasty if the septum is significantly deviated and will obstruct surgical access. Next the lacrimal system is assessed. The punctum is dilated with a dilator and then the Bowman

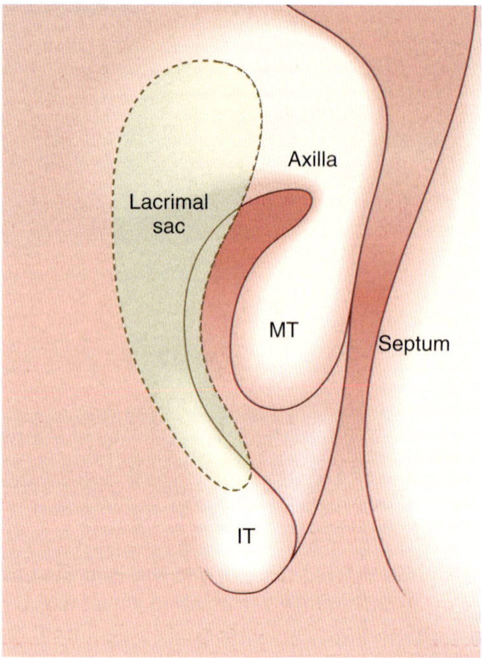

• **Fig. 14.1** The sac extends significantly above the axilla (8 to 10 mm) and lies anterior to the middle turbinate (*MT*). *IT*, inferior turbinate.

lacrimal probe (Integra LifeSciences, Cincinnati, OH) is used to assess the patency of the inferior and common canaliculus. As the probe is passed along the canaliculus, it enters the lacrimal sac and hits up against the side wall of the sac, resulting in a hard stop. This indicates patency of the canaliculus. If the probe stops before a hard stop is encountered, this is called a soft stop and usually indicates stenosis or obstruction of the canaliculus. These tests can be augmented by the Jones tests. A Jones I test is performed by injecting saline solution into the inferior canaliculus. If the nasolacrimal drainage pathway is patent, the saline solution will flow freely into the nose and then the nasopharynx. Checking for reflux via the superior or inferior canaliculus further elucidates the site of lacrimal path obstruction. Reflux through the irrigated punctum occurs when the canaliculus is stenosed (soft stop). Reflux through the upper punctum indicates obstruction of the nasolacrimal duct. The Jones II test is performed by injecting fluorescein-stained saline solution into the lacrimal system and then passing an endoscope into the nose to assess if there is fluorescein-stained saline solution in the nasal cavity.

Imaging: Dacrocystogram and Lacrimal Scintillography

Dacryocystography (DCG) is a diagnostic test for imaging the lacrimal apparatus. Contrast is injected into the lacrimal system, outlining the canaliculi and sac, and thereby identifying the site of obstruction. Dilation of the lacrimal sac often indicates a complete obstruction of the nasolacrimal duct. If the common canaliculus is obstructed, contrast agent will not fill the lacrimal sac. If the contrast agent passes easily into the nasolacrimal duct and nasal cavity, this indicates a functional obstruction. DCG is not an assessment of function of the lacrimal system as the dye is injected under pressure. To assess function, lacrimal scintillography is performed where a radioisotope is placed in the conjunctival fornix and its passage through the lacrimal system is assessed. This test is best used to ascertain function when DCG shows that the lacrimal system is patent. Failure of the isotope to penetrate the nasal cavity indicates a functional obstruction. A complete examination of the entire lacrimal system is mandatory to obtain a correct diagnosis and indication for surgery.

Surgical Technique

The patient should be positioned prone with the head neutral, the nasal cavity decongested, and the mucosa infiltrated with local anesthesia. A slow pulse rate and mild hypotension improves surgical visibility substantially.[22]

Surgical access is determined by the position of the septum; any deviation of the septum that obstructs access to the lacrimal area needs to be addressed with an endoscopic septoplasty.[23] Other anatomic obstructions such as nasal polyposis or a pneumatized middle turbinate should also be addressed.[6,12,24]

Exposure of the lacrimal sac begins with a horizontal incision (Fig. 14.2) made with a No. 15 scalpel blade 8 to 10 mm above and 10 mm anterior to the axilla. The superior incision is about 3 mm posterior to the insertion of the middle turbinate and extends 10 mm toward the frontal process of the maxilla. The second vertical incision is made 10 mm anterior toward the uncinate process and ends at the insertion of the inferior turbinate. The inferior horizontal incision starts at the uncinate joining the vertical incision. This flap is elevated with a suction Freer elevator (Martin, Tutligen, Germany) under visualization with a 30-degree endoscope. During flap elevation care should be taken to keep the elevator in the subperiosteal plane with the tip of the elevator in contact with the bone, especially as the frontal process of the maxilla dips away from the surgeon as the uncinate insertion is approached (Fig. 14.3). The orbit is located posterior to the

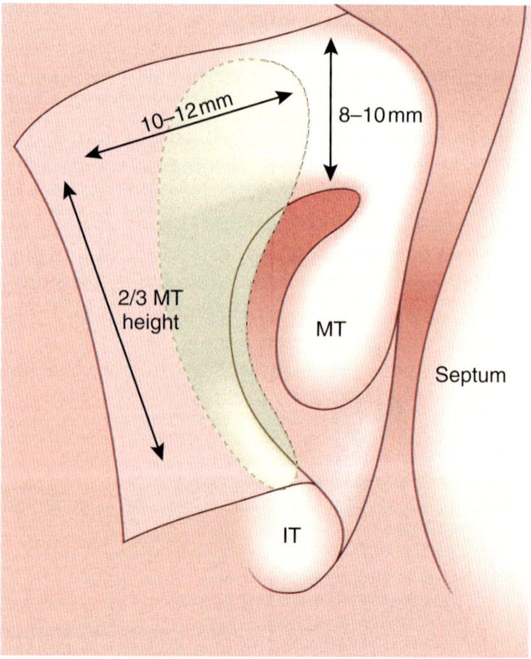

• **Fig. 14.2** A superior incision is made 8 to 10 mm above the axilla. The superior incision extends 10 mm onto the frontal process of the maxilla. The second vertical incision is made on the frontal process down to the insertion of the inferior turbinate. The inferior horizontal incision starts at the uncinate to join the vertical incision. *IT*, inferior turbinate; *MT*, middle turbinate.

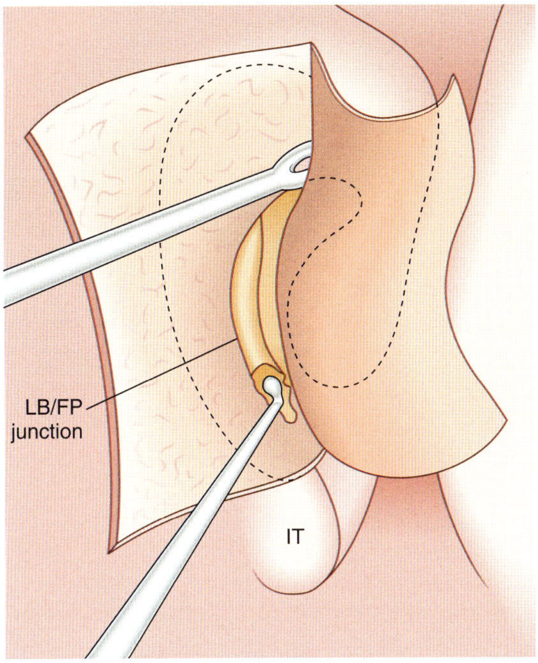

• **Fig. 14.3** The mucosal flap is elevated off the frontal process with a suction Freer elevator. A round knife is used to flake away the fine lacrimal bone at the junction between the frontal process (*FP*) and the lacrimal bone (*LB*) exposing the posteroinferior part of the lacrimal sac.

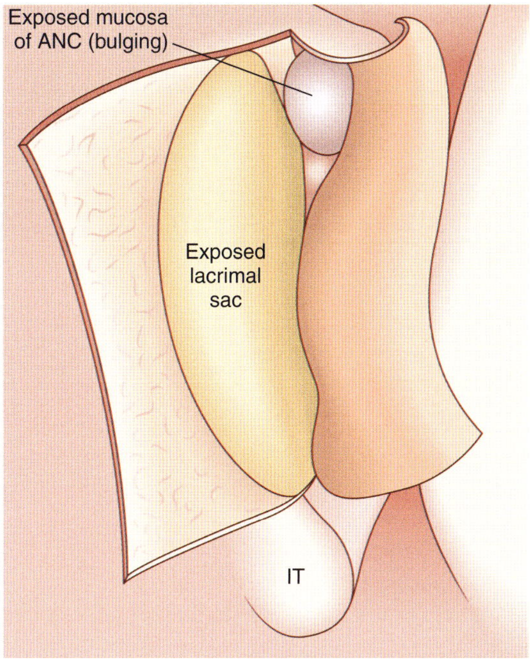

• **Fig. 14.4** A Hajek-Koefler punch and a diamond burr are used to remove the bone of the frontal process and above the axilla until the agger nasi cell is exposed. The lacrimal sac stands proud of the lateral wall of the nose and is fully exposed. *ANC,* agger nasi cell; *IT,* inferior turbinate.

lacrimal bone and the underlying sac and behind the insertion of the uncinate and should never need to be exposed. The most important landmark is the junction of the hard bone of the frontal process of the maxilla and the soft lacrimal bone. This junction is best identified just above the insertion of the inferior turbinate. The lacrimal bone can then be flaked away with a round knife, exposing the posteroinferior part of the lacrimal sac (see Fig. 14.3).

During removal of the lacrimal bone, the uncinate process should be kept intact, protecting the lamina papyracea. After removal of the lacrimal bone, the frontal process is removed with a Hajek-Koffler punch (Integra LifeSciences). Especially with the first few bites of the punch, it is important to open the jaws after each bite to avoid any inadvertent sac injury, as the sac wall often can be pinched by the punch against the bone of the frontal process. It is also useful to push the sac with the tip of the punch before the jaws are closed to grip the bone. As the bone is removed superiorly, it thickens until it is no longer possible to grip the bone with the punch. At this stage, the punch is replaced by a 25-degree curved 2.5-mm rough diamond burr (Medtronic ENT; Minneapolis, MN). The drill is used to continue exposure of the sac up to the superior border of the mucosal flap. When the burr is used, caution is needed to stay on the junction between the bone and the sac and not to let the burr slip under the edge of the bone, as this will result in the burr eroding the sac wall with a resultant hole in the sac.

As the bone is removed above the axilla of the middle turbinate, the agger nasi cell is exposed. The bone is removed from around the lacrimal sac until the sac stands proud of the lateral wall of the nose (Fig. 14.4). This allows the sac to be marsupialized into the lateral wall with the flaps lying flat on the lateral wall. To open the sac, a lacrimal probe is placed through the inferior canaliculus into the sac. The tip of the probe should be clearly visible behind the mucosa of the sac. If the tip of the probe is not clearly seen, then it is likely that the probe is still at the junction of the common canaliculus and the sac and not in the sac; cutting down onto the probe in this position can result in damage to the common canaliculus. With the probe clearly visible through the mucosa of the tented sac wall, a vertical incision is made with a DCR mini–spear knife (Integra LifeSciences). The sac is opened from top to bottom. To create an anterior flap, the mini–sickle knife (Integra LifeSciences) is used to make horizontal incisions superiorly and inferiorly to allow the anterior flap to be rolled out and to sit up against the frontal process of the maxilla without any tension. A Bellucci scissors (Integra LifeSciences) is used to make superior and inferior cuts in the posterior flap to allow this flap to be rolled posteriorly with resultant complete marsupialization of the sac into the lateral nasal wall (Fig. 14.5).

The initially raised lateral nasal wall flap is placed over the sac and the size of the exposed bone is measured so that the center of the flap can be removed, leaving an upper and lower thin flap to cover any exposed bone (Fig. 14.6). The posterior edge of the lacrimal sac is matched with the posterior edge of the raised mucosal flap. The approximation of these edges ensures first-intention healing with a minimum of granulomatous tissue and subsequent scarring. The agger nasi cell is opened vertically and the mucosa is carefully approximated to the mucosa of the superoposterior portion of sac (Fig. 14.7).

To decide whether O'Donaghue tubes need to be placed, the tightness of the common canaliculus opening into the lacrimal sac needs to be assessed. A Bowman canaliculi probe (Integra LifeSciences) is advanced into the common canaliculus. The common canaliculus opening is observed as the probe passes through the valve into the sac. If the valve of Rosenmüller grips the tube tightly, then we recommend stenting with placement of O'Donghue tubes.[25] Silastic lacrimal tubes (O'Donoghue tubes) are passed through the upper and lower puncta. A small piece of Gelfoam (Pharmacia, Piscataway, New Jersey, USA) is now moved over

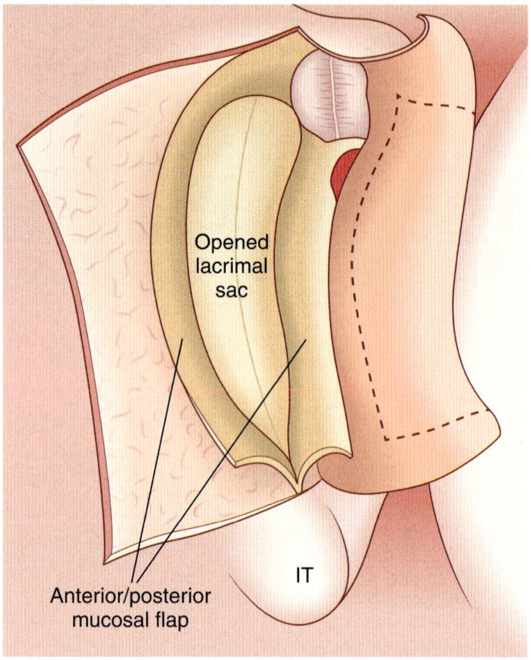

• **Fig. 14.5** The lacrimal sac is tented with a lacrimal probe through the inferior canaliculus and a vertical incision is made with a dacryocystorhinostomy mini–spear knife to open the sac from top to bottom. An anterior flap is created to allow the flap to be rolled out flat on the lateral wall of the nose (frontal process of the maxilla). The posterior flap is created and is then rolled posteriorly with complete marsupialization of the sac into the lateral nasal wall. *IT,* interior turbinate.

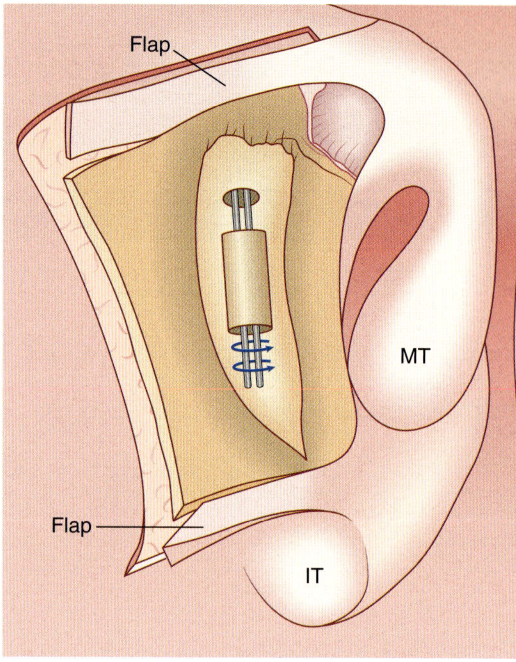

• **Fig. 14.7** Upper and lower mucosal flaps are created by removing the center of the initially raised lateral wall flap. This flap is trimmed until the posterior edge of the mucosa of the sac is matched with the posterior edge of the nasal mucosal flap. The vertically opened agger nasi cell mucosa is then approximated to the mucosa of the posterosuperior region of the sac. *IT,* inferior turbinate; *MT,* middle turbinate.

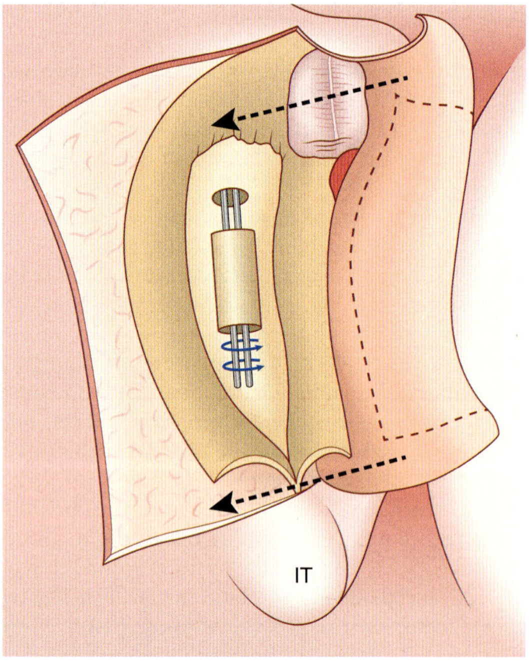

• **Fig. 14.6** If needed, O'Donaghue tubes are placed and secured with a spacer and Ligar clips. The lateral nasal wall mucosal flap is placed over the sac to measure the size of the exposed bone that will be covered by the flaps. *IT,* inferior turbinate.

the silastic tubes and a 4-mm silastic tubing cut to about 5 mm in length (or a 5-mm length of a nasogastric feeding tube) is slid over the tubes and used to push the Gelfoam onto the opened lacrimal sac. A loop of silastic tubing is pulled in the medial canthal area to ensure there is no tension on the tubes, and two titanium Liga clips (Ethicon, Cincinatti, Ohio, USA) are placed below the tubing to secure the tubes. Pulling the loop into the medial canthal region prevents cheese-wiring of the tubes through the lacrimal puncta. Postoperatively systemic (5 days) and topical (10 days) antimicrobial therapy is given. Nasal saline solution irrigation is begun the next day until patient review 2 weeks later. If O'Donoghue tubes were placed, they are usually removed at 4 weeks unless there is a perceived common canaliculus stenosis. If this is the case, they are left in place for 6 months.

Results of Powered Dacryocystorhinostomy

Endoscopic DCR as performed with the described technique has a technical success rate between 95% and 97%.[26] It is important to provide an adequate follow-up period of at least a year as the success rate might drop with late failures 6 to 12 months postoperatively.[27] Recently published data support the excellent long-term outcomes: 283 powered endoscopic DCRs were performed in 214 patients between 2002 and 2013.[15] Of these, 196 (91.6%) patients had a primary DCR and 18 (8.4%) underwent revision DCR. The mean follow-up was 17.1 months. Results show that both primary and revision powered endoscopic DCR offer reliable long-term results comparable with the best outcomes of external DCR procedures ranging from 94% to 98%.

Various authors use different criteria to define successful DCR. There are two major criteria that need to be fulfilled: (1) an asymptomatic patient and (2) postoperative anatomic patency endonasally confirmed by a positive fluorescein test result. If these requirements are met, anatomic as well as functional successful outcome is achieved. In our series of 214 patients, successful *anatomic* outcome was achieved in 96.9% of primary DCRs and 91.3% cases of revision DCRs throughout the past decade. *Functional* success has been observed in in 93% cases of primary DCRs and 86.9% cases of revision DCRs.[14,15] Twenty-three revisions were conducted in 18 patients with failed primary DCR. Data prove that revision surgery is beneficial in improving symptoms.

Some authors propose an evaluation of surgical success by means of validated quality-of-life measure for outcome assessment. *Questionnaires* assessing quality of life such as the Lac-Q or the Glasgow Benefit Inventory might help to evaluate postoperative symptom control.[28–30] These tools for subjective patient assessment after endoscopic DCR are currently investigated to indicate whether this validation method becomes clinically relevant.[31] Success of intervention is also dependent on the surgeon's *level of experience*. During a mean follow-up of 4 years in experienced hands the success rate is about 94%, whereas it drops to 58% in inexperienced hands.[32] In our series of 260 primary powered endoscopic DCRs performed by consultants and residents, a comparison revealed that in the group with less-experienced surgeons, there were 9 cases of complications (ostium granulomas, postoperative bleeding, stent prolapse, and turbinoseptal synechiae). In contrast, 3 mild complications were observed in the group with 160 DCRs performed by consultants at a long-term mean follow-up of 14.2 months. However, comparison of success rates showed a good surgical success rate, even in the less-experienced fellow group, for anatomic (98.1% vs. 95%) and functional (95.6% vs. 89%) outcomes.[33] These outcomes are a result of intensive supervised surgical training and an efficient transfer of knowledge.

Revisions

Even though primary endoscopic DCR results in very good outcome rates,[34] there is a trend toward lower success rates in revision procedures.[13] A majority of failure is due to the formation of granulation tissue or scarring over the rhinostomy site.[35] Additionally, bone neogenesis, obstructive septal deviations, inadequate osteotomy, and insufficient opening of the lacrimal sac contribute to failure. However, long-term results show that stable outcomes can be achieved even in revision surgery with a rate of 86.9% functional and 91% anatomic success at a minimum of 12 months' follow-up.[14]

Complications

Endoscopic DCR is a well-proven surgical procedure with a low complication rate. The most common complication is intraoperative or postoperative hemorrhage. In addition, silicone tubing loss, punctal erosion with cheese-wiring related to too-tight silicone tubing, and canalicular obstruction have been described.[34] Complications might occur when anatomic landmarks are not recognized. An incision posterior to the uncinate might result in an opening of the orbit. This can lead to orbital injury with consecutive herniation of orbital fat or orbital emphysema, conjunctival fistula formation, retrobulbar hematoma, and even temporary ophthalmoplegia.[34] Prolapsed periorbital fat should not be manipulated and the patient should be instructed to avoid blowing of the nose. In these cases, the use of the drill should be avoided to prevent further uncontrollable damage to the orbit. Very rarely a damage of the skull base with cerebrospinal fluid leaks occurs during endoscopic DCR.

Additional Surgery

Simultaneous adjunctive nasal procedures are commonly performed in endoscopic DCR. In our series adjunctive nasal procedures were performed in 53.4% of 269 consecutive powered endoscopic DCRs performed over a period of 10 years.[23] Ancillary procedures aim to the improve outcome of endoscopic DCR by improving access to the lacrimal sac and to resolve coexistent disease.[36]

Key Points

The literature clearly indicates that endoscopic DCR has comparable and even better results than traditional external DCR with regard to safety, success rate, and long-term outcomes. Furthermore, the endoscopic approach circumvents lacrimal pump disruption, causes less intraoperative bleeding, provides a shorter operative time, and enables the surgeon to simultaneously address nasal pathologies during the intervention. Patient satisfaction is high as there is no external scarring.[37]

An interdisciplinary approach and with close liaison with ophthalmologists is emphasized.[6] The expertise of the ophthalmologist is important in the clinical assessment, differential diagnosis, and surgical approach. Within the framework of a functional team approach, both disciplines can complement each other. Otorhinolaryngologists and oculoplastic surgeons on our team perform a preoperative patient assessment together. Whereas the sinus surgeon can endoscopically assess potential nasal ancillary disease, the oculoplastic surgeon can addresses differential diagnoses for epiphora, such as entropion, extropion, blepharitis, or lid laxity. During surgery there are excellent opportunities to develop synergies to achieve optimal surgical results. The sinus surgeon can optimize access to the lacrimal sac and correct concomitant sinus disease. Probing of the lacrimal system or placement of the O'Donoghue tube is often conducted by the oculoplastic surgeon. Thus the joint work between the disciplines can benefit the patient.

There are a broad variety of different DCR techniques, but endoscopic DCR is now considered the gold standard for the management of nasolacrimal duct obstruction. [6] However, not all endonasally performed DCR procedures result in equivalent outcomes. We propagate a powered endoscopic approach with a large osteotomy to entirely expose the lacrimal sac to completely marsupialize it onto the lateral nasal wall. Mucosa sparing in combination with creation of a lacrimal sac–to–nasal mucosa approximation is the key to optimize healing by primary intention and provide the best possible outcome.

References

1. Ali, M. J., Murphy, J., Wormald, P. J., & Psaltis, A. J. (2015). Bony nasolacrimal duct dehiscence in functional endoscopic sinus surgery: Radiological study and discussion of surgical implications. *Journal of Laryngology and Otology*, *129*(Suppl 3), S35–S40.
2. Busse, H., Hollowich F. (1978). Diseases of the tear duct system and treatment options; *Library of the Ophtalmologist*, 74, 1–155
3. Toti, A. (1904). New conservative method for the treatment of chronic infection of the lacrimal sac (dacrocystorhinostomy). *Clin Mod Firenze*, 10, 385–387.

4. Caldwell, G. W. (1893). Two new operations for obstruction of the nasal duct with preservation of canaliculi and incidental description of a new lacrimal probe. *American Journal of Ophthalmology, 10*, 189–193.
5. Horn, I. S., Tittmann, M., Fischer, M., Otto, M., Dietz, A., & Mozet, C. (2014). Endonasal nasolacrimal duct surgery: A comparative study of two techniques. *European Archives of Oto-Rhino-Laryngology, 271*, 1923–1931.
6. Wormald, P. J., & Roithmann, R. (2012). Endoscopic and external dacryocystorhinostomy (DCR): Which is better? *Brazilian Journal of Otorhinolaryngology, 78*, 2.
7. Hartikainen, J., Antila, J., Varpula, M., Puukka, P., Seppa, H., & Grenman, R. (1998). Prospective randomized comparison of endonasal endoscopic dacryocystorhinostomy and external dacryocystorhinostomy. *Laryngoscope, 108*, 1861–1866.
8. Metson, R. (1991). Endoscopic surgery for lacrimal obstruction. *Otolaryngology–Head and Neck Surgery, 104*, 473–479.
9. McDonogh, M., & Meiring, J. H. (1989). Endoscopic transnasal dacryocystorhinostomy. *Journal of Laryngology and Otology, 103*, 585–587.
10. Welham, R. A., & Wulc, A. E. (1987). Management of unsuccessful lacrimal surgery. *British Journal of Ophthalmology, 71*, 152–157.
11. Wormald, P. J. (2002). Powered endoscopic dacryocystorhinostomy. *Laryngoscope, 112*, 69–72.
12. Wormald, P. J., Kew, J., & Van Hasselt, A. (2000). Intranasal anatomy of the nasolacrimal sac in endoscopic dacryocystorhinostomy. *Otolaryngology–Head and Neck Surgery, 123*, 307–310.
13. Tsirbas, A., Davis, G., & Wormald, P. J. (2005). Revision dacryocystorhinostomy: A comparison of endoscopic and external techniques. *American Journal of Rhinology, 19*, 322–325.
14. Ali, M. J., Psaltis, A. J., Bassiouni, A., & Wormald, P. J. (2014). Long-term outcomes in primary powered endoscopic dacryocystorhinostomy. *British Journal of Ophthalmology, 98*, 1678–1680.
15. Ali, M. J., Psaltis, A. J., Murphy, J., & Wormald, P. J. (2015). Powered endoscopic dacryocystorhinostomy: A decade of experience. *Ophthalmic Plastic and Reconstructive Surgery, 31*, 219–221.
16. Linberg, J. V., Anderson, R. L., Bumsted, R. M., & Barreras, R. (1982). Study of intranasal ostium external dacryocystorhinostomy. *Archives of Ophthalmology, 100*, 1758–1762.
17. Shams, P. N., Wormald, P. J., & Selva, D. (2015). Anatomical landmarks of the lateral nasal wall: Implications for endonasal lacrimal surgery. *Current Opinion in Ophthalmology, 26*, 408–415.
18. Wormald, P. J., & Tsirbas, A. (2004). Investigation and endoscopic treatment for functional and anatomical obstruction of the nasolacrimal duct system. *Clinical Otolaryngology & Allied Sciences, 29*, 352–356.
19. Tsirbas, A., & Wormald, P. J. (2003). Endonasal dacryocystorhinostomy with mucosal flaps. *American journal of ophthalmology, 135*, 76–83.
20. Tsirbas, A., & Wormald, P. J. (2003). Mechanical endonasal dacryocystorhinostomy with mucosal flaps. *British Journal of Ophthalmology, 87*, 43–47.
21. Wormald, P. J. (2006). Powered endoscopic dacryocystorhinostomy. *Otolaryngologic Clinics of North America, 39*(539–549), ix.
22. Ha, T. N., van Renen, R. G., Ludbrook, G. L., & Wormald, P. J. (2016). The effect of blood pressure and cardiac output on the quality of the surgical field and middle cerebral artery blood flow during endoscopic sinus surgery. *International Forum of Allergy & Rhinology, 6*, 701–709.
23. Ali, M. J., Psaltis, A. J., & Wormald, P. J. (2015). The frequency of concomitant adjunctive nasal procedures in powered endoscopic dacryocystorhinostomy. *Orbit, 34*, 142–145.
24. Ali, M. J., Psaltis, A. J., & Wormald, P. J. (2014). Long-term outcomes in revision powered endoscopic dacryocystorhinostomy. *International Forum of Allergy & Rhinology, 4*, 1016–1019.
25. Callejas, C. A., Tewfik, M. A., & Wormald, P. J. (2010). Powered endoscopic dacryocystorhinostomy with selective stenting. *Laryngoscope, 120*, 1449–1452.
26. Coumou, A. D., Genders, S. W., Smid, T. M., & Saeed, P. (2017). Endoscopic dacryocystorhinostomy: Long-term experience and outcomes. *Acta Ophthalmologica, 95*, 74–78.
27. Khalifa, M. A., Ragab, S. M., Saafan, M. E., & El-Guindy, A. S. (2012). Endoscopic dacryocystorhinostomy with double posteriorly based nasal and lacrimal flaps: A prospective randomized controlled trial. *Otolaryngology–Head and Neck Surgery, 147*, 782–787.
28. Green, R., Gohil, R., & Ross, P. (2017). Mucosal and lacrimal flaps for endonasal dacryocystorhinostomy: A systematic review. *Clinical Otolaryngology, 42*, 514–520.
29. Mistry, N., Rockley, T. J., Reynolds, T., & Hopkins, C. (2011). Development and validation of a symptom questionnaire for recording outcomes in adult lacrimal surgery. *Rhinology, 49*, 538–545.
30. Knisely, A., Harvey, R., & Sacks, R. (2015). Long-term outcomes in endoscopic dacryocystorhinostomy. *Current Opinion in Otolaryngology & Head and Neck Surgery, 23*, 53–58.
31. Penttila, E., Smirnov, G., Seppa, J., Tuomilehto, H., & Kokki, H. Validation of a symptom-score questionnaire and long-term results of endoscopic dacryocystorhinostomy. *Rhinology, 52:* 84–89.
32. Onerci, M., Orhan, M., Ogretmenoglu, O., & Irkec, M. (2000). Long-term results and reasons for failure of intranasal endoscopic dacryocystorhinostomy. *Acta Oto-Laryngologica, 120*, 319–322.
33. Ali, M. J., Psaltis, A. J., Murphy, J., & Wormald, P. J. (2014). Outcomes in primary powered endoscopic dacryocystorhinostomy: Comparison between experienced versus less experienced surgeons. *American Journal of Rhinology & Allergy, 28*, 514–516.
34. Leong, S. C., Macewen, C. J., & White, P. S. (2010). A systematic review of outcomes after dacryocystorhinostomy in adults. *American Journal of Rhinology & Allergy, 24*, 81–90.
35. Kominek, P., Cervenka, S., Pniak, T., Zelenik, K., Tomaskova, H., & Matousek, P. (2011). Revison endonasal dacryocystorhinostomies: analysis of 44 procedures. *Rhinology, 49*, 375–380.
36. Hull, S., Lalchan, S. A., & Olver, J. M. (2019). Success rates in powered endonasal revision surgery for failed dacryocystorhinostomy in a tertiary referral center. *Ophthalmic Plastic and Reconstructive Surgery, 29*, 267–271.
37. Gauba, V. (2014). External versus endonasal dacryocystorhinostomy in a specialized lacrimal surgery center. *Saudi Journal of Ophthalmology, 28*, 36–39.

15

Revision Endoscopic Dacryocystorhinostomy and Conjunctivodacryocystorhinostomy

NYSSA FOX FARRELL, MD, ERIC HINK, MD, AND TODD T. KINGDOM, MD

Pearls

- Outcomes after revision endoscopic dacryocystorhinostomy (endoscopic DCR) are excellent and the preferred approach when possible.
- Endoscopic DCR allows the surgeon to thoroughly evaluate the neo-ostium and address concomitant nasal pathology at the time of surgery in a minimally invasive fashion
- Understanding the critical endonasal anatomic relationships is essential to successful revision endoscopic DCR
- If patients have concomitant severe canalicular stenosis, conjunctivodacryocystorhinosotomy (CDCR) should be considered independently or in conjunction with endoscopic DCR

Nasolacrimal duct obstruction (NDLO) is commonly managed through dacryrocysorhinostomy (DCR). Historically, this has been performed via an external approach with excellent outcomes. Although intranasal techniques for DCR were first introduced in the early 1900s, modern endoscopic DCR was not described until 1989.[1] After its initial introduction, endoscopic DCR acceptance was limited because of inconsistent success rates within the literature. Initially reports of poor visualization, limited understanding of intranasal anatomy, and suboptimal surgical instrumentation were cited as factors leading to inferior outcomes after endoscopic DCR compared with external DCR. However, technological advances in both videoscopic visualization and rhinologic instrumentation, in combination with a rapid growth in clinical experience, have mitigated these concerns in recent years. In fact, recent literature now demonstrates that endoscopic DCR has success comparable to external DCR.[2] Advantages of the endoscopic approach include the avoidance of a cutaneous incision, preservation of the orbicularis oculi pump function, decreased operative time, and the ability to address concomitant intranasal pathology that may be contributing to the NLDO, such as septal deviation or nasal polyposis. Additional information about primary endoscopic DCR and management of NLDO is discussed in more detail in Chapters 13 and 14.

Causes of Dacryocystorhinostomy Failure

Regardless of the chosen approach, both external and endoscopic DCR have failure rates of up to 10%.[2–5] Patients with a prior history of facial trauma, craniofacial abnormalities, or prior DCR are at greater risk for recurrence of symptoms.[6–8] There are two primary categories of DCR failure: anatomic, indicating a physical obstruction; and functional, which describes patients who experience persistent symptoms of epiphora despite evidence of a patent neo-ostium on objective testing.[9] For a complete list of common causes of failure, see Box 15.1.[4,10–12]

Inadequate Bony Osteotomy

Many studies have demonstrated primary DCR failure secondary to inadequately or inappropriately placed osteotomies. When performing a DCR, it is vital that the surgeon have a thorough knowledge of the lacrimal anatomy and its relationship to nasal anatomy. Fig. 15.1 demonstrates a patient whose external DCR failed as the result of inappropriate placement of the osteotomy. The lacrimal sac rests in an ovoid fossa measuring approximately 15 × 10 mm along the maxillary line. The frontal process of the maxilla contributes the anterior half of the fossa and the thin lacrimal bone provides the posterior half. In 2000 Wormald, Kew, and Van Hasselt performed a radiographic analysis of cadavers that demonstrated that the lacrimal sac often is located higher on the lateral nasal wall than previously thought. In this study, the location of the lacrimal sac was found to extend to a mean height of 8.8 mm above the middle turbinate insertion and approximately 5.3 mm above the common canaliculus.[13]

When placing the osteotomy, it is important that it is not only in an adequate position but also of sufficient size. One prospective study demonstrated ostium shrinkage of approximately 35%, with the majority of size change occurring in the first 4 weeks postoperatively.[14] After 4 weeks the ostium size does not appear to change significantly.[15,16] Linberg et al. were the first to endoscopically examine the size the postoperative intranasal ostium after external DCR but did not find correlation between the final and the intraoperative osteotomy size.[17] More recent studies using internal ostium photography have shown a correlation between larger intraoperative osteotomy size and postoperative intranasal neo-ostium size.[18] Although the overall size of the osteotomy may not directly correlate with surgical success, it is believed that osteotomy size must be sufficiently large initially to prevent complete closure with known postoperative contraction. Therefore if

• BOX 15.1 Common Causes of Primary DCR Failure[4,10–12]

Surgeon inexperience
Inappropriately placed osteotomy
Incomplete bony removal
Soft-tissue obstruction of the osteotomy (cicatricial ostium closure, granuloma, synechiae)
Concomitant nasal pathology or anatomic obstruction (i.e., septal deviation, concha bullosa of the middle turbinate)
Functional failure (lacrimal pump failure, eyelid laxity)
Upper system/canalicular stenosis

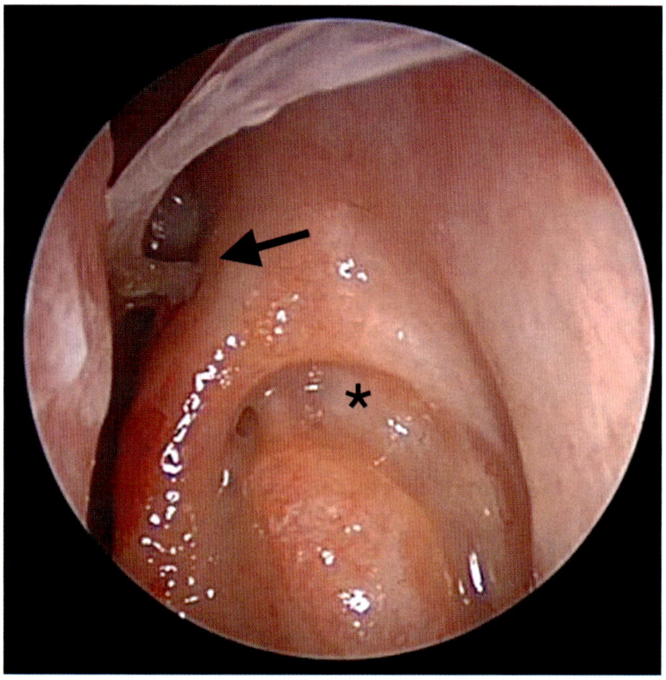

• Fig. 15.1 A thorough understanding of the anatomic relationship of the lacrimal sac within the nasal cavity is vital for successful dacryocystorhinostomy (DCR). In this example after external DCR, the osteotomy was positioned posterior to the lacrimal sac *(arrow)*, through the axilla of the middle turbinate, resulting in failure. In addition, there is polypoid change evident in the middle meatus *(asterisk)* that could not have been addressed during an external approach (view via 0-degree endoscope).

the initial bony osteotomy is not large enough to expose the entirety of the lacrimal fossa after the ostium contracture occurred, failure may ensue. The primary objective is adequate exposure of the common internal punctum (canaliculus).

Mucosal Scarring

Mucosal contracture is a common cause of DCR failure. Evaluations of failed primary DCRs, both external and endonasal, have demonstrated that approximately 50% of failures are due to cicatricial scarring of the neo-ostium (Fig. 15.2).[4,10] After bony osteotomy is created, the entirety of the medial wall of the lacrimal sac should be exposed and then incised sufficiently so that the entirety of the sac is marsupialized and the common canaliculus is exposed. If during this process there is excessive mucosal injury, either to the

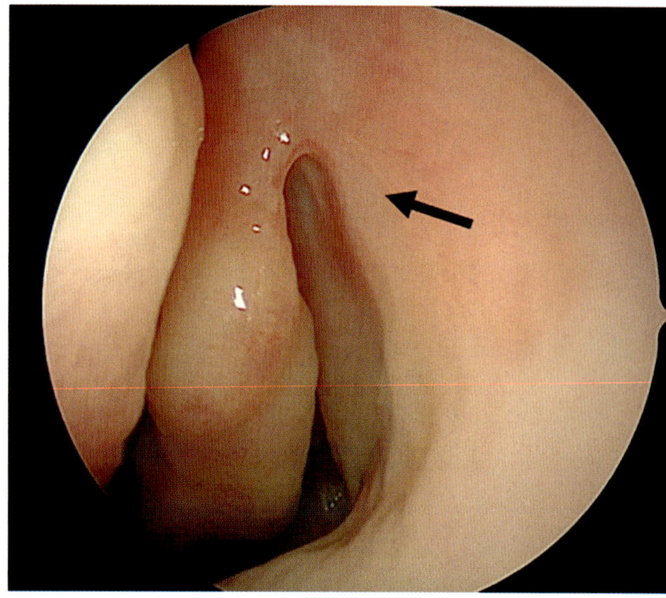

• Fig. 15.2 During the postoperative healing phase, the mucosa around the neo-ostium may scar and form complete occlusion of the neo-ostium *(arrow)*. This can be a common cause of failure (view via 0-degree endoscope).

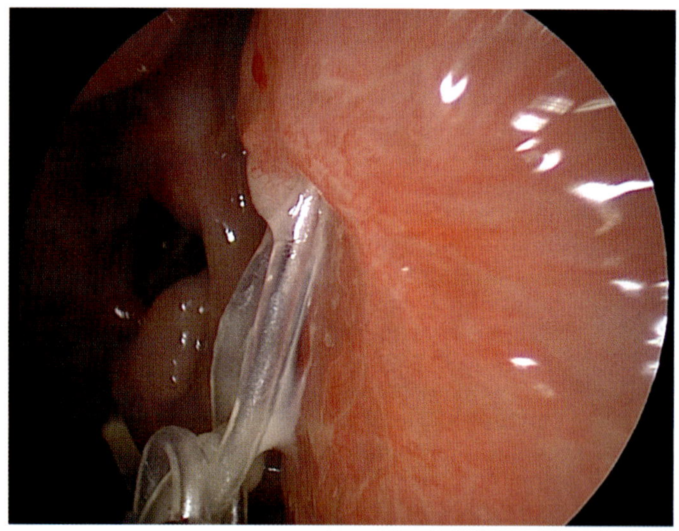

• Fig. 15.3 This example shows a small neo-ostium with a stent in place surrounded by inflammation. Persistent epiphora developed in this patient within 4 weeks of surgery (view via 30-degree endoscope).

nasal or lacrimal mucosa, it could contribute to more scarring and increased ostial shrinkage.[4] In addition, inflammation during healing could lead to the formation of granulomas or intranasal synechiae, which can contribute to ostium obstruction (Fig. 15.3). Some groups advocate for apposition of nasal and lacrimal mucosa (preservation of mucosal flaps), encouraging primary wound healing and thus decreasing scar formation.[19] It is our belief that the presence of redundant mucosa may contribute to excess scar formation in certain cases and thus should be trimmed, if present, to allow for optimized healing by secondary intention. We have found this technique of not preserving the mucosal flaps to produce comparable outcomes.[20,20a]

Concomitant Nasal Pathology or Anatomic Variations

It is important for the surgeon performing DCR to recognize the potential implications of intranasal pathology and anatomic variations. Abnormalities, such as a deviated septum, lateralized middle turbinate, or concha bullosa of the middle turbinate, can cause a physical obstruction of the osteotomy. In addition, if those structures have any mucosal injury at the time of primary DCR, synechiae may form, causing additional obstruction. Other nasal pathologies, such as the presence of nasal polyps, may also contribute to neo-ostium obstruction postoperatively and should be addressed at the time of DCR. Although concomitant nasal pathology contributing to anatomic failure is more common after external DCR, it may also serve as a source of failure after endoscopic DCR.[4]

It is also important to note that normal anatomic variations may result in obstruction of the neo-ostium. In their review of 25 revision DCRs, Liang et al. evaluated the anatomic relationship of the agger nasi cell with the lacrimal fossa. They found that, when present, 95% of agger nasi cells overlap the lacrimal fossa.[21] Similarly, Soyka, Treumann, and Schlegel noted that if this relationship is not recognized, then the neo-ostium may be partially or completely obstructed by the agger nasi, thereby causing DCR failure.[22] In other words, failure to adequately open the agger nasi cell may lead to poorer outcomes.

Functional Failure

Despite meticulous surgical technique, studies frequently describe a subset of patients in whom functional failure develops after both external and endoscopic DCR. Functional failure—the persistence of epiphora—despite a patent neo-ostium, is not fully understood. However, it is thought to be secondary to proximal problems with the lacrimal system, such as dysfunctional lacrimal pump mechanism, eyelid laxity, or canalicular stenosis.[9] It is important to recognize proximal dysfunction of the lacrimal system, such as eyelid laxity, before performing DCR to limit functional failure.[5,9]

Although endoscopic DCR does not disrupt the bony or soft tissues that support that lacrimal system, external DCR requires an external incision through these support systems. Damage to the peripheral fibers of the facial nerve that innervate the medial orbicularis oculi, leading to poor eyelid closure and poor lacrimal pump function, has been demonstrated after external DCR.[23] In the study of 247 external DCRs by Vagefi et al., there was a 7.4% incidence of temporary orbicularis weakness after surgery.[23] Eyelid laxity, punctal position, punctal size, and canalicular tortuosity or stenosis may also contribute to poor tear film drainage and functional obstruction. In addition, Lee et al. examined the endoscopic features associated with functional failure after 50 external DCRs. Their study demonstrated that, despite anatomic success, 16% of patients demonstrated functional failure. Examination of the neo-ostium shape of those with functional failure demonstrated that a neo-ostium that healed in the cavernous shape, described as a large osteotomy with preservation of the lacrimal sac, were more likely to have functional failure. They hypothesized that this remnant sac, which was not incised fully during the primary surgery, obstructed the drainage pathway.[24]

Upper System/Canalicular Stenosis

Proximal stenosis of the canalicular system may also contribute to failure after primary DCR. It is important for surgeons to recognize proximal obstruction before performing a primary DCR because if it is present, DCR alone would not be sufficient. Instead, conjunctivodacryocystorhinostomy (CDCR) would be required to properly address the stenosis. If CDCR were not performed, either alone or in conjunction with DCR, it is likely that the patient will continue to have symptoms of epiphora postoperatively.

Proximal stenosis may also develop after primary DCR. Trauma or inflammation induced by canalicular manipulation at the time of primary DCR can contribute to the development of common canalicular obstruction. This has been noted to be a frequent cause of failure, both independently and in conjunction with ostium closure.[3,7,25] Failure to properly identify proximal system obstruction or causes of epiphora is one of the more important causes of poor outcomes after endoscopic DCR. This highlights the need for accurate preoperative assessment and diagnostic tests.

Indications for Revision Surgery

Similar to patients presenting for primary DCR, patients with previous failed DCRs present with bothersome tearing and/or dacryocystitis. When considering revision surgery for patients in whom recurrent symptoms develop, the surgeon must carefully determine the etiology of the failure. Most of the workup is similar to that performed before primary DCR: evaluation for midfacial trauma, systemic inflammatory conditions, and abnormalities of the lacrimal system, as described in other chapters of this text. In addition, a thorough endoscopic endonasal evaluation should be completed by an otolaryngologist to assess the neo-ostium and to evaluate for concomitant nasal pathology that could be contributing to recurrence of symptoms. If chronic sinusitis is suspected, computed tomography imaging of the paranasal sinuses should be performed. Ultimately, a thorough understanding of the source of primary failure is required to drive the approach for revision surgery.

If an obstruction distal to the common canaliculus is identified, revision DCR is the best surgical option. Although revision DCR can be performed externally, endoscopic DCR, performed in a collaborative fashion with otolaryngology and ophthalmology colleagues, has distinct advantages. Endoscopic DCR allows the surgeon to directly visualize the neo-ostium under high magnification to address any intranasal pathology that has contributed to failure, such as synechiae, granulomas, or anatomic obstruction. In addition, there is no external incision or disruption of the lacrimal pump apparatus. Endoscopic DCR also has shorter operative times, decreased blood loss, and earlier rehabilitation.[3]

It is also important to note that if patients have canalicular stenosis, DCR will likely be insufficient to address the patient's symptoms. In cases of proximal lacrimal duct stenosis or severe common canalicular stenosis, stent placement at the time of revision DCR may be an option. However, if the stenosis is severe, the patient may benefit instead from CDCR alone or in combination with DCR. During CDCR, a Jones tube (glass tube) is placed from the tear lake at the caruncle directly into the middle meatus. This ultimately bypasses the lacrimal system, creating a new tear outflow tract.

Surgical Technique

Revision Endoscopic DCR

More detailed description of the technique for endoscopic DCR is included in other chapters in this textbook; thus we will focus on the highlights unique to revision endoscopic DCR.

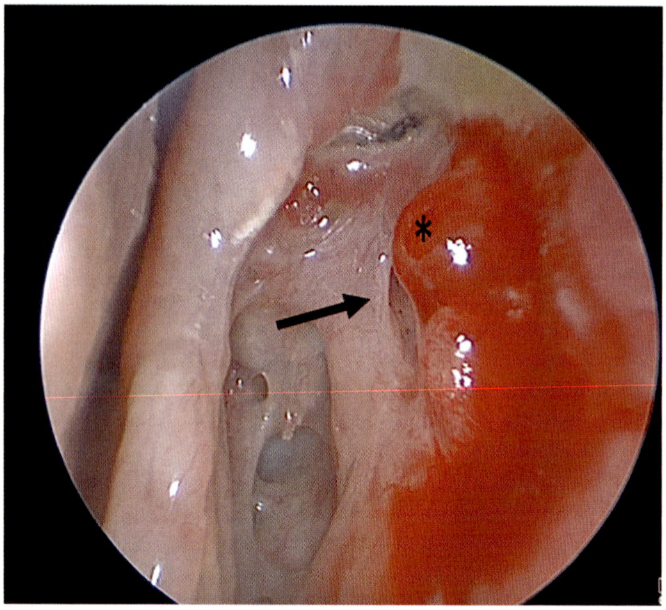

• **Fig. 15.4** Development of granulation tissue (*asterisk*) can be a consequence of exposed bone around the neo-ostium after drilling. Often this resolves with topical steroid irrigations and oral steroids. This picture shows only partial obstruction of the neo-ostium (*arrow*), but complete obstruction is a possible reason for failure (view via 30-degree endoscope).

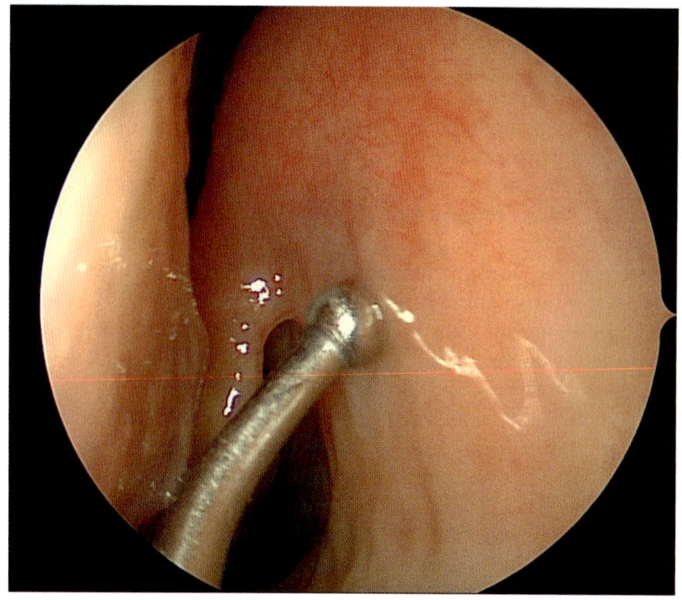

• **Fig. 15.5** The patient in this example presented with persistent epiphora after left endoscopic dacryocystorhinostomy. Palpation of the lateral nasal wall is performed to define the limits of the prior osteotomy to help direct the soft-tissue and bone dissection during the revision procedure (view via 30-degree endoscope).

Revision endoscopic DCR can be performed using either local or general anesthesia, although our preference is for it to be done with the patient under general anesthesia. The challenge in the revision setting, however, is appreciating the anatomic factors that have led to failure and then approaching them with a plan to address each of them. Most commonly this includes looking for mucosal scarring or obstruction of the neo-ostium, inadequate bone removal and exposure of the lacrimal sac, lateralization of the middle turbinate, or a residual septal deviation limiting access. Granulation tissue, such as that demonstrated in Fig. 15.4, may be one source of neo-ostium obstruction.

Revision surgery is begun by addressing obvious sources of scarring or anatomic obstruction. Any synechiae present between the DCR site and middle turbinate or septum are sharply divided. Next, the middle turbinate is medialized to optimize surgical access. Curved probes are then used to palpate the lateral nasal wall and neo-ostium to determine if the prior osteotomy was performed in the proper position or of adequate size (Fig. 15.5). The lacrimal sac lies along the anterior maxillary line, at the junction of the frontal process of the maxilla and lacrimal bone just above the attachment of the middle turbinate. The prior osteotomy should be present along the maxillary line, completely exposing the lacrimal sac and the common internal punctum. In some cases, it is difficult to identify the location of the prior DCR. In this situation, we find it helpful to have the oculoplastic surgery team join the case early to perform lacrimal system probing and dilation to aid in defining the altered anatomy. We have found this approach to be of great value in such challenging revision cases.

After identifying the position of the lacrimal sac and defining the limits of the prior osteotomy, attempts are made to carefully elevate the mucosa from the underlying bone and lacrimal sac. This can be a hazardous step because mucosa will be lying directly in apposition with the lateral wall of the lacrimal sac. Consequently, the common internal punctum and lateral sac wall is at risk for injury. Meticulous elevation of the mucosa is important and is typically best started from the neighboring bone edges of the prior osteotomy (Fig. 15.6). Inadequate removal of the frontal process of the maxilla is the most common situation we encounter; thus beginning the elevation of mucosa from this area posteriorly toward the mucosal scar and lacrimal sac is ideal. The mucosa is then elevated with a Freer or suction elevator, exposing the frontal

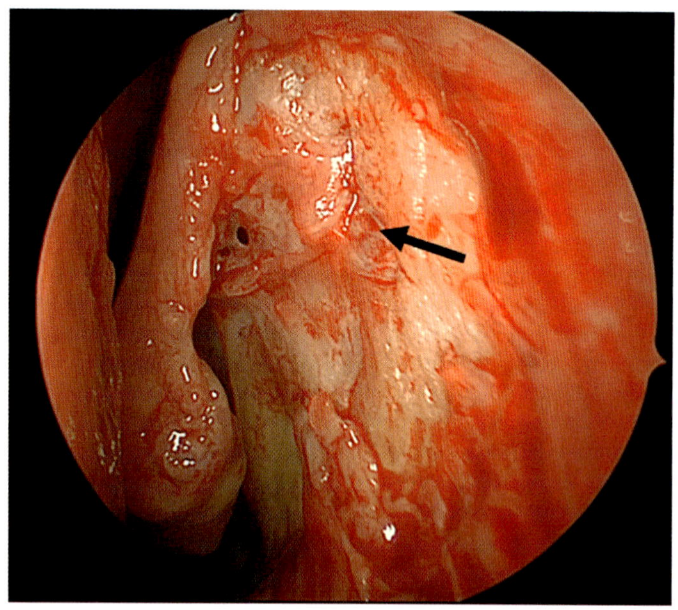

• **Fig. 15.6** After careful elevation of the mucosa in a patient with persistent epiphora after left endoscopic dacryocystorhinostomy, the prior limited osteotomy and dense scar (*arrow*) are evident (view via 30-degree endoscope).

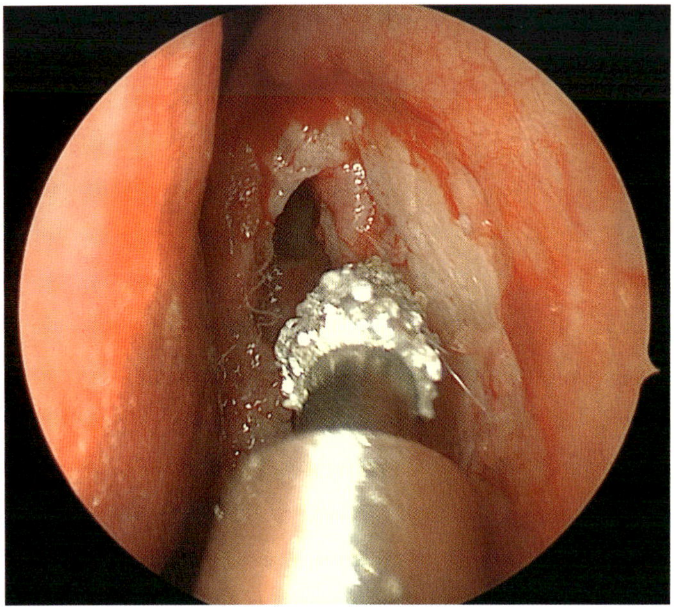

• **Fig. 15.7** Once the residual bone around the lacrimal sac has been exposed, a high-speed irrigating drill is used in a controlled fashion to expose the medial wall of the lacrimal sac (view via 30-degree endoscope).

process of the maxilla and lacrimal bone. In revision cases, this mucosa is often significantly scarred, making elevation challenging, so care must be taken to elevate the entirety of the scar and mucosa. Ultimately, the goal is to define and protect the common internal punctum during this dissection. If there is a small opening present, this can be used to help identify the lacrimal sac, which should be opened sharply during the mucosal elevation. If there is complete mucosal scarring and obstruction, then passing the lacrimal probe will help "tent" the residual medial lacrimal sac wall to orient the surgeon.

In contrast to a primary endoscopic DCR, during revision cases we strive to open the medial wall sooner rather than later to safely identify the lateral sac wall and common internal punctum. Once achieved, mucosal scar and bone are then removed to widely open the entire lacrimal sac using the standard techniques described for powered endoscopic DCR. Once the neo-ostium has been completely exposed, any residual frontal process bone overlying the region of the lacrimal sac is removed using a high-speed irrigating diamond burr, taking care not to induce any collateral soft-tissue injury (Fig. 15.7). We do not attempt to save mucosal flaps, as it is often not possible or helpful, in our opinion. Once again, having the common internal punctum clearly identified by your oculoplastic surgery colleagues by using a lacrimal probe is of great value (Figs. 15.8 and 15.9). Finally, any scarring of the anterior ethmoid, a retained agger nasi cell, or concurrent disease must be addressed. Placement of lacrimal intubation stents and application of mitomycin C is not routinely done, but there are specific indications that favor their use selectively (see the section Mitomycin C later in this chapter).

Certain techniques are keys to success in performing a revision endoscopic DCR. First, although wide bony exposure is vital to maintaining patency, meticulous bony dissection should be used so there is minimal exposed bone at the conclusion of the procedure. In addition, care should be taken to minimize redundant mucosal edges, as this could contribute to web formation and

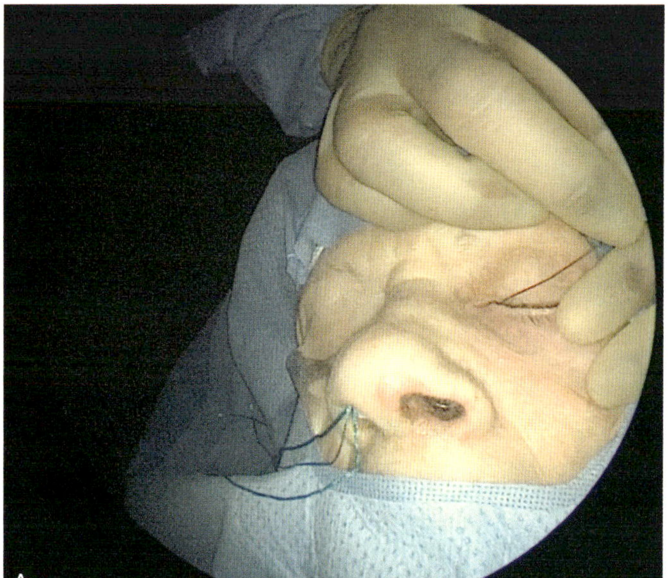

A

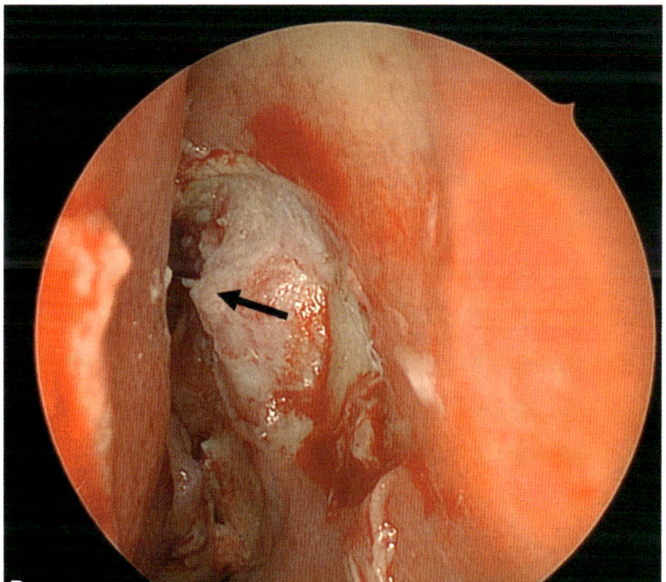

B

• **Fig. 15.8** After the medial wall of the lacrimal sac has been exposed, the canalicular system is probed to confirm adequate bone removal. A. Lacrimal probe is placed via the interior canaliculus. B, Endoscopic view of tenting of the medial wall of the lacrimal sac (*arrow*) (view via 30-degree endoscope).

scarring. Finally, it is important to analyze the surrounding structures after creating a wide neo-ostium. The middle turbinate should be examined carefully to ensure that it is stable enough to remain in a position that will not obstruct the neo-ostium, and the septum should be evaluated to ensure that any deviated portion will not cause neo-ostium obstruction. If there is a question of middle turbinate stability, it should either be partially resected or sutured to the septum. If the septum is deviated toward the neo-ostium, septoplasty should be performed.

Conjunctivodacryocystorhinostomy

In patients with severe common canalicular stenosis or obstruction of both the superior and inferior canaliculi, CDCR can be used

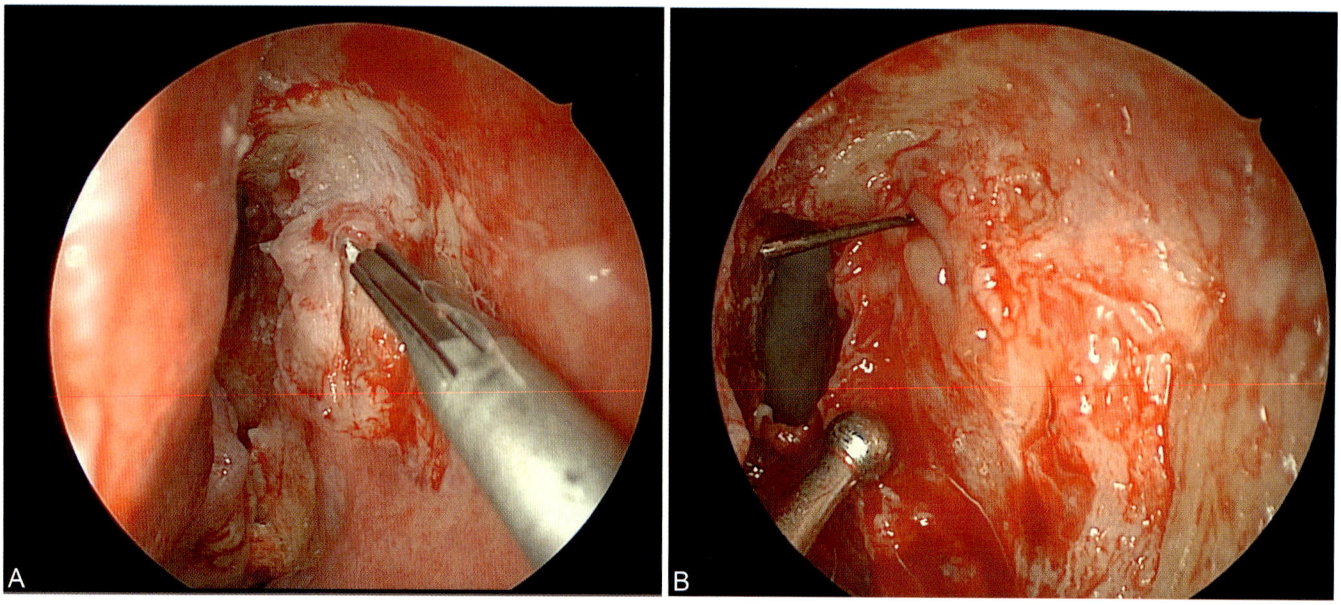

• Fig. 15.9 A, The lacrimal sac is incised sharply, while tented, with an endoscopic sickle knife. B, View of the lacrimal probe passing through the common internal punctum after removal of redundant flap edges and wide exposure of the entire lacrimal sac (view via 30-degree endoscope).

alone or in combination with endoscopic revision DCR. Similar to endoscopic DCR, CDCR can be performed using general or local anesthesia. Again, the nasal cavity is decongested with oxymetazoline-soaked cottonoids. Additionally, 1% lidocaine with 1:100,000 epinephrine is infiltrated into the region of the caruncle and, under endoscopic guidance, infiltrated into the nasal mucosa overlying the region of the lacrimal sac, as described previously. Using endoscopic guidance, a neo-ostium is created in a fashion similar to endoscopic DCR. The inferior half of the caruncle is excised. Next a guide needle is passed through the now debulked inferior caruncle and into the center of the intranasal neo-ostium. A 1.5-mm trephine (Henderson trephine) is then used to cut a cylindrical track around the guide wire. The trephine is removed while leaving the guide wire in position, and then the glass (Jones) tube can be passed down the guide wire. The Jones tube can be affixed by suturing it to the caruncle with 6-0 prolene sutures. Numerous modifications to the Jones tube have been developed (frosted, angled, flanged, with a suture hole, porous polyethylene-coated, and with a silicone intranasal flange) to lessen the incidence of postoperative extrusion.

Additional Considerations

Lacrimal Stents

The use of silicone lacrimal stents has been debated after primary DCR. In a recent meta-analysis of 12 randomized controlled trials, it was determined that there was no significant difference in success after primary DCR with or without lacrimal stenting.[26] However, several authors report using stents often when performing revision endoscopic DCR. No randomized controlled trials have been performed to analyze the utility of stents in revision DCR. The length of time in which lacrimal stents are kept in place is highly variable according to the literature. The goal is to keep lacrimal stents in place until inflammation around the ostium has resolved, which ranges widely.[a] Another concern with stent placement is the development of biofilms, leading to postoperative stent-associated infections.[29] Although there is concern that long-term placement of lacrimal stents can result in the development of granulomas and synechiae, frequent endoscopic evaluation postoperatively can address these developments early before significant complications could arise, decreasing the risk of long-term sequelae. In our practice, we largely reserve the use of stents for common canalicular stenosis or upper system obstruction.

Mitomycin C

Application of mitomycin C at the time of revision surgery has also been a controversial topic. Mitomycin C is an antineoplastic chemotherapeutic agent that blocks DNA synthesis. It has been demonstrated to be safe in ophthalmology and has been used for the prevention of pterygium recurrence and to increase the success of glaucoma filtering procedures. Kao et al. demonstrated that mytomycin C was effective in maintaining a larger osteotomy size after external DCR.[30] In 2013, a meta-analysis of mitomycin C use during DCR demonstrated significantly higher success of revision DCR after application of mitomycin C.[31] It is thought that this is due to mitomycin C preventing the formation of scarring and granulation tissue over the neo-ostium. Unfortunately, although the literature does appear to support the use of mitomycin C in revision DCR, the optimal dose and exposure times are still unknown, with doses ranging from 0.2 to 0.5 mg/mL and exposure times ranging from 2 to 15 minutes.[31] Although we do not routinely use mitomycin C in our practice, its use can be considered in cases when there is higher concern for scar formation, such as in patients with autoimmune processes, such as sarcoidosis or granulomatosis with polyangiitis, as well as in those patients in whom revision surgery has previously failed.

[a]References 3, 6, 7, 9, 25, 27, 28.

Postoperative Care

After revision endoscopic DCR or CDCR, meticulous postoperative care is vital. All patients should be discharged with ophthalmic antibiotic and steroid drops to be used for 1 week as well as nasal saline solution irrigations to reduce intranasal crusting and inflammation. Oral steroids and oral antibiotics are not routinely used. Patients should have regular postoperative follow-up with both otolaryngologists and ophthalmologists. Routinely our patients follow up with an otolaryngologist at 1, 4, and 12 weeks postoperatively, at which time the neo-ostium is examined and any crusting, granulation, or synechiae is removed. Additionally, oral steroids or intranasal steroids can be applied if significant inflammation or granulation is noted. During follow-up with an ophthalmologist, care is taken to ensure that no extrusion of either the stents or Jones tubes has occurred. If migration is noted, they can be adjusted in the office. Silicone stents are typically removed between 4 to 12 weeks postoperatively.

Outcomes

In the past decade, a number of studies have been performed to evaluate the efficacy of revision endoscopic DCR. Overall, revision DCR has been shown to have a high success rate—79% to 91%—although it is still lower than the success of primary DCR.[b] A recent review of our experience with 16 revision endoscopic DCR procedures in 11 patients at the University of Colorado demonstrated a 91% success rate based on improvement in epiphora with 100% anatomic patency at a mean follow-up of 37 months.[20a]

The causes of failure after revision endoscopic DCR are similar to those of primary DCR. In fact, if failure occurs with revision, it is likely due to the same source as the primary failure; the common causes of failure are scar formation, ostial stenosis, inappropriate osteotomy location, and intranasal anatomic obstruction.[25] As such, success of the revision surgery is dependent on the surgeon successfully analyzing and addressing the source of primary failure, while also ensuring the creation of a wide osteotomy that completely exposes the medial wall of the lacrimal sac. It is also vital to use meticulous surgical technique to precisely remove all membrane or scar formation while ensuring minimal bony exposure and limiting mucosal injury that could ultimately lead to synechiae and scar formation.[3,27] If significant canalicular stenosis or unknown causes of functional failure are found in patients, using a CDCR may aid in long-term success, with success rates of primary and revision CDCR ranging from 60% to 91%.[34,35] Failure after CDCR is most commonly secondary to inappropriate tube length or position, so endoscopic evaluation of the tube position at the time of placement is essential.[35]

Although revision DCR can be performed endoscopically or externally, endoscopic revision is highly preferred because it allows the surgeon to concomitantly manage intranasal pathologies as well as to closely evaluate the neo-ostium, ensuring that it is of adequate size and in appropriate position. In addition, endoscopic DCR preserves the lacrimal pump, is associated with less intraoperative bleeding, has a lower morbidity rate, and prevents the creation of an external scar.[3,9] Another important feature of performing revision DCR endoscopically is that it does not preclude the surgeon from performing an external approach at a later date, if needed.

[b]References 6, 7, 9, 25, 28, 32, 33.

Complications

The complication rates of revision endoscopic DCR are very low. The actual complication rates are hard to determine, given the small sample sizes reported in the literature. In fact, most reports of revision endoscopic DCRs have no complications. In the description by Hull, Lalach, and Olver of 19 revision endoscopic DCRs, there was only 1 report of mild epistaxis.[9] Similarly, in a review of 43 patients, Korkut et al. noted only three cases of periorbital ecchymosis. Other, more serious theoretical risks include prolapse of orbital fat, orbital hematoma, and severe epistaxis.[33]

As with revision endoscopic DCR, complications after CDCR are very low. Potential complications include medial migration of the Jones tube, resulting in septal irritation or epistaxis, tube extrusion with corneal abrasion or ulceration, and infection. Regular ophthalmology follow-up is vital so that if tube migration occurs, it can be addressed before the development of corneal or septal injury.[36] It is also vital that, at the time of placement, the Jones tube be of optimal length to minimize complications and optimize success.[34]

Conclusion

Revision DCR is an important tool after failure of primary DCR. Although revisions can be performed externally or endoscopically, endoscopic DCR is preferred because it (1) allows the surgeons to closely examine the neo-ostium and address any concomitant nasal pathology at the time of revision, (2) has lower morbidity, and (3) does not require an external incision. CDCR can be performed independently or in conjunction with endoscopic DCR at the time of revision surgery if patients have significant canalicular stenosis. Overall, meticulous surgical technique combined with a thorough knowledge of the anatomy of the nasolacrimal system is essential to optimize success.

References

1. McDonogh, M., & Meiring, J. H. (1989). Endoscopic transnasal dacryocystorhinostomy. *Journal of Laryngology and Otology, 103*(6), 585–587.
2. Huang, J., Malek, J., Chin, D., Snidvongs, K., Wilcsek, G., Tumuluri, K., et al. (2014). Systematic review and meta-analysis on outcomes for endoscopic versus external dacryocystorhinostomy. *Orbit, 33*(2), 81–90.
3. Ali, M. J., Psaltis, A. J., Bassiouni, A., & Wormald, P. J. (2014). Long-term outcomes in primary powered endoscopic dacryocystorhinostomy. *British Journal of Ophthalmology, 98*, 678–1680.
4. Lin, G. C., Brook, C. D., Hatton, M. P., & Metson, R. (2017). Causes of dacryocystorhinostomy failure: External versus endoscopic approach. *American Journal of Rhinology & Allergy, 31*, 181–185.
5. Jung, S., Kim, Y., Cho, W., Paik, J., & Yang, S. (2015). Surgical outcomes of endoscopic dacryocystorhinostomy: Analysis of 1083 consecutive cases. *Canadian Journal of Ophthalmology, 50*, 466–470.
6. Paik, J., Cho, W., & Yang, S. (2013). Comparison of endoscopic revision for failed primary external versus endoscopic dacryocystorhinostomy. *Clinical and Experimental Ophthalmology, 41*, 116–121.
7. Kominek, P., Cervenka, S., Pniak, T., Zelenik, K., Tomaskova, H., & Matousek P. Revision endonasal dacryocystorhinostomies: Analysis of 44 procedures. *Rhinology, 49*, 375–380.
8. Ben Simon, G. J., Joseph, J., Lee, S., Schwarcz, R. M., McCann, J. D., & Goldberg, R. A. (2005). External versus endoscopic dacryocystorhinostomy for acquired nasolacrimal duct obstruction in a tertiary referral center. *Ophthalmology, 112*, 1463–1468.

9. Hull, S., Lalchan, S., & Olver, J. M. (2013). Success rates in powered endonasal revision surgery for failed dacryocystorhinostomy in a tertiary referral center. *Ophthalmic Plastic & Reconstructive Surgery, 29*, 267–271.
10. Dave, T. V., Mohammed, F. A., Ali, M. J., & Naik, M. N. (2016). Etiologic analysis of 100 anatomically failed dacryocystorhinostomies. *Clinical Opthalmology, 10*, 1419–1422.
11. Welham, R. A. N., & Wulc, A. E. (1987). Management of unsuccessful lacrimal surgery. *British Journal of Ophthalmology, 71*, 152–157.
12. Ali, M. J., Psaltis, A. J., Murphy, J., & Wormald, P. J. (2015). Powered endoscopic dacryocystorhinostomy: A decade of experience. *Ophthalmic Plastic and Reconstructive Surgery, 31*, 219–221.
13. Wormald, P. J., Kew, J., & Van Hasselt, A. (2000). Intranasal anatomy of the nasolacrimal sac in endoscopic dacryocystorhinostomy. *Otolaryngology Head–Neck Surgery, 123*, 307–310.
14. Chan, W., & Selva, D. (2013). Ostium shrinkage after endoscopic dacryocystorhinostomy. *Opthalmology, 20*, 1693–1696.
15. Mann, B. S., & Wormald, P. J. (2006). Endoscopic assessment of the dacryocystorhinostomy ostium after endoscopic surgery. *Laryngoscope, 116*, 1172–1174.
16. Rose, G. E. (2004). The lacrimal paradox: Toward a greater understanding of success in lacrimal surgery. *Ophthalmic Plastic Reconstructive Surgery, 20*(4), 262–265.
17. Linberg, J. V., Anderson, R. L., Bumsted, R. M., & Barreras, R. (1982). Study of intranasal ostium external dacryocystorhinostomy. *Archives of Ophthalmolology, 100*, 1758–1762.
18. Simon, G. B., Brown, C. L., & McNab, A. A. (2012). Larger osteotomies result in larger ostia in external dacryocystorhinostomies. *Archives of Facial Plastic Surgery, 14*(2), 127–131.
19. Knisely, A., Harvey, R., & Sacks, R. (2015). Long-term outcomes in endoscopic dacryocystorhinostomy. *Currrent Opinion in Otolaryngology & Head Neck. Surgery, 23*, 53–58.
20. Ramakrishnan, V. R., Durairaj, V. D., & Kingdom, T. T. (2008). Revision endoscopic dacryocystorhinostomy. *Operative Techniques in Otolaryngology, 9*, 177–181.
20a. Kingdom, T. K., Barham, H. P., & Durairaj, V. D. (2020). Long-term outcomes after endoscopic dacryocystorhinostomy without mucosal flap preservation. *Laryngoscope, 130*, 12–17.
21. Liang, J., Hur, K., Merbs, S., & Lane, A. (2014). Surgical and anatomic considerations in endoscopic revision of failed external dacryocystorhinostomy. *Otolaryngology–Head Neck Surgery, 150*(5), 901–905.
22. Soyka, M. B., Treumann, T., & Schlegel, C. T. The agger nasi cell and uncinate process, the keys to proper access to the nasolacrimal drainage system. *Rhinology, 48*, 364–367.
23. Vagefi, M. R., Winn, B. J., Lin, C. C., Sires, B. S., LauKaitis, S. J., Anderson, R. L., et al. (2009). Facial nerve injury during external dacryocystorhinostomy. *Ophthalmology, 116*(30), 585–590.
24. Lee, M. J., Khwarg, S. I., Choung, H., & Kim, N. (2014). Associated factors of functional failure of external dacryocystorhinostomy. *Canadian Journal of Ophthalmology, 49*(1), 40–44.
25. Baek, J. S., Jeong, S. H., Lee, J. H., Choi, H. S., Kim, S. J., & Jang, J. W. (2017). Cause and management of patients with failed endonasal dacryocystorhinostomy. *Clinical and Experimental Otorhinolaryngology, 10*(1), 85–90.
26. Kang, M. G., Shim, W. S., Shin, D. K., Kim, J. Y., Lee, J., & Jung, H. J. (2018). A systematic review of benefit of silicone intubation in endoscopic dacryocystorhinostomy. *Clinical and Experimental Otorhinolaryngology, 11*(2), 81–88.
27. Korkut, A. Y., Teker, A. M., Ozsutcu, M., Askiner, O., & Gedikli, O. (2011). A comparison of endonasal with external dacryocystorhinostomy in revision cases. *European Archives of Oro-Rhino-Laryngology, 268*, 377–381.
28. Demarco, R., Strose, A., Araujo, M., Valera, F. B. P., Moribe, I., & Anselmo-Lima, W. T. (2007). Endoscopic revision of external dacryocytorhinostomy. *Otolaryngology Head–Neck Surgery, 137*, 497–499.
29. Samimi, D. B., Ediriwickrema, L. S., Bielory, B. P., Miller, D., Lee, W., & Johnson, T. E. (2016). Microbiology and biofilm trends of silicone lacrimal implants: Comparing infected versus routinely removed stents. *Ophthalmic Plastic and Reconstructive Surgery, 32*(6), 452–457.
30. Kao, S. C., Liao, C. L., Tseng, J. H., Chen, M. S., & Hou, P. K. (1997). Dacryocystorhinostomy with intraoperative mitomycin C. *Ophthalmology, 104*(1), 86–91.
31. Cheng, S., Feng, Y., Xu, L., & Huang, J. (2013). Efficacy of mitomycin C in endoscopic dacryocystorhinostomy: A systematic review and meta-analysis. *PLoS One, 8*(5). e67237.
32. Yarmohammadi, M. E., Ghasemi, H., Jafari, F., Izadi, P., Nadoushan, M. J., & Chin, N. S. (2016). Teamwork endoscopic endonasal surgery in failed external dacryocystorhinostomy. *Journal of Ophthalmic and Vision Research, 11*(3), 282–286.
33. Korkut, A. Y., Teker, A. M., Yazici, M. Z., Kahya, V., Gedihli, O., & Kayhan, F. T. (2010). Surgical outcomes of primary and revision endoscopic dacryocystorhinostomy. *Journal of Craniofacial Surgery, 21, 1706–1708.*
34. Chang, M., Lee, H., Park, M., & Baek, S. (*2015*). Long-term outcomes of endoscopic endonasal conjunctivodacryocystorhinostomy with Jones tube placement: A thirteen year experience. *Journal of Cranio-Maxillo-Facial Surgery, 2015*, 43,7–10.
35. Park, M. S., Chi, M. J., & Baek, S. H. (2007). Clinical study of endoscopic endonasal conjunctivodacryocystorhinostomy with Jones tube placement. *Ophthalmologica, 221*, 36–40.
36. Barrett, R., & Meyer, D. (2008). Endoscopic conjunctivodacryocystorhinostomy. *Operative Techniques in Otolaryngology, 19*, 192–194.

16

Endoscopic Management of Pediatric Nasolacrimal Obstruction

JAMIE LEA SCHAEFER, MD, HABIB ZALZAL, MD, JOHN NGUYEN, MD, AND HASSAN RAMADAN, MD

Epiphora in the pediatric population often originates from a disorder of the lacrimal drainage system.[1,2] In most cases, the cause is congenital nasolacrimal duct obstruction (CNLDO), which often presents during the first year of life, with a prevalence ranging from 1.2% to 6% (Fig. 16.1).[2,3] Additional symptoms and signs of CNLDO may include a high tear meniscus, positive dye disappearance test result, recurrent mucopurulent discharge, and reflux of lacrimal sac contents with digital pressure.[4]

The nasolacrimal drainage system arises during the third month of fetal development.[5,6] A rudimentary drainage system initially forms from the cord of epithelium between the maxillary and frontonasal recesses. Canalization then occurs uniformly throughout its entire length. The lateral portion of the cord differentiates into the ocular end with the creation of the superior and inferior canaliculi. In the sixth month of fetal development, the medial portion of the cord canalizes to create a drainage communication with the inferior nasal meatus. Incomplete canalization leading to a residual membranous barrier between the nasolacrimal duct and the nasal cavity at the level of the valve of Hasner is the most common cause CNLDO.[1,5,6] Jones and Wobig[7] have also described seven other anatomic variations that cause obstruction of the lower nasolacrimal duct system (Box 16.1). These variations constitute a significant cause of failure for spontaneous CNLDO resolution and are theorized to contribute to cases of failed nasolacrimal duct probing.

Because neonatal tear secretion does not reach adult volume until 4 weeks after birth, CNLDO symptoms are not typically seen in newborns.[2,4] Symptomatic infants may attain spontaneous absorption of the membranous obstruction at the valve of Hasner up to 6 to 8 months of age. Nasolacrimal duct probing and irrigation are typically used for persistent obstruction. Endoscopy is a powerful addition to the typically blind nasolacrimal duct probing, as it minimizes nasal mucosa trauma, decreases the chance of creating a false passage, and provides an optimum management option of different congenital variants of CNLDO.[1,4]

Simple Congenital Nasolacrimal Duct Obstruction

Spontaneous resolution of CNLDO is seen in 85% to 96% of children by 1 year of age, so conservative management is recommended with lid hygiene, topical antibiotic drops, and a hydrostatic massage known as a Crigler massage.[1,2] Digital pressure is applied on the common canaliculus with firm downward pressure onto the lacrimal sac to increase hydrostatic pressure, leading to the rupture of the membranous obstruction. There is no definitive consensus on the timing of intervention for children with persistent CNLDO, and probing and irrigation with the patient under general anesthesia is often delayed until 12 months of age and has a success rate of 55% to 95%. Nasolacrimal duct probing is a reliable primary management of CNLDO; however, this blind procedure mainly depends on the surgeon's knowledge of anatomy and feel of metal-on-metal contact, or proprioceptive intuition, to determine the location and severity of the obstruction and to confirm the passage of the probe through the inferior meatus.[8] Metal-on-metal contact may traumatize the nasal mucosa surrounding the delicate valve of Hasner. The leading factors implicated in the failure of probing include improper technique, anatomic variations, complex NLDO, inferior turbinate impaction or hypertrophy, or associated nasal pathology.[3] Even with positive metal-on-metal touch, false passages can be created, especially in cases of "buried probe" with the nasolacrimal duct extends into the nose down the submucosa for several millimeters or even to the floor without opening into the meatus, or the duct may end in the medial wall of the maxillary sinus blindly. Adjunctive use of the nasal endoscope has revealed a high incidence of false passage creation with this technique; thus nasal endoscopy is now increasingly used with nasolacrimal duct probing to improve the unexplained variable success rate, anatomic anomalies causing difficulty in probe advancement, and difficulty in accurately identifying the variants of CNLDO. In cases of obstruction caused by collapse of the inferior turbinate onto the nasolacrimal duct ostium, medialization, or fracturing, of the turbinate is also required in addition to probing to improve the outflow tract.[4]

The success rate for the first nasolacrimal probing after 13 months of age is 54.7%.[2,4] Many recommend probing before 13 months of age, as it is theorized that the risk of infection and scarring increases if probing is postponed. Conversely, other studies on conservative treatment have shown that the timing of probing can be postponed while still achieving a safe, satisfactory outcome with comparable success rates until the child reaches the age of 36 months. Additional factors associated with decreased success are severity of symptoms, bilateral symptoms, canalicular stenosis, atony of the lacrimal sac, and nonmembranous obstruction of the

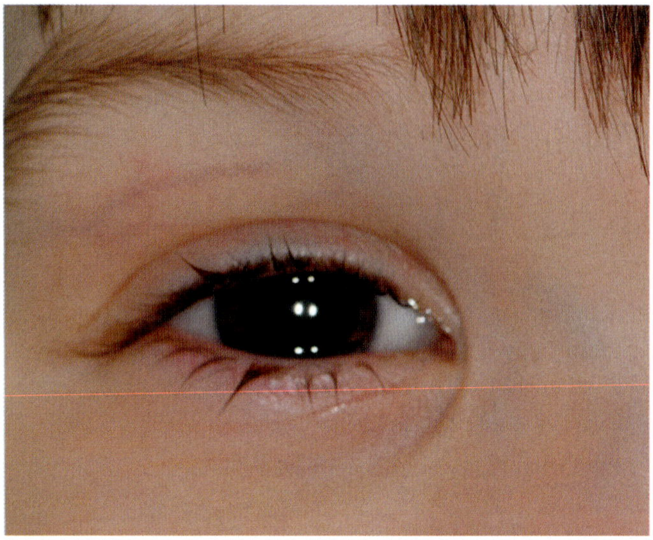

• **Fig. 16.1** Congenital nasolacrimal duct obstruction with epiphora and periocular matting of lashes.

• BOX 16.1 Seven Variations That Cause Obstruction of the Lower Nasolacrimal Duct System

1. The duct extends to the floor of the nose lateral to the nasal mucosa.
2. The duct extends several millimeters down lateral to the nasal mucosa without an opening.
3. The duct fails to canalize owing to failure of osseous nasolacrimal canal formation
4. An impacted inferior turbinate blocks the duct meatus.
5. The duct ends blindly in the anterior end of the inferior turbinate.
6. The duct ends blindly in the medial wall of the maxillary sinus.
7. A bony nasolacrimal duct extends to the floor of the nose without an opening (Fig. 16.2).

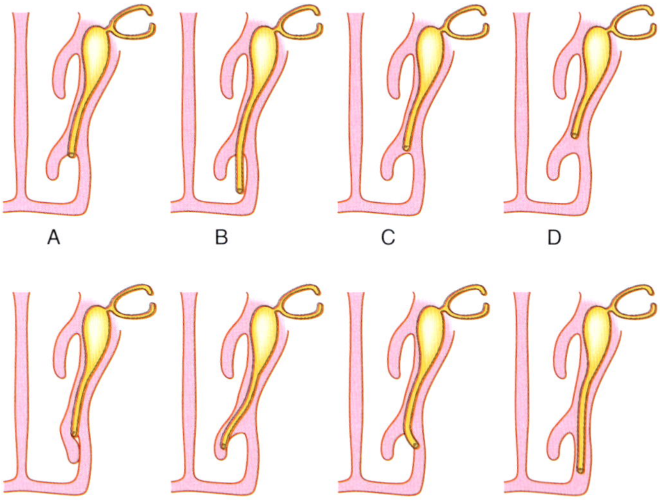

• **Fig. 16.2** Anatomic variations of the lower nasolacrimal system. A. Persistent membrane blockage at the valve of Hasner. B. Extension of the nasolacrimal duct to the nasal floor along the lateral nasal wall. C. Extension of the nasolacrimal duct a few millimeters down the lateral nasal wall without an opening. D. Failure of the duct to canalize. E. Blockage of the nasolacrimal duct from an impacted inferior turbinate. F. The duct ends blindly in the anterior end of the inferior turbinate. G. The duct ends blindly in the medial wall of the maxillary sinus. H. Bony nasolacrimal duct extends to the floor of the nose without an opening.

nasolacrimal duct (NLD).[4,5,9] Repeat probing with intubation of a silicone stent and sometimes balloon catheter dilation are reserved for cases of failure. When the obstruction is refractory to such measures, or in those children with a more proximal NLDO, dacryocystorhinostomy (DCR) is needed. DCRs have been reported in children as young as 12 to 18 months without disturbance of bone growth; it is recommended that this procedure be deferred until the patient is 2 to 5 years old.

Complex Congenital Nasolacrimal Duct Obstruction

Complex CNLDO can results from other causes of obstruction, including bony obstruction, craniofacial deformities such as congenital facial cleft syndrome, cyclopia, and cryptophthalmos.[2,7,8,10] As clefting can causes abnormalities of the soft tissues and bony structures, Tessier cleft types 2, 3, 4 are located in the lower medial canthal and nasolacrimal area and can lead to abnormalities of the nasolacrimal drainage system. Preoperative imaging with computed tomography scanning can be advantageous for surgical planning. The open cleft may preclude the need for endoscopic visualization.

Dacryocele/Dacryocystocele, and Dacryocystitis

Dacryocele typically appears as a bluish cystic mass just below the medial canthal tendon at birth or, as tear production increases, within the first few weeks of life[5] (Fig. 16.3). Epidemiologically, dacryoceles have a female predominance with a possible genetic predilection and occur more frequently in Caucasians than other racial groups. They may be unilateral or bilateral, although bilateral symptomatic presentation is infrequent.

Dacryoceles result from a concomitant upper functional obstruction at the valve of Rosenmüller and a lower anatomic obstruction of the valve of Hasner.[11] The upper functional obstruction occurs at the junction of the common canaliculus and lacrimal sac with a proximal valve-like or trapdoor-like blockage. The distal membranous obstruction results from redundant membranous tissue or imperforation of the nasolacrimal duct with the

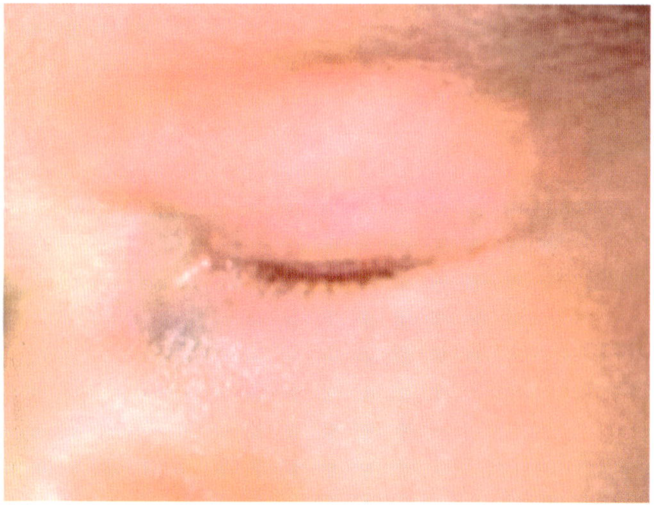

• **Fig. 16.3** An infant with a blue cystic mass below the left medial canthus, dacryocystocele.

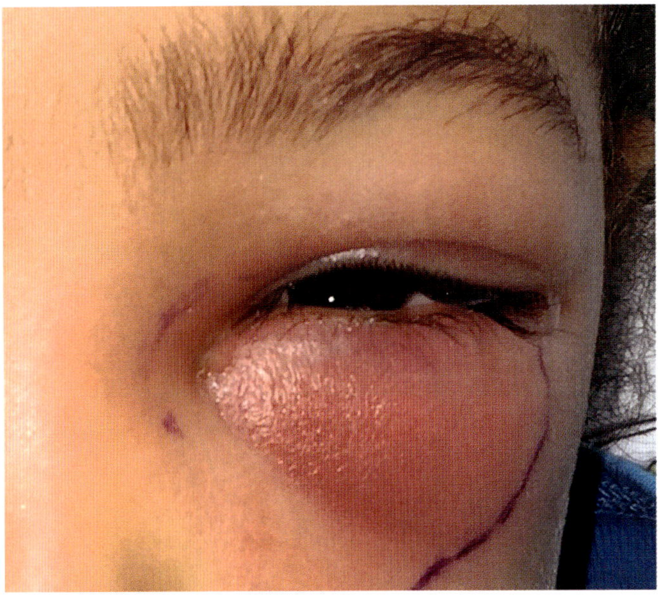

• **Fig. 16.4** A child with an acute dacryocystitis and preseptal cellulitis.

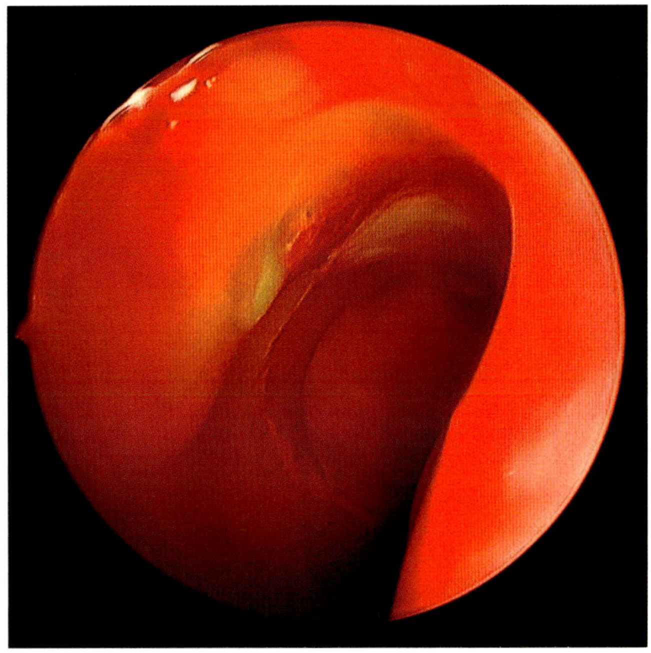

• **Fig. 16.5** The right inferior meatus with fluorescein dye drainage from irrigation of the nasolacrimal duct.

nasal cavity. The nasolacrimal duct system then becomes distended with an accumulation of tears, mucoid material, and debris to cause the gray-blue cystic swelling at the medial canthus. Affected children are at risk of secondary infection. Dacryocystitis and preseptal cellulitis may develop within days or weeks and require intravenous antibiotics to prevent sepsis (Fig. 16.4). Extension of the dacryocele intranasally may form a cyst below the inferior turbinate and cause nasal congestion.[5] A large cyst can cause respiratory distress during feeding and sleeping, and is potentially life-threatening from airway compromise because neonates are nasal breathers.

In the absence of complicating factors such as infection or airway compromise, initial treatment includes warm compresses, hydrostatic digital massage, and topical antibiotics.[3,5] In-office digital massage to reduce the cyst can expedite the resolution of a dacryocele. Transcutaneous needle or incisional aspiration is not recommended because of the risk of lacrimocutaneous fistula formation and does not address the underlying etiology. Endoscopic- assisted nasolacrimal probing and irrigation are successful mostly for the treatment of a congenital dacryocele. Direct visualization under endoscopic guidance assists with the removal of redundant mucosa from the lateral wall of the inferior meatus as well as marsupialization and excision of the medial wall of an intranasal cyst. Intubation with silicone stents may also be performed to minimize the postoperative scarring.

Technique of Nasal Endoscopic-Assisted Probing and Irrigation

After administration of general anesthesia, the patient is positioned in a standard surgical fashion for sinus surgery.[1] The patient is prepped and draped in sterile fashion for proper exposure of both the nose and the affected eye within the operative field.[8] Nasal packing with nasal decongestant, such as oxymetazoline hydrochloride 0.05% or xylometazoline hydrochloride 0.025%, is usually applied. The 2.7-mm 0-degree or 30-degree rigid endoscope is optimal for use in the pediatric nasal cavity because the small caliber of the endoscope with the angled view provides better visualization of the NLD opening under the inferior turbinate. Examination of the structures in the nasal cavity and appearance of the interior turbinate and nasal mucosa are initiated during the first pass of the endoscope. As the endoscope is passed along the nasal floor for examination, the NLD outflow tract underneath the inferior meatus can be identified as a small dimple in the mucosa of the lateral wall (Fig. 16.5).

Nasolacrimal Duct Irrigation and Probing

The initial surgical management of CNLDO has not significantly changed since probing was first described by Petrus Camper in the 18th century.[1,12] The evolution of endoscopic-assisted nasolacrimal duct probing has led to a success rate of 94% to 97%. About 23% of cases with associated nasal anomalies with CNLDO would not be detected and treated without the use of nasal endoscopy.[9] This direct visualization highlights the nature of the CNLDO and optimizes management options according to the nature of the obstruction, such as the use of a sickle knife to perforate or increase the size of the distal NLD ostium in the nasal cavity.

During endoscopic examination of the inferior meatus, the superior punctum is simultaneously enlarged with a punctal dilator. A lacrimal cannula attached to a 3-mL syringe containing fluorescein solution is then advanced through the punctum and canaliculus into the lacrimal sac. Gentle irrigation with the fluorescein solution may reveal swelling of the nasal mucosa without dye drainage of the meatus to indicate an imperforate valve of Hasner, and probing is then performed with a 00-Bowman probe (Jedmed Instrument Company, St. Louis, MO) after dilation of the upper punctum. The probe is advanced through the punctum and canaliculus into the lacrimal sac. The probe is rotated inferolaterally into the duct. A tenting of the lateral mucosal wall underneath the inferior turbinate indicates the imperforate valve of Hasner

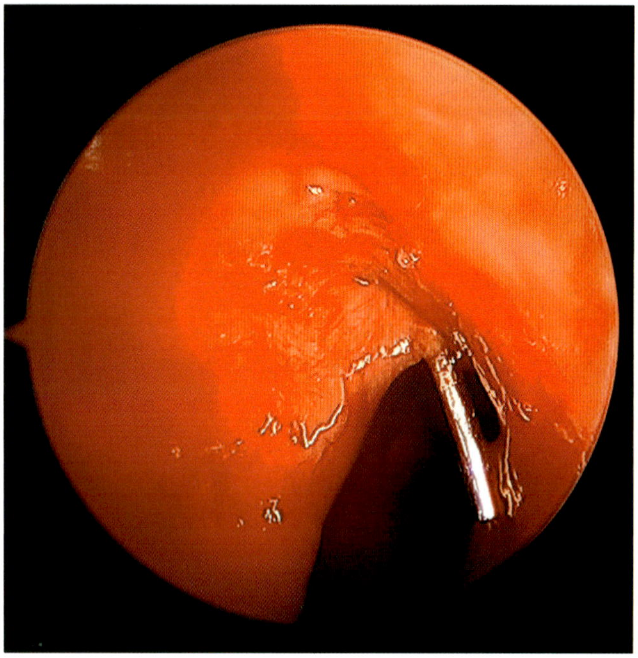

• **Fig. 16.6** A 00-Bowman probe is passed through the inferior meatus to imperforate the soft-tissue membrane.

for which gentle pressure is needed to open the obstruction, revealing the probe is in the nasal cavity (Fig. 16.6). In rare cases, the use of a sickle knife on the probe tip can widen the mucosal opening.[1,4,9] A hard stop may indicate bony obstruction, for which the success rate may be lower. A buried probe can be found by careful advancement and gentle directing of the probe medially toward the inferior meatus apex to allow for revelation of the ostium. Marsupialization of the mucosa may be necessary to relieve the obstruction, and excision of redundant mucosal tissue with endoscopic forceps minimizes scar formation. Complete excision of the dacryocele cyst is required to prevent recurrence of nasolacrimal duct obstruction and to relieve nasal congestion. Repeat irrigation is performed to confirm patency.

In patients with a narrow inferior meatus from a collapsed inferior turbinate or inferior turbinate hypertrophy, medialization of the inferior turbinate is useful to enhance the success of nasolacrimal duct irrigation and probing.[10] A Freer elevator is typically used to medialize the turbinate, and nasolacrimal duct irrigation and probing then proceed in similar manner earlier.

Stenting

Endoscopic-assisted retrieval of the stent's probe during silicone intubation increases visualization of the procedure and thereby decreases damage to the mucosa.[8,10] Placement of a stent such as a Crawford or a Bika stent (FCI Ophthalmics, Pembroke, MA) is introduced using a techniques similar to the one previously described, and the lacrimal stent is retrieved with its respective hook and removed from the nasal cavity in an atraumatic manner (Fig. 16.7). The Ritleng intubation system (FCI Ophthalmics, Pembroke, MA) is designed to reduce time and trauma to the nasal mucosa. The Ritleng intubation probe is first inserted though the superior punctum and fed down the length of the NLD through the valve of Hasner. The Ritleng stent, which is a silicone stent with a polyetheretherketon thread guide, consisting of two varying diameters, is then fed down the intubation probe and retrieved in the inferior meatus. The thinner portion of the guide, which is adjacent to the tube, is then slid through a slit in the Ritleng intubation probe so that the probe can be removed while the tube remains in place. The polyetheretherketone portion is removed. The stent is tied to itself in similar fashion of the Crawford stents and Bika stents. The lacrimal stent is typically retained for 6 months and is removed in the office.

Bicanalicular stenting has been the standard for nasolacrimal duct intubation; however, monocanalicular stents have gained traction as an alternative option since their introduction more than 10 years ago.[1,13] Extrusion risks are comparable between the two types of stent. The monocanalicular stent has the advantage of quicker placement and easier removal. Various studies found a success rate for monocanalicular stents to bicanalicular stents of 67.7% versus 62.4%.

Ballooning

Balloon catheter dilation is a comparatively newer procedure and is a viable surgical adjunct to nasolacrimal duct probing.[2,10] Ballooning enables a more confident dilation of the lacrimal system that

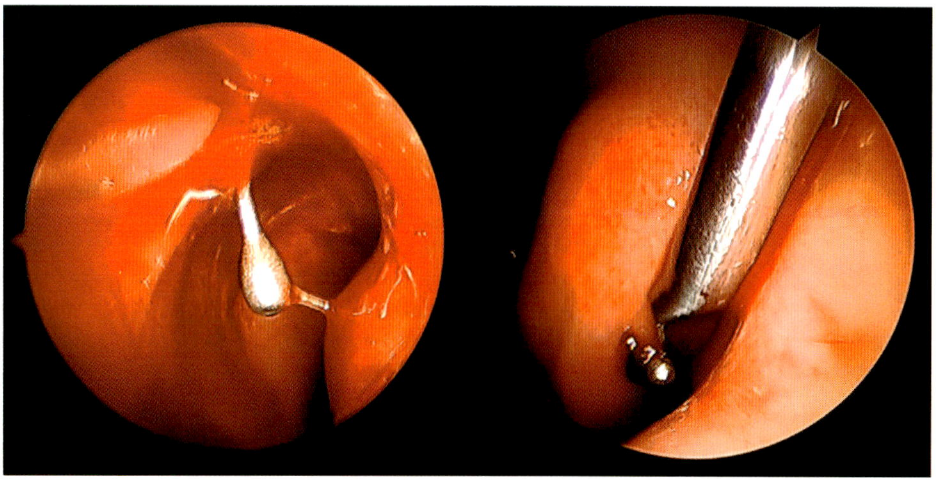

• **Fig. 16.7** A Crawford stent is passed through the inferior meatus and retrieved with a hook.

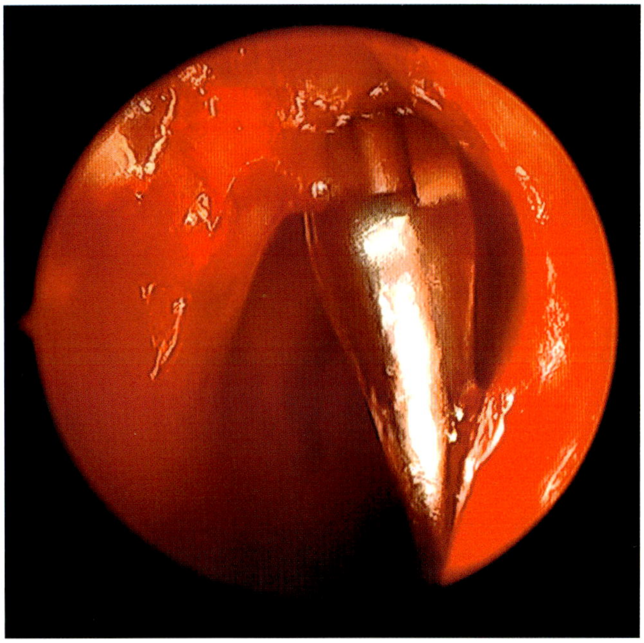

• **Fig. 16.8** Inflated balloon dacryoplasty catheter straddling the nasolacrimal duct ostium.

aids in cases of severe diffuse stenosis or significant mucosal stenosis. The success rates have been found to range from 74% to 94%. Uninflated, the balloon catheter has a diameter similar to a No. 1 Bowman probe. The balloon comes in two inflated diameters: 2 mm and 3 mm (Quest Medical Inc., Allen, TX). The end of the catheter has a 10- to 15-mm balloon. The balloon catheter is inserted through the puncta of the upper lacrimal system and advanced into the distal NLD through the valve of Hasner. When performing the procedure, the balloon is inflated to 8 atm for 90 seconds (Fig. 16.8). The balloon is then deflated for a short period before reinflation for an additional 60 seconds. The balloon catheter is then retracted 10 mm proximally, theoretically at the valve of Rosenmüuller, and is then inflated in a similar fashion. The system is then irrigated with 1 mL of an antibiotic steroid solution. Success rates are reported at 82% in primary cases, similar to that of bicanalicular intubation.

Endoscopic Dacryocystorhinostomy

Endoscopic DCR is reserved for children in whom nasolacrimal duct probing and stenting have failed, and this approach has the advantage of avoiding an external approach that may result in scarring.[5] There is not an optimal time for surgery, as DCR surgery can have effects on the growth of the sinus cavity. Extra care is warranted to balance the desired boundaries of the bony osteotomy in the presence of a lower skull base and the narrow nasal cavity. Success rates for pediatric endoscopic DCR ranges from 58% to 100%, whereas those for external DCR range from 89% to 97.5%.

With the patient under general anesthesia, the endoscopic DCR is performed using rigid scopes and endoscopic sinus instruments.[5] An incision is made to remove the uncinate bone, which will then expose the lacrimal bone anteriorly. An incision is made anterior to the lacrimal bone and elevated, exposing the maxillary line and the posterior lacrimal sac. A drill is then used to remove the thick bone of the frontal process of maxilla, exposing the sac. Afterward a dilator is used and a lacrimal probe is passed through the punctum of the sac. Under endoscopic view, the sac is then incised and probes are passed through into the nose. At this point, dilation, ballooning, and even stenting can be performed under endoscopic guidance.

Summary

The management of CNLDOs is evolving, and endoscopy contributed significantly to the understanding and treatment of CNLDO with visualization of the anatomy in the inferior meatus area and any potential anatomic variants, thereby decreasing the risk for false passage of the nasolacrimal duct probing, facilitating resident training and enhancing the surgeon's confidence in lacrimal surgery.

References

1. Al-Faky, Y. H. (2014). Nasal endoscopy in the management of congenital nasolacrimal duct obstruction. *Saudi Journal of Ophthalmology, 28*, 6–11.
2. Casady, D. R., Meyer, D. R., Simon, J. W., Stasior, G. O., & Zobal-Ratner, J. L. (2006). Stepwise treatment paradigm for congenital nasolacrimal duct obstruction. *Ophthalmic Plastic and Reconstructive Surgery, 22*(4), 243–247.
3. Yagci, A., Karci, B., & Ergerzen, F. (2000). Probing and bicanalicular silicone tube intubation under nasal endoscopy in congenital nasolacrimal duct obstruction. *Ophthalmic Plastic and Reconstructive Surgery, 16*(1), 58–61.
4. Grover, A. K. (2017). Management of nasolacrimal duct obstruction in children: How is it changing? *Indian Journal of Ophthalmology, 65*(10), 910–911.
5. Cunningham, M. J. (2006). Endoscopic management of pediatric nasolacrimal anomalies. *Otolaryngologic Clinics of North America, 39*, 1059–1074.
6. Takahashi, Y., Matsuda, H., Nakamura, Y., & Kakizaki, H. (2013). Dacryoendoscopic findings of lacrimal passage with congenital punctal atresia. *Orbit, 32*(5), 338–340.
7. Jones, J. T., & Wobig, J. L. (Eds.). (1976). *Surgery of the eyelids and lacrimal system* (pp 157–163). Birmingham, AL: Aesculapius.
8. Lueder, G. T. (2004). Endoscopic treatment of intranasal abnormalities associated with nasolacrimal duct obstruction. *Journal of the American Association for Pediatric Ophthalmology and Strabismus, 8* (2), 128–132.
9. Prabhakaran, V. C., & Selva, D. (2008). Orbital endoscopic surgery. *Indian Journal of Ophthalmology, 56*(1), 5–8.
10. Takahashi, Y., Kakizaki, H., Chan, W. O., & Selva, D. (2010). Management of congenital nasolacrimal duct obstruction. *Acta Ophthalmologica, 88*, 506–513.
11. Kakizaki, H., Takahashi, Y., Sa, H. S., Ichinose, A., & Iwaki, M. (2012). Congenital dacryocystocele: Comparative findings of dacryoendoscopy and histopathology in a patient. *Ophthalmic Plastic and Reconstructive Surgery, 28*(4), e85–e86.
12. Takahashi, Y., Nakamura, Y., & Kakizaki, H. (2013). Dacryoendoscopic findings in the lacrimal passage in failed dacryocystorhinostomy. *Ophthalmic Plastic and Reconstructive Surgery, 29*, 373–375.
13. Goldstein, S. M., Goldstein, J. B., & Katowitz, J. A. (2004). Comparison of monocanalicular stenting and balloon dacryoplasty in secondary treatment of congenital nasolacrimal duct obstruction after failed primary probing. *Ophthalmic Plastic and Reconstructive Surgery, 20*(5), 352–357.

17

Outcomes of Endoscopic Dacryocystorhinostomy

Enhancing the Patency of the Rhinostomy

ERIC M. DOWLING, MD AND JANALEE K. STOKKEN, MD

Dacryocystorhinostomy (DCR) is the definitive treatment for epiphora caused by nasolacrimal duct obstruction (NLDO). The procedure creates a functioning passageway for tears from the lacrimal sac into the nasal cavity by bypassing the obstructed nasolacrimal duct. The cause of NLDO can be idiopathic, as in primary acquired NLDO, or it can be secondary to other disease entities. Secondary causes include infectious, inflammatory, neoplastic, traumatic, and mechanical processes.[1]

A common cause of DCR failure is mucosal scarring around or over the ostium. Many techniques for preventing or limiting fibrosis and scarring around the surgical ostium have been described. These include various surgical techniques, placement of postoperative stents, and application of anti-inflammatory or antiproliferative mediations. As surgical techniques have been described in the previous chapters, this section reviews the adjunct procedures and medications that have been used to optimize outcomes.

Outcomes of Endoscopic Dacryocystorhinostomy

Endoscopic DCR has been compared to external DCR in various studies. Advocates for the endonasal approach offer the benefits of addressing comorbid sinonasal disease and septal deviation as well as the avoidance of an external scar. A Cochrane review published in 2017 reports no difference in anatomic success between the two groups when mechanical endonasal DCR was compared to the external approach (90% both groups; relative risk 1.00; 95% confidence interval 0.81 to 1.23; 40 participants); however, the endonasal group did not achieve patency as often when the laser-assisted technique was used (63% vs. 91%; relative risk 0.69; 95% confidence interval 0.52 to 0.92; 64 participants).[2]

Two recent retrospective case series report data from 624 and 120 cases of endoscopic, endonasal DCRs. Coumou et al. reported an anatomic success rate in 90.1% and a functional success rate in 90.1% of adults with the use of silicone stenting, removed 3 months after surgery. They had a 3.2% complication rate and average follow-up time between 3 and 21 months.[3] Ciger et al. reported an anatomic success rate of 92.5% and functional success rate of 92.5% without the use of silicone stenting with mean follow-up of 46.5 months. Similarly, they had a 3.3% complication rate. Both of these studies discuss postoperative scarring (fibrosis, granulation, and synechiae) at the rhinostomy site as the primary cause for failure. Further, Ciger et al. reported that the scarring was identified in the 3- to 4-month postoperative time frame.[4]

Outcome data for patients who undergo revision DCR for either failed external or endoscopic DCR are also available. Ali, Psaltis, and Wormald report 91.3% anatomic and 86.9% functional success rates after revision endoscopic DCR with a mean follow-up of 26.4 months. Moreover, they report the causes of primary failure, including cicatricial ostium closure (55%), scarred internal common opening (27%), and organized granuloma over the common canaliculus (16.7%). In addition, 39% of patients underwent adjunctive septoplasty and 5.5% had endoscopic sinus surgery at the time of revision.[5]

The published rate of success for patency in endoscopic DCR ranges from 78% to 100% and is approximately 90% in the studies reviewed previously.[4] These rates are comparable to those of the open approach, but both approaches continue to leave an approximate 10% risk of failure, primarily from the formation of scar tissue. This provides an opportunity for the discovery of an adjunctive therapy or procedure to improve the overall outcome of this procedure.

Nasolacrimal Stent Type

Since the development of nasolacrimal stents, a number of different materials have been used, including organic materials, metals, and synthetic materials. Stents are designed to promote longer retention and prevent inflammation. Stenting materials should be inert, pliable, smooth, and readily available. Silicone and polyethylene meet many of these qualifications and are the material of choice for most modern stents.

The decision regarding whether or not to insert a stent is made, by some, based on the tightness of the common canaliculus. This can be assessed by passing a Bowman probe (Integra LifeSciences,

Cincinnati, OH) through the canaliculus, and if significant resistance is met, a stent is placed. Bicanalicular stents, which traverse the superior and inferior canaliculi and meet in the common canaliculus, are the most common type used for DCR. Silicone material is used most often, but alternative stent materials have also been used, including small red rubber catheters and C-flex lacrimal catheters (Consolidated Polymer Technologies, Clearwater, FL).[6–8] A study by Woog, Metson, and Puliafito et al. used traditional silicone tubing, 10-Fr red rubber urinary catheters, and C-flex catheters for stenting purposes.[8] A segment of either red rubber catheter or C-flex catheter was used at the stoma site to aid with patency. They demonstrated success in all 10 cases when the red rubber catheter was used, with no need for revision. The use of this catheter was abandoned later in the study, however, as placement and securement of this catheter type were found to be tedious. They instead opted for a C-flex catheter made of highly biocompatible thermoplastic for the remainder of the study. This catheter was easier to place, as the silicone stent could be placed through the center of the C-flex catheter rather than next to it, as was done with the red rubber catheter. Patency was maintained in all five cases stented with the C-flex stent, but follow-up in this group was shorter. In comparison, only a 68% success rate was found when the silicone stent was used alone. The authors endorse that the earlier cases, which used silicone stenting alone, may have been subjected to increased failure rates related to the learning curve for using the device.[8]

Studies have reported that the silicone stent itself may cause tissue granulation, predisposing the site to postoperative infection, adhesions, and punctal lacerations, resulting in surgical failure and complications.[9] A meta-analysis by Kang et al. found no significant difference in the surgical success rate between endoscopic DCR with silicone intubation and that without stenting. Complications of DCR without stenting can also include synechiae formation and granulation tissue surrounding the stoma.[10]

Modifications to stent materials have also been proposed to improve the success rate in DCR. Applications of antimicrobial substances can, in theory, prevent biofilm formation and prevent stent occlusion. However, these substances create irregularities on the stent surface, which allows for easier adherence and colonization by disruptive bacteria. Uncoated devices have been found to develop similar surface irregularities after exposure to normal living conditions for 3 months.[11] This may suggest a negligible change in risk of biofilm development owing to the physical characteristics of coating materials. Nevertheless, no effective method to prevent formation of biofilms on nasolacrimal stents has been identified. Future endeavors should seek to design materials with nonstick properties and material coatings that can prevent formation of polysaccharide biofilms.

Nasolacrimal Stent Timing

The duration of stenting remains a topic of debate. Some clinicians recommend leaving stents in place for 6 to 9 months if the common canaliculus is markedly stenosed.[12] The logic behind this strategy is that mature scar formation is not complete until several months postoperatively.[7] The recent literature suggests that the majority of mucosal healing is complete at 4 to 6 weeks and a longer duration of stenting may promote granuloma formation and subsequent stenosis.[5] Literature directly comparing duration of stenting with outcomes is lacking. Studies using stenting for an average of 4 to 6 weeks have shown success in 85% to 94% of cases, whereas stenting for longer durations demonstrates success rates between 84% and 96%.[10] A survey conducted in 2016 of members of the American Rhinologic Society demonstrates that nasolacrimal stents are most commonly left in place for 6 to 8 weeks.[12]

Topical Mitomycin C

Antimetabolite medications are also considered by some surgeons as an adjuvant therapy. The medication is applied topically to the rhinostomy site with a goal of scar prevention. These medications have a comparatively well-established role in treatment of tracheal and esophageal stenosis. They are also commonly used after strabismus surgery to prevent fibrosis. The most common antimetabolite used in DCR is mitomycin C. This medication, derived from the broth of *Streptomyces caespitosus,* creates single-strand breaks in DNA. Mitomycin C preferentially affects rapidly dividing cells, resulting in inhibition of fibroblast and modulation of postoperative fibrosis. This is thought to prevent excessive shrinkage of the ostium and canalicular obstruction. Mitomycin C is applied to the rhinostomy site in a concentration of 0.1 to 0.5 mg/mL with a cotton-tipped applicator. This is applied from 2 to 30 minutes before being flushed with saline solution.

Mitomycin C application has not been shown to provide consistent significant symptomatic benefit, and the majority of surgeons do not routinely use this in DCR.[13,14] There may be a role, however, in cases of chronic dacryocystitis with external lacrimal fistula, repeated acute dacryocystitis, scar prone situations, and failed DCR cases.[15–17] Sweeney et al. suggest adjuvant use of mitomycin C in cases of obvious intranasal inflammation at the time of surgery or in cases with a high likelihood of failure, such as in granulomatosis with polyangiitis.[1] Meta-analysis by Xu, Mellington, and Norris demonstrated nearly half the failure rate in revision cases when mitomycin was used compared with cases in which it was not used.[14] The side effects of antimetabolites include maculopathy, wound infection, scleral ulceration, and corneal epithelial defects.[18–20] Currently the use of topical antimetabolites has not been adopted for routine use in DCR.

Anti-Inflammatory Medications

Topical corticosteroid medications have a variety of applications and are commonly used for their innate anti-inflammatory properties. Corticosteroids are known to suppress inflammation and fibroblast recruitment, resulting in reduced scar formation. The role of steroids in DCR is to prevent abnormal wound healing and prevent ostium granuloma formation. The most common application in DCR is in the form of corticosteroid nasal sprays. The downfall of this delivery method is that nasal sprays distribute the drug mainly on the anterior edges of the inferior and middle turbinates, with only a small amount reaching the rhinostomy site. A few studies advocate steroid injection into the nasolacrimal sac wall for more direct application to the nasal mucosa and theoretically providing a stronger and longer therapeutic effect than topical medications.[21] Injection of 1-mg betamethasone into the nasolacrimal sac intraoperatively has shown good results with improved success rates without introducing new complications.[21] Jo et al. found good response to injection of 0.3 mL of 40 mg/mL of triamcinolone acetonide into granulomas identified in the postoperative period.[22] In fact, the granulomas regressed after steroid injection and the final outcomes were similar to cases without granuloma formation. Complications related to intranasal steroid injection are uncommon, but precautions should be used to prevent catastrophic events such as blindness. Measures taken to mitigate the risk of retinal embolization include thorough mixing to prevent particle clumping, application of topical vasoconstrictors, and slow, gradual injection.[23]

Conclusion

DCR is a safe and effective method for treatment of NLDO. A variety of surgical techniques have been adopted without a clear consensus on the most effective method. The most common reasons for the failure of endoscopic DCR include adhesions, restenosis, and obstruction of the common canaliculus. Stenting is a strategy used to circumvent these complications that is used in most revision cases. However, the role of stenting in primary DCR has been evaluated more recently, and surgical outcomes do not differ in the stented and nonstented cohorts. Additional modifications to DCR include application of antimetabolites and anti-inflammatory medications. These treatments have been shown to have minimal side effects and potentially reduce failure rates, especially in revision cases. Future studies should seek to better elucidate the effectiveness of these medications and standardize the manner in which they are applied.

References

1. Sweeney, A. R., Davis, G. E., Chang, S. H., & Amadi, A. J. (2018). Outcomes of endoscopic dacryocystorhinostomy in secondary acquired nasolacrimal duct obstruction: A case-control study. *Ophthalmic Plastic and Reconstructive Surgery*, *34*(1), 20–25.
2. Jawaheer, L., MacEwen, C. J., & Anijeet, D. (2017). Endonasal versus external dacryocystorhinostomy for nasolacrimal duct obstruction. *Cochrane Database of Systematic Reviews*, *2*. CD007097 doi:10.1002/14651858.CD007097.pub3.
3. Coumou, A. D., Genders, S. W., Smid, T. M., & Saeed, P. (2017). Endoscopic dacryocystorhinostomy: Long-term experience and outcomes. *Acta Ophthalmologica*, *95*(1), 74–78. https://doi.org/10.1111/aos.13217.
4. Ciger, E., Balci, M. K., Arslanoglu, S., & Eren, E. (2018). Endoscopic-powered dacryocystorhinostomy without stenting: Long-term outcomes of 120 procedures. *American Journal of Rhinology & Allergy*, *32*(4), 303–309. https://doi.org/10.1177/1945892418773638.
5. Ali, M. J., Psaltis, A. J., & Wormald, P. J. (2014). Long-term outcomes in revision powered endoscopic dacryocystorhinostomy. *International Forum of Allergy & Rhinology*, *4*(12), 1016–1019. https://doi.org/10.1002/alr.21398.
6. Unlü, H. H., Oztürk, F., Mutlu, C., Ilker, S. S., & Tarhan, S. (2000). Endoscopic dacryocystorhinostomy without stents. *Auris Nasus Larynx*, *27*(1), 65–71, 2000.
7. Griffiths, J. D. (1991). Nasal catheter use in dacryocystorhinostomy. *Ophthalmic Plastic and Reconstructive Surgery*, *7*, 177–186.
8. Woog, J. J., Metson, R., & Puliafito, C. A. (1993 Jul 1). Holmium: YAG endonasal laser dacryocystorhinostomy. *American journal of ophthalmology*, *116*(1). 1-0.
9. Feng, Y. F., Cai, J. Q., Zhang, J. Y., & Han, X. H. (2011). A meta-analysis of primary dacryocystorhinostomy with and without silicone intubation. *Canadian Journal of Ophthalmology*, *46*(6), 521–527.
10. Kang, M. G., Shim, W. S., Shin, D. K., Kim, J. Y., Lee, J. E., & Jung, H. J. (2018). A systematic review of benefit of silicone intubation in endoscopic dacryocystorhinostomy. *Clinical and Experimental Otorhinolaryngology*, *11*(2), 81–88. https://doi.org/10.21053/ceo.2018.00031.
11. Backman, S., Björling, G., Johansson, U. B., Lysdahl, M., Markström, A., Schedin, U., et al. (2009). Material wear of polymeric tracheostomy tubes: A six-month study. *Laryngoscope*, *119*(4), 657–664.
12. Chen, S., Le, C. H., & Liang, J. (2016). Practice patterns in endoscopic dacryocystorhinostomy: Survey of the American Rhinologic Society. *International Forum of Allergy & Rhinology*, *6*(9), 990–997.
13. Ali, M. J., Psaltis, A. J., Ali, M. H., & Wormald, P. J. (2015). Endoscopic assessment of the dacryocystorhinostomy ostium after powered endoscopic surgery: Behaviour beyond 4 weeks. *Clinical and Experimental Ophthalmology*, *43*(2), 152–155.
14. Xue, K., Mellington, F. E., & Norris, J. H. (2014). Meta-analysis of the adjunctive use of mitomycin C in primary and revision, external and endonasal dacryocystorhinostomy. *Orbit*, *33*, 239–244.
15. Deka, A., Bhattacharjee, K., Bhuyan, S. K., Barua, C. K., Bhattacharjee, H., & Khaund, G. (2006). Effect of mitomycin C on ostium in dacryocystorhinostomy. *Clinical and Experimental Ophthalmology*, *34*(6), 557–561.
16. Goldberg, R. A. (2000). Expert commentary—Standard endonasal dacryocystorhinostomy. In J. A. Mauriello (Ed.), *Unfavorable results of eyelid and lacrimal surgery: Prevention and management* (pp. 535–336). Boston, MA: Butterworth Heinemann.
17. Mauriello, J. J., & Vadehra, V. K. (1997). Dacryocystectomy: Surgical indications and results in 25 patients. *Ophthalmic Plastic and Reconstructive Surgery*, *13*(3), 216–220.
18. Hayasaka, S., Noda, S., Yamamoto, Y., & Setogawa, T. (1989). Postoperative instillation of mitomycin C in the treatment of recurrent pterygium. *Ophthalmic Surgery*, *20*, 580–583.
19. Shields, M. B., Scroggs, M. W., Sloop, C. M., & Simmons, R. B. (1993). Clinical and histopathologic observations concerning hypotony after trabeculectomy with adjunctive mitomycin C. *American Journal of Ophthalmology*, *116*, 673–683.
20. Skuta, G. L., Beeson, C. C., Higginbotham, E. J., Lichter, P. R., Musch, D. C., Bergstrom, T. J., et al. (1992). Intraoperative mitomycin versus postoperative 5-fluorouracil in high-risk glaucoma filtering surgery. *Ophthalmology*, *99*, 438–444.
21. Zeldovich, A., & Ghabrial, R. (2009). Revision endoscopic dacryocystorhinostomy with betamethasone injection under assisted local anaesthetic. *Orbit*, *28*(6), 328–331.
22. Jo, A., Lee, S. H., Song, W. C., & Shin, H. J. (2018). Effects of ostium granulomas and intralesional steroid injections on the surgical outcome in endoscopic dacryocystorhinostomy. *Graefe's Archive for Clinical and Experimental Ophthalmology*, *256*(10), 1–8.
23. Mabry, R. L. (1981). Visual loss after intranasal corticosteroid injection: Incidence, causes, and prevention. *Archives of Otolaryngology*, *107*(8), 484–486.

PART 4

Endoscopic Orbital and Optic Nerve Decompression

18 Thyroid Eye Disease

KYLE J. GODFREY, MD AND MICHAEL KAZIM, MD

Thyroid eye disease (TED) is an autoimmune inflammatory disorder that affects the periocular soft tissues. TED is associated with Graves disease (GD) and is synonymous with Graves orbitopathy/ophthalmopathy and thyroid-related orbitopathy/ophthalmopathy, among other names. The term TED is used by the authors because it is simple, universal, and understandable to patients and multidisciplinary clinicians. Although the majority of patients with TED experience mild disease, marked primarily by expansion of orbital fat volume and eyelid retraction, approximately one-third of patients experience more aggressive disease. In these cases, rapidly progressive expansion of the extraocular muscles can deliver compressive forces to the vasculature and optic nerve, threatening vision, and causes patients to have dry, bulging eyes, orbital pain, and double vision[1] (Fig. 18.1).

TED generally follows a biphasic course, with an active, inflammatory phase lasting 6 to 18 months, followed by a durable inactive, fibrotic phase. In patients who smoke, the active phase can be prolonged. This conceptual framework for the natural history of TED was first informed by Rundle's detailed observations of two patients in 1945, and TED clinical severity over time is referred to as following Rundle's curve.[2] Whereas mild cases may have a barely perceptible worsening curve, more aggressive disease has a steep curve. Furthermore, after a prolonged period of quiescence and inactivity, disease reactivation may occur years later.[3] Treatment options for active TED include immunomodulatory agents, radiation therapy, and orbital decompression surgery. Treatment options for inactive disease are primarily surgical. Because appropriate therapy, both modality and timing, is informed by an accurate understanding of disease severity and activity phase, detailed assessment and observation over time are essential.

This chapter reviews TED pathogenesis, risk factors, clinical manifestations, differential diagnosis, and disease activity classification, and includes a brief overview of TED management with consideration for the role of endoscopic surgical approaches.

Epidemiology

In the United States, the incidence of TED has been reported as 16 in 100,000 women and 3 in 100,000 men.[4] There is a bimodal age distribution in women, peaking at 40 to 44 and 60 to 64 years. In men this bimodal distribution shifts slightly older with peaks at 45 to 49 and 65 to 69 years. Among patients diagnosed with TED, approximately 90% have hyperthyroidism, 5% are euthyroid, 3% have Hashimoto thyroiditis with hypothyroidism, and 1% have primary hypothyroidism. Of patients with Graves hyperthyroidism, 30% to 50% will experience TED, depending on diagnostic criteria.[5] TED symptoms and signs begin at approximately the same time that hyperthyroidism is diagnosed in almost a third of patients with TED; TED onset precedes the diagnosis of hyperthyroidism in 7.5% of patients and follows it in 63%. Overall, TED and the dysthyroid state occur within 18 months of each other in 85% of cases.[6]

Pathophysiology

The clinical signs and symptoms of TED are due to inflammation, expansion, and fibrosis of the orbital soft tissues, primarily orbital fat and the extraocular muscles.[7] Because these soft-tissue changes occur acutely within the fixed volume of the bony orbit, their expansion displaces the globe anteriorly and can impede venous outflow, causing congestion and further expansion of orbital soft tissues. The immunologic drivers of this process include elements of both cellular and humoral immunity, including $CD4^+$ and $CD8^+$ T cells, mononuclear cells, and resident macrophages, which infiltrate the orbit and secrete cytokines and other mediators of inflammation.

Stimulated by autoimmune attack, orbital fibroblasts are thought to play a central role in TED (Fig. 18.2). Developmentally plastic, neural crest–derived orbital fibroblast precursors can differentiate into adipocytes, causing an expansion of orbital adipose tissue. Additionally, orbital fibroblasts can produce hyaluronan, a hydrophilic, osmotically active glycosaminoglycan that accumulates locally and further exacerbates orbital edema.[8] The extraocular muscle bodies are enlarged in early, active stages of the disease, whereas the muscle cells themselves are intact and widely separated by locally secreted hyaluronan.[9] However, as the disease becomes inactive, the resolving inflammatory process within the muscles may result in fibrosis and strabismus.

The central role of the orbital fibroblast in TED is due to its surface expression of thyroid-stimulating hormone receptor (TSHR).[7] The hyperthyroidism of GD is caused by autoantibodies directed against the TSHR on thyroid follicular cells, and orbital fibroblasts share this antigenic epitope. In addition, activation of helper T cells recognizing TSHR peptides presented by orbital fibroblasts or resident antigen-presenting cells leads to the local secretion of inflammatory cytokines and chemokines. Further, ligation of TSHR on orbital fibroblasts by circulating autoantibodies results in increased hyaluronan production and enhanced adipogenesis within the orbital fibroblast population.[10,11] The ensuing connective tissue remodeling leads to varying degrees of extraocular muscle enlargement and orbital fat expansion. Recent studies have also described a subset of orbital fibroblasts that

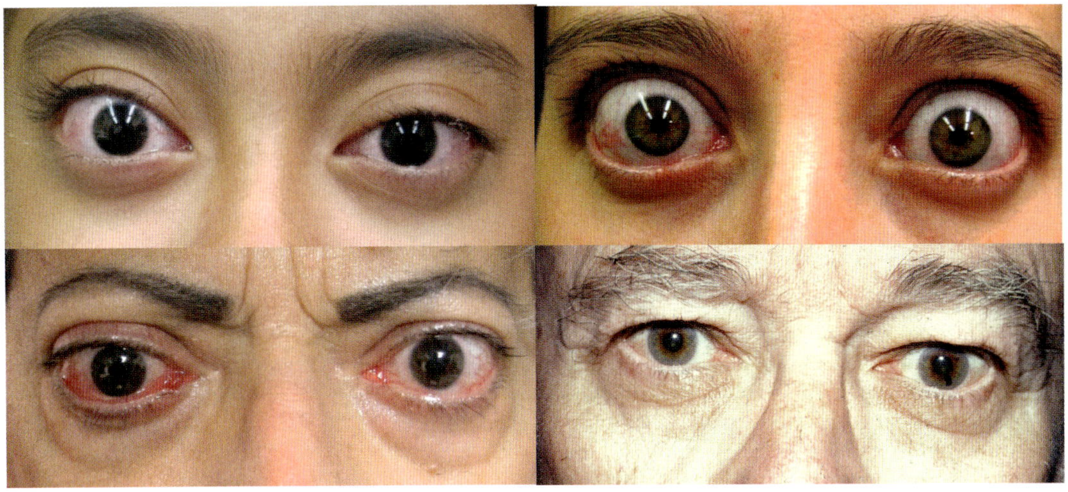

• **Fig. 18.1** Active TED demonstrating phenotypic variance at different ages. Counterclockwise from top left: pediatric, young adult, older adult, middle-aged adult. Note the relative absence of congestive, inflammatory features in the youngest and oldest patients.

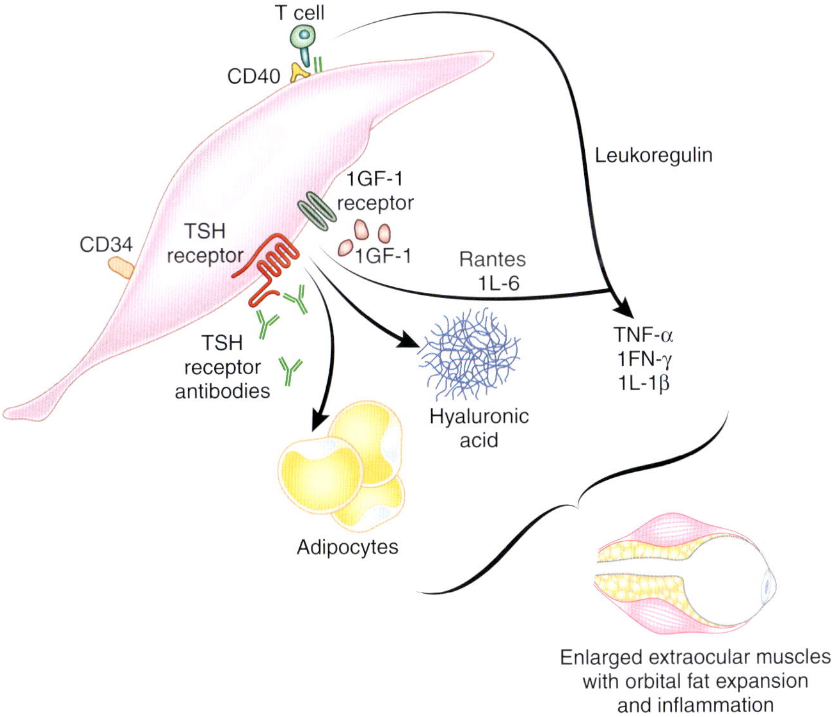

• **Fig. 18.2** Hypothesized pathogenesis of TED in which orbital fibroblasts expressing CD34, CD40, IGF-1 receptor, and TSH receptor, activate helper T cells, and stimulate the production of inflammatory cytokines, chemokines, hyaluronan, and adipogenesis. Subsequent connective tissue remodeling produces characteristic orbital fat expansion and extraocular muscle enlargement. Figure reproduced with permission from Bahn RS, *Current Insights into the Pathogenesis of Graves' Ophthalmopathy*, 2015, Publisher: Georg Thieme Verlag KG.

express CD34 are derived from bone marrow and reach the orbit and other sites of inflammation via the circulation.[12] As these cells express particularly high levels of TSHR and are capable of producing copious cytokines and chemokines, they may represent an important subpopulation. In addition to TSHR, orbital fibroblasts from patients with TED express high levels of insulin-like growth factor 1 receptor[13] Early studies suggested that these receptors may engage in cross-talk induced by TSHR ligation to synergistically enhance TSHR signaling, hyaluronan production, adipogenesis, and the secretion of inflammatory mediators.[14]

Sibling and twin studies have identified the major histocompatibility complex class II as an important genetic factor involved in the development of GD. More recently, other immune regulatory or thyroid-specific genes have been implicated, including cytotoxic T-lymphocyte–associated protein 4 (*CTLA-4*), *PTPN22*, *FOXP3*, *CD40*, *CD25*, thyrotropin receptor (*TSHR*), and thyroglobulin.[15]

Despite these findings, no consistent genetic associations have been found to be more prevalent in patients with GD and TED than in those with GD alone.[16] Accordingly, TED likely possesses a multifactorial etiology with environmental factors contributing to epigenetic modification.[17]

Modifiable Risk Factors

Smoking

Smoking is the most significant modifiable risk factor and may double the risk of TED.[18–20] TED risk is proportional to the number of cigarettes smoked per day, and former smokers have significantly lower risk than do current smokers.[19] In addition, patients who smoke are less responsive to therapeutic intervention.[21] Although mechanisms underlying the association between smoking and TED are unclear, contributors may include hypoxia or the free radical production, both of which promote orbital fibroblast proliferation.[22] A recent genome-wide expression study also found that gene expression differences, including genes affecting the immune system, may be attributable to smoking and are largely reversible after smoking cessation.[23] With this overwhelming evidence, smoking cessation or reduction should be actively encouraged.

Radioactive Iodine Therapy

Radioactive iodine therapy (RAI) therapy has also been extensively studied as a risk factor for the development and progression of TED. Risks of 33% to 39% for RAI, 10% to 21% for antithyroid drugs, and 16% for thyroidectomy have been reported.[20,24] In a large randomized study, methimazole therapy was compared with RAI treatment either with or without concurrent corticosteroids.[25] Within 6 months of treatment, TED progression was seen in 15% of patients treated with RAI alone, in 3% of patients treated with methimazole, and in no patient treated simultaneously with RAI and corticosteroids. Patients with inactive TED do not experience this risk.[26] These data suggest that alternative modalities for controlling hyperthyroidism should be considered during the active phase of TED for patients with moderate to severe disease. In appropriate, low-risk cases, such as nonsmokers with mild active TED, RAI with prophylactic corticosteroids may be considered and should include prophylactic corticosteroids. The best-studied regimen is oral prednisone (0.4-0.5 mg/kg per day) started 1 to 3 days after RAI therapy, continued for 1 month and tapered over the subsequent 2 months.[26] However, lower doses of prednisone (0.2 mg/kg per day) for 6 weeks may be equally effective.[27] Absolute contraindications to RAI include pregnancy, lactation, suspicion of thyroid cancer, or females planning pregnancy within 4 to 6 months.[28]

Thyroid Dysregulation

Abnormal thyroid levels may increase TED risk and severity. In a retrospective study, an odds ratio of 2.8 was found for patients with more severe TED who had current thyroid dysfunction compared with patients who had milder eye disease.[29] In a prospective study, the beneficial impact on TED of early levothyroxine supplementation beginning 2 weeks after RAI therapy was demonstrated.[24] These data suggest that persistent hyperthyroidism or iatrogenic hypothyroidism after RAI therapy or methimazole should be avoided. The optimal thyroxine replacement protocol for prevention of hypothyroidism after RAI is presently unknown.

Hyperlipidemia

Hyperlipidemia is an emerging potential risk factor in TED. In a review of 8404 patients with GD, the use of oral statin pharmacotherapy was associated with a 40% decreased hazard for the development of TED.[30] However, in the same study, non-statin cholesterol-lowering medication did not affect the development of TED. A subsequent cross-sectional study of 250 patients with GD found in a multivariate analysis that hyperlipidemia, both total cholesterol and low-density lipoprotein cholesterol, correlated with the presence of TED.[31] In this analysis, TED severity did not correlate with serum lipid levels but did correlate with elevated total cholesterol. Additionally, a small, prospective, case-control study of six patients analyzed orbital adipose tissue in severe TED and identified differential expression of genetic transcripts that included upregulation of very-low-density lipoprotein and low-density lipoprotein receptor relative to control samples.[32] These upregulated genes may reflect cellular activities central to orbital adipogenesis, including fatty acid uptake. Overall, these data suggest that cholesterol may play a role in the development and severity of TED, but additional confirmatory investigations are needed.

Obstructive Sleep Apnea

Obstructive sleep apnea (OSA) has also emerged as a possible additional modifiable risk factor in TED. In a recent retrospective study, patients with TED were screened with an OSA risk assessment tool. In these patients, the prevalence of high risk of OSA was significantly higher in patients with compressive optic neuropathy (59.2%) compared to those with noncompressive TED, controlling for sex (32.8%; $P = .006$).[33] Presently unpublished data by the authors also suggest that risk of OSA in TED may be associated with worse color vision, visual fields, proptosis, and double vision. Similar to smoking, the exact pathophysiologic mechanism is unknown but is hypothesized to be related to elevated serologic and tissue inflammatory mediators, including interleukin (IL)-6, IL-8, IL-1, and tumor necrosis factor alpha.[34–36] Although this hypothesis follows logically and mechanistically, additional prospective and interventional data are needed to validate this association.

Diagnosis and Clinical Workup

No single clinical finding or laboratory test is universally diagnostic of TED or its activity phase. The diagnosis is made on the basis of a careful history, physical examination, laboratory studies, and imaging studies. In cases of suspected TED, it is helpful to consider three elements that aid in establishing the diagnosis. The diagnosis of TED can be reliably established when at least two of these elements are present:

1. Typical *clinical* features
2. History of Graves hyperthyroidism or *serologic* evidence of autoimmune thyroidopathy
3. Typical *radiographic* findings

Typical clinical features of TED include the classic triad of unilateral or bilateral upper eyelid retraction, exophthalmos, and extraocular motility restriction in a pattern consistent with TED (most commonly restrictive supraduction or abduction deficits). Retraction of the upper and lower eyelids is the most common and specific manifestation of TED and is present in more than 90% of patients. Other common features include lid lag in downgaze and dull orbital pain. Nonspecific symptoms include tearing, sensitivity to light, blurred vision, and ocular surface irritation. The dermal and bony manifestations of GD, dermopathy and acropachy, are relatively rare and almost never develop in patients with mild orbitopathy.

If neither current nor past hyperthyroidism can be identified, the presence of either TSHR-binding or TSHR-stimulating antibodies in a patient with a clinical presentation compatible with TED is suggestive of the diagnosis.[37] In contrast, thyroid peroxidase (TPO) antibodies may not support the diagnosis, as the prevalence of anti-TPO antibodies in the general population is high. Although the absence of elevated TSHR autoantibodies does not rule out the diagnosis of TED, it necessitates further evaluation and/or observation over time.

Inconstancy or inadequacy of the clinical features or endocrine history warrants further investigation with imaging. The radiographic hallmarks of TED have been well described and include fusiform enlargement of the rectus muscles with relative sparing of the tendinous insertions (Fig. 18.3). The most commonly enlarged rectus muscles are, in order, superior rectus/levator complex, inferior rectus, medial rectus, and lateral rectus.[38] The oblique muscles are less commonly involved.[39] It is important to examine the superior rectus/levator complex carefully, as the magnitude of enlargement is relatively small, but the apical volume may be disproportionately consequential to the development of compressive optic neuropathy.[40,41]

Diagnostically, computed tomography (CT) and magnetic resonance imaging are equivalent and contrast is not required. Accordingly, considerations of surgical planning, radiation exposure, claustrophobia, and facility quality and location should be considered. For surgical planning, CT is preferred, as the bony walls are more clearly defined for possible decompression.

Pediatric TED may be particularly difficult to diagnose. In this setting, the clinical manifestations are often limited to progressive proptosis. The typical inflammatory signs and symptoms of the older phenotypes of the disease are strikingly absent[42] (see Fig. 18.1). Proptosis in children typically results from orbital fat expansion alone. Accordingly, imaging may not be helpful diagnostically, as the typical fusiform enlargement of the rectus muscles is absent. Fat enlargement is inconspicuous when imaged by CT or magnetic resonance imaging, as there is no well-validated algorithm for assessing pathologic fat volume expansion. Similarly, very early-phase TED can present clinically with nonspecific manifestations of inflammation (i.e., conjunctival or lid injection and ocular surface irritation).

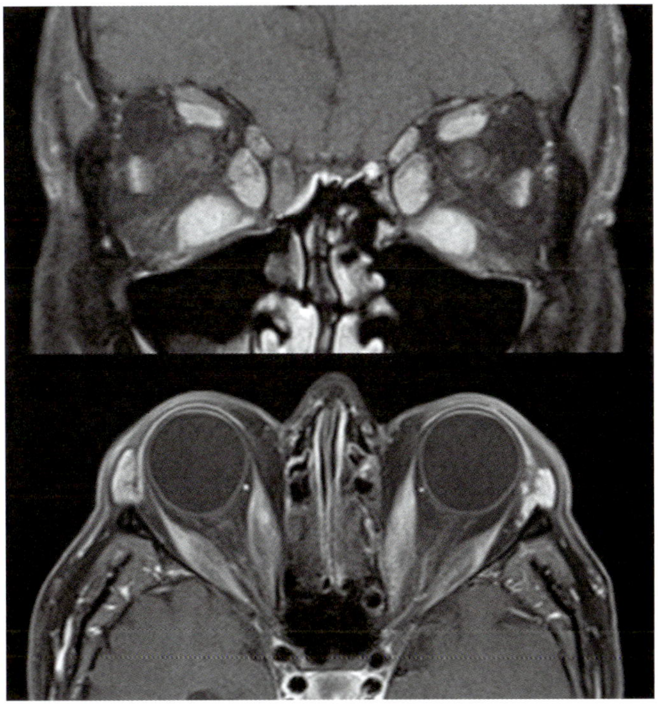

• **Fig. 18.3** Post-contrast T1 fat suppressed computed tomography scans (top—coronal view, bottom—axial view) demonstrating fusiform enlargement of the extraocular muscles sparing the tendinous insertion in TED.

Differential Diagnosis

Despite the effectiveness of the aforementioned diagnostic approach, in a small subset of outliers in which the imaging results may be inconclusive or when there is coexisting disease, diagnosis can sometimes be difficult. The differential diagnosis of TED broadly overlaps with other conditions that may produce orbital inflammation or congestion, eyelid malposition, strabismus, and optic neuropathy.

Interpretation of the orbital imaging can also be challenging. Similar patterns of extraocular muscle enlargement can result from cavernous sinus fistula, metastatic disease, lymphoma, prior strabismus surgery, and other inflammatory pathologies. In these cases, a combined analysis of the clinical and radiographic features is required to establish the correct diagnosis. Moreover, the diagnostic picture can be further complicated by the coincidence of TED and other orbital diseases. These have included optic nerve meningioma, orbital tumors, ocular myasthenia gravis, primary open-angle glaucoma, and various retinal disorders.

Classification and Disease Activity

Given the implication of TED severity and activity on the appropriateness and effectiveness of medical and surgical intervention, accurate and reproducible disease classification is desirable. Historically, several attempts have been made to classify TED over the past 60 years. Although each system has addressed a particular clinical question, none is perfect in fulfilling all clinical and research requirements. These classification systems include NOSPECS, EUGOGO (EUropean Group on Graves' Orbitopathy) Atlas, CAS (Clinical Activity Score), and VISA (Vision, Inflammation, Strabismus, Appearance) Classification.

The NOSPECS classification system is an acronym that describes and grades the clinical features of TED (*N*: no signs or symptoms, *O*: only signs, *S*: soft-tissue signs and symptoms, *P*: proptosis, *E*: extraocular muscle involvement, *C*: corneal involvement, *S*: sight loss).[43] Although useful as a descriptive tool in individual cases, the system does not correlate well with disease severity or activity and has been of limited use in research studies. The EUGOGO Atlas of TED is a valuable and comprehensive research tool but is time consuming to use in clinical settings.[44] A companion to the EUGOGO Atlas is the CAS. Initially developed as a predictor of response to corticosteroid therapy, the CAS features a binary scale to describe seven clinical signs and symptoms. These include eye pain at rest, eye pain with motion, lid erythema, lid swelling, conjunctival erythema, chemosis, and caruncular edema. Although the first visit is scored out of a total of 7, follow-up visits also include an additional point for significant progression in motility restriction, proptosis, or onset of optic neuropathy.

Although the CAS is useful in predicting the response to corticosteroids, it may be misleading in the patient with persistent orbital congestion, improving clinical symptoms that have not fully resolved, and in young patients and individuals of East Asian ancestry in whom compressive optic neuropathy without inflammatory signs often develops. Furthermore, its only measure of optic nerve function is Snellen visual acuity, an insensitive and nonspecific measure of optic neuropathy, and as with NOSPECS, the CAS fails to weigh appropriately the importance of optic neuropathy.

In an attempt to address these limitations, the VISA classification was introduced in 2006 by Dolman and Rootman and has been more recently adopted by the International Thyroid Eye Disease Society.[45] The VISA classification grades severity and activity for both subjective and objective measures of TED. The recording form is a single page and data entry rows from a routine clinical examination. At the end of the form, there is a summary grade for severity and progression of each of the disease parameters individually instead of a summed grade to include all of the parameters, including quality of life. This facilitates detailed assessment and surveillance of patients with TED.

Management of Thyroid Eye Disease

When evaluating a patient with TED, differentiating between active and quiescent disease is preeminently important. Generally speaking, active inflammatory disease is managed with immunomodulation, and inactive disease is managed surgically. An exception is orbital decompression surgery, which may be considered in the active phase to relieve orbital congestion, proptosis, and optic nerve compression in the most severely affected cases. Whenever possible, surgery is postponed until the quiescent phase, when necessary interventions can be performed more safely, effectively, and predictably. The overall goal of managing a patient with TED is to support the patient, treat symptoms, monitor progression, and intervene when indicated. The goal of any medical intervention should be to improve morbidity, prevent the development of vision-threatening sequelae, and decrease the surgical rehabilitation necessary once the active phase has resolved.

The clinical evaluation and management of TED is optimally accomplished in a multidisciplinary fashion that involves endocrinologists and ophthalmologists with consultation from other specialties (e.g., radiology, otolaryngology, and radiation oncology) when indicated.[46] Although care roles often overlap, endocrinologists typically manage the patient's thyroid function and address the reversible risk factors for TED. The ophthalmologist monitors TED progression and intervenes with medical or surgical therapy when indicated. Management of TED should include a full discussion with the patient regarding his or her concerns and priorities.

Mild Disease

In both active and inactive mild TED, symptom relief may be achieved using supportive measures.[26] Ocular lubrication with artificial tears or gels addresses corneal symptoms of dryness, photophobia, and foreign body sensation. The application of viscous gels or ointment at bedtime is particularly useful for patients with nocturnal lagophthalmos who may have prominent symptoms on awakening. In these cases, tape tarsorrhaphy, Glad Press and Seal wrap, or moisture chambers may also be useful.[47] Approximately 60% of patients with mild disease experience spontaneous improvement within about 6 months, 40% remain stable, and only a few percent worsen during that period.[5] Accordingly, most patients with mild TED can be treated with supportive care and observation. However, in some patients with mild disease, the quality of life is significantly diminished and additional intervention may be warranted.[26]

An additional consideration is selenium supplementation. Selenium is an oral antioxidant that was studied in a prospective trial in which patients with mild TED were randomly assigned to receive selenium (100 μg twice daily), pentoxifylline (another antioxidant), or a placebo.[48] Greater improvement in several ocular parameters as well as in quality of life was found at 6 and 12 months in patients in the selenium group. No adverse effects were identified. However, the patients in this study were from a population with marginally decreased selenium levels, leaving it unclear whether selenium supplementation is beneficial to selenium-sufficient patients or those with moderate to severe disease.

Moderate to Severe Active Disease

The goal of intervention in the active phase of disease is to decrease disease burden and reduce the magnitude or necessity of surgical rehabilitation in the subsequent inactive phase. Accordingly, immunomodulatory therapy consisting of glucocorticoids, nonsteroidal immunomodulatory agents, orbital radiotherapy, and thyroidectomy can be considered in patients with progressive TED with significant inflammatory scores and evidence of extraocular muscle involvement.

Corticosteroids

Although oral glucocorticosteroids (GCs) are commonly used in TED management, evidence from several prospective clinical trials suggests that GCs given intravenously (IVGCs) are more effective with fewer side effects. In the largest trial comparing oral GC and IVGCs, 70 patients with severe and active TED were randomly assigned to receive either oral prednisone (starting at 100 mg/day and tapered by 10 mg daily at weekly intervals for a total dose of 4.0 g) or intravenous methylprednisolone (500 mg weekly × 6 weeks then 250 mg weekly × 6 weeks for a total dose of 4.5 g).[49] After 3 months, the composite outcome (improvement in three or more of the following: intraocular pressure, diplopia, muscle size, proptosis, lid fissure width, and visual acuity) was met in 77% of patients treated with IVGCs but in only 51% of those treated with oral GCs. However, 10% to 20% of patients experienced relapse after a course of IVGCs, and optic neuropathy may still develop in them.[50] Compared with oral GC therapy, IVGC is associated with fewer adverse events, improved quality of life, and fewer subsequent ocular surgeries. Severe hepatotoxicity is a potential complication of IVGC therapy, but it appears to be dose dependent and is thought to occur only in patients receiving a cumulative dose greater than 8 g of methylprednisolone.[51] Other severe complications of IVGC include cardiovascular or cerebrovascular events, autoimmune encephalitis, and liver test abnormalities greater than fourfold the upper limit of normal.[52] Therefore relative contraindications for IVGC therapy include chronic viral infections, autoimmune diathesis, and preexisting hepatic abnormalities. Liver function should be monitored during therapy.[26]

Nonsteroidal Immunomodulatory Agents

Nonsteroidal immunosuppressant agents have also been studied in TED, both in combination with corticosteroids and as steroid-sparing monotherapy. These agents inhibit specific points in the immunopathologic pathway of TED. Those that have demonstrated efficacy in treating TED in vivo include agents targeting T lymphocytes (e.g., teplizumab, cyclosporine), B lymphocytes (e.g., rituximab), IL-6 (e.g., tocilizumab), tumor necrosis factor (e.g., infliximab), and insulin-like growth factor 1 receptor (e.g., teprotumumab).[53–57] Agents that have demonstrated in vitro efficacy target platelet-derived growth factors (e.g., imatinib), TSHR, and IL-1 (e.g., anakinra).[58,59] Although these treatments may ultimately represent significant therapeutic advances, many have been studied only in small pilot studies or in case series, and true efficacy and long-term safety are yet to be determined. Additionally, intravenous immunoglobulin therapy has been found to be as effective as oral GCs with a low rate of adverse effects.[60] However, the high cost limits its use as a first-line therapy. Somatostatin analogs were studied in four placebo-controlled trials that demonstrated no benefit and troublesome gastrointestinal side effects.[61] There is also evidence that nonsteroidal anti-inflammatory agents may be of benefit.[62]

Orbital Radiotherapy

Orbital radiotherapy, or ORT, has been used in treating TED for more than 80 years.[63] Typically external beam radiation is used, but there may be a role for brachytherapy.[64] The efficacy of ORT in TED is hypothesized to be related to the modulation of the permanent resident components of the autoimmune process.[65] It has also been appreciated that ORT induces terminal differentiation of progenitor fibroblasts, decreases adhesion of blood-borne lymphocytes to activated endothelial cells, and reduces the secretion of proinflammatory cytokines from activated lymphocytes.[66–68] Given the immunomodulatory mechanism of ORT, ideal candidates for ORT are patients in the early, active phase of TED with moderate to severe or rapidly progressive disease, including patients with significant motility deficits and thyroid eye disease–compressive optic neuropathy (TED-CON). ORT should generally be used in conjunction with corticosteroid therapy when a response to corticosteroids demonstrates the immunomodulatory therapeutic potential of ORT.[69] Patients with mild or inactive disease will not benefit from ORT compared to the natural history of the disease.[70] ORT has the largest effect on dysmotility, some effect on soft-tissue swelling, and minimal effect on exophthalmos.[71–74,75] ORT may be particularly useful in cases of TED-CON and may obviate the need for surgical decompression.[76] A large body of evidence accumulated over time suggests that ocular and systemic sequelae of ORT may be minimal when used judiciously.[77,78]

Thyroidectomy

It has been observed that treatment of hyperthyroidism with either antithyroid drugs or thyroidectomy is followed by a gradual decrease in TSHR antibody levels, with disappearance in most patients after 18 months.[79] In contrast, RAI therapy leads to an increase in TSHR antibody levels that may span a year and decline only slowly thereafter. A retrospective study compared near-total thyroidectomy with total thyroidectomy plus RAI (total thyroid ablation) in patients with active TED. Both patient groups received postoperative IVGCs as TED therapy. Using a composite outcome (proptosis, CAS, eyelid fissure height, diplopia), results at 9 months after surgery suggested that total thyroid ablation was superior to near-total thyroidectomy.[80] The previously referenced longitudinal cohort study of 8404 patients also found that surgical thyroidectomy alone or in combination with medical therapy was associated with a 74% decreased hazard for the development of TED compared with RAI alone.[30] Whether total thyroid ablation (or near-total thyroidectomy) is to be favored over methimazole therapy in patients with hyperthyroidism with significant TED awaits future prospective studies that directly compare these modalities.

Inactive Thyroid Eye Disease

The management of inactive TED is primarily surgical. After resolution of the active, inflammatory phase, patients often do not return to their predisease state and may be left with significant proptosis, eyelid retraction, and restrictive strabismus. It is during this period of stability that planned surgical rehabilitation can be considered. Most surgeons agree that, in the absence of vision-threatening complications, surgical intervention for TED should be performed only in patients whose disease has been inactive for at least 6 months, as demonstrated by stability of their clinical examination results, including orthoptic measurements. However, even during periods of apparent disease quiescence, reactivation of TED can occur. Recurrence of active phase orbitopathy may occur in up to 15% of cases and typically occurs at an interval of 10 years after initial onset.[3]

Before any surgical intervention medical therapy should be optimized and a thorough discussion regarding risks and anticipated benefits of any intervention should occur with the patient. The need for each procedure is considered in an attempt to restore the patient to his or her premorbid state from both the functional and aesthetic perspectives. In cases of elective intervention, surgical rehabilitation is typically staged, proceeding in the following sequence:

1. Orbital decompression surgery
2. Strabismus (eye muscle) surgery
3. Eyelid surgery

This progression attempts to optimize the effectiveness of each intervention and minimize the need for repeat surgery, as each procedure has an effect on the magnitude or necessity of the subsequent procedures. In the appropriate clinical context, unnecessary steps may be omitted from this surgical progression, and, occasionally, multiple steps may be combined.[81] The gold standard for any surgical intervention should be to return the patient to the predisease state as guided by prior photographs.

Surgical Decompression of the Orbit

Surgical decompression is used to address proptosis or optic nerve compression and can involve surgical removal of orbital fat or removal of the orbital walls. It is most effectively performed when customized to the individual patient, taking into account the amount of proptosis reduction desired, the nature of the soft-tissue expansion that produced the proptosis, and the relative risk associated with each surgical approach. The surgical effect of bone removal is additive; the more bone removed, the greater the proptosis reduction. Of note, endoscopic approaches to the medial wall and floor have the advantage of easier access to the most posterior air cells, which is particularly important when the surgical goal is apical decompression. In addition, sinus outflow can be managed from an endoscopic approach, as it provides superior visualization to the deeper spaces in the periorbital sinuses.

Strabismus Surgery

TED strabismus is caused by fibrosis of the rectus muscles. Therapeutic options for double vision include prism glasses, botulinum toxin injection to the extraocular muscles, and surgical repositioning of the extraocular muscles.[82] The goal is to provide a zone of single binocular vision in primary gaze and downgaze. Peripheral diplopia often persists but may improve after surgery.[83] Although the most commonly affected extraocular muscles are the inferior and medial recti, it is important to consider the role of the superior recti and the secondary effect of each of these muscles in the surgical plan. Intraoperatively, forced duction testing should guide the surgical plan and recession of the Tenon capsule from the conjunctiva may improve globe rotation.[84]

Eyelid Retraction Surgery

Upper and lower eyelid retraction can result from multiple mechanisms, including exophthalmos, fibrosis of the eyelid protractors and conjunctiva, overaction of the superior rectus–levator complex secondary to restriction of the ipsilateral inferior rectus muscle, and overaction of the Müller muscle secondary to persistent hyperthyroidism.[85] Recession of the inferior or superior rectus muscle can also create or worsen retraction of the associated eyelid. Upper lid retraction repair has been addressed historically by a variety of surgical procedures, but the recently described full-thickness blepharotomy has the advantages of simplicity, patient comfort, speed, limited intraoperative swelling, and good outcomes in terms of lid height and contour.[86,87] Lower eyelid retraction can be treated with release of the lower eyelid retractors in mild cases, but moderate to large retraction typically requires the use of spacer grafts. Options for spacer grafts include autografts (free tarsal/conjunctival, oral mucosa, nasal mucosa, or auricular cartilage), allografts (acellular dermal matrix), and xenografts (e.g., porcine acellular dermal matrix).

Considerations in Thyroid Eye Disease Optic Neuropathy

The most severe clinical manifestation of TED is vision loss due to TED-CON. Theoretical mechanisms for optic neuropathy are direct compression of the optic nerve by pathologically enlarged rectus muscles, generalized compression from enlargement of both the rectus muscles and the orbital fat resulting in annular pressure delivered to the optic nerve, and stretching of the optic nerve, typically caused by profound expansion of the orbital fat compartment.[88] Treatment of TED-CON can be surgical or nonsurgical. Surgical treatment is effective but has limitations, including increased risks and less predictable postoperative outcomes. Moreover, decompression surgery in the acute phase does not routinely shorten the course of the orbitopathy. When performed in the presence of enlarged extraocular muscles, decompression of the orbital apex is most important. In cases of annular compression or optic nerve stretch producing optic neuropathy in stable-phase cases, reversal of the optic neuropathy can be achieved by removal of orbital fat alone.[89]

Alternatively, when TED-CON is present in the active disease, corticosteroids can rapidly reduce inflammation and quickly improve optic nerve function. If response to corticosteroid therapy is evident in TED-CON, the addition of ORT can be considered. However, if a 2-week trial of prednisone (1 mg/kg) fails to reverse TED-CON, then the addition of ORT is unlikely to be effective. In such cases, the authors proceed to surgical decompression. The authors believe that treatment with ORT after corticosteroids favorably shortens the active phase of TED and reverses TED-CON in a high percentage of patients, allowing for corticosteroids to be discontinued without recurrence of CON.[76,90] The effect of ORT is first appreciated by 4 weeks, but the full benefit may not be seen until 3 months. The dose of corticosteroids can be tapered during this period at a rate titrated against the response of the optic neuropathy. After ORT and corticosteroids reverse TED-CON and stabilize patients with TED, orbital decompression surgery can be performed electively in the stable phase, if indicated. Furthermore, the administration of ORT in moderate to severe, noncompressive disease may prevent TED-CON in a patient in who it might otherwise develop.[76,90]

Conclusions

TED is an autoimmune inflammatory disease that causes significant discomfort, disfigurement, and threat to visual function. A complete understanding of the immunologic mechanisms is evolving, but the process likely involves both cellular and humoral immunity targeting developmentally plastic orbital fibroblast precursors. In patients with active TED, smoking cessation should be encouraged, RAI should generally be avoided, and patients should be screened for OSA and hyperlipidemia. Medical optimization should be achieved in conjunction with an endocrinologist, and surgical thyroidectomy can be considered in appropriate cases. Given its biphasic disease course—with the active, inflammatory phase preceding the inactive, fibrotic phase—accurate assessment of disease activity is preeminent in guiding appropriate therapy, which may be aided by use of the VISA classification system. Active-phase treatments, when indicated by rapidly progressive disease or by vision-threatening sequelae such as optic neuropathy, are typically immunomodulatory in nature and may include corticosteroids, ORT, and other immunosuppressive agents. With the exception of orbital decompression surgery, which may be considered in the active phase, surgical intervention should be deferred to the inactive phase of the disease when interventions are more safe, predictable, and effective. Although there are some exceptions, surgical rehabilitation generally should follow the sequence of orbital decompression surgery, strabismus surgery, and eyelid surgery. Future studies of immunomodulatory agents may eventually move them to the forefront of therapy for this debilitating disease.

References

1. Dolman, P. (2012). Evaluating Graves' orbitopathy. *Best Practice & Research Clinical Endocrinology & Metabolism, 26*, 229–348.
2. Rundle, F., & Wilson, C. W. (1945). Development and course of exophthalmos and ophthalmoplegia in Graves' disease with special reference to the effect of thyroidectomy. *Clinical Science, 5*, 177–1794.
3. Patel, P., Khandji, J., & Kazim, M. (2015). Recurrent thyroid eye disease. *Ophthalmic Plastic and Reconstructive Surgery, 32*, 445–458.
4. Bartley, G. (1994). The epidemiologic characteristics and clinical course of ophthalmopathy associated with autoimmune thyroid disease in Olmsted County. *Minnesota Transactions of the American Ophthalmological Society, 92*, 477–588.
5. Tanda, M., Piantanida, E., Liparulo, L., Veronesi, G., Lai, A., Sassi, L., et al. (2013). Prevalence and natural history of Graves' orbitopathy in a large series of patients with newly diagnosed Graves' hyperthyroidism seen at a single center. *Journal of Clinical Endocrinology and Metabolism, 98*, 1443–1449.
6. Laurberg, P., Berman, D. C., Bülow Pedersen, I., Andersen, S., & Carlé. (2012). Incidence and clinical presentation of moderate to severe Graves' orbitopathy in a Danish population before and after iodine fortification of salt. *Journal of Clinical Endocrinology and Metabolism, 97*, 2325–2332.

7. Bahn, R. (2010). Graves' ophthalmopathy. *New England Journal of Medicine, 362*, 726–738.
8. Bahn, R. (2003). Clinical review 157: Pathophysiology of Graves' ophthalmopathy: The cycle of disease. *Journal of Clinical Endocrinology and Metabolism, 88*, 1939–1946.
9. Smith, T., Bahn, R. S., & Gorman, C. A. (1990). Connective tissue, glycosaminoglycans, and diseases of the thyroid. *Endocrine Reviews, 10*, 366–391.
10. Kumar, S., Iyer, S., Bauer, H., Coenen, M., & Bahn, R. S. (2012). A stimulatory thyrotropin receptor antibody enhances hyaluronic acid synthesis in Graves' orbital fibroblasts: Inhibition by an IGF-1 receptor blocking antibody. *Journal of Clinical Endocrinology and Metabolism, 97*, 1681–1687.
11. Kumar, S., Nadeem, S., Stan, M. N., et al. (2011). A stimulatory TSH receptor antibody enhances adipogenesis via phosphoinositide 3-kinase activation in orbital preadipocytes from patients with Graves' ophthalmopathy. *Journal of Molecular Endocrinology, 46*, 155–163.
12. Smith, T. (2015). TSH-receptor-expressing fibrocytes and thyroid-associated ophthalmopathy. *Nature Reviews Endocrinology, 11*, 171–181.
13. Wiersinga, W. (2011). Autoimmunity in Graves' ophthalmopathy: The result of an unfortunate marriage between TSH receptors and IGF-1 receptors? *Journal of Clinical Endocrinology and Metabolism, 96*, 2386–2394.
14. Krieger, C., Neumann, S., Place, R. F., Marcus-Samuels, B., & Gershengorn, M. C. (2015). Bidirectional TSH and IGF-1 receptor cross talk mediates stimulation of hyaluronan secretion by Graves' disease immunoglobulins. *Journal of Clinical Endocrinology and Metabolism, 100*, 1071–1077.
15. Jacobson, E., & Tomer, Y. (2007). The CD40, CTLA-4, thyroglobulin, TSH receptor, and PTPN22 gene quintet and its contribution to thyroid autoimmunity: Back to the future. *Journal of Autoimmunity, 28*, 85–98.
16. Yin, X., Latif, R., Bahn, R., Tomer, Y., & Davies, T. F. (2008). Influence of the TSH receptor gene on susceptibility to Graves' disease and graves' ophthalmopathy. *Thyroid, 11*, 1201–1206.
17. Tomer, Y., & Menconi, F. (2009). Type 1 diabetes and autoimmune thyroiditis: The genetic connection. *Thyroid, 19*, 99–102.
18. Wiersinga, W., & Bartalena, L. (2004). Epidemiology and prevention of Graves' ophthalmopathy. *Thyroid, 12*, 855–860.
19. Thornton, J., Kelly, S. P., Harrison, R. A., & Edwards, R. (2007). Cigarette smoking and thyroid eye disease: A systematic review. *Eye (London, England), 21*, 1135–1145.
20. Traisk, F., Tallstedt, L., Abraham-Nordling, M., Andersson, T., Berg, G., Calissendorff, J., et al. (2009). Thyroid-associated ophthalmopathy after treatment for Graves' hyperthyroidism with antithyroid drugs or iodine-131. *Journal of Clinical Endocrinology and Metabolism, 94*, 3700–3707.
21. Bartalena, L., Marcocci, C., Tanda, M. L., Manetti, L., Dell'Unto, E., Bartomei, M. P., et al. (1998). Cigarette smoking and treatment outcomes in Graves' ophthalmopathy. *Annals of Internal Medicine, 129*, 632–635.
22. Cawood, T., Moriarty, P., O'Farrelly, C., & O'Shea, D. (2007). Smoking and thyroid-associated ophthalmopathy: A novel explanation of the biological link. *Journal of Clinical Endocrinology and Metabolism, 92*, 59–64.
23. Vink, J., Jansen, R., Brooks, A., Willemsen, G., van Grootheest, G., de Geus, E., et al. (2017). Differential gene expression patterns between smokers and non-smokers: Cause or consequence? *Addiction Biology, 22*, 550–560.
24. Tallstedt, L., Lundell, G., Tørring, O., Wallin, G., Ljunggren, J. G., Blomgren, H., et al. (1992). Occurrence of ophthalmopathy after treatment for Graves' hyperthyroidism: The Thyroid Study Group. *New England Journal of Medicine, 326*, 1733–1738.
25. Bartalena, L., Marcocci, C., Bogazzi, F., Panicucci, M., Lepri, A., & Pinchera, A. (1989). Use of corticosteroids to prevent progression of Graves' ophthalmopathy after radioiodine therapy for hyperthyroidism. *New England Journal of Medicine, 321*, 1349–1352.
26. Bartalena, L., Baldeschi, L., Dickinson, A. J., Eckstein, A., Kendall-Taylor, P., Marcocci, C., et al. (2008). Consensus statement of the European group on Graves' orbitopathy (EUGOGO) on management of Graves' orbitopathy. *Thyroid, 18*, 333–346.
27. Lai, A., Sassi, L., Compri, E., Marino, F., Sivelli, P., Plantanida, E., et al. (2010). Lower dose prednisone prevents radioiodine-associated exacerbation of initially mild or absent Graves' orbitopathy: A retrospective cohort study. *Journal of Clinical Endocrinology and Metabolism, 95*, 1333–1337.
28. Bahn Chair, R. S., Burch, H. B., Cooper, D. S., Garber, J. R., Greenlee, M. C., Klein, I., et al. (2011). Hyperthyroidism and other causes of thyrotoxicosis: Management guidelines of the American thyroid association and American association of clinical endocrinologists. *Thyroid, 21*, 593–646.
29. Prummel, M. F., Wiersinga, W. M., Mourits, M. P., Koorneef, L., Berghout, A., & van der Gaag, R. (1998). Effect of abnormal thyroid function on the severity of Graves' ophthalmopathy. *Archives of Internal Medicine, 150*, 1098–1101.
30. Stein, J., Childers, D., Gupta, S., Talwar, N., Nan, B., Lee, B. J., et al. (2015). Risk factors for developing thyroid associated ophthalmopathy among individual with Graves disease. *JAMA Ophthalmology, 133*, 290–296.
31. Sabini, E., Mazzi, B., Profilo, M. A., Mautone, T., Casini, G., Rocchi, R., et al. (2018). High serum cholesterol is a novel risk factor for Graves orbitopathy: Results of a cross sectional study. *Thyroid, 28*, 386–394.
32. Lee, B., Kumar, V. B., Biswas, P., Ko, A. C., Alameddine, R. M., Granet, D. B., et al. (2018). Transcriptome analysis of orbital adipose tissue in active thyroid eye disease using next generation RNA sequencing technology. *Open Ophthalmology Journal, 12*, 41–52.
33. Habib, L., Godfrey, K. J., Mathews, P., De Rojas, J., & Kazim, M. (2019). Association of risk of obstructive sleep apnea with thyroid eye disease compressive optic neuropathy. *Ophthalmic Plastic and Reconstructive Surgery, 35*(3), 232–234.
34. Metcalfe, R., & Weetman, A. P. (1994). Stimulation of extraocular muscle fibroblasts by cytokines and hypoxia: Possible role in thyroid-associated ophthalmopathy. *Clinical Endocrinology, 40*, 67–72.
35. Perrini, S., Cignarelli, A., Quaranta, V. N., Falcone, V. A., Kounaki, S., Porro, S., et al. (2017). Correction of intermittent hypoxia reduces inflammation in obese subjects with obstructive sleep apnea. *Journal of Clinical Investigation Insight, 2*(17). pii.94379.
36. de Lima, F., Mazzotti, D. R., Tufik, S., & Bittencourt, L. (2015). The role inflammatory response genes in obstructive sleep apnea syndrome: A review. *Sleeping & Breathing, 20*, 331–338.
37. Khoo, D., Eng, P. H., Ho, S. C., Tai, E. S., Morgenthaler, N. G., Seah, L. L., et al. (2000). Graves' ophthalmopathy in the absence of elevated free thyroxine and triiodothyronine levels: Prevalence, natural history, and thyrotropin receptor antibody levels. *Thyroid, 2000, 10*, 1093–1100.
38. Nugent, R., Belkin, R. I., Neigel, J. M., Rootman, J., Robertson, W. D., Spinelli, J., et al. (1990). Graves orbitopathy: Correlation of CT and clinical findings. *Radiology, 177*, 675–682.
39. Thacker, N., Velez, F. G., Demer, J. L., & Rosenbaum, A. L. (2005). Superior oblique muscle involvement in thyroid ophthalmopathy. *J AAPOS, 9*, 174–178.
40. Davies, M., & Dolman, P. J. (2017). Levator muscle enlargement in thyroid eye disease-related upper eyelid retraction. *Ophthalmic Plastic and Reconstructive Surgery, 33*, 35–39.
41. Oropesa, S., Dunbar, K. E., Godfrey, K. J., Callahan, A. B., Campbell, A. A., & Kazim, M. (2018). Predominant contribution of superior rectus-levator complex enlargement to optic neuropathy and inferior visual field defects in thyroid eye disease. *Ophthalmic Plastic and Reconstructive Surgery.* doi: https://doi.org/10.1097/IOP.0000000000001224 (web archive link).
42. Durairaj, V., Bartley, G. B., & Garrity, J. A. (2006). Clinical features and treatment of Graves ophthalmopathy in pediatric patients. *Ophthalmic Plastic and Reconstructive Surgery, 22*, 7–12.

43. Werner, S. (1969). Classification of the eye changes of Graves' disease. *Journal of Clinical Endocrinology and Metabolism, 29*, 982–984.
44. Mourits, M., Koornneef, L., Wiersinga, W. M., Prummel, M. F., Berghout, A., & van der Gaag, R. (1989). Clinical criteria for the assessment of disease activity in Graves' ophthalmopathy: A novel approach. *British Journal of Ophthalmology, 73*, 639–644.
45. Dolman, P., & Rootman, J. (2006). Visa classification for Graves orbitopathy. *Ophthalmic Plastic and Reconstructive Surgery, 22*, 319–324.
46. Wiersinga, W. (2007). Management of Graves' ophthalmopathy. *Natural Clinical Practice, Endocrinology & Metabolism, 3*, 396–404.
47. Scofield-Kaplan, S., Dunbar, K., & Kazim, M. (2017). Glad Press'n Seal for the treatment of chronic exposure keratopathy. *Ophthalmic Plastic and Reconstructive Surgery, 33*, 152–153.
48. Marcocci, C., Kahaly, G. J., Krassas, G. E., Bartalena, L., Prummel, M., Stahl, M., et al. (2011). Selenium and the course of mild Graves' orbitopathy. *New England Journal of Medicine, 364*, 1920–1931.
49. Kahaly, G., Pitz, S., Hommel, G., & Dittmar, M. (2005). Randomized, single blind trial of intravenous versus oral steroid monotherapy in Graves' orbitopathy. *Journal of Clinical Endocrinology and Metabolism, 90*, 5234–5240.
50. Bartalena, L., Krassas, G. E., Wiersinga, W., Marcocci, C., Salvi, M., Daumerie, C., et al. (2012). Efficacy and safety of three different cumulative doses of intravenous methylprednisolone for moderate to severe and active Graves' orbitopathy. *Journal of Clinical Endocrinology and Metabolism, 97*, 1–10.
51. Marino, M., Morabito, E., Brunetto, M. R., Bartalena, L., Pinchera, A., & Marocci, C. (2004). Acute and severe liver damage associated with intravenous glucocorticoid pulse therapy in patients with graves' ophthalmopathy. *Thyroid, 14*, 403–406.
52. Marcocci, C., Watt, T., Altea, M. A., Rasmussen, A. K., Feldt-Rasmussen, U., Orgiazzi, J., et al. (2012). Fatal and non-fatal adverse events of glucocorticoid therapy for Graves' orbitopathy: A questionnaire survey among members of the European thyroid association. *European Journal of Endocrinology, 166*, 247–253.
53. Smith, T. J., Kahaly, G. J., Ezra, D. G., Fleming, J. C., Dailey, R. A., Tang, R. A., et al. (2017). Teprotumumab for thyroid-associated ophthalmopathy. *New England Journal of Medicine, 376*, 1748–1761.
54. Khanna, D., Chong, K. K., Afifiyan, N. F., Lee, D. K., Garneau, H. C., Goldberg, R. A., et al. (2010). Rituximab treatment of patients with severe, corticosteroid-resistant thyroid-associated ophthalmopathy. *Ophthalmology, 117*, 133–139.
55. Perez-Moreiras, J., Alvarez-Lopez, A., & Gomez, E. C. (2014). Treatment of active corticosteroid-resistant Graves orbitopathy. *Ophthalmic Plastic and Reconstructive Surgery, 30*, 162–167.
56. Weetman, A., McGregor, A. M., Ludgate, M., Beck, L., Mills, P. V., Lazarus, J. H., et al. (1983). Cyclosporine improves Graves ophthalmopathy. *Lancet, 27*, 486–489.
57. Durrani, O., Reuser, T. Q., & Murray, P. I. (2005). Infliximab: A novel treatment for sight-threatening thyroid associated ophthalmopathy. *Orbit, 24*, 117–119.
58. van Steensel, L., Paridaens, D., Schrijver, B., Dingian, G. M., van Daele, P. L., van Hagen, P. M., et al. (2009). Imatinib mesylate and AMN107 inhibit PDGF-signaling in orbital fibroblasts: A potential treatment for Graves ophthalmopathy. *Investigative Ophthalmology & Visual Science, 50*, 3091–3098.
59. Tan, G., Dutton, C. M., & Bahn, R. S. (1996). Interleukin-1 (IL-1) receptor antagonist and soluble IL-1 receptor inhibit IL-1 induced glycosaminoglycan production in cultured human orbital fibroblasts from patients with graves ophthalmopathy. *Journal of Clinical Endocrinology and Metabolism, 81*, 449–452.
60. Kahaly, G., Pitz, S., Müller-Forell, W., & Hommel, G. (1996). Randomized trial of intravenous immunoglobulins versus prednisolone in Graves' ophthalmopathy. *Clinical and Experimental Immunolology, 106*, 197–202.
61. Stiebel-Kalish, H., Robenshtok, E., Hasanreisoglu, M., Ezrachi, D., Shimon, I., & Leibovici, L. (2009). Treatment modalities for Graves ophthalmopathy: systematic review and metaanalysis. *Journal of Clinical Endocrinology and Metabolism, 94*, 2708–2716.
62. Vondrichova, T., de Capretz, A., Parikh, H., Frenander, C., Asman, P., Aberg, M., et al. (2007). COX-2 and SCD, markers of inflammation and adipogenesis, are related to disease activity in Graves' ophthalmopathy. *Thyroid, 17*, 511–517.
63. Juler, F. (1913). Diseases of the orbit acute purulent keratitis in exophthalmos goiter treated by repeated tarsorrhaphy, resection of cervical sympathetic and x-rays: Retention of vision in one eye. *Transactions of the American Ophthalmological Society, 33*, 55–62.
64. Hao, H., Wang, Y., Wang, X., Lua, S., Cui, J., Chen, Y., et al. (2017). Treatment of Graves' ophthalmopathy with an in-house phosphorous-32 source: Initial clinical observations. *Experimental and Therapeutic Medicine, 14*, 2795–2800.
65. Trott, K., & Kamprad, F. (1999). Radiobiological mechanisms of anti-iflammatory radiotherapy. *Radiotherapy and Oncology, 51*, 197–203.
66. Bumann, J., Santo-Höltje, L., Löffer, H., Bamberg, M., & Rodemann, H. P. (1995). Radiation-induced alterations of the proliferative dynamics of human skin fibroblasts after repeated irradiation in the subtherapeutic dose range. *Strahlentherapie und Onkologie, 171*, 35–41.
67. Herskind, C., & Rodemann, H. P. (2000). Spontaneous and radiation-induced differentiation of fibroblasts. *Expimental Gerontology, 25*, 747–755.
68. Lowenthal, J., & Harris, A. W. (1985). Activation of mouse lymphocytes inhibits induction of rapid cell death by x-irradiation. *Journal of Immunolology, 135*, 1119–1125.
69. Marcocci, C., Bartalena, L., Tanda, M. L., Manetti, L., Dell'Unto, E., Rocchi, R., et al. (2001). Comparison of the effectiveness and tolerability of intravenous or oral glucocorticoids associated with orbital radiotherapy in the management of severe Graves' ophthalmopathy: Results of a prospective, single-blind, randomized study. *Journal of Clinical Endocrinology and Metabolism, 86*, 3562–3567.
70. Gorman, C., Garrity, J. A., Fatourechi, V., Bahn, R. S., Petersen, I. A., Stafford, S. L., et al. (2001). A prospective randomized, double-blind, placebo-controlled study of orbital radiotherapy for Graves' ophthalmopathy. *Ophthalmology, 108*, 1523–1534.
71. Bradley, E., Gower, E. W., Bradley, D. J., Meyer, D. R., Cahill, K. V., Custer, P. L., et al. (2008). Orbital radiation for Graves' ophthalmopathy: A report by the American Academy of Ophthalmology. *Ophthalmology, 115*, 398–409.
72. Prummel, M., Mourits, M. P., Blank, L., Berghout, A., Koorneef, L., & Wiersinga, W. M. (1993). Randomized double-blind trial of prednisone versus radiotherapy in Graves' ophthalmopathy. *Lancet, 342*, 949–954.
73. Tsujino, K., Hirota, S., Hagiwara, M., Fukada, S., Takada, Y., Hishikawa, Y., et al. (2000). Clinical outcomes of orbital radiation combined with or without systemic high-dose or pulse corticosteroids for Graves' ophthalmopathy. *International Journal of Radiation Oncology, Biology, Physics, 48*, 857–864.
74. Ng, C., Yuen, H. K., Choi, K. L., Chan, M. K., Yue, K. T., Ng, Y. W., et al. (2005). Combined orbital irradiation and systemic steroids compared with systemic steroids alone in the management of moderate-to-severe Graves' ophthalmopathy: A preliminary study. *Hong Kong Medical Journal, 11*, 322–330.
75. Prummel, M. F., Terwee, C. B., Gerding, M. N., Baldeschi, L., Mourits, M. P., Blank, L., et al (2004). A randomized controlled trial of orbital radiotherapy versus sham irradiation in patients with mild Graves' ophthalmopathy. *Journal of Clinical Endocrinology and Metabolism, 89*, 15–20.
76. Kazim, M., & Trokel, S. (1991). Treatment of acute Graves' orbitopathy. *Ophthalmology, 98*, 1443–1448.
77. Marcocci, C., Bartalena, L., Rocchi, R., Marinò, M., Menconi, F., Morabito, E., et al. (2003). Long-term safety of orbital radiotherapy for Graves' ophthalmopathy. *Journal of Clinical Endocrinology and Metabolism, 88*, 3561–3566.
78. Wakelkamp, I., Tan, H., Saeed, P., Schlingemann, R. O., Verbraak, F. D., Blank, L. E., et al. (2004). Orbital irradiation for

Graves' ophthalmopathy: Is it safe? A long-term follow-up study. *Ophthalmology, 111*, 557–562.

79. Laurberg, P., Wallin, G., Tallstedt, L., et al. (2008). TSH-receptor autoimmunity in Graves' disease after therapy with anti-thyroid drugs, surgery, or radioiodine: A 5-year prospective randomized study. *European Journal of Endocrinology, 158*, 69–75.
80. Menconi, F., Marinò, M., Pinchera, A., Rocci, Mazzi, B., Nardi, M., et al. (2007). Effects of total thyroid ablation versus near-total thyroidectomy alone on mild to moderate Graves' orbitopathy treated with intravenous glucocorticoids. *Journal of Clinical Endocrinology and Metabolism, 92*, 1653–1658.
81. McCracken, M., del Prado, J. D., Granet, D. B., Levi, L., & Kikkawa, D. O. (2008). Combined eyelid and strabismus surgery: Examining conventional surgical wisdom. *Journal of Pediatric Ophthalmology & Strabismus, 45*, 220–224.
82. Granet, D., Hodgson, N., Godfrey, K. J., Ventura, R., Kikkada, D. O., Levi, L., et al. (2016). Chemodenervation of extraocular muscles in thyroid eye disease. *Graefe's Archive for Clinical and Experimental Ophthalmology, 254*, 999–1003.
83. Scofield-Kaplan, S., Dunbar, K., Stein, G., & Kazim, M. (2018). Improvement in both primary and eccentric ocular alignment after thyroid eye disease strabismus surgery with Tenon's recession. *Ophthalmic Plastic and Reconstructive Surgery, 34*, S85–S89.
84. Zoumalan, C., Lelli, G. J., & Kazim, M. (2011). Tenon recession: A novel adjunct to improve outcome in the treatment of large-angle strabismus in thyroid eye disease. *Ophthalmic Plastic and Reconstructive Surgery, 27*, 287–292.
85. Cruz, A., Ribeiro, S. F., Garcia, D. M., Akaishi, P. M., & Pinto, C. T. (2013). Graves' upper eyelid retraction. *Survey of Ophthalmology, 58*, 63–76.
86. Demirci, H., Hassan, A. S., Reck, S. D., Frueh, B. R., & Elner, V. M. (2007). Graded full-thickness anterior blepharotomy for correction of upper eyelid retraction not associated with thyroid eye disease. *Ophthalmic Plastic and Reconstructive Surgery, 23*, 39–45.
87. Nimitwongsakul, A., Zoumalan, C. I., & Kazim, M. (2013). Modified full-thickness blepharotomy for treatment of thyroid eye disease. *Ophthalmic Plastic and Reconstructive Surgery, 29*, 44–47.
88. Neigel, J., Rootman, J., Belkin, R. I., Nugent, R. A., Drance, S. M., Beattie, C. W., et al. (1988). Dysthyroid optic neuropathy: The crowded orbital apex syndrome. *Ophthalmology, 95*, 1515–1521.
89. Kazim, M., Trokel, S. L., Acaroglu, G., & Elliott, A. (2000). Reversal of dysthyroid optic neuropathy following orbital fat decompression. *British Journal of Ophthalmology, 84*, 600–605.
90. Gold, K., Scofield, S., Isaacson, S. R., Stewart, M. D., & Kazim, M. (2018). Orbital radiotherapy for thyroid eye disease compressive optic neuropathy. *Ophthalmic Plastic and Reconstructive Surgery, 34*, 172–177.

19

Surgical Indications and Outcomes of Orbital Decompression Surgery

VICTORIA S. LEE, MD AND ANDREW P. LANE, MD

Orbital decompression surgery is being increasingly used in the treatment of urgent and nonurgent complications related to Graves ophthalmopathy. An understanding of the specific indication for pursuing surgery is critical in deciding the optimal timing of the surgery, formulating the surgical plan, and determining the most relevant clinical outcomes. Quality-of-life (QOL) outcomes are also gaining increasing importance in assessing surgical success.

Surgical Indications

Graves Ophthalmopathy

Graves ophthalmopathy, also known as thyroid eye disease (TED), is the most common indication for orbital decompression surgery.

Urgent Indications

Dysthyroid (compressive) optic neuropathy (DON), which has an estimated incidence of 3% to 9% in patients with TED, is an urgent indication for orbital decompression surgery.[1,2] Extraocular muscle enlargement restricting the vascular supply to the optic nerve is the most well-accepted mechanism of DON. The diagnosis is challenging and controversial. It is considered primarily a clinical diagnosis, evidenced by decreased visual acuity, a relative afferent pupillary defect, altered color vision, optic disc abnormalities, and visual field defects. Studies have also investigated the diagnostic role of imaging, in particular computed tomography (CT), in assessing features associated with DON, including muscle enlargement, crowding of the orbital apex, and prolapse of fat through the superior orbital fissure. Magnetic resonance imaging may also be useful to evaluate changes in the optic nerve. Once the diagnosis is made, first-line treatment typically consists of pulsed high-dose intravenous steroids. Orbital radiation therapy, which can be used alone or in combination with steroid treatment, has been shown to be particularly useful in the treatment of mild to moderate active TED and in improving extraocular movements. Orbital decompression surgery is considered if the response to these interventions is poor and/or if there is clinical worsening. Surgical approaches and the extent of bony wall removal vary and are covered in detail in Chapters 20 and 21, but it is worth noting that in DON, decompression of the medial orbital wall is particularly critical, as this can be achieved most completely along the length of the intraorbital portion of the optic nerve.[2]

Severe corneal exposure can also lead to vision loss. In TED, persistent eyelid retraction related to inflammation and scarring of the eyelid retractors and the Whitnall ligament commonly results in lagophthalmos, increasing corneal exposure. Worsening proptosis can further increase corneal exposure and predispose patients to ulceration and subsequent vision compromise. If this exposure proves refractory to conservative measures, such as lubrication, lid taping, and botulinum toxin injections, orbital decompression surgery is urgently indicated.[3]

Nonurgent Indications

Medical therapy, including oral and intravenous steroids, is generally pursued initially in the absence of immediate surgical indications. In a recent survey of the American Society of Ophthalmic Plastic and Reconstructive Surgery, 83% of respondents preferred steroids as first-line treatment compared with only 10% of respondents who preferred orbital decompression surgery. As second-line and third-line treatment, 39% and 61% of respondents, respectively, preferred orbital decompression surgery.[4] Most patients respond well to conservative measures, but an estimated 5% undergo orbital decompression surgery in the first year after diagnosis and up to 20% in the first 10 years after diagnosis.[1]

Nonurgent indications for orbital decompression surgery include diplopia, proptosis, orbital and retrobulbar pain, and ocular hypertension. Surgery may also be indicated to improve cosmesis in TED.[1] It is generally recommended to avoid performing surgery in the inflammatory phase of TED, as studies have shown that surgical manipulation during this phase may significantly worsen orbital inflammation.[1,5,6] Orbital decompression surgery is typically recommended to be performed first before addressing the extraocular muscles and eyelid surgically.[1]

Additional Indications

Although TED is the most common indication for orbital decompression surgery, it may be indicated for other reasons. These include iatrogenic complications, such as orbital hematomas, trauma-related issues, neoplasms, and for cosmesis in patients with proptosis for other reasons.[7]

Surgical Contraindications

There are no absolute contraindications to orbital decompression surgery specifically. The surgery, however, does require the use of a general anesthetic, and patients may have comorbid conditions that affect their candidacy as in any other surgery. Patients taking anticoagulants should ideally discontinue them perioperatively, as bleeding can limit intraoperative visualization and increase the risk of postoperative hemorrhage. Patients with concurrent chronic sinusitis should receive appropriate medical therapy to treat chronic sinusitis, e.g. oral steroids and/or antibiotics, to optimize healing after surgery. The surgical plan may also involving opening diseased sinuses such as the frontal and sphenoid that are not necessarily required in orbital decompression surgery.

Patient Selection

The ophthalmologist typically identifies patients who meet indications for orbital decompression surgery, subsequently referring them to the otolaryngologist if an endoscopic approach is being considered. In a study of factors associated with greater quality of improvements after surgery, only nonwhite ethnic background was identified as a positive predictor, indicating that the benefit after surgery may be difficult to predict based on a patient's characteristics, history, and clinical presentation and evaluation. This study also found possible concurrent clinical depression and anxiety in 26% and 37% of patients, respectively, lending support to addressing comorbid psychiatric conditions to optimize outcomes.[8]

Decompression can include fat and/or bone removal, and patient selection also involves deciding whether the risk/benefit ratio is optimal with fat removal alone, bone removal alone, or fat and bone removal. Recent data have shown that fat removal achieves particularly reliable results in patients with proptosis secondary to either expansion of the fat compartment or enlargement of extraocular muscles, but not both, suggesting that in these patients it may be considered as a stand-alone option.[9]

Outcomes

The relevant outcomes of orbital decompression depend on the specific surgical indications. They can generally be divided into the following categories: clinical outcomes, radiographic-based outcomes, and QOL outcomes (Table 19-1).

Clinical Outcomes

For urgent orbital decompression in the setting of DON, visual acuity is a key outcome. Studies have demonstrated high success rates, with visual acuity improving in 82% to 88% of patients. The remainder of the patients had lack of improvement in their vision—not worsening—with stabilization of their visual loss.[1,10,11] For patients without DON, the rates of visual acuity improvement may be lower.[1,11] In patients with DON, intraocular pressure (IOP) is also assessed. Orbital decompression surgery has been shown to result in decreased IOPs 2 months postoperatively but may also result in slightly increased IOPs immediately after surgery.[7]

For nonurgent orbital decompression surgery, proptosis is an important outcome. Orbital fat removal alone has been shown to reduce proptosis by 1.8 to 4.7 mm.[10] Decompression of the medial, inferior, and/or lateral walls has been shown to reduce proptosis by 3.2 to 7.4 mm.[1,10,12] The presence of diplopia preoperatively may affect the reduction in proptosis, with one study demonstrating a greater reduction in patients with diplopia at

TABLE 19.1 Summary of Reported Outcomes in the Literature After Orbital Decompression Surgery

Outcomes	Quoted Values	References
Clinical		
Rate of visual acuity improvement (%)	82 to 88	1, 10, 11
Reduction in proptosis (mm)		
Fat only	1.8 to 4.7	10
Bony walls	3.2 to 7.4	1, 10, 12
Rate of new diplopia (%)	0 to 64	10
Quality of Life		
GO-QOL scale		
Vision-related mean change score (0-100)	8	8
Appearance-related mean change score (0-100)	19.5	8
SNOT-22 questionnaire		
Total mean change score (0-110)	-13.7	19

GO-QOL, Graves' Ophthalmopathy Quality of Life (positive change scores indicate improvement postoperatively); *SNOT-22*, Sinonasal Outcomes Test-22 (negative change scores indicate improvement postoperatively).

presentation compared with patients without diplopia.[10] The recommended extent of bone removal and whether fat removal is recommended instead or adjunctively is controversial. Based on recent systematic reviews, several nonrandomized studies suggest that three-wall decompression achieves the greatest reduction in proptosis but that the complication rates are higher; therefore more conservative decompression, such as balanced medial and lateral wall, may be preferred. Some studies have also suggested that fat removal, when combined with bone removal, results in an even greater improvement. The current literature suffers from lack of randomization and heterogeneity in design, techniques, and methods, making drawing summative conclusions difficult.[13–15]

Diplopia can be considered both an outcome to evaluate and a complication in orbital decompression surgery for any indication. Rates of new diplopia after orbital decompression surgery, with broadly varying indications and approaches, have been quoted to be anywhere from 0 to 64%. In a recent study of 77 patients undergoing orbital decompression surgery at a large academic center, the incidence of postoperative diplopia was low, with no patients reporting new diplopia and only 2 patients reporting worsening of their preoperative diplopia. This study postulated that preservation of the inferomedial strut may be critical in minimizing postoperative diplopia.[10] Further research using standardized indications and approaches is needed to truly assess rates of postoperative diplopia.

Radiographic-Based Outcomes

Imaging measurements may provide more objective outcome evaluation after orbital decompression surgery. Recent research has been focused on developing and establishing the validity of quantitative algorithms to objectively determine various imaging measurements, including the angle of the orbital apex, diameter of the extraocular muscles, exophthalmos, and orbital volume.[16–18] These measurements can be drawn from a CT scan and assessed preoperatively and postoperatively to more objectively evaluate the success of orbital decompression surgery and supplement clinical outcomes. The use of radiographic-based outcomes is not standardly assessed and its specific role in outcome evaluation is yet to be determined.

Quality-of-Life Outcomes

QOL instruments are not currently widely used to assess outcomes after orbital decompression surgery but do evaluate arguably the most relevant outcome: the patient's point of view. A recent study sought to evaluate a patient's QOL changes after orbital decompression surgery using the Graves Ophthalmopathy Quality of Life (GO-QOL) scale. The scale provides vision-related and appearance-related scores, which were assessed before, 6 weeks after, and 6 months after surgery. Patients were included in the study if they had a diagnosis of TED. Interestingly, vision-related QOL did not change until 6 months after surgery, and even then did not reach the minimally clinically important difference. Appearance-related QOL, on the other hand, improved significantly at 6 weeks after surgery and continued to improve at 6 months after surgery, well exceeding the minimal clinically important difference. This study differed from previous studies that showed more improvement in vision-related QOL after surgery, which was potentially attributed to the lack of visual symptoms in the patients included in the study.[8]

A recent study has also examined the impact of orbital decompression surgery on sinonasal-specific QOL. The 22-item Sinonasal Outcomes Test (SNOT-22) was given to patients preoperatively and at least 1 year after surgery. There was a statistically and clinically significant improvement in sinonasal-specific QOL as assessed by the SNOT-22 after orbital decompression surgery, which was primarily driven by improvements in domains 4 and 5 of the questionnaire, which evaluate psychological and sleep dysfunction, respectively.[19] These studies emphasize the importance of QOL outcomes assessment in a variety of areas after orbital decompression surgery and the need for further research in this area.

Pearls

- TED is the most common indication for orbital decompression surgery and is generally considered after medical treatment fails.
- Optic neuropathy and severe corneal exposure are urgent surgical indications. Nonurgent surgical indications include diplopia, proptosis, orbital and retrobulbar pain, and ocular hypertension.
- There are no absolute contraindications to orbital decompression surgery.
- The most relevant clinical outcomes depend on the indication for surgery and can include visual acuity, proptosis, and/or post-operative diplopia.
- Recent research has been focused on the development of imaging measurements obtained from CT scans to more objectively evaluate the success of surgery. QOL instruments are gaining increasing recognition as well.

References

1. Braun, T. L., Bhadkamkar, M. A., Jubbal, K. T., Weber, A. C., & Marx, D. P. (2017). Orbital decompression for thyroid eye disease. *Seminars in Plastic Surgery*, *31*(1), 40–45.
2. Saeed, P., Tavakoli Rad, S., & Bisschop, P. (2018). Dysthyroid optic neuropathy. *Ophthalmic Plastic and Reconstructive Surgery*, *34*(4 Suppl 1), S60–S67.
3. Dagi, L. R., Elliott, A. T., Roper-Hall, G., & Cruz, O. A. (2010). Thyroid eye disease: Honing your skills to improve outcomes. *Journal of the American Association for Pediatric Ophthalmology and Strabismus*, *14*(5), 425–431.
4. Perumal, B., & Meyer, D. R. (2015). Treatment of severe thyroid eye disease: A survey of the American Society of Ophthalmic Plastic and Reconstructive Surgery (ASOPRS). *Ophthalmic Plastic and Reconstructive Surgery*, *31*(2), 127–131.
5. Rao, R., MacIntosh, P. W., Yoon, M. K., & Lefebvre, D. R. (2015). Current trends in the management of thyroid eye disease. *Current Opinion in Ophthalmology*, *26*(6), 484–490.
6. Pletcher, S. D., Sindwani, R., & Metson, R. (2006). Endoscopic orbital and optic nerve decompression. *Otolaryngologic Clinics of North America*, *39*(5), 943–958.
7. Wehrmann, D., & Antisdel, J. L. (2017). An update on endoscopic orbital decompression. *Current Opinion in Otolaryngology & Head and Neck Surgery*, *25*(1), 73–78.
8. Wickwar, S., McBain, H., Ezra, D. G., Hirani, S. P., Rose, G. E., & Newman, S. P. (2015). The psychosocial and clinical outcomes of orbital decompression surgery for thyroid eye disease and predictors of change in quality of life. *Ophthalmology*, *122*(12), 2568–2576.e1.
9. Prat, M. C., Braunstein, A. L., Dagi Glass, L. R., & Kazim, M. (2015). Orbital fat decompression for thyroid eye disease: Retrospective case review and criteria for optimal case selection. *Ophthalmic Plastic and Reconstructive Surgery*, *31*(3), 215–218.
10. Kingdom, T. T., Davies, B. W., & Durairaj, V. D. (2015). Orbital decompression for the management of thyroid eye disease: An analysis of outcomes and complications. *Laryngoscope*, *125*(9), 2034–2040.
11. Jernfors, M., Valimaki, M. J., Setala, K., Malmberg, H., Laitinen, K., & Pitkaranta, A. (2007). Efficacy and safety of orbital decompression in treatment of thyroid-associated ophthalmopathy: Long-term follow-up of 78 patients. *Clinical Endocrinology*, *67*(1), 101–107.
12. Chu, E. A., Miller, N. R., Grant, M. P., Merbs, S., Tufano, R. P., & Lane, A. P. (2009). Surgical treatment of dysthyroid orbitopathy. *Otolaryngology–Head and Neck Surgery*, *141*(1), 39–45.
13. Boboridis, K. G., & Bunce, C. (2011). Surgical orbital decompression for thyroid eye disease. *Cochrane Database of Systematic Reviews*. *2011*(12). CD007630. https://doi.org/10.1002/14651858.CD007630.pub2.
14. Boboridis, K. G., Uddin, J., Mikropoulos, D. G., Bunce, C., Mangouritsas, G., Voudouragkaki, et al. (2015). Critical appraisal on orbital decompression for thyroid eye disease: A systematic review and literature search. *Advances in Therapy*, *32*(7), 595–611.
15. European Group on Graves Orbitopathy (EUGOGO), Mourits, M. P., Bijl, H., Altea, M. A., Baldeschi, L., Boboridis, K., et al. (2009). Outcome of orbital decompression for disfiguring proptosis in patients with Graves' orbitopathy using various surgical procedures. *British Journal of Ophthalmology*, *93*(11), 1518–1523.
16. Kang, E. M., & Yoon, J. S. (2015). Clinical and radiological characteristics of Graves' orbitopathy patients showing spontaneous decompression. *Journal of Cranio-Maxillo-Facial Surgery*, *43*(1), 48–52.
17. Thapa, S., Gupta, A. K., Gupta, A., Gupta, V., Dutta, P., & Virk, R. S. (2015). Proptosis reduction by clinical vs radiological modalities and medial vs inferomedial approaches: Comparison following endoscopic transnasal orbital decompression in patients with dysthyroid orbitopathy. *JAMA Otolaryngology–Head and Neck Surgery*, *141*(4), 329–334.
18. Schiff, B. A., McMullen, C. P., Farinhas, J., Jackman, A. J., Hagiwara, M., McKellop, J., et al. (2015). Use of computed tomography to assess volume change after endoscopic orbital decompression for Graves' ophthalmopathy. *American Journal of Otolaryngology*, *36*(6), 729–735.
19. Mueller, S. K., Miyake, M. M., Lefebvre, D. R., Freitag, S. K., & Bleier, B. S. (2018). Long-term impact of endoscopic orbital decompression on sinonasal-specific quality of life. *Laryngoscope*, *128*(4), 785–788.

20

Endoscopic Orbital Decompression

LEAH NOVINGER, MD, PhD, JONATHAN Y. TING, MD, MS, MBA, AND RAJ SINDWANI, MD, FACS, FRCS(C)

Endoscopic orbital decompression was developed soon after the advent of endoscopic sinus surgery. The technique was first described by Kennedy et al.[1] in 1990 and Michel et al.[2] in 1991 and has gained popularity over the past several decades, now representing about a quarter of orbital decompressions performed in the United States annually.[3] The major advantages of the endoscopic approach include avoidance of an external facial incision and resultant scar, as well as improved visualization of key anatomic structures, particularly in the region of the orbital apex,[4] a critical area of decompression in patients with optic neuropathy.

The major disadvantage of the procedure is coordination between an oculoplastic surgeon and an otolaryngologist and potential longer total operative time.[5] Although no significant difference in cost of the procedure was observed with bivariate analysis,[5] the need for coordination may contribute to the finding that the majority of oculoplastic surgeons surveyed perform the surgery alone via an external approach.[6]

Graves orbitopathy occurs in up to half of patients with Graves disease and is the most common indication for endoscopic orbital decompression. Graves orbitopathy can be associated with visual deficits from optic neuropathy and diplopia.[7] In patients with Graves disease, proptosis and exposure keratopathy are frequent indications for surgery.[8] Graves orbitopathy, also known as thyroid eye disease (TED), is characterized by an initial acute inflammatory phase followed by a chronic, fibrotic phase. Typically decompression is performed in the chronic phase of TED; however, severe symptoms with optic neuropathy during the acute phase may warrant immediate treatment. Other indications for orbital decompression techniques include access for drainage of orbital hematoma or subperiosteal abscess, resection of orbital and intracranial pathology, and transnasal endoscopic intraorbital ligation of the anterior ethmoid artery.

Postoperatively patients undergoing endoscopic orbital decompression for TED reported significantly improved mean scores for the 22-item Sinonasal Outcomes Test from preoperative baseline after 1 year.[9] When a Hertel exophthalmometer (Good-Lite, Elgin, IL) was used, a 3.2-mm reduction in proptosis was observed in patients with medial endoscopic decompression alone, with the addition of an external lateral decompression resulting in an additional 2.4-mm reduction in proptosis.[10] Several studies have used preoperative and postoperative computed tomography imaging to quantitatively assess volume change after decompression. In one study of seven patients, an average increase in volume was 7.3 cm^3 in patients for whom medial and inferior orbital wall decompression was performed while maintaining an inferomedial strut.[11] Another study, in which only medial decompression was performed, found an average increase in 6.08 cm^3 in volume on postoperative imaging of 12 patients.[12]

Anatomy

Several key surgical landmarks are important to safely perform endoscopic orbital decompression[13]; these are listed in Box 20.1. Fig. 20.1 illustrates the area of resection during an endoscopic orbital decompression. The lamina papyracea is the thin orbital plate of the ethmoid bone that forms the medial wall of the orbit that is removed during decompression surgery. It is often very attenuated, medially bowed, or even partially dehiscent in patients with Graves orbitopathy. The infraorbital nerve marks the lateral border of the inferior orbital wall (or floor), which is resected during an orbital decompression. The superior border of the medial wall decompression is defined by the skull base, frontal recess, and location of the anterior and posterior ethmoid arteries. The ethmoid skull base slopes downward in an antero-posterior vector and meets the anterior face of the sphenoid sinus posteriorly. This sphenoethmoid angle represents the posterior limit of orbital decompression.[14]

Appreciating the location of the medial rectus muscle within the surgical field is important to avoid injury and to create a periorbital sling if desired. The medial rectus is located reliably 1.5 cm above the crista ethmoidalis.[15] Preoperative evaluation of imaging is critical when available to review the surgical landmarks and may be supplemented with intraoperative surgical navigation.[16] Of particular importance is identification of sphenoethmoid (Onodi) cells as well as confirmation of the location of anterior and posterior ethmoid arteries and the opticocarotid recess when performing extended orbital procedures.[8]

Technique

Unilateral or bilateral orbital decompression may be performed in a staged fashion or simultaneously on both eyes, depending on surgeon preference. For severe disease, consideration should be given to a balanced three-wall decompression, which combines an endoscopic medial and inferior floor decompression with an external-approach lateral wall decompression via lateral cathotomy. The patient is positioned in the typical fashion for endoscopic sinus surgery after general anesthesia is induced. The eyes are left in the surgical field and are protected with scleral shells or taping. Intranasal vasoconstriction is obtained with oxymetazoline or topical

• BOX 20.1 Key Landmarks in Endoscopic Orbital Decompression

Maxillary Sinus
- Maxillary line
- Uncinate process
- Nasolacrimal canal
- Infraorbital nerve
- Orbital floor–maxillary sinus roof

Ethmoid Sinus
- Middle turbinate
- Skull base
- Lamina papyracea
- Anterior ethmoidal artery
- Sphenoethmoid cell (Onodi cell)

Sphenoid Sinus
- Sphenoid face
- Internal carotid artery within carotid canal
- Optic nerve within optic canal
- Opticocarotid recess

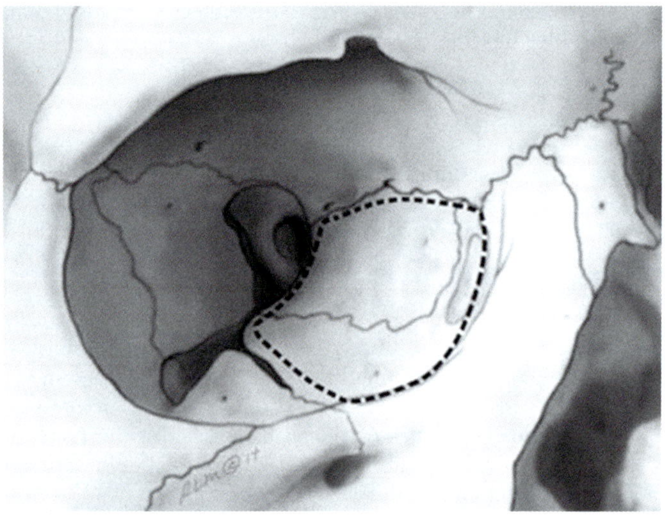

• **Fig. 20.1** Illustration of the boundaries of endoscopic orbital decompression. (Illustration by Robert Margulies. 2014. From Ting, J. Y., & Sindwani, R. [2014]. Endoscopic orbital decompression. *Operative Techniques in Otolaryngology–Head and Neck Surgery, 25*[2], 213–217.)

epinephrine-soaked pledgets and local anesthetic injection per the surgeon's preference. Intraoperative image guidance decreases the risk of complications in endoscopic sinus surgery and should be used during endoscopic orbital decompression if available.[16]

The first goal of the procedure is to obtain adequate visualization of the medial and inferior orbital walls for safe decompression. An uncinectomy is performed and a wide maxillary antrostomy is created to obtain adequate visualization of the posterior maxillary wall and orbital floor, as well as to avoid obstruction of the antrostomy by descendent orbital fat. Total sphenoethmoidectomy exposes the medial orbital wall, extending from the face of the sphenoid sinus down to the crista ethmoidalis and superiorly to the skull base. The middle turbinate may be resected for better visualization and postoperative monitoring. A good practice is to cauterize the posterolateral stump of the middle turbinate to prevent postoperative bleeding issues if the turbinate is resected. Mucosa over the medial orbital wall and medial floor is then removed often using an angled endoscope (Fig. 20.2).

Septoplasty may be performed to improve nasal airway obstruction postoperatively but did not significantly improve the 22-item Sinonasal Outcomes Test score after 1 year in one study of endoscopic orbital decompression.[9]

The second goal of the procedure is to remove bone from the medial and inferior orbital wall. The lamina papyrcea is carefully fractured in a controlled manner with a spoon curette and elevated away from intact periorbita deep to it (Fig. 20.3). Leaving the periorbita undisturbed is important at this stage of the operation. Bony fragments are removed to the level of the skull base superiorly, posteriorly to the sphenoethmoid angle, inferiorly to the orbital floor, and anteriorly to the maxillary line (Fig. 20.4).[8] Care is taken to avoid bony removal anteriorly in the region of the frontal recess to allow for drainage of the frontal sinus, as well as in the area of the anterior and posterior ethmoidal arteries to avoid bleeding.

Thick bone may be encountered posteriorly in the region of the orbital apex within 2 mm of the sphenoid face. This bone corresponds to the annulus of Zinn, from which four of six extraocular muscles originate and through which the optic nerve passes. This landmark represents the posterior limit of a standard medial orbital decompression.

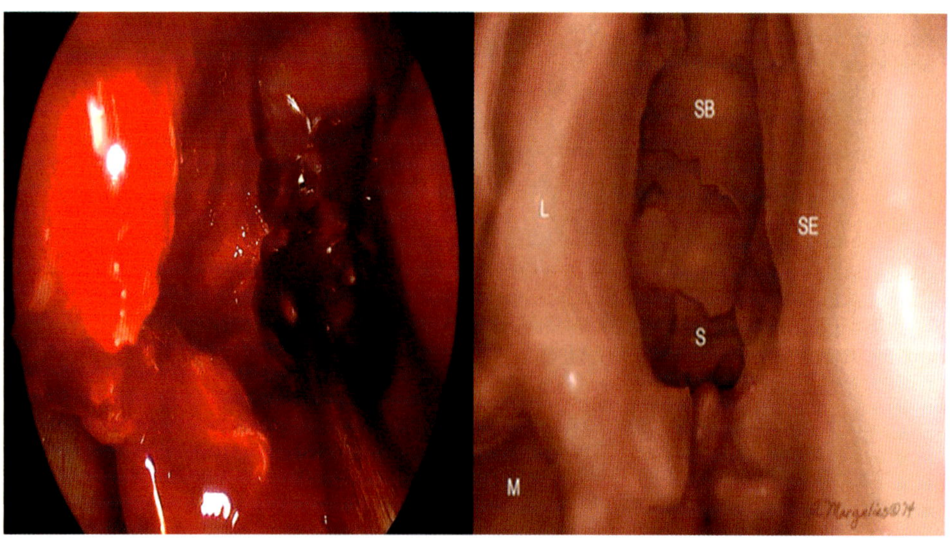

• **Fig. 20.2** Endoscopic image of maxillary antrostomy and sphenoethmoidectomy with middle turbinate resected. *L,* lamina papyracea; *M,* maxillary sinus; s, sphenoid sinus; *SB,* skull base; *SE,* septum). (B, Illustration by Robert Margulies, 2014. From Ting, J. Y., & Sindwani, R. [2014]. Endoscopic orbital decompression. *Operative Techniques in Otolaryngology–Head and Neck Surgery, 25*[2], 213–217.)

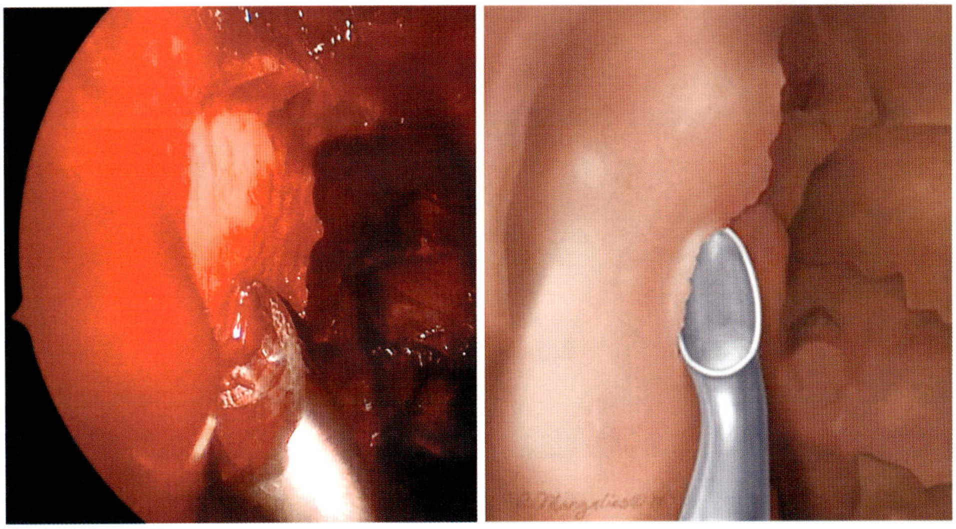

• **Fig. 20.3** Penetration of the medial orbital wall. (B, Illustration by Robert Margulies, 2014. From Ting, J. Y., & Sindwani, R. [2014]. Endoscopic orbital decompression. *Operative Techniques in Otolaryngology–Head and Neck Surgery, 25*[2], 213–217.)

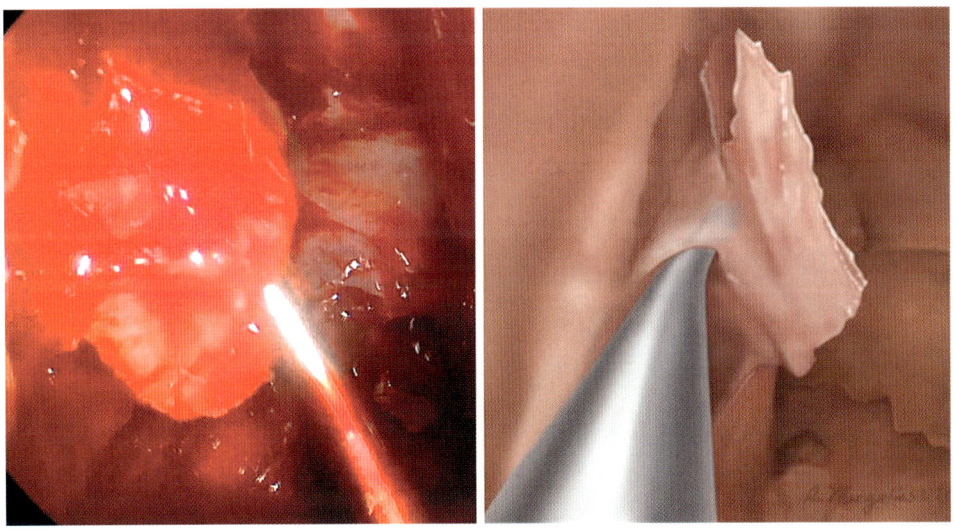

• **Fig. 20.4** Removal of medial orbital wall fragments. (B, Illustration by Robert Margulies, 2014. From Ting, J. Y., & Sindwani, R. [2014]. Endoscopic orbital decompression. *Operative Techniques in Otolaryngology–Head and Neck Surgery, 25*[2], 213–217.)

With the medial wall removed, the periorbita can be followed inferiorly and gently elevated off the bony floor of the medial orbit. A spoon curette or heavier mastoid curette is then insinuated into this plane and used to engage the orbital floor along its medial extent and down-fracture the medial orbital floor (Fig. 20.5). Only the portion of the floor that is medial to the infraorbital nerve is removed. A 30-degree endoscope and angled forceps may facilitate bone removal while preserving the infraorbital canal as the lateral limit of dissection. The infraorbital canal represents a natural cleavage plane. Alternatively, maintenance of a bony inferomedial strut may decrease new postoperative diplopia and improve proptosis.[17]

Once the bony decompression is completed, the final key step of decompression of the actual orbital contents is performed by incising the periorbita. Hemostasis is attained before visual obstruction of the surgical field occurs with dehiscent orbital fat, which can be expected once the investing layer of the periobita is incised. The periorbita can be either incised or removed with a sickle knife or arachnoid blade to enable fat and orbital content herniation into the ethmoid cavity (Fig. 20.6). Care must be taken to avoid "burying" the tip of the sickle knife and potentially injuring the underlying orbital contents, including the medial rectus muscle. This is performed in a posterior to anterior fashion owing to the visual obstruction caused by herniating orbital fat. Parallel axially oriented incisions are performed along the ethmoid roof and orbital floor. A ball-tipped probe and sickle knife may be used to identify and incise remaining fibrous bands that often course superficially between lobules of orbital fat (Fig. 20.7) to completely disrupt the investing periorbita. Upon completion of this portion of the procedure, a generous prolapse of fat into the ethmoid and maxillary cavities should be observed and can be confirmed by ballottement of the eye (Fig. 20.8). Maintenance of a periorbital sling that covers the medial rectus muscle, first described by Metson and Samaha,[18] may decrease postoperative diplopia.[18] A recent study

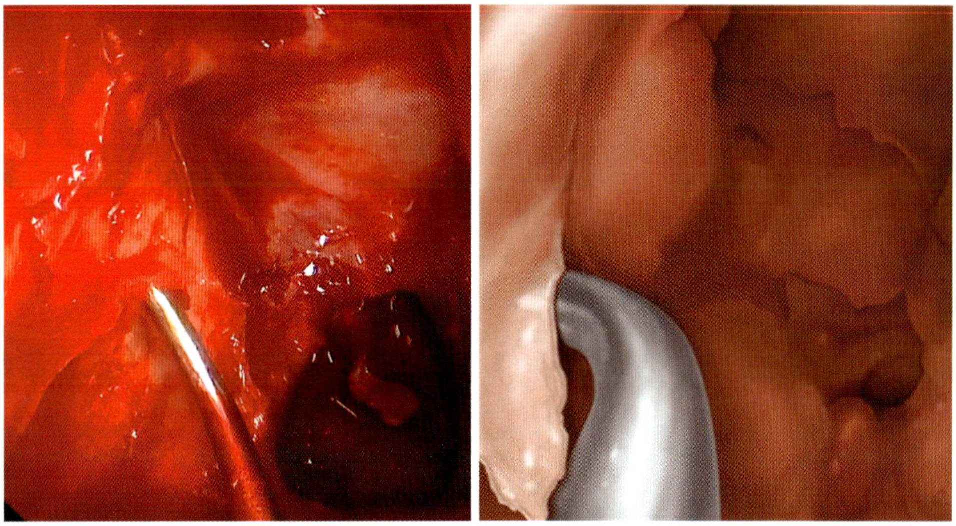

• **Fig. 20.5** Down-fracture of the medial orbital floor. (B, Illustration by Robert Margulies, 2014. From Ting, J. Y., & Sindwani, R. [2014]. Endoscopic orbital decompression. *Operative Techniques in Otolaryngology–Head and Neck Surgery, 25*[2], 213–217.)

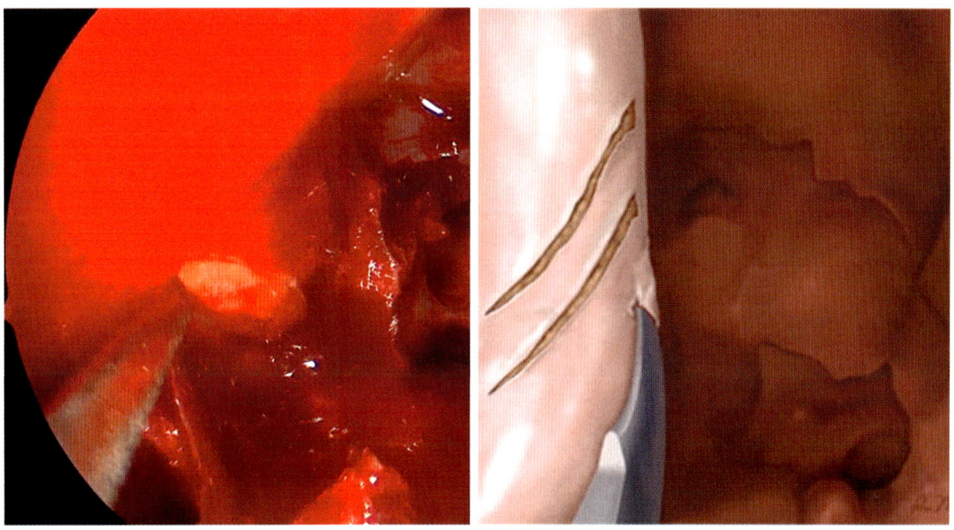

• **Fig. 20.6** Incision of periorbita. (B, Illustration by Robert Margulies, 2014. From Ting, J. Y., & Sindwani, R. [2014]. Endoscopic orbital decompression. *Operative Techniques in Otolaryngology–Head and Neck Surgery, 25*[2], 213–217.)

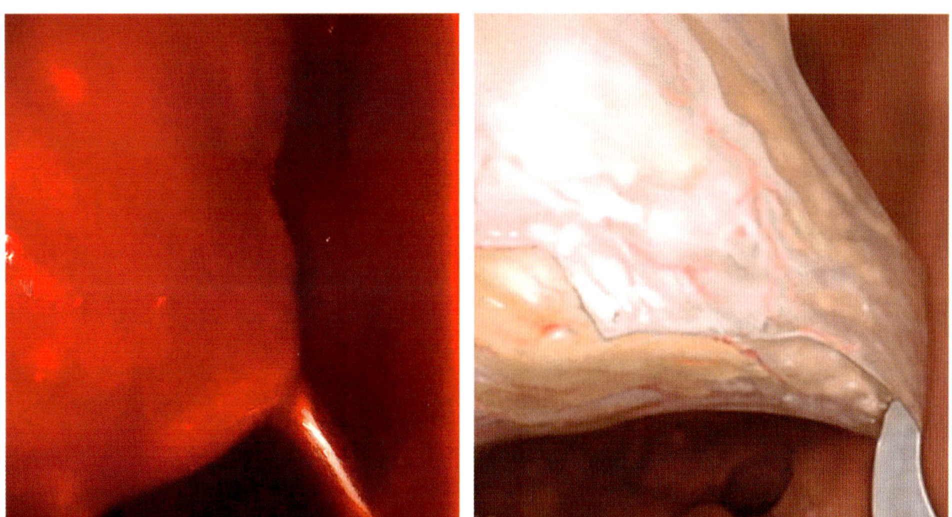

• **Fig. 20.7** Incision of periorbital fibrous bands. (B, Illustration by Robert Margulies, 2014. From Ting, J. Y., & Sindwani, R. [2014]. Endoscopic orbital decompression. *Operative Techniques in Otolaryngology–Head and Neck Surgery, 25*[2], 213–217.)

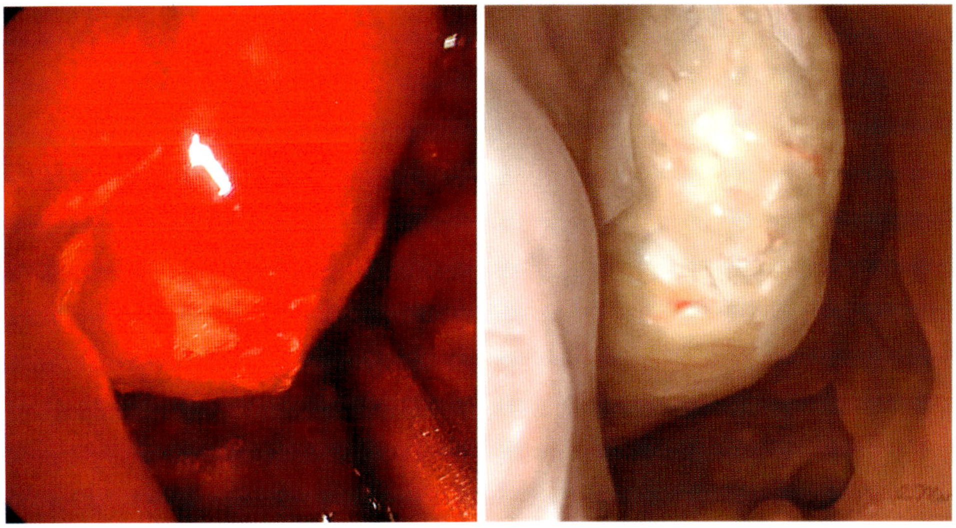

• **Fig. 20.8** Prolapse of orbital fat into maxillary and ethmoid cavities. (B, Illustration by Robert Margulies, 2014. From Ting, J. Y., & Sindwani, R. [2014]. Endoscopic orbital decompression. *Operative Techniques in Otolaryngology–Head and Neck Surgery, 25*[2], 213–217.)

demonstrated that the sling modification does not sacrifice reduction in proptosis while significantly improving preexisting diplopia.[19] Isolated orbital floor decompression and selective decompression (i.e., posterior medial wall alone) are all variants of the technique that have been described.[18,19] Balanced three-wall decompression using an external approach laterally may also help improve postoperative diplopia and provide a more "balanced" recession of orbital contents.

Complications

The most common complication after orbital decompression is worsening of preexisting diplopia or new-onset diplopia, which is thought to result from the altered vectors postoperatively in already abnormal extraocular muscles. Preoperative diplopia frequently does not resolve with surgery.[19] Injury to the optic nerve or ophthalmic artery and cerebrospinal fluid leak are quite rare. More common complications of surgery include epistaxis, nasal adhesions, and sinusitis. Postoperative sinusitis is significantly more likely in patients with preoperative chronic rhinosinusitis.[20]

References

1. Kennedy, D. W., Goodstein, M. L., Miller, N. R., & Zinreich, S. J. (1990). Endoscopic transnasal orbital decompression. *Archives of Otolaryngology–Head Neck Surgery, 116*, 275–282.
2. Michel, O., Bresgen, K., Rüssmann, W., Thumfart, W. F., & Stennert, E. (1991). Endoscopically-controlled endonasal orbital decompression in malignant exophthalmos. *Laryngorhinootologie, 70*, 656–662. https://doi.org/10.1055/s-2007-998119.
3. Svider, P. F., Arianpour, K., Nguyen, B., Hsueh, W. D., Langer, P. D., Eloy, J. A., et al. (2018). Endoscopic and external approaches for orbital decompression: an analysis of trends from a U.S. perspective. *International Forum of Allergy & Rhinology, 8*, 934–938. https://doi.org/10.1002/alr.22124.
4. Leung, M.-K., Platt, M. P., & Metson, R. (2009). Revision endoscopic orbital decompression in the management of Graves orbitopathy. *Otolaryngology–Head and Neck Surgery, 141*, 46–51. https://doi.org/10.1016/j.otohns.2009.04.007.
5. Ference, E. H., Sindwani, R., Tan, B. K., Chandra, R. K., Kern, R. C., Conley, D., et al. (2016). Open versus endoscopic medial orbital decompression: Utilization, cost, and operating room time. *American Journal of Rhinology & Allergy, 30*, 360–366. https://doi.org/10.2500/ajra.2016.30.4350.
6. Reich, S. S., Null, R. C., Timoney, P. J., & Sokol, J. A. (2016). Trends in orbital decompression techniques of surveyed American Society of Ophthalmic Plastic and Reconstructive Surgery Members. *Ophthalmic Plastic and Reconstructive Surgery, 32*, 434–437. https://doi.org/10.1097/IOP.0000000000000573.
7. Boboridis, K. G., & Bunce, C. (2011). Surgical orbital decompression for thyroid eye disease. *Cochrane Database of Systematic Reviews, 136* (2011), 11–22. https://doi.org/10.1002/14651858.CD007630.pub2.
8. Ting, J. Y., & Sindwani, R. (2014). Endoscopic orbital decompression. *Operative Techniques in Otolaryngology–Head and Neck Surgery, 25*, 213–217. https://doi.org/10.1016/j.otot.2014.02.013.
9. Mueller, S. K., Miyake, M. M., Lefebvre, D. R., Freitag, S. K., & Bleier, B. S. (2017). Long-term impact of endoscopic orbital decompression on sinonasal-specific quality of life. *Laryngoscope, 128*, 785–788. https://doi.org/10.1002/lary.26812.
10. Metson, R., Dallow, R. L., & Shore, J. W. (1994). Endoscopic orbital decompression. *Laryngoscope, 104*, 950–957. https://doi.org/10.1288/00005537-199408000-00008.
11. Park, S. M., Nam, S. B., Lee, J. W., Song, K. H., Choi, S. J., & Bae, Y. C. (2015). Quantitative assessment of orbital volume and intraocular pressure after two-wall decompression in thyroid ophthalmopathy. *Archives of Craniofacial Surgery, 16*, 53–55. https://doi.org/10.7181/acfs.2015.16.2.53.
12. Schiff, B. A., McMullen, C. P., Farinhas, J., Jackman, A. H., Hagiwara, M., McKellop, J., et al. (2015). Use of computed tomography to assess volume change after endoscopic orbital decompression for Graves' ophthalmopathy. *American Journal of Otolaryngology, 36*, 729–735. https://doi.org/10.1016/j.amjoto.2015.06.005.
13. Pletcher, S. D., Sindwani, R., & Metson, R. (2006). Endoscopic orbital and optic nerve decompression. *Otolaryngologic Clinics of North America, 39*, 943–958. https://doi.org/10.1016/j.otc.2006.06.003.
14. Chastain, J. D., & Sindwani, R. (2006). Anatomy of the orbit, lacrimal apparatus, and lateral nasal wall. *Otolaryngologic Clinics of North America, 39*, 855–864. https://doi.org/10.1016/j.otc.2006.07.003.
15. Gras-Cabrerizo, J., Martel-Martin, M., Garcia-Lorenzo, J., Rodríguez-Álvarez, F., Montserrat-Gili, J. R., Mirapeix-Lucas, R., et al. Surgical anatomy of the medial wall of the orbit in 14 human cadavers. *Journal of Neurological Surgery Part B, Skull Base, 77*, 439–444. https://doi.org/10.1055/s-0036-1579544.

16. Vreugdenburg, T. D., Lambert, R. S., Atukorale, Y. N., & Cameron, A. L. (2015). Stereotactic anatomical localization in complex sinus surgery: A systematic review and meta-analysis. *Laryngoscope*, *126*, 51–59. https://doi.org/10.1002/lary.25323.
17. Finn, A. P., Bleier, B., Cestari, D. M., Kazlas, M. A., Dagi, L. R., Lefebvre, D. R., et al. (2017). A retrospective review of orbital decompression for thyroid orbitopathy with endoscopic preservation of the inferomedial orbital bone strut. *Ophthalmic Plastic and Reconstructive Surgery*, *33*, 334–339. https://doi.org/10.1097/IOP.0000000000000782.
18. Metson, R., & Samaha, M. (2002). Reduction of diplopia following endoscopic orbital decompression: The orbital sling technique. *Laryngoscope*, *112*, 1753–1757. https://doi.org/10.1097/00005537-200210000-00008.
19. Yao, W. C., Sedaghat, A. R., Yadav, P., Fay, A., & Metson, R. (2016). Orbital decompression in the endoscopic age. *Otolaryngology–Head and Neck Surgery*, *154*, 963–969. https://doi.org/10.1177/0194599816630722.
20. Antisdel, J. L., Gumber, D., Holmes, J., & Sindwani, R. (2013). Management of sinonasal complications after endoscopic orbital decompression for Graves' orbitopathy. *Laryngoscope*, *123*, 2094–2098. https://doi.org/10.1002/lary.23948.

21

Endoscopic Optic Nerve Decompression: Intracanalicular Portion

NICOLE I. FARBER, MD, PETER F. SVIDER, MD, WAYNE D. HSUEH, MD, JAMES K. LIU, MD, FACS, FAANS, AND JEAN ANDERSON ELOY, MD, FACS, FARS

Optic Nerve Decompression

The Evolution of Optic Nerve Decompression

Although endoscopic transnasal surgery has become a widely used method for optic nerve decompression, its emergence would not be conceivable without technological advances in modern endoscopic surgery. Improvements in optics, instrumentation, and image-guided surgical navigation have transformed the approach to the optic nerve from an open craniotomy to the minimally invasive methodology of today. Historically, the route to the optic canal encompassed transcranial approaches (pterional, supraorbital, orbitozygomatic, and so on), which require both brain retraction and manipulation of critical neurovascular structures.[1-3] Other surgical approaches that have been described include a medial approach by external ethmoidectomy or an inferomedial approach via a transantral transethmoidal route.[4] The current purely endoscopic endonasal extended transsphenoidal approach provides a direct midline trajectory and immediate access to the base of both optic nerves, allowing for 270-degree decompression and bimanual microsurgical resection of associated pathology.

Since 1998, patients have benefited from the advantages of the endoscopic transnasal approach.[5] These advantages include lack of external incisions, early extradural decompression of both optic nerves, preservation of olfaction, superior visualization of the infrachiasmatic perforators, and access to the inferomedial aspect of the optic nerve, a site often involved in neoplastic extension.[6] In addition, a recent meta-analysis reported greater visual outcomes with the transnasal approach compared with the transcranial, with postoperative visual improvement in 75% and 58.4% of patients, respectively.[7] The endoscopic transnasal approach is often criticized for higher rates of cerebrospinal fluid (CSF) leak compared with the transcranial approach. However, recent advancements in techniques for the coverage of skull base defects have provided a valuable solution: a vascularized pedicle nasoseptal flap offers robust tissue for coverage of skull base defects and has been shown to significantly reduce the CSF leak rate to 5.4%.[8,9] Although this procedure is characterized by low invasiveness and wide exposure, endoscopic transnasal optic nerve decompression remains a procedure that is not yet practiced universally, a fact likely related to the close proximity of critical neurovascular structures localized in this portion of the skull.

Anatomy

The Orbital Apex

Composed of seven different bones, the orbit encompasses the eye, extraocular muscles, nerves, blood vessels, fat, and much of the lacrimal apparatus. The periorbita encases the extraconal space, which consists mostly of orbital fat. Located within the fascia of the extraocular muscles, the intraconal space contains the muscles, optic nerve, and ophthalmic artery. Situated at the intersection of the cranium and face, the orbit contains multiple intricate orifices that convey a vast network of neurovascular elements. The orbit communicates with the middle cranial fossa via the optic canal and superior orbital fissure, the infratemporal fossa and the pterygopalatine fossa via the inferior orbital fissure, the nasal cavity via the anterior and occasionally the posterior ethmoidal foramen, the inferior meatus of the nose via the nasolacrimal canal, and the face via the infraorbital and supraorbital foramen.[10,11]

The orbital apex, positioned at the posterior aspect of the pyramid-shaped orbit, exists at the craniofacial junction linking the orbit and anterior ventral skull base. Situated in the medial portion of the apex, the optic canal is neighbored laterally by the superior orbital fissure. These two channels are separated by a thin osseous wall known as the optic strut. The inferior orbital fissure lies in the inferolateral aspect of the apex, located between the lateral wall and floor of the orbit. The annulus of Zinn, another elemental landmark of the orbital apex, remains the site of attachment for the extraocular muscles. This fibrous thickening is the least expandable portion of the optic sheath and is usually located at the narrowest part of the optic canal.[5]

The Optic Nerve and Its Canal

Unlike other peripheral nerves, the optic nerve is a direct extension of the brain and has three meningeal layers as well as subarachnoid space containing CSF. There are four segments of the optic nerve: intracranial, intracanalicular, intraorbital, and intraocular. Once intraorbital, the dura of the optic nerve splits to form an outer layer, contributing to the periorbital, and an inner layer, which merges with the arachnoid. The intracanalicular optic nerve shares the optic canal with the ophthalmic artery, typically located inferomedially to the nerve, making it highly susceptible to injury from a midline approach.[12,13] The optic canal is bounded medially by the body of the sphenoid bone, superiorly by the anterior root of the lesser wing of the sphenoid, and inferolaterally by the optic strut.[11] The anterior clinoid process forms the lateral margins of the optic canal. Attached to this process is the falciform ligament, a dural fold that extends over the optic nerve to attach to the tuberculum sellae.[14]

Surrounding Structures

Optic nerve decompression remains a formidable challenge because of this structure's intimate involvement with critical neurovascular structures, such as the optic apparatus and the anterior cerebral artery complex and associated perforators. The paranasal sinuses provide surgical access to the optic canal without compromising critical surrounding structures and subsequent functionality. The ethmoid sinus, bounded by the middle and superior turbinates, anterior skull base, and lamina papyracea, can be traversed to access the sphenoid sinus.[15] The optic nerve impression can be found within the superolateral aspect of the sphenoid sinus, with the bulge of the internal carotid artery located just inferior (Fig. 21.1). The lateral opticocarotid recess (OCR), a critical landmark representing the pneumanization of the optic strut of the anterior clinoid process, is located at the 10-o'clock and the 2-o'clock points laterally to the sellar floor (Fig. 21.1).[15] It should be noted that there is wide variability in sphenoid sinus pneumatization, and knowledge of a patient's distinctive anatomy is essential when planning for optic nerve decompression.[16]

In about 10% of cases, the optic nerve travels through a sphenoidethmoidal cell, also known as an Onodi cell, which is a posterior ethmoid cell that has pneumatized superolaterally to the sphenoid sinus (Fig. 21.2).[6,17] The prevalence of Onodi cells among a cohort of patients has been cited as high as 65.3%.[18] This provides an opportunity for potential injury of the nerve if the appropriate attention is not given to identifying the nerve before entering the sphenoid sinus.

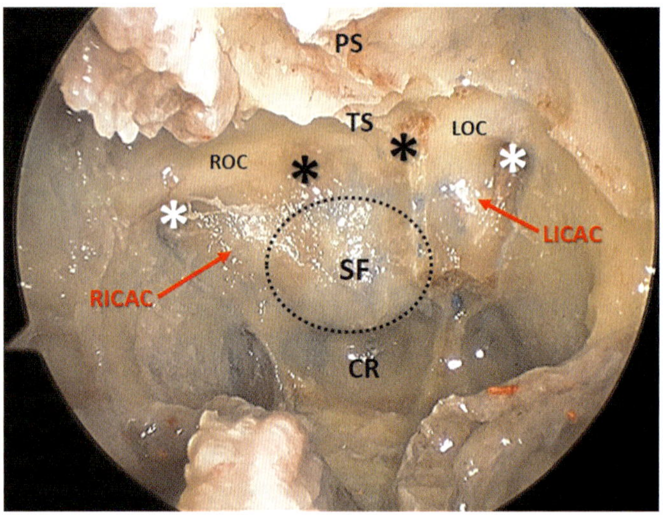

• **Fig. 21.1** Photograph of an endoscopic endonasal cadaveric dissection demonstrating the planum sphenoidale (*PS*), tubercullum sellae (*TS*), left optic canal (*LOC*), right optic canal (*ROC*), left internal carotid artery canal (*LICAC*), right internal carotid artery canal (*RICAC*), clival recess (*CR*), lateral opticocarotid recesses (*white asterisks*), and medial opticocarotid recesses (*black asterisks*). The *dashed circle* represents the area of the sellar floor (*SF*).

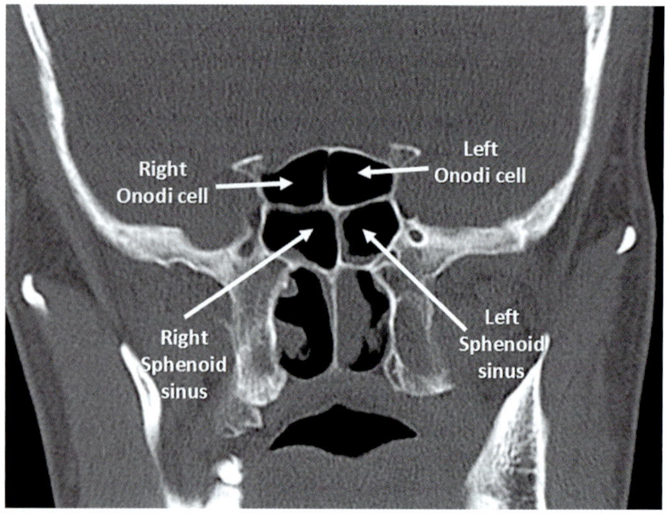

• **Fig. 21.2** Coronal computed tomography scan demonstrating a patient with bilateral Onodi cells (*arrows*).

Pathology Involving the Optic Nerve: Indications and Contraindications for Decompression

A variety of insults can inflict injury on the optic nerve, ranging from traumatic etiologies to neoplasia. Furthermore, each disease process has the capability to inflict injury on the optic nerve through a variety of mechanisms, including ischemia, compression, demyelination, and tumor invasion.[5] Although many of the mechanisms that cause optic neuropathy are irremediable, compressive insults are potentially reversible with timely surgical management.[6,19-21]

Traumatic optic neuropathy (TON), a consequence of blunt head trauma, is a well-described cause of optic neuropathy. TON results in indirect injury to the optic nerve via increased intracranial pressure and vascular ischemia.[22] Nontraumatic optic neuropathy is a less common disorder encompassing several etiologies, including endocrine orbitopathy, idiopathic intracranial hypertension, bone dysplasia, and infectious insults.[20] These processes result in direct or indirect mechanical compression of the optic nerve or its vascular supply, resulting in atrophy.[23]

In addition to the previously mentioned etiologies, surgical decompression of the optic nerve is useful in the resection of intracranial and extracranial tumors that invade the territory of the optic canal. Optic nerve decompression is indicated for both primary compressive processes, such as intraorbital tumors, or as a preliminary step in the pursuit to resect deeper pathology, such as pituitary adenomas.[24] The endoscopic endonasal approach has been shown to treat lesions of the sellar and parasellar regions, such as meningiomas, pituitary adenomas, craniopharyngiomas, and sinonasal malignancies.[25-29] Meningiomas commonly occur in this anatomically complex region, with anterior skull base meningiomas representing 40% of all intracranial meningiomas, and of these, 25% are tuberculum sellae tumors.[30] These tumors are often characterized by extension into the optic canals, displacing the optic chiasm backward and the optic nerves superolaterally. Intracanalicular tumor extension typically occurs on the inferomedial side of the optic canal, a position difficult to visualize from an ipsilateral anterolateral approach but readily accessible by an endoscopic endonasal approach.[31] This particular pathology highlights the benefits of wide exposure when working within the sellar region, especially within the optic canal, in regard to both the preservation of vision and avoidance of tumor recurrence.

In general, conservative management consisting of medical therapy should precede consideration of surgical decompression when appropriate. However, if there is no evidence of improvement, or if visual acuity deteriorates with the tapering of medical therapy, surgery should be performed.[5,13] Optic nerve decompression is a well-known therapeutic concept that is indicated for the pathologic conditions of traumatic optic neuropathy, Graves ophthalmopathy associated with optic neuropathy, vision loss secondary to idiopathic intracranial hypertension (pseudotumor cerebri), fibro-osseous lesions, and the neoplasms mentioned previously.[32-34] Considerable controversy exists regarding decompression for TON, particularly because of the high rate of spontaneous resolution without surgical intervention. The superiority of medical, surgical, or combination therapy remains a focus of current research endeavors.[5,22] A recent meta-analysis by Dhaliwal, Sowerby, and Rotenberg reported that endoscopic decompression for treatment of TON resulted in improved visual outcomes compared with medical therapy or observation alone.[21]

Contraindications for optic nerve decompression involve irreversible visual deficits resulting from complete disruption or atrophy of the nerve and/or chiasm before decompression. Another contraindication, specific to this procedure, is the presence of a carotid-cavernous fistula. As with all surgeries, other life-threatening problems or medical comorbidities making this surgical procedure hazardous will result in a lack of candidacy for surgical decompression.[5,13]

Preoperative Considerations

Preoperative Planning

Each patient considered for optic nerve decompression should undergo a thorough and complete ophthalmologic physical examination, including fundoscopic evaluation, measurement of intraocular pressure, visual field testing, visual acuity testing, and color vision testing as the perception of red is lost first.[13,20] If the patient is unable to cooperate or unconscious, monitoring of visual evoked potentials is of high value. Other causes of vision loss should be ruled out before proceeding with the procedure.[13]

Preoperative radiographic imaging should include fine-cut computed tomographic (CT) scans of the sinuses and orbits to evaluate the anatomy and extent of optic canal compression. This imaging modality offers information on the ethmoid and sphenoid sinus pneumatization and septation. Additionally, a fine-cut CT scan reveals dehiscence of the carotid artery. CT scans are also valuable in assessing bone density and thickness, noteworthy details in cases of spheno-orbital meningiomas or fibrous dysplasia. Review of coronal and axial magnetic resonance images (MRI) should follow to analyze the soft tissue contents of the orbital apex. Beyond traditional MRI sequences (T1- and T2-weighted), three-dimensional time-of-flight high-resolution sequences may be considered, as these demonstrate the relationship between the optic nerve, the ophthalmic artery, and underlying compressive pathologies.[20] Intraoperative navigation systems, coupling CT and MRI data, ensure identification of critical structures and anatomic landmarks, increasing the surgeon's ability to perform complete decompression and/or resection.

The relation of the lesion to the optic nerve should be considered. The superolateral and lateral aspects of the optic canal are relatively inaccessible from this inferomedial approach.[27,35] Furthermore, the ability to perform safe exposure and resection with the endoscopic endonasal approach is limited when the dural attachment of tumors extends beyond the lateral aspect of the optic canal and along the orbital roof and anterior clinoid process. Under these circumstances, complete lesion resection cannot be reasonably obtained.[6] If findings of lateral optic canal extension or vascular encasement are demonstrated on preoperative imaging, a transcranial approach is preferable.[27]

Preparation and Patient Positioning

Because of the complex anatomy of the optic canal, a multidisciplinary team should be involved in the planning and execution of this procedure. For the endoscopic endonasal approach to the ventral skull base, the surgical team should include, but not be limited to, a skull base neurosurgeon working simultaneously with an otolaryngologist specializing in endoscopic sinus and skull base surgery. Since the introduction of endoscopes in the 1980s, the involvement of otolaryngologists in surgery of the optic canal has increased.[36] Their expertise in endoscopic transnasal techniques is particularly valuable in cases that involve the inferomedial portion of the canal. Contrastingly, a neurosurgeon is essential in cases that involve the roof of the optic canal. Additionally, the management team should always involve an ophthalmologist, as visual assessment is critical both preoperatively and postoperatively.

After induction of general anesthesia, care should be taken to position and secure the endotracheal tube to the patient's left, out of the way of the operating surgeon positioned on the patient's right side. The decision to place a lumbar drain for temporary postoperative diversion of CSF varies depending on the surgeon; however, it should be noted that placement of a lumbar drain can lead to postoperative intracranial hypotension and other complications.[6,37] To ensure adequate venous return, the patient should be positioned supine with the head above the heart. The head is stabilized in a three-point Mayfield head frame (Integra LifeSciences, Plainsboro, NJ) and positioned to optimize the surgeon's comfort and ability in assessing both the nose and the deep anterior skull base: laterally bending the head gently toward the left shoulder, rotating it slightly toward the right shoulder, and extending it slightly. The draping should leave both eyes exposed in case perioperative evaluation of the globes is desired. Frameless stereotactic navigation provides continuous, three-dimensional information that facilitates both determining the extent of bone resection (sella, planum sphenoidale, tuberculum sellae, and so on) and creating the trajectory toward the optic canal and any associated pathology.[38] Visual evoked potentials are typically used to assess for intraoperative optic nerve injury. It is preferred to maintain mean arterial pressures above 90 mm Hg to prevent optic nerve ischemia. High-dose corticosteroids are also used intraoperatively and postoperatively.

Standard antiseptic protocols should be carried out to ensure the absence of surgical site infections. Betadine solutions should not only be applied to the nose and nares, but also to any extremity sites being used for harvesting autologous fascia lata in future dura repair and reconstruction. In our practice, preparation of the nose with Betadine solution (Purdue Pharma LP, Stamford, CT) is followed by packing with oxymetazoline-soaked pledgets. Both intravenous antibiotics (preferably ampicillin/sulbactam) and 10 mg of dexamethasone are given prior to beginning the operation. Because the endoscopic endonasal approach is extra-arachnoid in nature and lacks brain retraction, anticonvulsants are not routinely administered in patients without a preexisting history of seizures.[6]

Pearls and Potential Pitfalls

Pearls

- In challenging cases involving complex neoplastic extensions, a binostril technique lacking a nasal speculum allows the neurosurgeon and otolaryngologist to work simultaneously with up to three to four instruments in the field.[6]
- As recovery of visual deficits remains the primary pursued outcome of optic nerve decompression, substantial care should be taken to preserve visual function. The key to such preservation lies in minimizing direct manipulation or trauma to the optic nerve and in avoiding injury to the blood supply of the optic apparatus.[39-41] Evidence suggests that the posterior portion of the optic nerve circulation is most at risk of ischemia, as it is supplied solely by the perforating dural vessels. Additionally, it is not the compression of the apical circulation that causes sufficient vasospasm of these vessels, but rather the direct handling of the vessels and the postoperative accumulation of inflammatory mediators.[42]
- Visualization is critical throughout this procedure. Early identification of the lamina papyracea with complete ethmoidectomy, wide sphenoidotomy, and, if necessary, a middle turbinectomy or middle turbinate swing procedure should be performed to provide ease in instrument placement and optimal visualization.[6,20]
- Owing to the accumulation of irrigant in the sphenoid sinus, a drill with simultaneous suction and irrigation can be used.[43]

Potential Pitfalls

- Use of preoperative CT to identify the presence of an Onodi cell is necessary. Failure to recognize an Onodi cell leaves the nerve vulnerable to injury when entering the sphenoid sinus.[44]
- Special care should be taken to keep the periorbita intact. Accidental violation of such structures results in fat prolapse and bleeding with subsequent loss of visualization.[13,45]
- Extreme caution must be used when incising the optic nerve sheath to avoid transecting a medially arising ophthalmic artery (Fig. 21.3). The use of preoperative angiography may be invaluable for identifying the ophthalmic artery's course and relation to the optic nerve.[5,20,46]
- In case of tumor extending medially in the subchiasmatic region, using bipolar cautery in this area is not recommended; this should be avoided to preserve blood supply to the optic apparatus.[6,47]
- In cases requiring tumor debulking, adequately dissecting tumor free from all critical neurovascular structures (optic nerve, optic chiasm, anterior communicating artery complex) before removing it through the nose is essential. Avoid blind pulling of the tumor capsule, as this may result in arterial avulsion or optic nerve traction.[6,48]

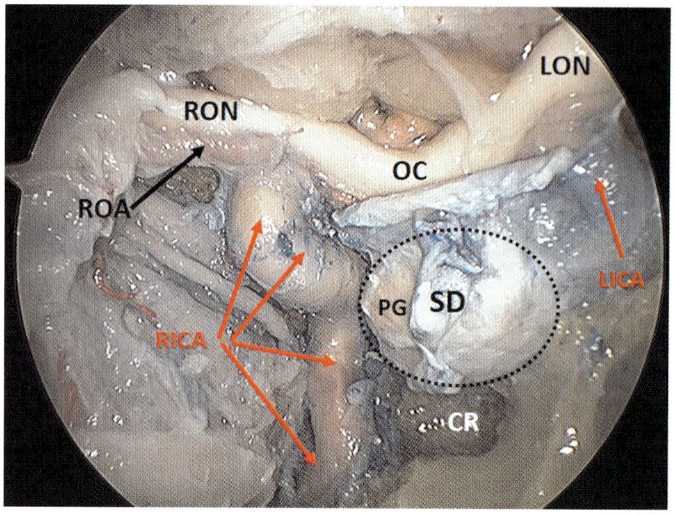

• **Fig. 21.3** Photograph of an endoscopic endonasal cadaveric dissection demonstrating an inferomedially arising right opthalmic artery (*ROA*) along the right optic nerve (*RON*). The *dashed circle* represents the sellar region showing a reflected sellar dura (*SD*) exposing the pituitary gland (*PG*). Also in view is the optic chiasm (*OC*), left optic nerve (*LON*), clival recess (*CR*), right internal carotid artery (*RICA*), and left internal carotid artery (*LICA*).

Surgical Technique

Approach: Endoscopic Endonasal Transsphenoidal

The nasal approach is typically performed with a 4-mm diameter, 0-degree rigid endoscope; however, the use of a 30-degree endoscope has demonstrated the benefit of additional angled viewing capabilities while maintaining the same degree of surgical exposure.[6] After injecting the nasal septum and anterosuperior attachment of the middle turbinates with 1% lidocaine and epinephrine (1:100,000 dilution), both inferior and middle turbinates are lateralized using a Goldman elevator. As stated previously, a middle turbinectomy can be performed to create adequate space for instrument placement in the nostril.[13] A posterior ethmoidectomy is performed before opening the anterior wall of the sphenoid sinus. In the subset of cases that contain an Onodi cell, care should be taken during the posterior ethmoidectomy to avoid damaging the optic nerve and/or carotid artery that course through the lateral aspect of the cell. After identifying the sphenoid ostium, a sphenoidotomy is performed using a mushroom punch or Kerrison rongeur to maximally widen the opening of the sinus. Ideally, all septa within the sinus are removed, allowing for optimal visualization of the optic nerve protuberance, the carotid protuberance, and the lateral opticocarotid recess (see Fig. 21.1). This step may be complicated by bleeding from the posterior nasal branch of the sphenopalatine artery, located in the inferior aspect of the sphenoid sinus, but can be controlled with adequate cauterization.

If the use of a pedicled nasoseptal flap for skull base dural repair is planned, it is preferable to obtain the flap at this interval so that further exposure of the skull base does not compromise the vascular pedicle of the flap. This flap has the potential to minimize postoperative CSF leak in patients with large dural defects of the anterior ventral skull base. The flap is harvested from the nasal septum mucoperichondrium and mucoperiosteum, as outlined by Hadad et al.,[49] and placed into the nasopharynx while leaving it pedicled to the posterior septal neurovascular bundle. Care should be taken to protect the vascular pedicle when exposing the sella, tuberculum sellae, and planum sphenoidale. Any additional efforts to remove bone or soft tissue should be pursued to ensure a direct line of vision to the planum sphenoidale and orbital apex region. An estimated 1.5 to 2 cm of the posterior septum is removed to provide adequate space for angulation of instrumentation through both nostrils in the pursuit of bimanual microsurgical dissection if necessary.[6]

Extradural Exposure: Transplanum Transtuberculum (Extended Transsphenoid)

When a meningioma or other skull base lesions extend to the optic canal, a transplanum transtuberculum approach may be necessary during optic nerve decompression. The extended transsphenoidal approach has the inherent advantage of optic canal opening occurring earlier in the surgical procedure. In the unroofing process, the sella, planum sphenoidale, tuberculum sellae, and both medial OCRs are removed. This feat is achieved using an endonasal diamond drill with an emphasis on substantial irrigation.[6] Equipment ideally provides simultaneous suction and irrigation, allowing for sufficient visualization, a factor that can be compromised by excess bone dust. Additionally, self-irrigation prevents overheating of the drill tip while near critical neurovascular structures. The bone overlying the sella is removed initially, immediately followed by a wide opening of the planum sphenoidale. This maneuver prevents bony hindrance to surgical freedom of dissecting instruments in both the intradural exposure and, if necessary, tumor dissection. Care should be taken to remove the planum anterior to the posterior cribriform, as this ensures adequate anterosuperior trajectory toward the anterior ventral skull base.[6]

After the removal of the sellae and planum, the remaining tuberculum strut and the medial OCR are removed to completely reveal the intracanalicular optic nerve. The strut and medial OCR are drilled down to eggshell thickness. What remains of the tuberculum strut is removed with an up-angled curette. The medial aspect of the optic nerve is revealed once the medial OCR is removed, allowing for extradural exposure of the optic nerve and paraclinoid carotid artery in the opticocarotid cistern.[6,9] We have found that using Gelfoam (Pharmacia, Kalamazoo, MI) or Surgiflo (Johnson & Johnson, New Brunswick, NJ), followed by gentle pressure with Cottonoid pledgets (American Surgical Company, Salem, MA), helps control venous bleeds from the cavernous and superior intercavernous sinuses. Bony decompression sets the stage for subsequent optic dural sheath opening. However, before proceeding with intradural exposure, the extent of skull base bone removal is assessed to ensure that the optic canal and potential tumor can be adequately reached without obstruction to the surgeon's line of vision or instrument maneuverability.

Intradural Exposure: Opening of the Optic Nerve Sheath

In addition to the osseous canal, the optic nerve sheath and the fibrous annulus of Zinn may need to be open to achieve adequate optic nerve decompression.[13,29] Although controversial, opening the optic nerve sheath is often indicated in cases with intracanalicular tumor extension or in specific patients with idiopathic intracranial hypertension.[13,50] This maneuver increases the risk of ophthalmic artery injury and CSF leaks, likely owing to the anatomy of the prechiasmatic cistern, which can often extend laterally to involve the intracranial portion of the optic nerves.[51] However, this particular maneuver has demonstrated improvements in vision in 78% to 80% of patients as the result of the immediate decompressive effects and subsequent alleviation of ischemia.[3] In addition to improving visual outcomes, intradural access to the optic canal is critical for ensuring complete tumor resection in some cases, as unaddressed residual tumor within the canal can be a source of recurrence.[52] The supraorbital approach was once the favored approach for removal of intracanalicular tumors because of its ability to unroof both optic canals and allow wide excision of the dura.[3] However, over the past few years, endoscopic transnasal approach has gained popularity as it has retained the ability to widely expose the intracanalicular optic nerve without necessitating brain retraction or manipulation.[6,53-55] Additionally, the endoscopic endonasal approach spares the falciform ligament from being dissected before opening the dural sheath, a maneuver that is essential in the traditional transcranial approach.[51]

If indicated, tumor resection should occur at this junction. Intracapsular tumor debulking is performed initially, followed by extracapsular dissection of the tumor away from the neurovascular structures using bimanual microsurgical dissection techniques.[56,57] If the tumor is strictly adherent to any critical structure (anterior cerebral artery, internal carotid artery, optic nerve, perforators, and so on), a small remnant should be left behind to avoid irreversible complications. Preservation of critical neurovascular structures should take precedence over complete tumor resection. Immediately after delivering the tumor capsule through the nose, the optic canal is inspected using a 30-degree endoscope. We use an angled hook to open the medial aspect of the optic dural sheath, thus exposing the previously encased optic nerve as it traverses the optic canal.

Closure and Skull Base Reconstruction

Although challenging, reconstructing the barriers between the arachnoid space and the sinonasal tract is paramount in preventing a postoperative CSF leak.[58] This feat remains a hindrance to the use and acceptance of the expanded endonasal approach to optic canal decompression. Recent studies have demonstrated great success in repairing the anterior skull base dural defects with an autologous fascia lata inlay graft followed by a vascularized pedicled nasoseptal flap.[9,49,59]

The fascia lata graft, harvested from the thigh, is placed as an inlay graft with the edges tucked underneath the dural edges. To temporarily secure the fascia graft in place, stamp-sized pieces of Surgicel (Ethicon, Cornelia, GA) are positioned over the bony defect. Previous studies have used a fat graft intradurally in an attempt to obliterate dead space within the resected cavity.[58,60] However, this technique has the potential consequence of visual impairment, secondary to fat graft swelling and mass effect on the optic apparatus.[61] Key to ensuring complete closure is coverage of the defect with the vascularized nasoseptal flap that was previously isolated during the surgical approach. When the vascularized flap is rotated superiorly to cover the dural closure, care should be taken to ensure the edges of the nasoseptal flap are in contact with the demucosalized bone. This small, but critical, component of the procedure is vital for flap adherence.[6,9,49]

A singular, thin layer of sealant (DuraSeal, Integra LifeSciences) or Tisseel fibrin glue (Baxter, Deerfield, Illinois) may be administered over the nasoseptal flap. However, previous studies have demonstrated that this practice does not decrease the incidence of CSF leaks and may increase surgical costs.[62] Avoidance of placing a sealant between the dural closure and the nasoseptal flap is important in ensuring flap adherence.[6] After placement of the sealant, a gentamicin-soaked Gelfoam pledget is used to secure the flap repair. A light nasal pack is placed in the nasal cavity for further stabilization and removed after 10 days.

Postoperative Complications, Considerations, and Management

An initial visual assessment should be performed in the recovery room, with monitoring of vision continued throughout the first 2 to 3 postoperative days. Postoperatively, our patients receive 60 mg of prednisone followed by a steroid taper. Additionally, the patient should continue to take antibiotics until the nasal packs are removed. Patients should be monitored for epistaxis during this time period. Nasal saline sprays can be helpful for both accelerating mucosal healing and maintaining patient comfort. Patients are typically discharged in 2 to 3 days with follow-up 1 week later for endoscopic examination and complete visual assessment.

Although opening the optic nerve sheath provides surgeons with great access to the optic nerve, it also opens up the subarachnoid space, increasing the likelihood of a CSF leak. Compared with transcranial approaches, endoscopic endonasal approaches have demonstrated higher rates of CSF leaks ranging from 10 to 28%, particularly in the resection of tuberculum sellae meningiomas.[7,60] However, these studies did not incorporate the novel reconstructive technique of a vascularized pedicled nasoseptal flap in skull base reconstruction,[49] which has demonstrated a significantly reduced CSF leak rate of 5.4%.[8,9,63] Other complications of this procedure include iatrogenic injury to the nerve fascicle or ophthalmic artery, resulting in irreversible visual deficits. Although a wide decompression is achieved with the transnasal approach, the risk of ophthalmic artery injury is greater owing to the intimate relationship between artery and nerve in the inferior portion of the optic canal. To prevent such injury, preoperative neuroimaging should be used to identify anatomic landmarks.[13] Furthermore, surgical disturbance through the nasal cavity and paranasal sinuses carries the increased risk of transmitting infection to the anterior ventral skull base.[64] These critical and life-threatening complications emphasize the prerequisite that this procedure be undertaken by an experienced endoscopic team.

The introduction of the endoscope has revolutionized the approach to the optic canal. Traditionally, the optic nerve was decompressed via a transcranial approach. Over the past two decades, this method has evolved into novel techniques characterized by a purely endoscopic endonasal transsphenoidal approach. The increased use of this approach has established several advantages, such as superior visualization of infrachiasmatic perforators, access to the inferomedial portion of the optic canal, and greater visual outcomes. Although the endoscopic endonasal approach has the potential for higher rates of CSF leaks, the use of a vascularized pedicle nasoseptal flap has provided a valuable solution. Further integration of this approach into surgical practice will solidify its advantageous role in optic nerve decompression.

References

1. Gogela, S. L., Zimmer, L. A., Keller, J. T., & Andaluz, N. (2017). Refining operative strategies for optic nerve decompression: A morphometric analysis of transcranial and endoscopic endonasal techniques using clinical parameters. *Operative Neurosurgery, 14*, 295–302.
2. Li, K. K., Teknos, T. N., Lai, A., Lauretano, A., Terrell, J., & Joseph, M. P. (1999). Extracranial optic nerve decompression: A 10-year review of 92 patients. *Journal of Craniofacial Surgery, 10*, 454–459.
3. Mahmoud, M., Nader, R., & Al-Mefty, O. (2010). Optic canal involvement in tuberculum sellae meningiomas: Influence on approach, recurrence, and visual recovery. *Operative Neurosurgery, 67*(3 Suppl Operative), ons108–ons119.
4. Anand, V. K., Sherwood, C., & Al-Mefty, O. (1991). Optic nerve decompression via transethmoid and supraorbital approaches. *Operative Techniques in Otolaryngology–Head and Neck Surgery, 2*, 157–166.
5. Luxenberger, W., Stammberger, H., Jebeles, J. A., & Walch, C. (1998). Endoscopic optic nerve decompression: The Graz experience. *Laryngoscope, 108*, 873–882.
6. Liu, J. K., Christiano, L. D., Patel, S. K., Tubbs, R. S., & Eloy, J. A. (2011). Surgical nuances for removal of tuberculum sellae meningiomas with optic canal involvement using the endoscopic endonasal extended transsphenoidal transplanum transtuberculum approach. *Neurosurgical Focus, 30*(5), E2.
7. de Divitiis, E., Esposito, F., Cappabianca, P., Cavallo, L. M., & de Divitiis, O. (2008). Tuberculum sellae meningiomas: High route or low route? A series of 51 consecutive cases. *Neurosurgery, 62*, 556–563.
8. Kanaan, H. A., Gardner, P. A., Yeaney, G., Prevedello, D. M., Monaco, E. A., 3rd, Murdoch, G., et al. (2008). Expanded endoscopic endonasal resection of an olfactory schwannoma. *J Neurosurg Pediatr, 2*, 261–265.
9. Kassam, A. B., Thomas, A., Carrau, R. L., Snyderman, C. H., Vescan, A., Prevedello, D., et al.(2008). Endoscopic reconstruction of the cranial base using a pedicled nasoseptal flap. *Neurosurgery, 63*, ONS44–52. discussion ONS52-43.
10. Turvey, T. A., & Golden, B. A. (2012). Orbital anatomy for the surgeon. *Oral and Maxillofacial Surgery Clinics, 24*, 525–536.
11. Daniels, D. L., Mark, L. P., Mafee, M. F., Massaro, B., Hendrix, L. E., Shaffer, K.A., et al. (1005). Osseous anatomy of the orbital apex. *American Journal of Neuroradiology, 16*, 1929–1935.
12. Lang, J. (1989). Anatomy of optic nerve decompression and anatomy of the orbit and adjacent skull base in surgical anatomy of the skull base. In *Surgery of the skull base: An interdisciplinary approach* (pp. 16–19). Berlin: Springer.
13. Lal, D., & Stankiewicz, J. A. (2009). Endoscopic optic nerve decompression. *Operative Techniques in Otolaryngology–Head and Neck Surgery, 20*, 96–100.
14. Akture, E., & Baskaya, M. K. (2014). Microsurgical anatomy and variations of the anterior clinoid process. *Turkish Neurosurgery, 24*, 484–493.
15. Sargi, Z. B., & Casiano, R. R. (2007). Surgical anatomy of the paranasal sinuses. In *Rhinologic and sleep apnea surgical techniques* (pp. 17–26). Berlin: Springer.
16. Tomovic, S., Esmaeili, A., Chan, N. J., Shukla, P. A., Choudhry, O. J., Liu, J. K., et al. (2013). High-resolution computed tomography analysis of variations of the sphenoid sinus. *Journal of Neurological Surgery Part B, Skull Base, 74*, 82–90.
17. Weinberger, D. G., Anand, V. K., Al-Rawi, M., Cheng, H. J., & Messina, A. V. (1996). Surgical anatomy and variations of the Onodi cell. *American Journal of Rhinology, 10*, 365–372.
18. Tomovic, S., Esmaeili, A., Chan, N. J., Choudhry, O. J., Shukla, P. A., Liu, J. K., et al. (2012). High-resolution computed tomography analysis of the prevalence of onodi cells. *Laryngoscope, 122*, 1470–1473.
19. Sleep, T., Hodgkins, P., Honeybul, S., Neil-Dwyer, G., Lang, D., & Evans, B. (2013). Visual function following neurosurgical optic nerve decompression for compressive optic neuropathy. *Eye (London, England), 17*, 571–578.
20. Berhouma, M., Jacquesson, T., Abouaf, L., Vighetto, A., & Jouanneau, E. (2014). Endoscopic endonasal optic nerve and orbital apex decompression for nontraumatic optic neuropathy: Surgical nuances and review of the literature. *Neurosurgical Focus, 37*, E19.

21. Dhaliwal, S. S., Sowerby, L. J., & Rotenberg, B. W. (2016). Timing of endoscopic surgical decompression in traumatic optic neuropathy: A systematic review of the literature. *International Forum of Allergy & Rhinology, 6*(6), 661–667.
22. Kountakis, S. E., Maillard, A. A., El-Harazi, S. M., Longhini, L., & Urso, R. G. (2000). Endoscopic optic nerve decompression for traumatic blindness. *Otolaryngology–Head and Neck Surgery, 123*, 34–37.
23. Miller, N. R., Walsh, F. B., & Hoyt, W. F. (2005). *Walsh and Hoyt's clinical neuro-ophthalmology.* Philadelphia: Lippincott Williams & Wilkins.
24. Metson, R., & Pletcher, S. D. (2006). Endoscopic orbital and optic nerve decompression. *Otolaryngologic Clinics of North America, 39*, 551–561.
25. Mathiesen, T., & Kihlström, L. (2006). Visual outcome of tuberculum sellae meningiomas after extradural optic nerve decompression. *Neurosurgery, 59*, 570–576.
26. Sade, B., & Lee, J. H. (2009). High incidence of optic canal involvement in tuberculum sellae meningiomas: Rationale for aggressive skull base approach. *Surgical Neurology, 72*, 118–123.
27. Kong, D.-S., Shin, H. J., Kim, H. Y., Chung, S. K., Nam, D. H., Lee, J. I., et al. (2011). Endoscopic optic canal decompression for compressive optic neuropathy. *Journal of Clinical Neuroscience, 18*, 1541–1545.
28. Bulters, D. O., Shenouda, E., Evans, B. T., Mathad, N., & Lang, D. A. (2009). Visual recovery following optic nerve decompression for chronic compressive neuropathy. *Acta Neurochirurgica, 151*, 325–334.
29. Acheson, J. (2004). Optic nerve disorders: Role of canal and nerve sheath decompression surgery. *Eye (London, England), 18*, 1169–1174.
30. Schick, U., & Hassler, W. (2005). Surgical management of tuberculum sellae meningiomas: Involvement of the optic canal and visual outcome. *Journal of Neurology, Neurosurgery & Psychiatry, 76*(7), 977–983.
31. Puchner, M., Fischer-Lampsatis, R., Herrmann, H.-D., & Freckmann, N. (1998). Suprasellar meningiomas—neurological and visual outcome at long term follow-up in a homogeneous series of patients treated microsurgically. *Acta Neurochirurgica, 140*, 1231–1238.
32. Trobe, J. D. (1981). Optic nerve involvement in dysthyroidism. *Ophthalmology, 88*, 488–492.
33. Sergott, R. C., Savino, P. J., & Bosley, T. M. (1988). Modified optic nerve sheath decompression provides long-term visual improvement for pseudotumor cerebri. *Archives of Ophthalmology, 106*, 1384–1390.
34. Pletcher, S. D., & Metson, R. (2007). Endoscopic optic nerve decompression for nontraumatic optic neuropathy. *Archives of Otolaryngology–Head & Neck Surgery, 133*, 780–783.
35. Roth, J., Fraser, J. F., Singh, A., Bernardo, A., Anand, V. K., & Schwartz, T. H. (2011). Surgical approaches to the orbital apex: Comparison of endoscopic endonasal and transcranial approaches using a novel 3D endoscope. *Orbit, 30*, 43–48.
36. Schaberg, M. R., Anand, V. K., Schwartz, T. H., & Cobb, W. (2010). Microscopic versus endoscopic transnasal pituitary surgery. *Current Opinion in Otolaryngology & Head and Neck Surgery, 18*, 8–14.
37. Samadani, U., Huang, J. H., Baranov, D., Zager, E. L., & Grady, M. S. (2003). Intracranial hypotension after intraoperative lumbar cerebrospinal fluid drainage. *Neurosurgery, 52*, 148–152.
38. Roth, M., Lanza, D. C., Kennedy, D. W., Yousem, D., Scanlan, K. A., & Zinreich, J. (1995). Advantages and disadvantages of three-dimensional computed tomography intraoperative localization for functional endoscopic sinus surgery. *Laryngoscope, 105*, 1279–1286.
39. Wang, Q., Lu, X.-J., Ji, W.-Y., et al. (2010). Visual outcome after extended endoscopic endonasal transsphenoidal surgery for tuberculum sellae meningiomas. *World Neurosurgery, 73*, 694–700.
40. Andrews, B. T., & Wilson, C. B. (1988). Suprasellar meningiomas: the effect of tumor location on postoperative visual outcome. *Journal of Neurosurgery, 69*, 523–528.
41. Kim, T.-W., Jung, S., Jung, T.-Y., Kim, I.-Y., Kang, S.-S., & Kim, S.-H. (2009). Prognostic factors of postoperative visual outcomes in tuberculum sellae meningioma. *British Journal of Neurosurgery, 22*, 231–234.
42. Rose, G. E. (2007). The "devil's touch"; visual loss and orbital surgery. A synopsis of the Mustardé Lecture, 2006. *Orbit, 26*, 147–158.
43. Kennedy, D. W. (2006). Technical innovations and the evolution of endoscopic sinus surgery. *Annals of Otology, Rhinology & Laryngology, 115*, 3–12.
44. Ogata, Y., Okinaka, Y., & Takahashi, M. (1998). Optic neuropathy caused by an isolated mucocele in an Onodi cell. *ORL Journal for Oto-rhino-laryngology and Its Related Specialties, 60*, 349–352.
45. Karligkiotis, A., Appiani, M. C., Verillaud, B., & Herman, P. (2014). How to prevent diplopia in endoscopic transnasal resection of tumors involving the medial orbital wall. *Laryngoscope, 124*, 2017–2020.
46. Rene, C., Rose, G., Lenthall, R., & Moseley, I. (*2001*). Major orbital complications of endoscopic sinus surgery. *British Journal of Ophthalmology, 2001*(*85*), 598–603.
47. Isolan, G. R., de Aguiar, P. H. P., Laws, E. R., Strapasson, A. C. P., & Piltcher, O. (2009). The implications of microsurgical anatomy for surgical approaches to the sellar region. *Pituitary, 12*, 360–367.
48. Kassam, A., Snyderman, C. H., Carrau, R. L., Gardner, P., & Mintz, A. (2005). Endoneurosurgical hemostasis techniques: Lessons learned from 400 cases. *Neurosurgical Focus, 19*, 1–6.
49. Hadad, G., Bassagasteguy, L., Carrau, R. L., Mataza, J. C., Kassam, A., Snyderman, C. H., et al.(2006). A novel reconstructive technique after endoscopic expanded endonasal approaches: Vascular pedicle nasoseptal flap. *Laryngoscope, 116*, 1882–1886.
50. Tarrats, L., Hernández, G., Busquets, J. M., et al. (2017). Outcomes of endoscopic optic nerve decompression in patients with idiopathic intracranial hypertension. *International forum of Allergy & Rhinology, 7*(6), 615–623.
51. Locatelli, M., Caroli, M., Pluderi, M., Motta, F., Gaini, S. M., Tschabitscher, M., et al. (2011). Endoscopic transsphenoidal optic nerve decompression: An anatomical study. *Surgical and Radiologic Anatomy, 33*, 257–262.
52. Nozaki, K., Kikuta, K.-I., Takagi, Y., Mineharu, Y., Takahashi, J. A., & Hashimoto, N. (2008). Effect of early optic canal unroofing on the outcome of visual functions in surgery for meningiomas of the tuberculum sellae and planum sphenoidale. *Neurosurgery, 62*, 839–846.
53. Frank, G., Pasquini, E., & Mazzatenta, D. (2001). Extended transsphenoidal approach. *Journal of Neurosurgery, 95*, 917–918.
54. Cavallo, L. M., de Divitiis, O., Aydin, S., Messina, A., Esposito, F., Iaconetta, G., et al. (2007). Extended endoscopic endonasal transsphenoidal approach to the suprasellar area: Anatomic considerations—part 1. *Operative Neurosurgery, 61*(3 Suppl), 24–33. 2007.
55. Cappabianca, P., Cavallo, L., Esposito, F., De Divitiis, O., Messina, A., & De Divitiis, E. (2008). Extended endoscopic endonasal approach to the midline skull base: The evolving role of transsphenoidal surgery. *Advances and Technical Standards in Neurosurgery, 33*, 151–199.
56. Kassam, A. B., Gardner, P. A., Snyderman, C. H., Carrau, R. L., Mintz, A. H., & Prevedello, D. M. (2008). Expanded endonasal approach, a fully endoscopic transnasal approach for the resection of midline suprasellar craniopharyngiomas: A new classification based on the infundibulum. *Journal of Neurosurgery, 108*(4), 15–128.
57. Kaptain, G. J., Vincent, D. A., Sheehan, J. P., & Laws, E. R., Jr. (2001). Transsphenoidal approaches for the extracapsular resection of midline suprasellar and anterior cranial base lesions. *Neurosurgery, 49*, 94–101.
58. Snyderman, C. H., Kassam, A. B., Carrau, R., & Mintz, A. Endoscopic reconstruction of cranial base defects following endonasal skull base surgery. *Skull Base, 17*, 73–78.
59. Zanation, A. M., Carrau, R. L., Snyderman, C. H., Germanwala, A. V., Gardner, P. A., Prevedello, D. M., et al. (2009). Nasoseptal flap reconstruction of high flow intraoperative cerebral spinal fluid leaks during endoscopic skull base surgery. *American Journal of Rhinology & Allergy, 23*, 518–521.

60. Laufer, I., Anand, V. K., & Schwartz, T. H. (2007). Endoscopic, endonasal extended transsphenoidal, transplanum transtuberculum approach for resection of suprasellar lesions. *Journal of Neurosurgery, 106*, 400–406.
61. Cook, S. W., Smith, Z., & Kelly, D. F. (2004). Endonasal transsphenoidal removal of tuberculum sellae meningiomas. *Neurosurgery, 55*, 239–246.
62. Eloy, J. A., Choudhry, O. J., Friedel, M. E., Kuperan, A. B., & Liu, J. K. (2012). Endoscopic nasoseptal flap repair of skull base defects: Is addition of a dural sealant necessary? *Otolaryngology–Head and Neck Surgery, 147*, 161–166.
63. Komotar, R. J., Starke, R. M., Raper, D. M., Anand, V. K., & Schwartz, T. H. (2012). Endoscopic endonasal compared with microscopic transsphenoidal and open transcranial resection of giant pituitary adenomas. *Pituitary, 15*, 150–159.
64. Harvey, R. J., Smith, J. E., Wise, S. K., Patel, S. J., Frankel, B. M., & Schlosser, R. J. (2008). Intracranial complications before and after endoscopic skull base reconstruction. *American Journal of Rhinology, 22*, 516–521.

22

Complications in Endoscopic Orbital Surgery

GUSTAVO COY, MD, JOÃO MANGUSSI-GOMES, MD, AND ALDO C. STAMM, MD, PhD

Orbital decompression has been performed for more than 100 years and is aimed at decompressing the orbital content by partially removing its bony boundaries. It has evolved from a transfrontal orbital roof approach to the classical external transantral approach.[1] The endoscopic orbital decompression (EOD) was first described by Kennedy et al. in the early 1990s as a surgical treatment for thyroid eye disease (TED), and it used the transnasal corridor to decompress the medial and inferior orbital walls.[2] Since then, indications for EOD have expanded and involve not only TED but also procedures for other orbital diseases including neoplastic, traumatic, vascular, inflammatory, and infectious ones.

Decompression of the optic nerve (ON) is indicated for reducing the pressure at its intracanalicular portion and was first performed through an external approach via craniotomy. Only 20 years ago, the endoscopic approach was described.[3,4] Its indications involve decompression of acute and subacute optic neuropathy, secondary to trauma, TED, neoplastic causes, fibrous dysplasia, and others.[5]

Although complications in orbital surgery can lead to serious consequences, they are uncommon when surgery is performed by experienced surgeons. The chances of complications and their severity rise considerably depending on the complexity of the disease and proposed orbital procedure. For instance, surgery for intraconal orbital tumors, especially those located lateral to the ON, are of greater risk.[6]

Because endoscopic orbital surgery is a relatively new surgical modality, there is a lack of reports and discussion in the literature of surgical complications specifically related to endoscopic orbital surgery. In didactic terms, complications of endoscopic orbital surgery can be categorized according to the time when they occur (intraoperative vs. postoperative; immediate, early, or late), the anatomic structure that is injured (neural, vascular, muscular, or cerebral), or the region where they manifest (orbital, sinonasal, or intracranial). In this chapter, complications are divided into two categories: immediate/early and late. Immediate/early complications are those easily identifiable in the intraoperative or early postoperative period, consisting mainly of vascular, muscular and neural injuries, and cerebral spinal fluid (CSF) leaks. Late complications, for their turn, consist of mainly orbital and sinonasal complications, such as diplopia, enophtalmos, nasal obstruction, and chronic rhinosinusitis.[6-8]

Immediate/Early Complications

Vascular Injuries

Vascular injuries occur especially when dealing with intraconal disease. Injury to orbital vessels can lead to catastrophic sequelae, including orbital hematomas and total blindness.

The ophthalmic artery (OA) provides the main blood irrigation to the orbit in most individuals. Fortunately, injury to this vessel is rare owing to its anatomic location, inferolateral to the ON. The ciliary arteries are branches of the OA that form a vascular network surrounding the ON, and their damage may cause important visual impairment. The central retinal artery is one of the first branches of the OA, and injury to this artery causes sudden blindness. Lesions to muscular branches are rare; however, they may occur when working in the posterior orbit. Arterial branches to the medial rectus muscle (MRM) are the most commonly injured.[6]

The anterior and posterior ethmoidal arteries are also at risk of injury during dissection of the ethmoidal cells and the lamina papyracea (LP). The superior limit of bone removal in EOD is traditionally the ethmoidal foramens.[1]

Epistaxis and orbital hematomas can manifest immediately or in the early postoperative period, secondary to inefficient hemostasis or injury to blood vessels, especially during removal of orbital fat (Fig. 22.1).[6,8] Injuries to minor vessels are usually easily controlled and managed but may cause periorbital hematomas (Fig. 22.2).

Neural Injuries

Neural injuries are infrequent and usually of a lesser degree of morbidity compared with vascular lesions. An exception to this would be ON injuries. Although uncommon, this complication usually leads to total blindness.[6]

Motor nerves may be iatrogenically damaged during surgery. The most commonly affected nerve are branches of the oculomotor nerve that innervate the MRM and the inferior rectus muscle. Because these nerves enter the muscles medially in the posterior orbit, lesions are rare, but when they occur, they can cause diplopia. The long ciliary nerves are also at risk of trauma during surgery. They are usually medial to the ON and have mostly sensory fibers to the sclera.[6]

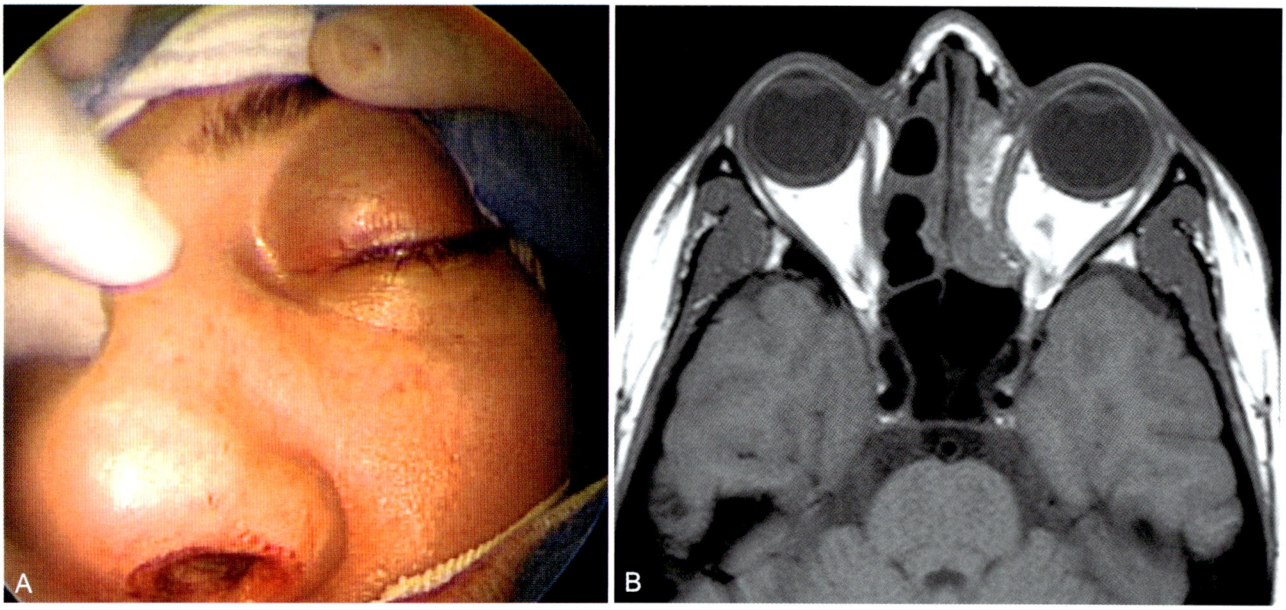

• **Fig. 22.1** A 33-year-old female patient was diagnosed with an orbital hematoma intraoperatively. A, Instant photo of the patient taken from the camera used for endoscopic surgery. B, T1-weighted magnetic resonance image of the patient after orbital decompression.

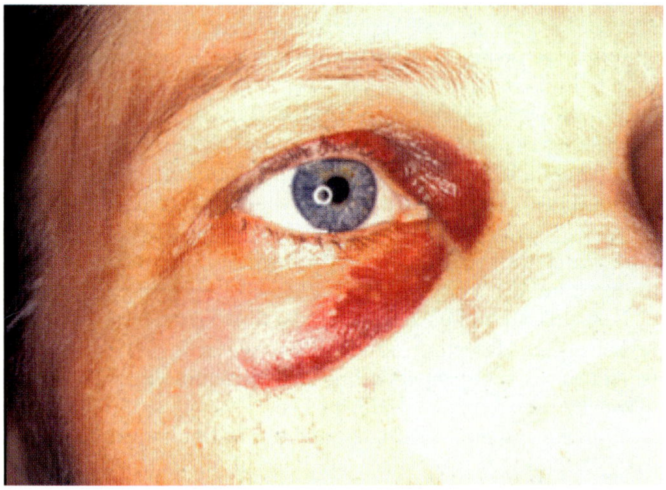

• **Fig. 22.2** A 54-year-old male patient after endoscopic orbital surgery was performed. Because of a minor vascular injury, the patient presented with periorbital hematoma immediately after surgery.

Muscular Injuries and Cerebrospinal Fluid Leaks

The most commonly injured muscle in the orbit is the MRM, either by direct surgical trauma or intense manipulation. Although usually temporary, diplopia may manifest for months.[1,6]

CSF leaks are another possible complication, and endonasal approaches offer the advantage of facilitating their prompt identification and management. These are exceedingly rare and can be accounted for less than 0.7% of all complications.[8]

Late Complications

Sinonasal Complications

Chronic rhinosinusitis, mucoceles, and nasal obstruction are some of the most frequent complications encountered after orbital surgery.[7,8] They can be avoided not only by performing an accurate and meticulous surgery but also by doing frequent postoperative endoscopic evaluations and nasal debridements to prevent synechia and blockage of paranasal sinuses ostia.[6] Hyposmia can also occur as a sinonasal complication secondary to orbital surgery.[7,8]

Orbital Complications

Enophtalmos occurs when there is excessive decrease in orbital volume, either by exaggerated removal of orbital fat or as a result of orbital fat herniation.[6]

Diplopia is usually transient and secondary to manipulation of the MRM. Persistent diplopia happens after important damage of extraocular muscles or displacement of the globe.[6,9]

Finally, subcutaneous emphysema may also occur when the periorbita is incised; therefore patients should be advised to avoid blowing their nose in the first postoperative weeks.[6-8]

Preventing Complications

Preoperative Evaluation

In aiming to prevent complications, it is imperative to correctly select patients or, at least, to understand which patients will benefit more from EOD. In Graves orbitopathy, for example, surgical timing is critical, as EOD should not be performed during the acute orbital inflammation period as the inflammatory process might worsen after surgery. In most cases of TED, it is feasible and advised to stabilize the condition before EOD is considered.[1,10,11] Furthermore, it has been suggested that the best results occur for patients with TED caused by orbital fat expansion (type 1) rather than muscular hypertrophy (type 2), which can be assessed through imaging studies. For type 1 patients, EOD with removal of orbital fat has been associated with better outcomes in terms of proptosis reduction.[11,12]

Preoperative imaging should be thoroughly studied and understood before attempting EOD. Correct knowledge of the anatomy of the anterior and posterior ethmoidal arteries, as they cross the orbit and nasal cavity from lateral to medial, is fundamental to avoid vascular damage and prevent epistaxis or orbital hematoma. Computed tomography scans assist in the identification of such anatomy.

The anatomic location of the MRM and its relationship to other structures are important; injury to this muscle may lead to transient or even permanent diplopia. In a retrospective study analyzing the position of the MRM in relation to the LP, Suh et al. identified that the distance between these two structures is larger anteriorly and permits safer dissection of the orbital content. Posteriorly, the MRM lays only 1 to 2 mm lateral to the periorbita, posing a greater risk of injury.[13]

When proceeding to ON decompression, it is mandatory to know the position of the OA in relation to the ON. In the majority of cases, the OA enters the optic canal inferomedially to the ON and runs laterally toward the orbit, entering it through the optic canal inferolaterally to the ON. Other anatomic variations of the OA should be expected as its localization in the orbit is highly variable. In 8% of patients the OA may enter the orbit through the superior orbital fissure. Therefore preoperative gadolinium-enhanced magnetic resonance imaging is mandatory before operating on the ON, superior orbital fissure, or orbital apex.[14]

Similarly, imaging studies are fundamental in identifying highly vascularized orbital malformations, such as ophthalmic artery aneurysms and arteriovenous malformations. These constitute a contraindication to orbital and optic canal decompression and must be identified before surgery. Injury to these vascular malformations might lead to serious complications.[6]

Intraoperative image guidance can improve identification and avoid injury of key structures. It has been shown to improve intraoperative time and enhance outcomes, as well as avoiding unexpected hemorrhages.[15] However, surgeons should use image guidance systems only to confirm their prior anatomic knowledge and to increase surgical safety.

Intraoperative Care

Before initiating endoscopic orbital surgery, it is important to have adequate instrumentation in the operation room. An endonasal kit should be sufficient for orbital decompression. For more delicate dissection, especially involving the ON or intraconal tumors, a skull base surgery kit might be necessary.

For hemostasis, a bipolar cautery must be readily available for careful cauterization and as a way to shrink extraconal fat to improve visualization when necessary. It should not be used intraconally, as there is risk of damage to critical neurovascular structures. Additionally, neuropathies soaked in saline solution are useful for hemostasis and can be helpful in removing blood from the surgical field as well as assisting in retraction of orbital fat. Irrigation with warm saline solution may also be used for hemostasis.[16,17]

With the LP exposed, a Freer elevator is used to enter it anteriorly to avoid trauma to the MRM, and blunt dissection is carried out to separate the LP from the periorbita. The LP adjacent to the frontal recess is left intact, and manipulation of the frontal recess is usually avoided to prevent disruption of the frontal sinus drainage pathway. The periorbita is then incised in a posterior to anterior fashion to avoid the prolapse of orbital fat into the surgical field. This maneuver might be assisted by navigation systems to prevent MRM injury.[1,5,6,14]

Drilling of the optic canal should be done carefully and with constant and abundant irrigation to avoid thermal injury to the ON and OA. Opening of the ON sheath may expose the patient to a CSF leak and OA injury and should be reserved for very specific indications. If there are any Onodi cells that must be dissected, this should be done with caution as the ON might be dehiscent. Having navigation available is helpful, especially in sphenoid sinuses that are not well pneumatized.[5,14]

When sinus dissection is carefully performed, sinonasal complications are rare. In a retrospective review, Antisdel et al. reviewed 86 orbital decompressions, with an incidence of complications of only 3.5%; complications were one case of hemorrhage that required intervention, three cases that demanded revision surgery owing to obstructive sinusitis, and one case of nasal obstruction secondary to adhesions. No patients had CSF leakage or orbital hemorrhage and all patients who underwent revision surgery had good outcomes. The authors attribute these results to creating a maximal antrostomy, preserving an intact rim of 2 mm of the LP superiorly, and prophylactically cauterizing the middle turbinate stump after resection.[7]

Special consideration has been made to reduce the risk of postoperative diplopia. Dissection of the medial and inferior orbital walls with preservation of the inferomedial orbital strut, which is the junction of the medial and inferior orbital walls that extend from the maxillary line anteriorly to the palatine bone posteriorly, has been shown to prevent diplopia. This technique seems to avoid inferomedial displacement of the globe, lowering the risk of diplopia after surgery.[18] Preservation of the periorbital sling, a strip of periorbita covering the MRM, also seems to prevent diplopia.[19] Borboridis et al., in a systematic review that evaluated EOD for TED, demonstrated that a balanced orbital wall decompression (medial and lateral walls) has been related to better surgical results with fewer complications.[20]

Conclusions

Endoscopic orbital surgery has evolved greatly over the years. The turning point for these procedures was the evolution of endoscopic approaches. Since then sinonasal surgery has become less morbid and more efficient. Endoscopic orbital surgery is a feasible and increasingly performed procedure, with a low incidence of complications when carried out by a team of experienced surgeons.

References

1. Wehrmann, D., & Antisdel, J. L. (2017). An update on endoscopic orbital decompression. *Current Opinion in Otolaryngology & Head and Neck Surgery, 25(1)*, 73–78.
2. Kennedy, D. W., Goodstein, M. L., Miller, N. R., & Zinreich, S. J. (1990). Endoscopic transnasal orbital decompression. *Archives of Otolaryngology–Head Neck Surgery, 116*(3), 275–282.
3. Kountakis, S. E., Maillard, A. A., & Stiernberg, C. M. (1995). Optic neuritis secondary to sphenoethmoiditis: Surgical treatment. *American Journal of Otolaryngology, 16*(6), 422–427.
4. Kountakis, S. E., Maillard, A. A., El-Harazi, S. M., Longhini, L., & Urso, R. G. (2000). Endoscopic optic nerve decompression for traumatic blindness. *Otolaryngology–Head and Neck Surgery, 123*(1 Pt 1), 34–37.
5. Choi, K. J., Jang, D. W., & Abi Hachem, R. (2018). Endoscopic endonasal approaches to the orbit. *International Ophthalmology Clinics, 58*(2), 85–99.
6. Castelnuovo, P., Turri-Zanoni, M., Battaglia, P., Locatelli, D., & Dallan, I. (2015). Endoscopic endonasal management of orbital pathologies. *Neurosurgery Clinics of North America, 26*(3), 463–472.

7. Antisdel, J. L., Gumber, D., Holmes, J., & Sindwani, R. (2013). Management of sinonasal complications after endoscopic orbital decompression for Graves' orbitopathy. *Laryngoscope*, *123*(9), 2094–2098.
8. Sellari-Franceschini, S., Dallan, I., Bajraktari, A., Fiacchini, G., Nardi, M., Rocchi, R., et al. (2016). Surgical complications in orbital decompression for Graves' orbitopathy. *Acta Otorhinolaryngologica Italica*, *36*(4), 265–274.
9. Curragh, D. S., Halliday, L., & Selva, D. (2018). Endonasal approach to orbital pathology. *Ophthalmic Plastic and Reconstructive Surgery*, *34*(5), 422–427.
10. Melcescu, E., Horton, W. B., Kim, D., Vijayakumar, V., Corbett, J. J., Crowder, K. W., et al. (2014). Graves orbitopathy: Update on diagnosis and therapy. *Southern Medical Journal*, *107*(1), 34–43.
11. Prat, M. C., Braunstein, A. L., Dagi Glass, L. R., & Kazim, M. (2015). Orbital fat decompression for thyroid eye disease: Retrospective case review and criteria for optimal case selection. *Ophthalmic Plastic and Reconstructive Surgery*, *31*(3), 215–218.
12. Wu, W., Selva, D., Bian, Y., Wang, X., Sun, M. T., Kong, Q., et al. (2015). Endoscopic medial orbital fat decompression for proptosis in type 1 graves orbitopathy. *American Journal of Ophthalmology*, *159*(2), 277–284.
13. Suh, J. D., Kuan, E. C., Thompson, C. F., Scawn, R. L., Feinstein, A. J., Barham, H. P., et al. (2016). Using fixed anatomical landmarks to avoid medial rectus injury: A radiographic analysis in patients with and without Graves' disease. *American Journal of Otolaryngology*, *37*(4), 334–338.
14. Berhouma, M., Jacquesson, T., Abouaf, L., Vighetto, A., & Jouanneau, E. (2014). Endoscopic endonasal optic nerve and orbital apex decompression for nontraumatic optic neuropathy: Surgical nuances and review of the literature. *Neurosurgical Focus*, *37*(4), E19.
15. Kazak, Z., Celik, S., Ozer, M. A., & Govsa, F. (2015). Three-dimensional evaluation of the danger zone of ethmoidal foramens on the frontoethmoidal suture line on the medial orbital wall. *Surgical and Radiologic Anatomy*, *37*(8), 935–940.
16. Yao, W. C., & Bleier, B. S. (2016). Endoscopic management of orbital tumors. *Current Opinion in Otolaryngology & Head and Neck Surgery*, *24*(1), 57–62.
17. Bleier, B. S., Castelnuovo, P., Battaglia, P., Turri-Zanoni, M., Dallan, I., & Metson, R., et al. Endoscopic endonasal orbital cavernous hemangioma resection: Global experience in techniques and outcomes. *International Forum of Allergy & Rhinology*, *6*(2), 156–161.
18. Kingdom, T. T., Davies, B. W., & Durairaj, V. D. (2015). Orbital decompression for the management of thyroid eye disease: An analysis of outcomes and complications. *Laryngoscope*, *125*(9), 2034–2040.
19. Yao, W. C., Sedaghat, A. R., Yadav, P., Fay, A., & Metson, R. (2016). Orbital decompression in the endoscopic age: The modified inferomedial orbital strut. *Otolaryngology–Head and Neck Surgery*, *154*(5), 963–969.
20. Boboridis, K. G., Uddin, J., Mikropoulos, D. G., Bunce, C., Mangouritsas, G., Voudouragkaki, I. C., et al. (2015). Critical appraisal on orbital decompression for thyroid eye disease: A systematic review and literature search. *Advances in Therapy*, *32*(7), 595–611.

23

Postoperative Care of the Endoscopic Orbital Decompression Patient

RAKESH CHANDRA, MD AND ERIC SUCCAR, MD

Postoperative treatment of patients undergoing endoscopic orbital decompression (EOD) shares many similarities with that of patients who have standard functional endoscopic sinus surgery. Important distinctions that must be accounted for relate to the herniation of orbital contents into the nose and specific potential complications. Potential orbital complications include corneal abrasion, epiphora, new or worsening diplopia, worsening vision, and vision loss.[1-5] Potential sinus complications include postoperative hemorrhage, obstructive sinusitis, nasal obstruction, anosmia, infraorbital nerve hypoesthesia, and cerebrospinal fluid (CSF) leak.[1,2,4-7] An understanding of these possible sequelae is essential to treating these patients postoperatively.

Perioperative considerations, postoperative management, and the rate of complications are influenced by the indication for EOD.[5] The majority of decompressions are performed for the sequelae of Graves ophthalmopathy, including proptosis with aesthetic concerns, exposure keratitis, strabismus/diplopia, and compressive optic neuritis (CON).[5,8] Other indications include orbital cellulitis/abscess, retrobulbar hematoma/hemorrhage, and traumatic optic neuropathy.[5,9] These patients are best managed through a multidisciplinary approach consisting of otolaryngology, ophthalmology, and endocrinology specialists.[3,8] The goals of surgery, expected outcomes, and risks for short- and long-term complications are determined based on the extent of disease and the indication for the procedure.[5]

Perioperative

Preoperative

A baseline preoperative assessment of corrected visual acuity, pupillary examination, ocular motility, intraocular pressure, fundus examination, and Hertel exopthalmometry is required to compare postoperative vision status and orbital outcomes.[2] A comprehensive assessment of sinonasal history, examination, and imaging is essential. The presence or history of sinonasal disease is associated with an increased likelihood of developing postoperative obstructive sinusitis.[1]

The preoperative period represents an opportunity to counsel patients regarding their specific surgical indication and to guide patient expectations for the postoperative course. The goal of EOD for proptosis is to improve cosmesis without causing diplopia, requiring a more balanced and less aggressive approach.[2] Patients with preoperative diplopia/strabismus should be counseled that this may worsen, remain the same, or improve postoperatively.[2] The chance of requiring future strabismus surgery is higher in this population.

Patients undergoing EOD for exposure keratitis require a greater degree of orbital regression, elevating their risk for postoperative diplopia. Continued conservative management of their exposure keratitis is required in the initial postoperative period until orbital swelling resolves. A temporary tarsorrhaphy may be required in these cases.

EOD for CON focuses on decompressing the posterior lamina papyracea and orbital apex.[10] These patients have less orbital regression and are less likely to develop postoperative diplopia.[2,10] The risks of worsening vision, vision loss, and CSF leak are higher in these patients, particularly if optic nerve decompression is performed.[6,10] CON patients require a multidisciplinary team to provide comprehensive medical management, including the optimization of postoperative steroid and thyroid disease management.[6,10]

Intraoperative

Specific intraoperative techniques can decrease the rate of postoperative obstructive sinusitis, new or worsening diplopia, and hemorrhage. Wide maxillary antrostomies and sphenoidotomies should always be performed, and the lamina papyracea near the frontal recess should be preserved.[1,5,6] Preservation of an inferior medial bony or periorbital strut has been shown to decrease the incidence of new or worsening postoperative diplopia.[2,11] A balance between obtaining maximal orbital regression without causing new or worsening diplopia should be the goal, particularly when the indication for surgery is proptosis or cosmesis.[2,3,11]

Meticulous intraoperative hemostasis with the assistance of bipolar cautery and absorbable hemostatic agents is essential. Rigid nonabsorbable packing should be avoided in the intraoperative and postoperative setting, as it can lead to excessive tamponade pressure on the exposed orbital soft tissues.[1,6] Emergence from anesthesia should be gentle, and positive-pressure ventilation should be avoided, as it can induce subcutaneous or intraorbital emphysema.[5,6]

Postoperative

Visual vital signs (acuity, pupillary reflex, motility, and intraocular pressure) should be obtained as soon as possible postoperatively and followed closely in the surgical recovery unit.[2] Any patient-reported change in vision should be investigated promptly. Cool compresses are used to assist with orbital swelling and improve patient comfort.

Patients with episodes of refractory severe postoperative hemorrhage should undergo definitive operative control with the assistance of bipolar cautery and absorbable hemostatic agents. Monopolar cautery has the potential to transmit electrical impulses to intraocular structures, potentially inducing myopathy or neuropraxia, whereas rigid nonabsorbable packing has the potential to tamponade the orbit and raise intraocular pressure. Both should be avoided when treating postoperative hemorrhage in the setting of EOD.[6]

Discharge

Patients are candidates for discharge once it is determined that their vision is stable, that they have adequate hemostasis, and that they do not have any other postoperative barriers to discharge.[1,2] Based on surgical team preference, orbital decompression patients can either be discharged later on the day of surgery or observed overnight. Those also undergoing optic nerve decompression are monitored overnight.[2] If a patient is sent home the same day, follow-up with ophthalmology should be scheduled the following morning for a formal vision examination.[2] The surgical team should be informed immediately of any vision changes or episodes of significant epistaxis that occur after discharge.

Discharge instructions should include sinus precautions (avoid nose blowing, sneeze with mouth open, and avoidance of heavy lifting or straining), initiation of a nasal saline regimen, and continuation of cool compresses for the eyes.[6] Although twice-daily gentle positive-pressure saline irrigations can be initiated, the authors' practice is to use saline mist (2 sprays every 1 to 2 hours while awake) for the first postoperative week.

A combination antibiotic and steroid ophthalmic ointment should be continued after discharge. Nasal steroids are not required.[2] Definitive data regarding the need for postoperative oral antibiotics in EOD patients have not been reported, and a consensus has not been developed.[1,2,6] The authors' practice is to empirically prescribe a single intraoperative intravenous antibiotic dose and a postoperative 10-day oral antibiotic course covering *Staphylococcus aureus*. Postoperative steroids are typically required for patients with CON and for patients undergoing optic nerve decompression.[1,2,6] Management of steroid dosages requires a multidisciplinary approach and should be based on individual patient factors.[1,2,6]

Follow-up

After discharge, patients continue close follow-up with their multidisciplinary team. Visual acuity, degree of recession, and diplopia are assessed by an ophthalmologist. The reported incidence of new or worsening postoperative diplopia has not been definitively defined owing to the variability of surgical indications and techniques.[2,3,8,10,12] Stable, new, or worsening postoperative diplopia is monitored for 9 to 10 months.[6] For patients in whom diplopia does not resolve, definitive strabismus surgery should be considered.[6]

Patients are seen by an otolaryngologist at 1 week postoperatively for an initial debridement. Early debridement requires great care and diligence to avoid injuring the intranasally exposed orbital contents.[2] Palpation of the orbit is performed during debridement to help delineate the intranasal orbital contents. The frequency of future debridement is determined based on the severity of crusting. During the natural healing process, the intranasal orbital fat begins to atrophy and the orbital contents eventually solidify and mucosalize (Figs. 23.1 and 23.2). Once the mass movement of the intranasal orbital contents stabilizes, more definitive debridement of crusting can be pursued. Gentle nasal saline irrigations, which are initiated after the first week postoperatively, should be continued until crusting stops.

The reported rates of postoperative sinonasal complications range from 3.5% to 20%.[1,3,8,10] Refractory cases of postoperative nasal obstruction and obstructive sinusitis may require surgical intervention.[1,5] During any revision for obstructive sinusitis, the intranasal orbital contents should not be manipulated, even if these tissues impede a traditional approach to the sinuses.[1] Definitive treatment of the maxillary sinuses may require a mega-antrostomy.[1] Obstructive frontal sinusitis can be managed with a transaxillary frontal sinusotomy with stent placement (Figs 23.3 and 23.4).[1] In select refractory cases, patients may require a Draf IIb or Draf III frontal sinus drill-out.[5] Postoperative epiphora, secondary to injury of the nasolacrimal duct, is treated with a dacryocystostomy.[6,13]

CSF leak may be identified intraoperatively, in the immediate postoperative period or in the delayed postoperative setting.[5,7,9,14] Patients undergoing EOD for CON, traumatic optic neuropathy,

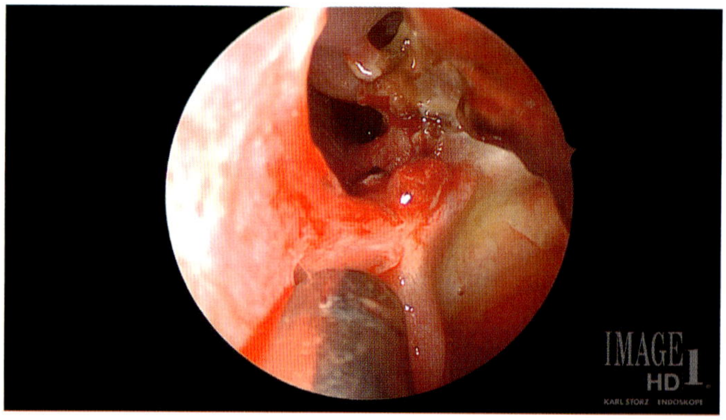

• **Fig. 23.1** Postoperative endoscopic orbital decompression nasal cavity before definitive debridement.

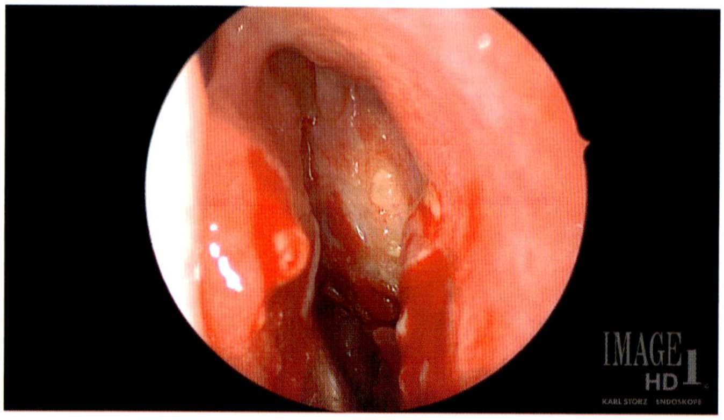

• **Fig. 23.2** Postoperative decompression nasal cavity before definitive debridement nasal cavity after definitive debridement displaying mucosalization and solidification of the intranasal orbital fat.

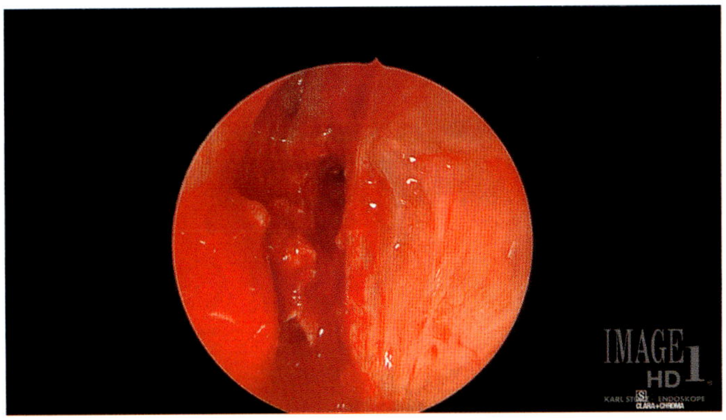

• **Fig. 23.3** Endoscopic frontal sinusotomy in a postoperative patient who underwent decompression nasal cavity surgery before definitive debridement.

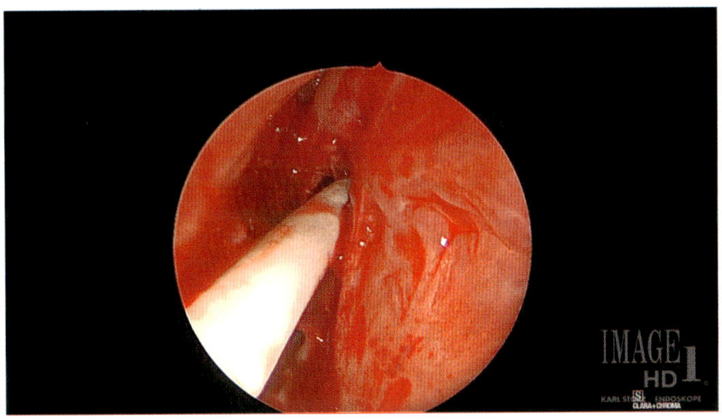

• **Fig. 23.4** Endoscopic frontal sinusotomy in a postoperative patient who underwent decompression nasal cavity surgery after placement of a nonabsorbable stent.

or those undergoing endoscopic optic nerve decompression are at higher risk.[7,9,14] Providers should investigate all symptoms consistent with CSF rhinorrhea promptly, and if identified, treat them definitively without delay.[5]

Despite the potential for complications, most EOD patients do well from a sinonasal perspective. A significant reduction in the 1-year postoperative 22-item Sino-nasal Outcome Test scores of patients with EOD was demonstrated by Mueller et al.[13] Although this study was limited by its small sample size, it supports the notion that most patients can expect an eventual return to normal sinonasal function.[13]

Conclusion

Postoperative management of EOD is nuanced by the presence of intranasal orbital contents. To achieve a successful outcome, surgeons must understand how this alters the natural course of healing and how it changes the management of potential complications. Similar to care after functional endoscopic sinus surgery, meticulous postoperative care of the EOD patient can mitigate complications while improving outcomes.

References

1. Antisdel, J. L., Gumber, D., Holmes, J., & Sindwani, R. (2013). Management of sinonasal complications after endoscopic orbital decompression for Graves' orbitopathy. *Laryngoscope*, *123*, 2094–2098.
2. Kingdom, T. T., Davies, B. W., & Durairaj, V. D. (2015). Orbital decompression for the management of thyroid eye disease: An analysis of outcomes and complications. *Laryngoscope*, *125*, 2034–2040.
3. Leong, S. C., Karkos, P. D., Macewen, C. J., & White, P. S. (2009). A systematic review of outcomes following surgical decompression for dysthyroid orbitopathy. *Laryngoscope*, *119*, 1106–1115.
4. Kennedy, D. W., Goodstein, M. L., Miller, N. R., & Zinreich, S. J. (1990). Endoscopic transnasal orbital decompression. *Archives of Otolaryngology–Head Neck Surgery*, *116*, 275–282.
5. Sellari-Franceschini, S., Dallan, I., Bajraktari, A., Fiacchini, G., Nardi, M., Rocchi, R., et al. (2016). Surgical complications in orbital decompression for Graves' orbitopathy. *Acta Otorhinolaryngologica Italica*, *36*, 265–274.
6. Pletcher, S. D., Sindwani, R., & Metson, R. (2006). Endoscopic orbital and optic nerve decompression. *Otolaryngologic Clinics of North America*, *39*, 943–958. vi.
7. Cohen, L. M., Jiménez Pérez, J. C., Holbrook, E. H., Curry, W. T., & Yoon, M. K. (2018). Meningoencephalocele and cerebrospinal fluid leak complicating orbital decompression. *Ophthalmic Plastic and Reconstructive Surgery*, *34*, e79–e81.
8. Leong, S. C., & White, P. S. (2010). Outcomes following surgical decompression for dysthyroid orbitopathy (Graves' disease). *Current Opinion in Otolaryngology & Head and Neck Surgery*, *18*, 37–43.
9. Yu, B., Ma, Y., Tu, Y., & Wu, W. (2016). The outcome of endoscopic transethmosphenoid optic canal decompression for indirect traumatic optic neuropathy with no-light-perception. *Journal of Ophthalmology*, *2016*, 6492858.
10. Chu, E. A., Miller, N. R., & Lane, A. P. (2009). Selective endoscopic decompression of the orbital apex for dysthyroid optic neuropathy. *Laryngoscope*, *119*, 1236–1240.
11. Tyler, M. A., Zhang, C. C., Saini, A. T., & Yao, W. C. (2018). Cutting-edge endonasal surgical approaches to thyroid ophthalmopathy. *Laryngoscope Investigative Otolaryngology*, *3*, 100–104.
12. Bleier, B. S., Lefebvre, D. R., & Freitag, S. K. (2014). Endoscopic orbital floor decompression with preservation of the inferomedial strut. *International Forum of Allergy & Rhinology*, *4*, 82–84.
13. Mueller, S. K., Miyake, M. M., Lefebvre, D. R., Freitag, S. K., & Bleier, B. S. (2019). Long-term impact of endoscopic orbital decompression on sinonasal-specific quality of life. *Laryngoscope 2018*, *128*, 785–788.
14. Massoud, V. A., Fay, A., & Yoon, M. K. (2014). Cerebrospinal fluid leak as a complication of oculoplastic surgery. *Seminars in Ophthalmology*, *29*, 440–449.

PART 5

Endoscopic Intraorbital Surgery and Tumor Resection

24

Endoscopic Endonasal Approaches to the Orbit and Skull Base in the Coronal Plane

CARL H. SNYDERMAN, MD, MBA, PAUL A. GARDNER, MD, AND ERIC W. WANG, MD

Endoscopic endonasal approaches to the skull base are classified by their orientation in the sagittal and coronal planes.[1] The anterior coronal plane corresponds with the anterior cranial fossa and extends laterally from the midline sagittal corridor across the floor of the anterior cranial base and roof of the orbit. Access to the roof of the orbit is limited medially by the medial orbital wall, ethmoidal arteries, and orbital contents.[2] Tumors that involve the roof of the orbit or extend laterally over the orbit can be accessed endonasally by sacrificing the ethmoidal arteries, decompressing the medial orbit, and displacing the orbital contents. The endonasal approach may be combined with other transcranial and transorbital approaches depending on the location and extent of the pathology.[3,4]

Anatomy

The anterior cranial base is composed of the frontal, ethmoid, and sphenoid bones.[5] The orbital roof is part of the frontal bone and articulates with the sphenoid bone posteriorly and the ethmoid bone medially (Fig. 24.1A). The optic canal and anterior clinoid are part of the sphenoid bone. The medial wall of the orbit consists primarily of the lamina papyracea of the ethmoid bone (Fig. 24.1B). This paper-thin bone articulates with the frontal bone along the frontoethmoidal suture.

Bony foramina for the anterior ethmoid artery (AEA) and posterior ethmoidal artery (PEA) are located along the frontoethmoidal suture line. A middle ethmoidal artery is also present in approximately one-third of patients.[6] The AEA is between the second and third lamellae of the ethmoid bone just posterior to the nasofrontal recess and is in a coronal plane tangential to the posterior surface of the globe. Owing to variability in the pneumatization of the ethmoid and sphenoid sinuses, the PEA may be anterior or posterior to the first bony wall anterior to the optic canal.[6] Both vessels course across the roof of the ethmoid sinus and may be prominent or embedded within the bone (Fig. 24.2).

The optic canal is within the sphenoid bone medial and superior to the superior orbital fissure.[5] It is bounded by the anterior clinoid superolaterally. The lateral optic-carotid recess is between the optic canal and superior orbital fissure and represents pneumatization of the optic strut (Fig. 24.3). Extensive pneumatization can extend into the anterior clinoid.

Indications

An endonasal approach in the anterior coronal plane provides access to the roof of the orbit posterior to the globe. With sacrifice of the ethmoidal arteries and displacement of the orbital contents, the midsagittal plane of the orbital roof can be reliably reached (see Fig. 24.1). The most common indications for this approach include primary tumors of the bone (osteoma, ossifying fibroma, fibrous dysplasia), sinonasal tumors with medial orbital or lateral dural involvement, or intracranial tumors that extend laterally (meningioma) (Fig. 24.4).[4] With meningiomas, there is often a dural tail that extends beyond the margin of the main tumor mass. Complete resection (Simpson grade I or II) requires removal of all involved bone and excision or coagulation of involved dura. Endonasal resection of sinonasal malignancies such as olfactory neuroblastoma can be reliably performed with clear oncologic margins in most cases. Complete resection of involved dura may require extending the skull base defect beyond the medial orbital wall. If clear dural margins cannot be achieved with resection up to the midsagittal plane of the orbit, the endonasal approach can be supplemented with a transorbital or transcranial approach; alternatively, the entire skull base resection can be performed via a transcranial approach.

Tumors may also involve the anterior clinoid, often in the presence of optic nerve compression. When the optic canal is decompressed, drilling of the roof of the optic canal and a small portion of the medial aspect of the anterior clinoid provides a more complete decompression of the optic nerve. Hypertrophy of the anterior clinoid is usually associated with primary bone pathology (osteoma, ossifying fibroma, fibrous dysplasia) or tuberculum meningiomas (Fig. 24.5). The anterior clinoid cannot be completely removed endonasally and, as noted previously, an endonasal approach may be combined with a transorbital or transcranial approach depending on the location of the tumor.[4]

Rarely a cerebrospinal fluid (CSF) leak may result from a pneumatized optic strut and anterior clinoid following transcranial

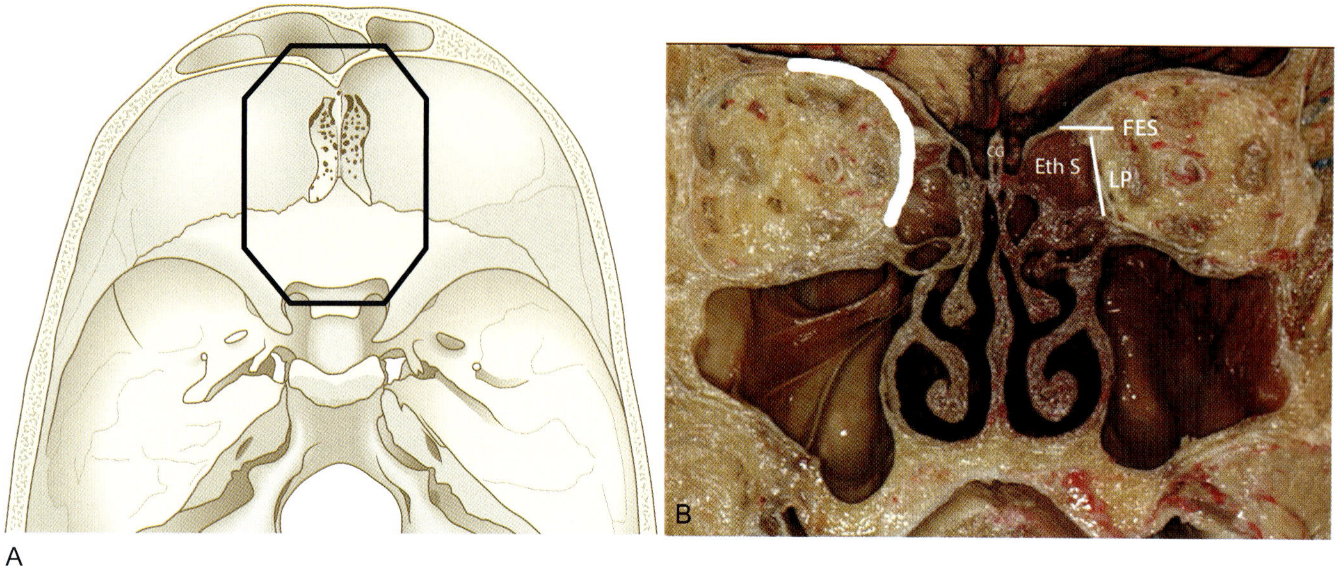

• **Fig. 24.1** A, In the anterior coronal plane, the orbital roof (frontal bone) articulates with the ethmoid bone medially and the sphenoid bone posteriorly. The *black outline* is a rough approximation of the limits of bone removal using an endoscopic endonasal approach. B, In the coronal plane, the medial wall of the orbit (lamina papyracea [*LP*]) articulates with the frontal bone along the frontoethmoidal suture (*FES*). Medial orbital decompression allows removal of the orbital roof to the midsagittal plane of the orbit (*white line*). ethmoid sinus (*Eth S*), crista galli (CG).

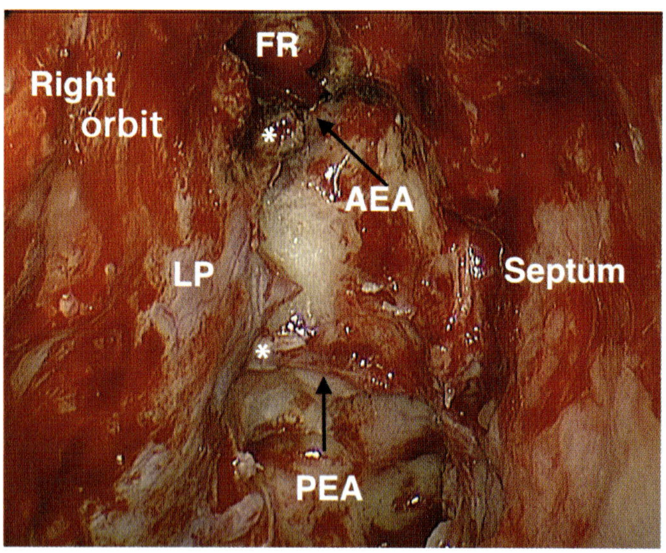

• **Fig. 24.2** The ethmoidal arteries diverge as they cross the roof of the ethmoid sinus from lateral to medial. The anterior ethmoidal artery (*AEA*, coagulated in this image) is located just posterior to the frontal recess (*FR*). The posterior ethmoidal artery (*PEA*) is in proximity to the anterior wall of the sphenoid sinus. The vessels are accessed on the orbital side of the skull base by removing the lamina papyracea (*LP*). *Asterisks* mark the proximal ends of cauterized ethmoidal arteries.

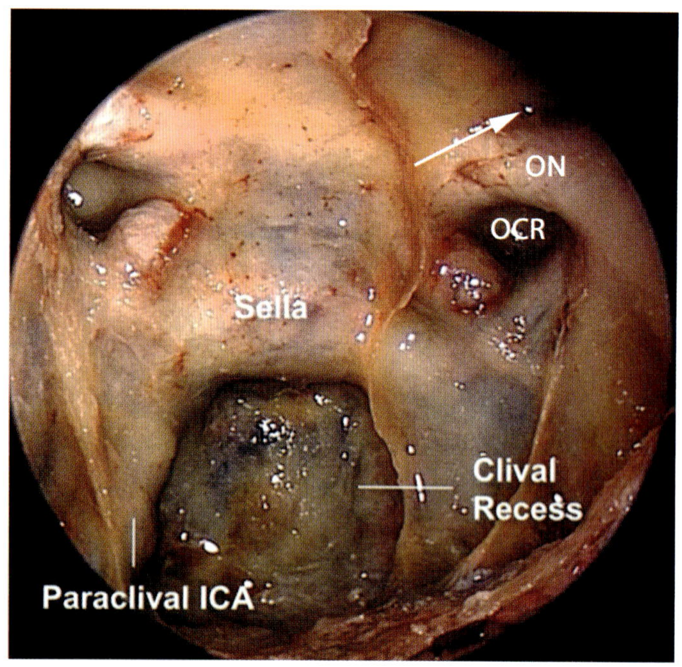

• **Fig. 24.3** Posteriorly the anterior cranial base is composed of the sphenoid bone. The anterior clinoid (*arrow*) extends laterally superior to the optic nerve (*ON*). The lateral opticocarotid recess (*OCR*) separates the optic canal from the internal carotid artery (*ICA*) and superior orbital fissure. In a well-pneumatized sinus, the OCR represents pneumatization of the optic strut and may extend to the anterior clinoid.

surgery with drilling of the anterior clinoid. An endoscopic endonasal approach allows repair of the CSF leak without resorting to re-exploration of the craniotomy site.

Inflammatory disease of the orbit may present with a subperiosteal orbital abscess. Subperiosteal abscesses located medially in the orbit are ideally suited to endoscopic drainage via an endonasal approach with medial orbital decompression. Subperiosteal abscesses in the superior orbit often arise from the frontal sinus and can often be drained with an endonasal approach to the orbital roof (Fig. 24.6).[7] For collections that are more lateral, an external approach may be necessary.

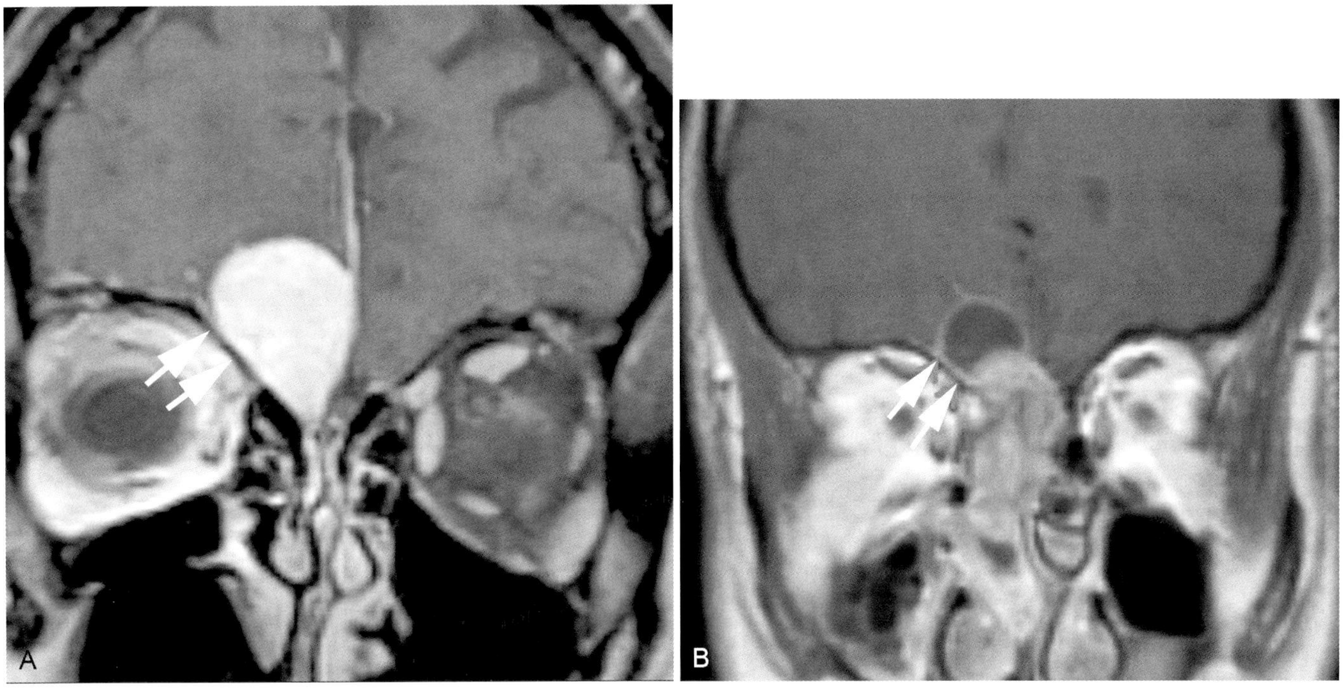

• **Fig. 24.4** Common indications for an endoscopic endonasal approach to the orbital roof include benign tumors such as meningioma (A) and malignant tumors such as olfactory neuroblastoma (B) that extend laterally over the orbital roof (*arrows*).

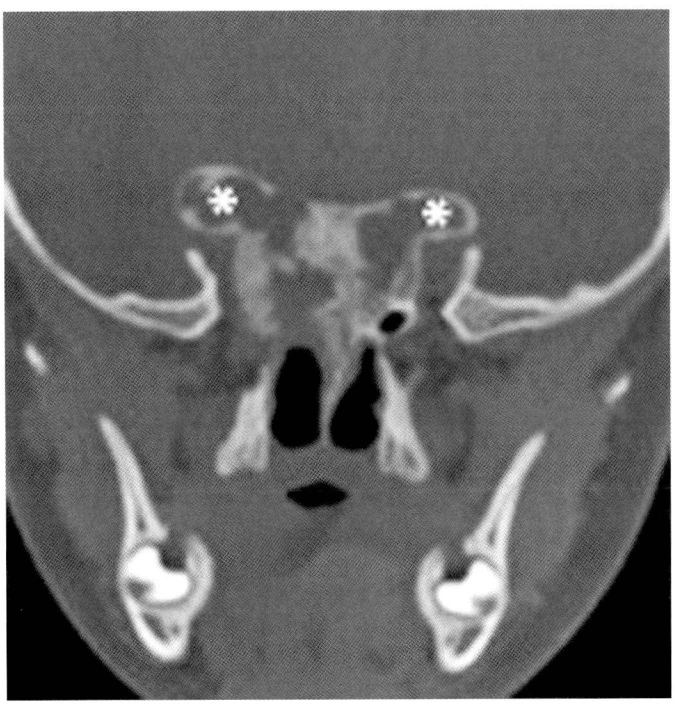

• **Fig. 24.5** The anterior clinoid may be involved by primary bone pathology (osteoma, ossifying fibroma, fibrous dysplasia) or tuberculum meningiomas. This extensive ossifying fibroma has expanded the bone of the anterior clinoids (*asterisks*).

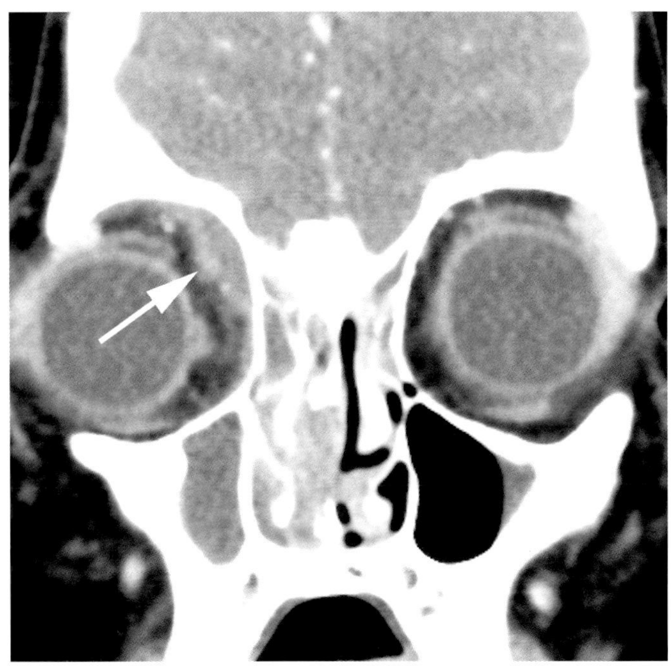

• **Fig. 24.6** Subperiosteal abscesses in the superior orbit (*arrow*) often extend from the frontal sinus and can often be drained with an endonasal approach to the orbital roof.

Orbital tumors, such as hemangiomas or schwannomas, can be accessed endonasally if they involve the medial or inferior orbit. A window can be created between the medial and inferior rectus muscles for access into the orbital cone. This may be combined with a transconjunctival approach to help localize or retract the muscles and/or access the anterior aspect of tumors.[8] The endoscopic endonasal approach also provides a good option for decompression of the orbit, orbital apex, and optic canal for tumors that cannot be safely resected, such as optic nerve sheath meningiomas extending into the orbit.

Technique

The patient is positioned in a Mayfield head holder (Integra Lifesciences, Plainsboro, NJ) with the head slightly rotated and angulated toward the surgeon. This provides ergonomic comfort for the surgeon, stabilizes the head for drilling, and facilitates the use of intraoperative navigation. The nasal cavity is decongested with 0.05% oxymetazoline and antibiotic prophylaxis (third-generation cephalosporin) is administered. The nasal aperture and midface are prepped with povidone-iodine (Betadine) solution. No cleaning of the nasal cavity and sinuses is necessary.

A complete ethmoidectomy is performed on the side of the tumor with resection of the pneumatized portion of the middle turbinate. The sphenoid sinus is maximally opened on one or both sides. For unilateral osseous tumors, a uninarial approach may be sufficient. A transseptal incision anterior to the cartilaginous nasal septum can be used for passage of instruments if a uninarial approach is insufficient. A binarial approach (bilateral sphenoidotomies with resection of the sphenoid rostrum) is preferred when posterior access with decompression of the optic canal is necessary.

For olfactory groove meningiomas and sinonasal malignancies, complete resection of the anterior cranial base (transfrontal, transcribriform, and transplanum approaches) is often necessary (Fig. 24.7). Resection of the superior nasal septum provides additional binarial access with improved angulation for drilling of the skull base.

The lamina papyracea is gently fractured with a Cottle elevator and elevated from the periorbita to the plane of the skull base. The AEA and PEA are localized with the aid of navigation if prominent bony mesenteries are not present (see Fig. 24.2). As noted previously, the AEA is in a coronal plane tangential to the posterior surface of the globe. This is easily visualized with intraoperative navigation. Once the orbit is exposed, the periorbita is elevated from the bone of the orbital roof with the Cottle elevator and "tenting" of the periorbita on the orbital side reveals the location of the AEA and PEA. The vessels are thoroughly cauterized with bipolar electrocautery and transected with microscissors, leaving a stump of the vessel to prevent retraction into the orbital tissues with risk of retrobulbar hematoma (Fig. 24.8). It is easier to cauterize and transect the vessels on the orbital side of the skull base where the vessels traverse the space between the orbital tissues and bone. Additional elevation of the periorbita is now possible with exposure to the midsagittal plane of the orbit. Access to the orbital roof anterior to the AEA is limited owing to the angle of the approach and orbital contents.

Bimanual dissection (two surgeons, dynamic endoscopy) allows safe drilling of the orbital roof while a suction tube retracts and protects the orbital contents (superomedial orbitotomy). A 4-mm coarse diamond drill bit is used for most bone drilling. Alternatively, an ultrasonic bone curette may be used. Once the bone is thinned, angled Kerrison rongeurs are introduced to remove the bone of the orbital roof (see Fig. 24.8). Curved Kerrison rongeurs are particularly useful when standard rongeurs have reached their limit. After resection of tumor, the additional access provided by removal of bone over the orbit is evident (Fig. 24.9).

Access to even a small portion of the anterior clinoid requires decompression of the optic canal. Optic canal decompression is discussed in greater detail in other chapters. Briefly, the medial orbital wall is removed posteriorly to the orbital apex and the bone of the optic canal is carefully thinned with a 3-mm or 4-mm coarse diamond drill bit and the bone fragments are then elevated from

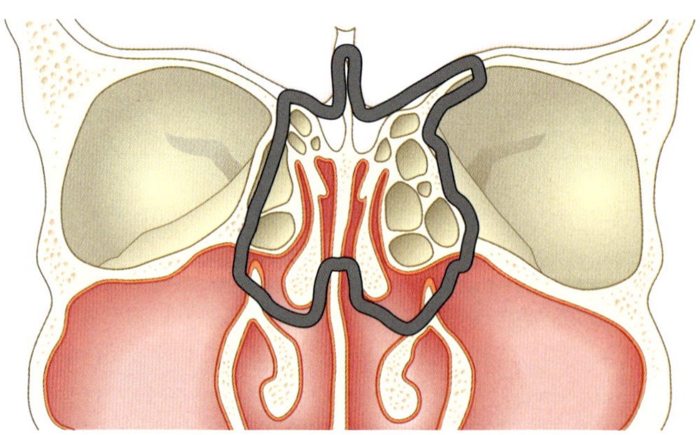

• Fig. 24.7 The extent of bone resection of the anterior cranial base depends on the location and type of pathology. For a sinonasal malignancy, the extent of resection (outlined in *black*) may include the medial orbital wall and roof on the predominant side of the tumor.

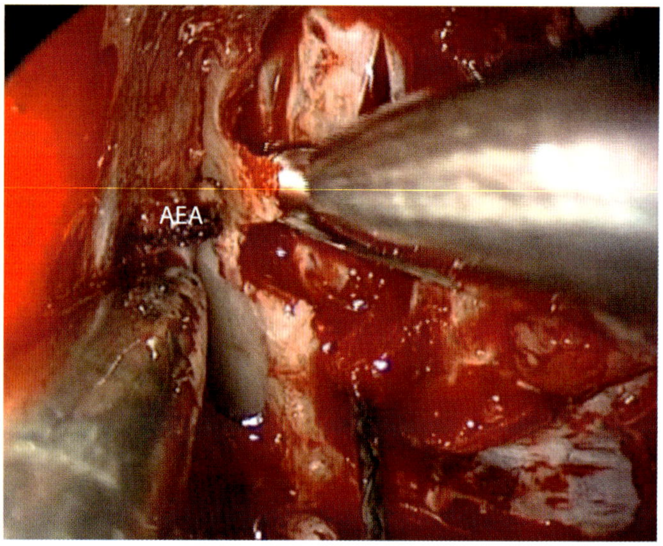

• Fig. 24.8 After decompression of the medial orbit and transection of the ethmoidal arteries (anterior ethmoidal artery [*AEA*]), the periorbita and soft tissues of the orbit are retracted and angled Kerrison rongeurs are introduced to remove the bone of the medial orbital roof.

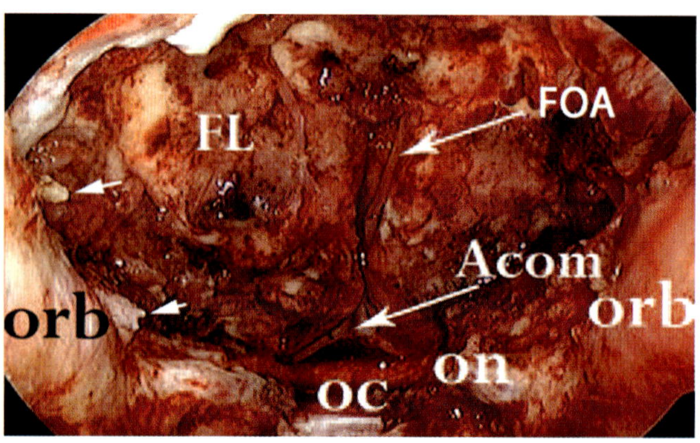

• Fig. 24.9 Panoramic view of surgical field after endoscopic endonasal surgery for a large olfactory grove meningioma. Note the access laterally above the right orbit (*orb*). The proximal stumps of the transected ethmoidal arteries are visible (*short arrows*). *Acom,* anterior communicating artery; *FL,* frontal lobe; *FOA,* fronto-orbital artery; *oc,* optic chiasm; *on,* optic nerve.

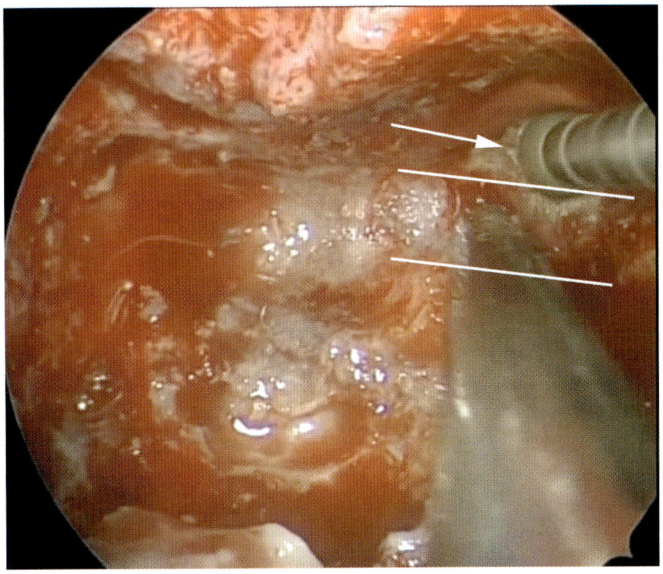

• **Fig. 24.10** The optic nerve (*parallel lines*) is first decompressed. Working between the planum dura and optic nerve, the anterior clinoid (*arrow*) is drilled with a 2-mm or 3-mm coarse diamond burr.

the optic sheath with dissecting instruments. Constant irrigation during drilling is necessary to prevent thermal injury to the nerve. The bone of the posterior planum is thinned with the drill to expose the dura. Working between the planum dura and optic nerve, the optic canal roof and medial aspect of the anterior clinoid are drilled with a 2-mm or 3-mm coarse diamond bit (Fig. 24.10). If there is tumor lateral to the nerve or significant anterior clinoid involvement, an alternative surgical approach is indicated.

If there is no resection of dura, no reconstruction is necessary. If the periorbita is violated, it may be covered with fibrin glue or a free mucosal graft. Significant periorbital resection may require reconstruction with allograft or autograft (fascia lata, temporal fascia). If a dural defect requires reconstruction, a multilayer reconstruction is performed with inlay and onlay collagen and fascial grafts (Fig. 24.11). The extradural fascial graft may be placed between the dura and anterior skull base/orbital roof or between the periorbita and orbital roof, helping to secure the graft. If necessary (large defect, planned or prior radiation), the reconstruction is supplemented with a vascularized nasoseptal flap or pericranial flap.[9] Nasal packing may be performed using nonresorbable (Merocel tampon [Medtronic, Minneapolis, MN]) or resorbable (NasoPore [Polyganics, Groninger, Netherlands], PosiSep, Hemostasis LLC, St. Paul, MN) dressing materials. Antibiotic prophylaxis should be continued as long as nasal packing is in place. A lumbar spinal drain is placed for 3 days when there is reconstruction of a large dural defect of the anterior cranial base.[10] For an example of this technique, see Chabot et al.[11]

Case Example

A patient with a giant olfactory groove meningioma presented with anosmia, emotional lability, memory and concentration problems, and several years of progressive personality change resulting in loss of job and social support system. Preoperative imaging (Fig. 24.12) demonstrated a large meningioma occupying the entire anterior cranial fossa with a maximum diameter of 8 cm. The A2 arteries were partially encased by tumor (arrows). Treatment options including endonasal resection were discussed with the patient and family, and they elected to proceed with surgery. Medial orbital decompression with sacrifice of the ethmoidal arteries and resection of the anterior cranial base helped to decrease the vascularity of the tumor. Removal of the medial orbital roof on each side was necessary to gain access to the lateral limits of the tumor via a superomedial orbitotomy. This large tumor required two stages to achieve gross total resection with preservation of cerebral vessels. Postoperative imaging (Fig. 24.13) demonstrated gross tumor resection with enhancement of the reconstructive nasoseptal flap. With 31 months of follow-up, the patient has no radiographic evidence of recurrence and is neurologically intact with significant improvement in cognitive function and emotional lability.

Complications

Informed consent includes discussion of the risks of orbital injury with diplopia or visual loss, intraoperative hemorrhage or stroke from the internal carotid artery (ICA) or anterior cerebral arteries, postoperative epistaxis, CSF leak, and postoperative infection.

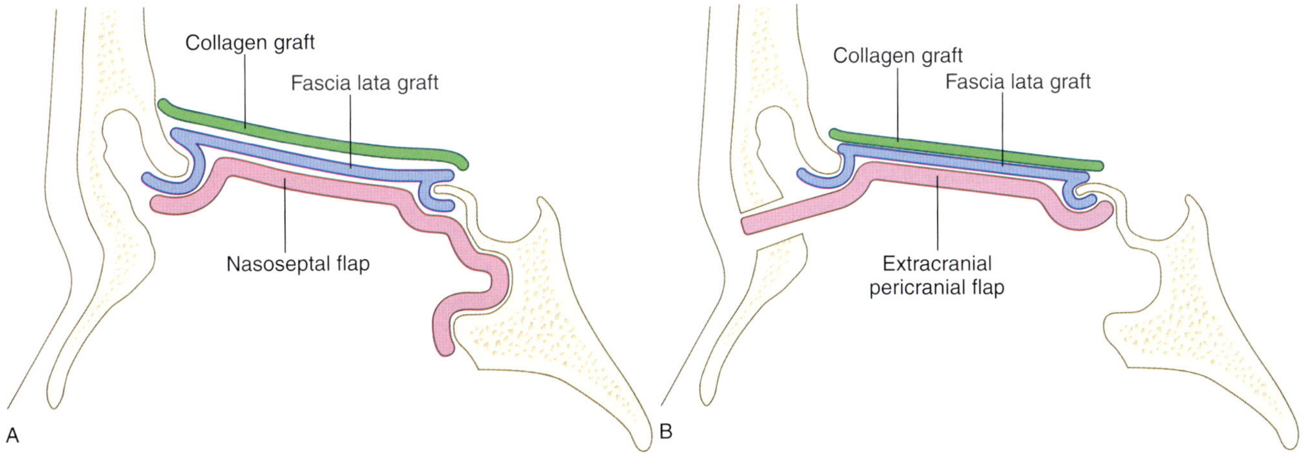

• **Fig. 24.11** Large dural defects of the anterior cranial base are reconstructed with multiple layers, including inlay and onlay fascial grafts, and a vascularized flap, either a nasoseptal flap (A) or extracranial pericranial flap (B).

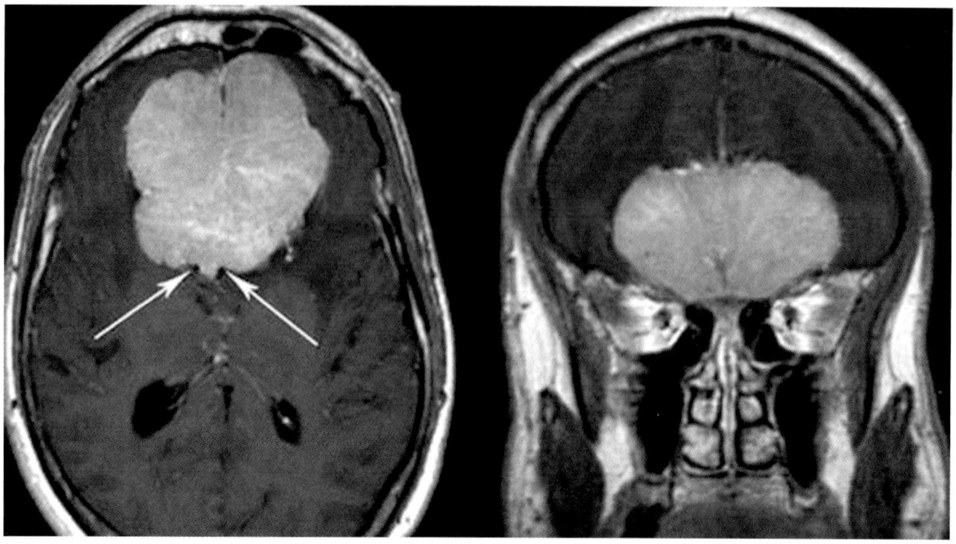

• **Fig. 24.12** Preoperative, postcontrast axial and coronal T1-weighted magnetic resonance imaging with contrast demonstrates a large meningioma occupying the entire anterior cranial fossa with a maximum diameter of 8 cm. The A2 arteries are partially encased by tumor (*arrows*).

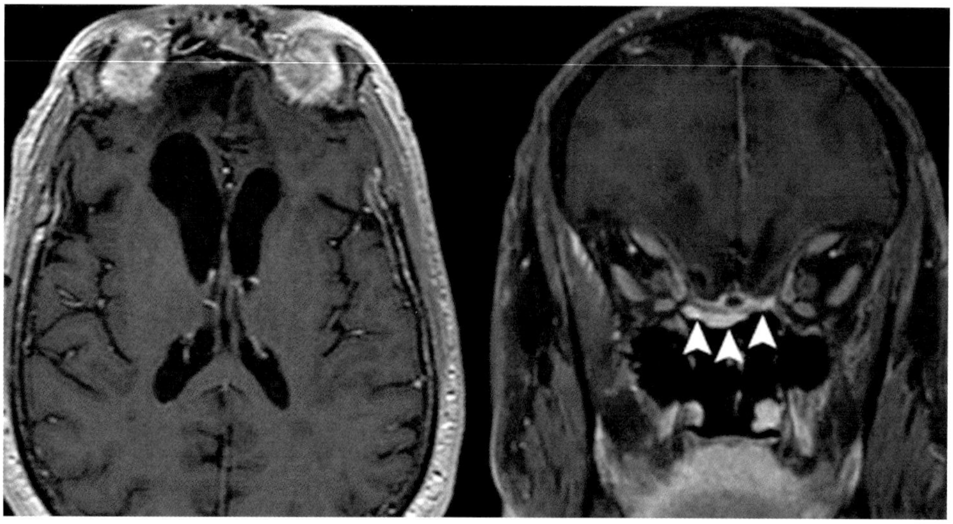

• **Fig. 24.13** Postoperative axial and coronal T1-weighted magnetic resonance imaging with contrast demonstrates gross total resection with enhancement of the reconstructive nasoseptal flap (*arrowheads*). The arteries are preserved.

Potential orbital complications include retrobulbar hematoma, orbital muscle or nerve injury, enophthalmos, and visual loss. Retrobulbar hemorrhage can be avoided by thorough bipolar cauterization of the AEA and PEA before transection. The stumps of the transected vessels are then cauterized a second time. Surgeons should be prepared to deal with a retrobulbar hematoma if it develops. Violation of the periorbita results in herniation of orbital fat into the surgical field and exposure of the extraocular muscles. Traction or removal of fat should be avoided because of the risk of injuring small vessels. Rather, exposed fat can be shrunk with gentle bipolar electrocautery or, if dramatic, retracted via a transconjunctival approach. Diplopia can result from direct injury to the extraocular muscles or their nerve supply, which enters the muscle on its deep aspect. Muscles or the optic nerve may be displaced by large bony tumors and are at increased risk of injury with drilling of the bony lesion. An ultrasonic bone curette can provide precise directional removal of bone in such situations. The medial rectus muscle is most susceptible to injury because of its superficial location. Temporary diplopia can result from postoperative swelling of orbital tissues and relief of proptosis from large bony tumors. Enophthalmos is unlikely as long as the orbital floor and periorbita remain intact. The greatest risk of visual loss is with decompression of the optic canal and may result from direct nerve trauma, thermal injury from drilling or electrocautery, or injury to the ophthalmic artery. Complications are increased with intraconal orbital dissection.

The ICA is susceptible to injury with decompression of the optic canal. The parasellar segment of the ICA is dehiscent in up to 20% of patients and may be injured with sharp instruments or drilling.[12] Postoperative epistaxis is usually from branches of the sphenopalatine artery, especially the posterior septal branches. These branches should be thoroughly cauterized if injured when performing a sphenoidotomy.

Risk factors for CSF leak are the same as for other sites but are increased with increased lateral exposure and defect size. With combined approaches, drilling of a pneumatized anterior clinoid could result in a CSF leak. The risk of a leak at the orbital roof is minimized by tucking an onlay fascial graft between the dura and periorbita.

Postoperative infection, including orbital cellulitis, may result with nasal packing. Patients are cautioned not to blow their nose owing to the risk of orbital emphysema and infection.

Conclusions

The endonasal transorbital approach in the anterior coronal plane provides access to the orbital roof for osseous lesions as well as intracranial and extracranial tumors. Mobilization of the orbital tissues requires sacrifice of the AEA and PEA. Maximal exposure is achieved in the midorbital region between the ethmoidal arteries. Resection of the orbital roof allows resection of lateral extension of tumor-involved dura. Removal of the orbital roof can be extended posteriorly to the anterior clinoid for lesions superior to the optic canal.

References

1. Snyderman, C. H., Wang, E. W., Fernandez-Miranda, J. C., & Gardner, P. A. (2019). Endoscopic transnasal approaches to the skull base and brain: Classifications and its applications. In A. C. Stamm (Ed.), *Transnasal endoscopic skull base surgery: Surgical anatomy and its applications* (2nd ed.). New York: Thieme.
2. Cárdenas Ruiz-Valdepeñas, E., Kaen, A., Gonzalez-Mártinez, E., Gardner, P. A., Wang, E. W., Snyderman, C. H., et al. (2019). Endoscopic endonasal superomedial orbitectomy: How far is safe and possible? *Laryngoscope*. Advance online publication. https://doi.org/10.1002/lary.28080.
3. Gardner, P. A., Paluzzi, A., Fernandez-Miranda, J. C., Tormenti, M., Stefko, S. T., Snyderman, C. H., et al. (2015). "Round-the-clock" surgical access to the orbit. *Journal of Neurological surgery Part B, Skull Base*, *76*(1), 12–24.
4. Borghei-Razavi, H., Truong, H. Q., Fernandes-Cabral, D. T., Celtikci, E., Chabot, J. D., Stefko, S. T., et al. (2018). Minimally invasive approaches for anterior skull base meningiomas: Supraorbital eyebrow, endoscopic endonasal, or a combination of both? Anatomic study, limitations, and surgical application. *World Neurosurgery*, *112*, e666–e674.
5. Patel, C. R., Fernandez-Miranda, J. C., Wang, W. H., & Wang, E. W. (2016). Skull base anatomy. *Otolaryngologic Clinics of North America*, *49*(1), 9–20.
6. Yamamoto, H., Nomura, K., Hidaka, H., Katori, Y., & Yoshida, N. (2018). Anatomy of the posterior and middle ethmoidal arteries via computed tomography. *SAGE Open Med.*, *6*. 2050312118772473.
7. Gavriel, H., Jabrin, B., & Eviatar, E. (2016). Management of superior subperiosteal orbital abscess. *European Archives of Oto-Rhino-Laryngology*, *273*(1), 145–150.
8. Koutourousiou, M., Gardner, P. A., Stefko, S. T., Paluzzi, A., Fernandez-Miranda, J. C., Snyderman, C. H., et al. (2012). Combined endoscopic endonasal transorbital approach with transconjunctival-medial orbitotomy for excisional biopsy of the optic nerve: Technical note. *Journal of Neurological Surgery Reports*, *73*(1), 52–56.
9. Mangussi-Gomes, J., Stamm, A. C., Snyderman, C. H., Fernandez-Miranda, J. C., Gardner, P. A., & Wang, E. W. (2019). Skull base reconstruction: An overview. In A. C. Stamm (Ed.), *Transnasal endoscopic skull base surgery: Surgical anatomy and its applications* (2nd ed.). New York: Thieme.
10. Zwagerman, N. T., Wang, E. W., Shin, S. S., Chang, Y. F., Fernandez-Miranda, J. C., Snyderman, C. H., et al. (2018). Does lumbar drainage reduce postoperative cerebrospinal fluid leak after endoscopic endonasal skull base surgery? A prospective, randomized controlled trial. *Journal of Neurosurgery*, 2019 Oct;131(4): 1172–1178.
11. Chabot, J. D., Stefko, S. T., Snyderman, C., & Fernandez-Miranda, J. C. (2017). Multicorridor endoscopic endonasal and supraorbital approach for orbital roof meningioma: 3-dimensional operative video. *Opererative Neurosurgery (Hagerstown, MD)*, *13*(3), 401.
12. Gardner, P. A., Tormenti, M. J., Pant, H., Fernandez-Miranda, J. C., Snyderman, C. H., & Horowitz, M. B. (2013). Carotid artery injury during endoscopic endonasal skull base surgery: Incidence and outcomes. *Neurosurgery*, *73*(S Suppl Operative), ons261–ons270.

25

Intraorbital Pathology (Tumors) and Management Strategies

ARUN D. SINGH, MD, ANAIS L. CARNICIU, MD, AND ROXANA Y. RIVERA, MD

Orbital tumors encompass a heterogenous range of lesions, from congenital cystic masses to both benign and malignant neoplasms, and can originate from a variety of tissue types. In a large 30-year study of orbital tumors, 64% of masses were benign and 36% were malignant. The most common orbital tumors by category are vascular, secondary or metastatic, and lymphoid. Rhabdomyosarcoma is the most common malignancy in children (3% of cases), and lymphoma is the most common malignancy in older patients (10% of cases). The percentage of malignant orbital tumors increases with age, with malignancies three times more common in older patients owing to the higher incidence of lymphoma and metastasis in this population.[1]

This chapter reviews the most important and common intraorbital tumors and simulating lesions that are encountered in clinical practice. We review the associated demographics, clinical presentation, diagnosis, and management of each tumor.

Lymphoproliferative Tumors

The majority (>90%) of orbital lymphoproliferative tumors are B-cell non-Hodgkin lymphoma, with increasing incidence in the United States. The most common subtype is extranodal marginal zone lymphoma of mucosa-associated lymphoid tissue, a low-grade B-call malignancy that represents 40% to 50% of all orbital lymphomas. High-grade (large cell) lymphoma is far less likely to present in the orbit.[2,3] Orbital lymphoma tends to occur in older patients and may be associated with systemic lymphoma, with a 10-year systemic incidence of 33% for patients with unilateral disease and 72% for those with bilateral disease.[4,5]

Orbital lymphoma usually presents as a painless, slowly progressive mass in the anterior orbit that may feel rubbery to palpation. Conjunctival involvement may have a salmon-patch appearance. Orbital imaging demonstrates a moderately enhancing ovoid mass that tends to mold to adjacent structures without bone involvement (Fig. 25.1). If orbital lymphoma is suspected, open biopsy is preferred to adequately sample the lesion, and a systemic evaluation by an oncologist is indicated to rule out remote lymphoma.[5] When biopsy is performed biopsy, fresh tissue should be sent for flow cytometry analysis in addition to formalin-fixed tissue study. Histopathologic analysis reveals a characteristic polymorphous appearance of small round lymphocytes and plasma cells with mitotically active germinal centers.[6] Hypercellular proliferation with sparse stroma may be similarly seen in benign lesions; molecular studies can be useful to further characterize the lesion as benign, intermediate, or malignant in these cases. Molecular analysis revealing a monoclonal proliferation is consistent with a malignant process.

Management depends on the extent and nature of the histopathologic subtype of lymphoma. In patients with localized ocular adnexal involvement with extranodal marginal zone lymphoma, low-dose radiotherapy (25 Gy) is the treatment of choice. Given the infiltrative nature of lymphoid tumors, a surgical cure is usually not achieved. More aggressive diffuse large B-cell lymphoma requires a combination of radiation and chemotherapy.[2] Co-management with a medical oncologist is crucial.

Burkitt Lymphoma

Burkitt lymphoma is a rare orbital non-Hodgkin B-cell lymphoma that typically presents in the jaw or abdomen of African children.[7,8] Orbital involvement usually occurs secondary to spread from the maxillary bone and may also extend into the globe. A particularly aggressive form of Burkitt lymphoma may develop in patients with AIDS.[9] A clinical presentation of a proptotic child with an abdominal and orbital mass and upward globe displacement is typical. Diagnostic orbital imaging demonstrates a maxillary bone or paranasal sinus lesion with secondary orbital invasion. Histopathology shows B-lymphocyte proliferation and a classic "starry-sky" appearance. Other features include translocation of chromosomes 8 and 14 as well as an association with Epstein-Barr virus. Burkitt lymphoma is typically chemosensitive. As such, management involves attempted debulking and chemotherapy, with external radiation for chemoresistant cases.[10]

Plasma Cell Tumors

Tumors composed of mature plasma cells include plasmacytoma (monoclonal proliferation of plasma cells) and localized plasma cell–rich pseudotumor.[2] Plasmacytoma may rarely present as a primary orbital tumor involving bone (solitary plasmacytomas of bone) or soft tissue (extramedullary plasmacytoma). Secondary orbital plasmacytoma is more common and is associated with multiple myeloma.[11] Systemic workup to rule out multiple myeloma is crucial before the diagnosis of primary orbital plasmacytoma can be

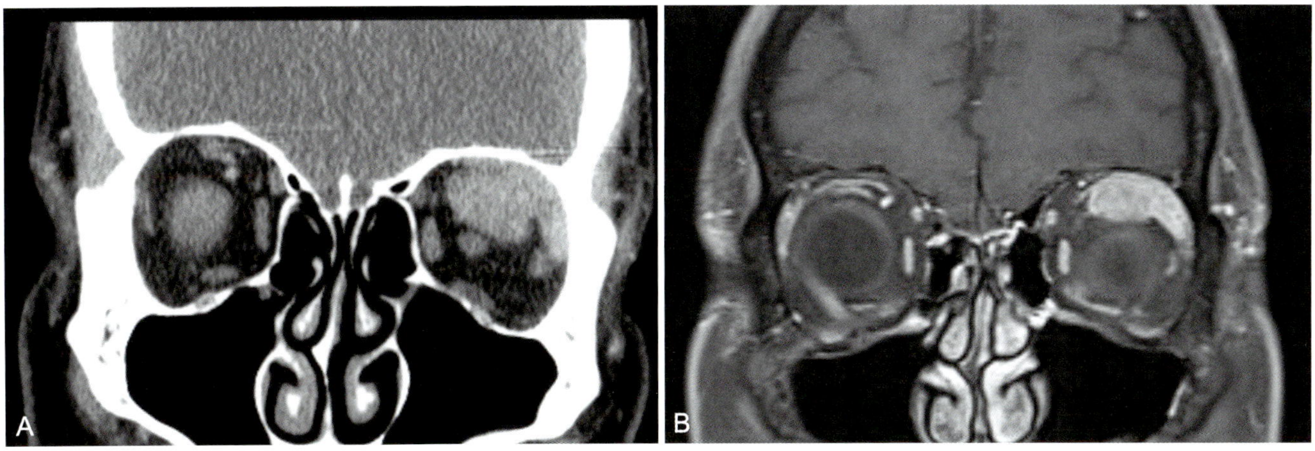

• **Fig. 25.1** A, Computed tomography scan of orbits with contrast showing a homogenous mass in the left orbit, involving the superior rectus, lateral rectus, and the lacrimal gland. The mass molds along the bony orbit without destroying bone. B, Magnetic resonance imaging of orbits with contrast. Coronal image showing an enhancing superotemporal orbital mass involving the superior rectus/levator complex and the lacrimal gland. The mass measures 24.1 mm horizontally × 11.2 mm vertically. Histopathology revealed a mucosa-associated lymphoid tissue lymphoma.

made. Patients typically present with nonspecific orbital signs, including painless proptosis, ptosis, and eyelid swelling. Orbital imaging shows a posterior extraconal orbital mass with possible bony destruction. Multiple myeloma–associated masses tend to occur in the superotemporal quadrant.[12,13] Definitive diagnosis requires histopathologic analysis of tumor tissue. Treatment is usually external beam radiation or chemoradiation. Underlying multiple myeloma is treated by a medical oncologist with chemoradiation and/or stem cell transplant.[13]

Histiocytic Tumors

Histiocytic disorders can be divided into two broad categories: Langerhans cell histiocytosis (LCH) and non-LCH.[14]

Juvenile Xanthogranuloma

Juvenile zanthogranuloma (JXG), the most common form of non-LCH, is a predominantly benign cutaneous disorder. Lesions typically appear during the first year of life as reddish-yellow cutaneous nodules that resolve spontaneously. The head and neck are the most common sites of involvement. Extracutaneous JXG occurs in a minority of patients and is most frequent, and potentially blinding, in the eye. It can also involve the brain, lungs, liver, spleen, and other sites. Management involves topical or periocular corticosteroids for ocular involvement and corticosteroids or excisional biopsy for periocular JXG. Conservative globe-sparing treatment leads to tumor control and satisfactory visual outcome in the majority of patients.[14]

Adult Xanthogranuloma

Adult xanthogranuloma may present in isolated forms in the eyelid or anterior orbit (necrobiotic xanthogranuloma, adult-onset xanthogranuloma) or in an aggressive, potentially lethal systemic form (Erdheim-Chester disease). Xanthogranuloma presents with fibrosclerosis of the orbital tissues. In Erdheim-Chester disease, the mediastinum, pericardium, pleura, bone, and retroperitoneum may be involved, and orbital disease is more diffuse with potential for vision loss. Local lesions are treated with systemic corticosteroids and other immunosuppressants. Vemurafenib, tocilizumab, and sirolimus have shown promising results in systemic disease.[2,15]

Langerhan Cell Histiocytosis

LCH is a rare condition characterized by the abnormal accumulation of proliferating dendritic histiocytes. It most often presents in children between the ages of 5 and 10 years with upper eyelid swelling. The disease spectrum ranges from acute disseminated form (Letterer-Siwe syndrome) with lethal outcomes to chronic, more benign forms (Hand-Schüller-Christian disease and eosinophilic granuloma).[16] Clinically episodes of orbital inflammation may occur recurrently and can involve soft tissue. On orbital imaging, lytic defects of the temporal fossa or sphenoid wing can help differentiate the lesion from orbital cellulitis. Management involves a systemic workup to evaluate for extraorbital involvement, confirmatory biopsy with debulking, followed by intralesional steroid injection or low-dose radiation. Systemic disease requires chemotherapy.[2]

Lacrimal Gland Tumors

The majority of lacrimal gland masses involve dacryoadenitis, or nonspecific inflammation. A smaller portion of lacrimal fossa masses are consistent with lymphoproliferative disease, as discussed earlier. A minority of lacrimal gland tumors are of epithelial origin: 50% are pleomorphic adenomas and 50% are carcinomas.[2]

Dacryops

Dacryops is a lacrimal gland fluid–filled cyst of epithelial origin associated with normal lacrimal tissue. It typically presents in young adults and middle-aged patients. Dacryops most frequently arises from the palpebral lobe of the lacrimal gland and presents as a slow-growing conjunctival mass in the superotemporal fornix. Although typically painless, dacryops may become inflamed or infected and cause pain. Imaging reveals a localized cystic mass in the lacrimal fossa. In symptomatic cases, localized resection may be performed through a superotemporal conjunctival approach, taking care to avoid damaging additional lacrimal ductules and thereby causing dry eye.[17]

Pleomorphic Adenoma

Pleomorphic adenoma (benign mixed tumor) is the most frequently occurring lacrimal gland epithelial tumor. It is slightly more common in men and typically presents during the fourth or fifth decade of life. Clinically the patient presents with painless proptosis from a slowly growing, progressive mass that displaces the globe inferonasally (Fig. 25.2). A firm, potentially nodular mass may be palpated in the lacrimal gland region. Imaging reveals a well-circumscribed mass that may be nodular in appearance. Diagnosis is confirmed by histopathologic analysis of the excised mass, which demonstrates benign-appearing epithelial cells in a spindle-shaped cellular stroma with components of cartilage, osseous, and/or mucin material present. Management involves complete excision of the tumor and its surrounding pseudocapsule without initial biopsy because the tumor frequently recurs (32% of cases) with potential for malignant degeneration.[18,19]

Malignant Mixed Tumor

Malignant mixed tumor, or pleomorphic adenocarcinoma, may arise from an incompletely excised pleomorphic adenoma. Microscopically this tumor demonstrates localized areas of malignant degeneration with otherwise similar histopathologic features as pleomorphic adenoma. Surgical management is typically followed by radiotherapy and/or chemotherapy.[2]

Adenoid Cystic Carcinoma

Adenoid cystic carcinoma is the most common lacrimal gland malignancy. Axial proptosis and inferonasal globe displacement are common, as is posterior orbital extension owing to the lack of encapsulation. In contrast to pleomorphic adenoma, patients present with a characteristic painful and rapid-growing mass over the course of less than 1 year. Histologic diagnosis reveals cells arranged in tubular, nets, or Swiss-cheese pattern with possible perineural invasion. Basaloid cellular morphology portends a poorer prognosis than cribriform morphology.[2]

Malignant lacrimal gland tumors have been associated with notoriously poor outcomes. Surgical debulking combined with radiation therapy is the recommended management strategy, as

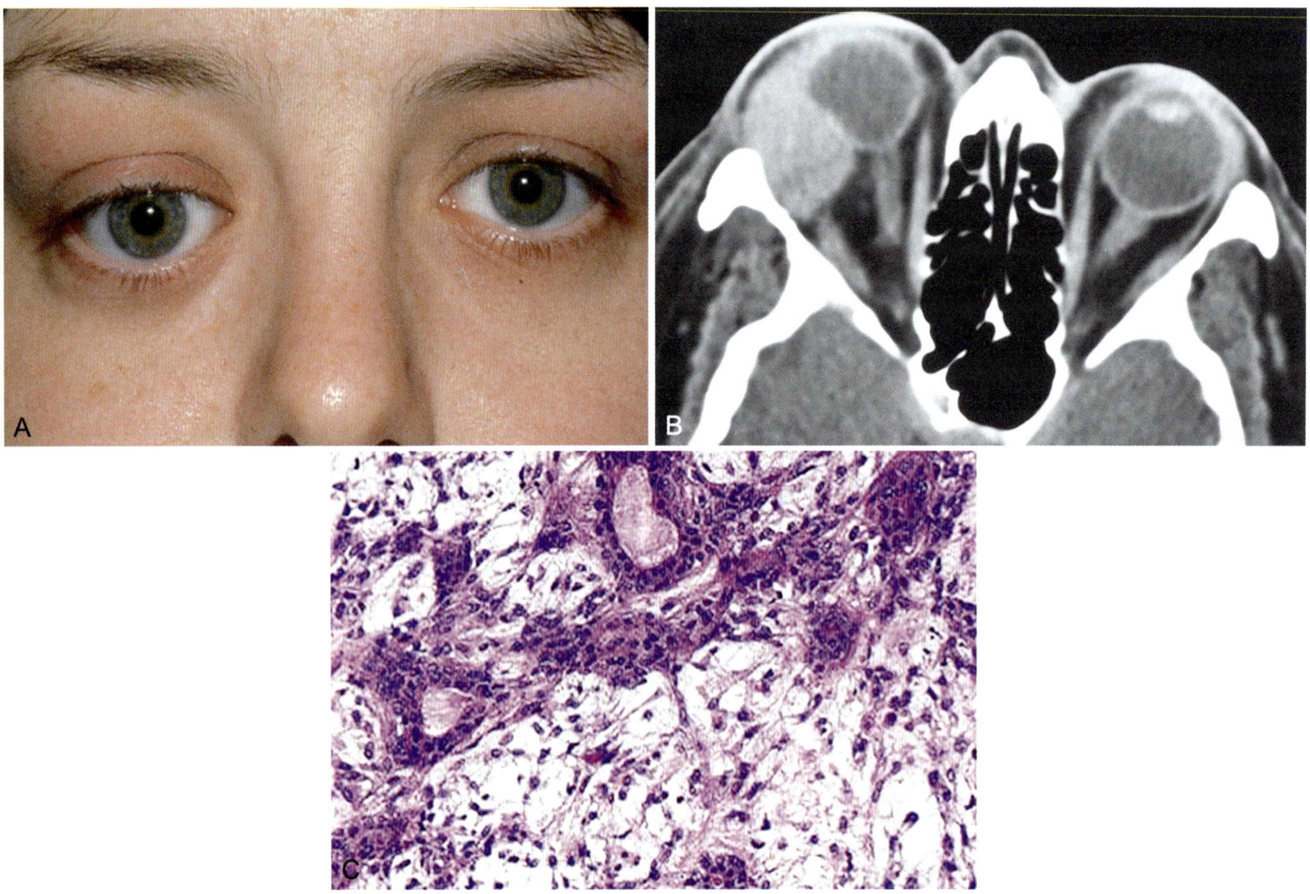

• **Fig. 25.2** A, Facial asymmetry caused by pleomorphic adenoma of the right lacrimal gland. B, Computed tomography scan showing marked enlargement of the right lacrimal gland with indentation of the globe. Epithelial cells centrally with eosinophilic cytoplasm and myoepithelial cells surrounding ducts showing clear lumen. C, Hematoxylin-eosin stain. (Reproduced with permission from Verity, D. H., & Rose, G. E. [2014]. Lacrimal gland tumors. In J. D. Perry & A. D. Singh [Eds.], *Clinical ophthalmic oncology* [pp. 105–113]. Berlin: Springer.)

exenteration has failed to demonstrate improvement in survival rates.[20,21] Neoadjuvant chemotherapy is under active investigation.[22] Unfortunately, mortality from intracranial extension typically occurs within years after a series of recurrences.[23,24]

Neurogenic Tumors

Meningioma

Meningiomas are invasive tumors originating from the arachnoid villi and represent the most common primary brain tumor. Orbital involvement may involve the optic nerve sheath or the sphenoid wing.[2,25]

Sphenoid Wing Meningioma

Orbital involvement typically occurs secondarily from spread of an intracranial meningioma along the sphenoid wing. Patients are typically Caucasian women older than 50 years and present with temporal fullness, proptosis, globe dystopia, eyelid edema, and/or chemosis. Tumors near the optic nerve can cause decreased visual acuity, visual field loss, and relative afferent pupillary defect (RAPD). Cavernous sinus infiltration may lead to diplopia from cranial neuropathy. An enhancing temporal fossa mass with hyperostosis of the sphenoid wing is seen on orbital imaging (Fig. 25.3). The diagnosis is secured by biopsy for histopathologic analysis, which shows whorls of meningothelial cells composed of epithelioid type cells with eosinophilic cytoplasm and calcium deposition (psammoma bodies). Sphenoid wing meningioma is usually observed unless functional deterioration occurs, at which point tumor debulking with or without postoperative radiotherapy is performed.[2,25]

Optic Nerve Sheath Meningioma

Primary meningioma may arise in the orbit from the arachnoid of the optic nerve sheath. Optic nerve sheath meningioma has a gradual, painless presentation with gradual loss of vision and RAPD. The typical patient is a woman in her third or fourth decade of life. Ophthalmic examination can show a normal optic nerve head or disc edema with optociliary shunt vessels. Orbital imaging is generally diagnostic and demonstrates tubular enlargement of the optic nerve with contrast enhancement. Computed tomography (CT) may show characteristic calcification of the optic nerve sheath, known as tram-tracking. Optic nerve sheath meningioma is observed with serial magnetic resonance imaging (MRI) scans if vison is minimally affected and intracranial extension is absent. In the setting of progressive or profound vision loss, radiation therapy is administered. Surgery is typically avoided because of the risk of permanent vision loss from optic nerve blood supply compromise.[2]

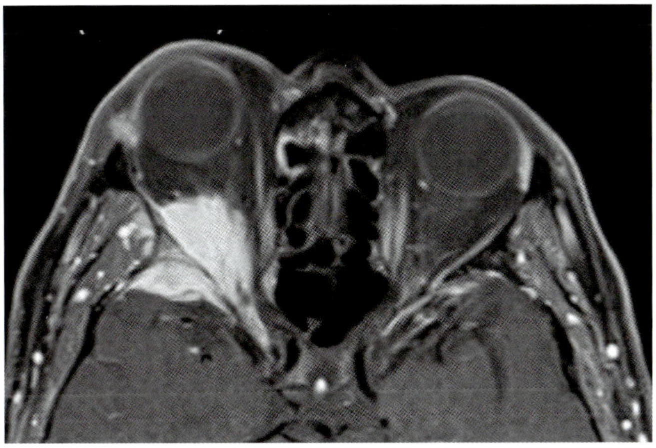

• **Fig. 25.3** Post-gadolinium–enhanced magnetic resonance image of a right sphenoid wing meningioma showing extension into the middle cranial fossa and posterior orbit.

Optic Nerve Glioma

Optic nerve glioma is a type of juvenile pilocytic astrocytoma that usually occurs in children younger than 10 years and may be associated with neurofibromatosis in up to 50% of cases.[26] Patients present with gradual, painless, unilateral axial proptosis and ipsilateral vision loss with RAPD. Optic atrophy, disc edema, strabismus, and/or nystagmus may be seen on ophthalmic examination.[2,27] Diagnosis can usually be made by imaging studies, which show fusiform enlargement and kinking of the optic nerve. Biopsy is typically avoided because of the risk of additional vision loss. Optic nerve gliomas may be observed with serial MRI unless vision loss is progressive and extraorbital involvement is present. When treatment is indicated, chemotherapy is usually considered the first-line therapy.[28] In the setting of progressive symptoms despite chemotherapy, radiation therapy can be used. Surgical debulking is considered only in exceptional cases with extreme proptosis.[29] The rare, malignant variant (glioblastoma) is fatal within 6 to 14 months despite chemotherapy and radiation.[2]

Neurofibroma

Neurofibroma is a Schwann cell tumor that may be discrete or associated with neurofibromatosis type 1 (plexiform neurofibroma). The patient presents with a stereotypical S-shaped lateral eyelid deformity and ptosis.[30] In cases associated with neurofibromatosis, multiple neurofibromas may cause diffuse facial disfigurement. On examination, the mass may have a "bag of worms" consistency to palpation. Surgical management is limited to tumors that cause disfigurement or visual compromise, although recurrence is common in plexiform tumors. In contrast, discrete tumors may be excised without recurrence.[2]

Schwannoma

Schwannoma (neurolemmoma) is a benign, slow-growing encapsulated tumor that arises from proliferation of Schwann cells. Affected patients are between the second and sixth decade of life.[31] Schwannomas typically occupy the superior orbit and rarely undergo malignant transformation (Fig. 25.4). Microscopically, tumors demonstrate a distribution of nuclear palisading (Antoni A) and myxoid (Antoni B) areas, and the appearance on MRI has a variable degree of heterogeneity.[32] Primary treatment is complete excision with maintenance of capsular integrity.[2]

Vascular Tumors and Malformations

Capillary Hemangioma

Capillary hemangioma is a benign childhood tumor that is typically presents at birth or develops soon thereafter. These lesions enlarge in the first year of life and spontaneously involute between the ages of 5 and 10 years. Risk factors include female sex, low birth weight, prematurity, and maternal chorionic villus sampling. Clinical examination is usually diagnostic, as the tumor often appears as a superficial, soft red mass of the medial upper eyelid; deeper

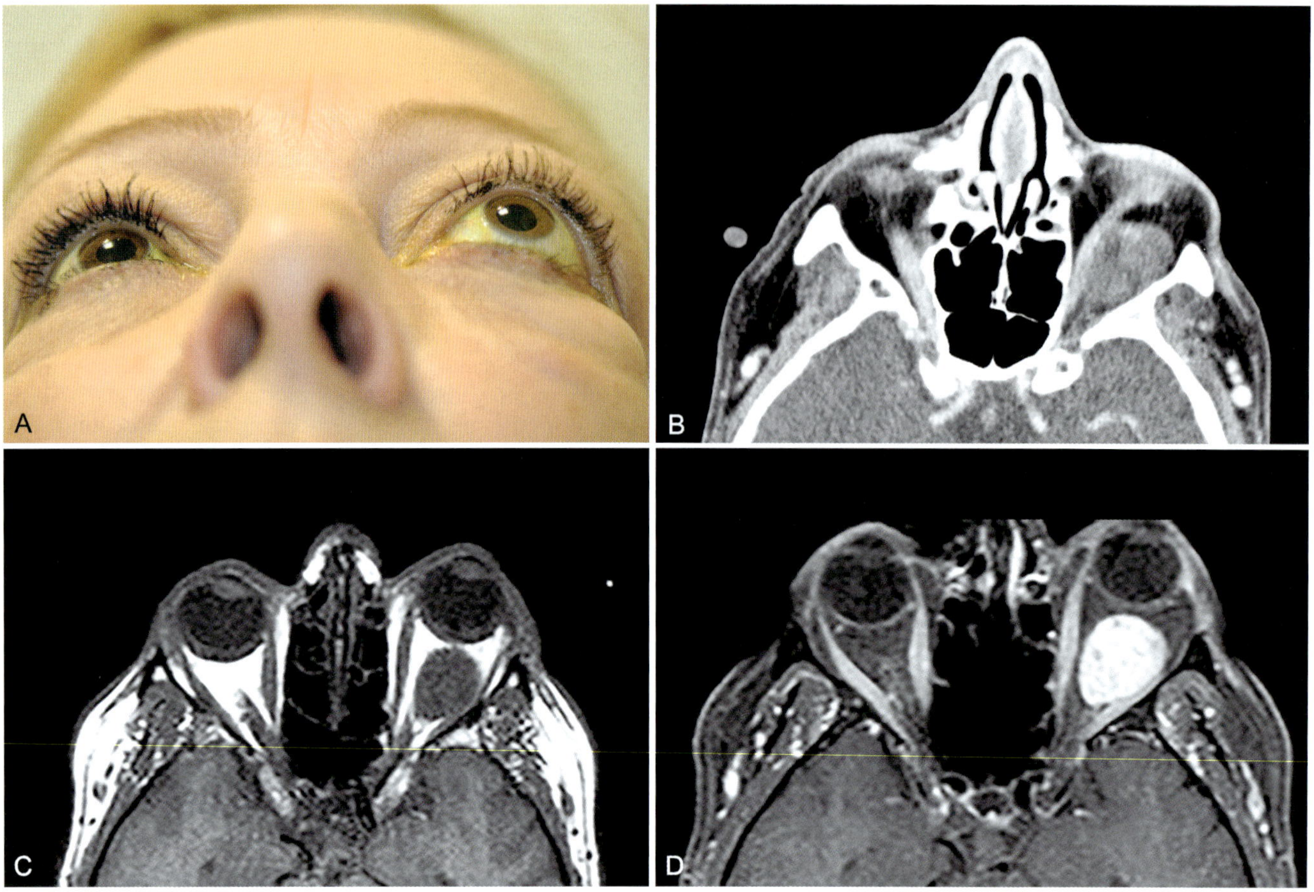

• **Fig. 25.4** A 66-year-old woman presented with a fullness of the left eye with visual acuity of 20/25 in both eyes. External examination revealed axial proptosis of 5 mm. A, External motility was full. Fundus evaluation showed normal optic disc and macula bilaterally. B, Previously performed computed tomography scan had indicated an intraconal mass located in the inferotemporal quadrant. C, Magnetic resonance imaging showed an intraconal well-circumscribed left orbital mass measuring 2.5 cm in the anteroposterior dimension, 1.8 cm in width, and 1.8 cm in the craniocaudal dimension. Mild heterogeneity of the mass with areas of microcystic change and predominantly hypointense appearance on T1 with (D) fairly avid enhancement on postgadolinium imaging was suggestive of schwannoma. Atypical cavernous malformation and other neoplasms could not be excluded. The tumor could be removed completely via anterior orbitotomy (lower lid swing approach). Orbital schwannoma was confirmed by histopathology and immunohistochemistry (SOX10).

lesions in the superonasal orbit may appear blue-tinged. Imaging can further characterize the lesion, which demonstrates high blood flow on dynamic magnetic resonance angiography (MRA). Ophthalmic complications include amblyopia, strabismus (ocular misalignment), and refractive error. Treatment is required when tumors compromise vision and do not involute.[2] Superficial lesions are treated with timolol gel,[33] whereas deeper orbital lesions respond to oral propranolol.[34] Refractory lesions are treated with topical, local, or oral steroids. Surgical excision is reserved for nonresponsive, amblyogenic lesions. Systemic evaluation is recommended, as associated systemic hemangiomas may be present and cause respiratory compromise, cardiac problems, or thrombocytopenia.[2,35]

Cavernous Venous Malformation (Cavernous Hemangioma)

Cavernous malformation is the most common benign orbital tumor in adults and more frequently occurs in middle-aged females. Patients typically present with slowly progressive axial proptosis.[36] Growth of a preexisting tumor may occur in pregnancy. Associated ophthalmic findings include retinal striae, hyperopia (far-sightedness), disc edema, increased intraocular pressure, and strabismus (Fig. 25.5). Imaging reveals an encapsulated and enhancing intraconal orbital mass with slow flow.[2,37] The tumor is composed of large endothelium-lined cavities that contain red blood cells. Symptomatic tumors that cause visual disturbance or diplopia may be excised with a cryoprobe with ease given their encapsulated nature. However, the approach to the orbit may be more challenging than the tumor removal itself. Given their intraconal location, coronal imaging is helpful for localizing the tumor before planned surgical excision.[2]

Lymphatic Malformation (Lymphangioma)

Lymphatic malformations are congenital lesions that arise from vascular dysgenesis and may often have both venous and lymphatic components. The typical patient is a child who presents with an enlarging mass or increased proptosis during an upper respiratory tract infection. MRI is diagnostic and demonstrates a nonenhancing grape-like septate cyst with fluid levels or, in the case of acute presentation, a possible intralesional hemorrhage.[38,39] These lesions respond well to percutaneous sclerotherapy.[40]

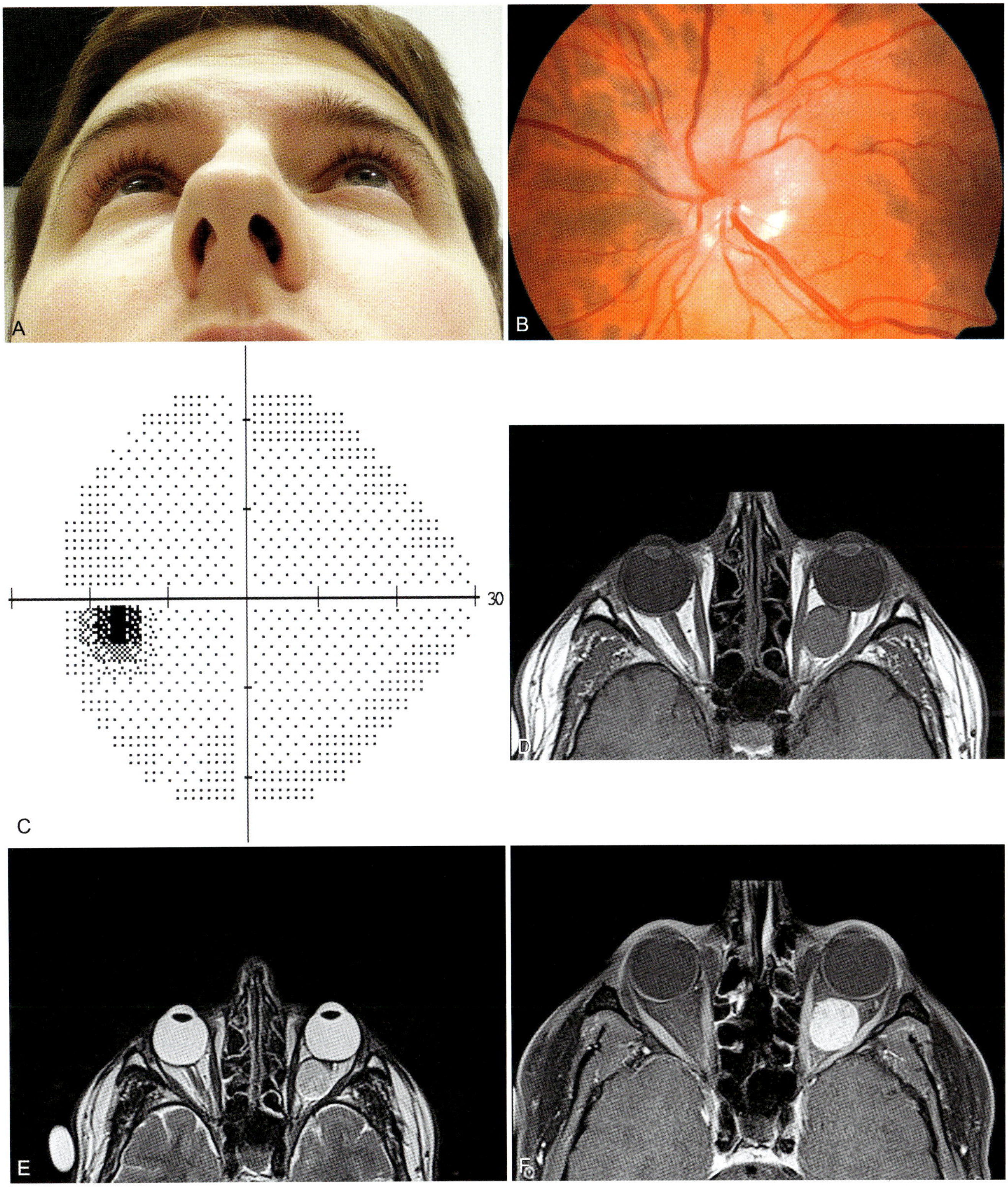

• **Fig. 25.5** A 28-year-old man presented with a prominence of the left eye with normal visual acuity of 20/20 in both eyes. A, External examination revealed left axial proptosis of 3 mm. External motility was full. Fundus evaluation showed disc edema (B) with normal visual field (C). Magnetic resonance imaging showed a well-circumscribed ovoid intraconal mass measuring 18 mm in maximal diameter. Precontrast (D) T1 images and (E) T2 images demonstrate intermediate signal intensity. F, Postcontrast images demonstrate intense lobulated enhancement. The left optic nerve is noted to be displaced superolaterally. The tumor could be removed completely via anterior orbitotomy (lower lid swing approach). Orbital cavernous malformation (hemangioma) was confirmed by histopathology and immunohistochemistry.

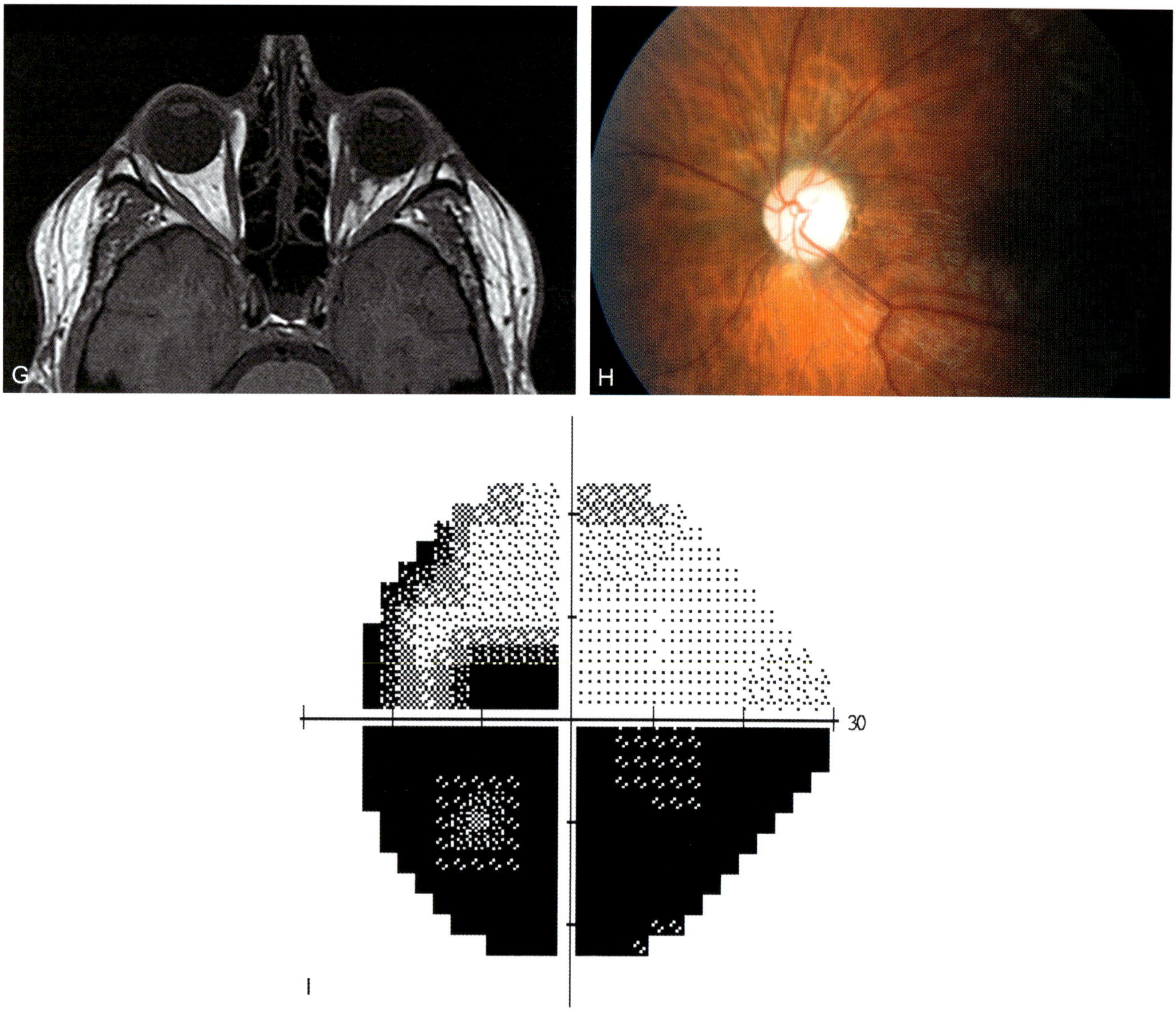

• **Fig. 25.5—cont'd** Although there was no intraoperative complication, and the tumor had been completely removed (G), a few weeks after the surgery, the patient had visual acuity of 20/100, inferior visual field defect (H), and optic atrophy (I).

Arteriovenous Anomalies

Arteriovenous Malformation

Arteriovenous malformations are congenital, high-flow lesions composed of a direct connection between the arterial and venous systems without an intervening capillary bed. Children may present with prominent episcleral vessels in a corkscrew pattern. Management involves targeted endovascular embolization with possible microsurgical excision.[2,41]

Arteriovenous Fistula

Arteriovenous fistulas are acquired low- or high-flow direct connections between the arterial and venous systems that form secondary to a degenerative or traumatic process, respectively. Direct carotid-cavernous fistulas are formed by a direct connection between the internal carotid artery and cavernous sinus, usually secondary to trauma. Patients may present with tortuous ocular surface vessels, bruit, increased intraocular pressure), extraocular muscle palsy, and/or pulsatile proptosis. CT imaging demonstrates an enlarged superior ophthalmic vein. Indirect (dural) carotid-cavernous fistulas are degenerative lesions that form in older patients with hypertension, vascular disease, or atherosclerosis. Clinical features include chronic red eye and ipsilateral elevated intraocular pressure with possible optic nerve damage (glaucoma). Although the gold standard test is x-ray angiogram, noninvasive MRA is typically diagnostic. As in arteriovenous malformations, endovascular treatment with glue or coils is usually successful. Orbitotomy may be required for canalization of the superior ophthalmic vein.[2,42,43]

Venous Malformation (Orbital Varix)

Venous malformation is caused by orbital vascular dysgenesis that results in a low-flow lesion. Proptosis upon Valsalva maneuver or dependent head positioning is characteristic, and diagnostic CT imaging during the Valsalva maneuver often shows venous enlargement. Biopsy and primary surgical excision, particularly in asymptomatic patients, are avoided because of the risk of hemorrhage and poorly defined lesion margins. Embolization can improve symptoms, and surgery may rarely be needed in cases of compressive optic neuropathy.[2]

Fibrous Connective Tissue Tumors

Hemangiopericytoma is a benign mass of mesenchymal origin with potential for malignant transformation. It shares many characteristics with fibrous histiocytoma; as such, these lesions have recently all been classified as solitary fibrous tumor.[44] This tumor is usually limited to the eyelids or orbit but may be locally aggressive.[45] Patients are often middle-aged and present with a firm, encapsulated mass of the eyelids or orbit. Progressive proptosis, diplopia, and orbital pressure/pain may be present. [46] If the lacrimal sac is involved, bloody epiphora may be observed. On imaging, a well-circumscribed typically intraconal mass is seen that may resemble cavernous hemangioma. Bony remodeling is possible in chronic tumors.[47] Definitive diagnosis is made by histopathology, which demonstrates pericytes in a rich capillary network with fibroblastic and histiocytic cells in a classic storiform pattern that may show CD34 positivity.[2,48] Complete surgical excision is advised owing to malignant potential.[46,49–51] Complex lesions may benefit from high-resolution CT/MRI or dynamic contrast-enhanced MRA (time-resolved imaging of contrast kinetics [TRICKS]) for surgical planning.[52]

Myogenic Tumors

Rhabdoyosarcoma

Rhabdomyosarcoma is the most common primary orbital malignancy in children and the most common mesenchymal tumor of the orbit. Typical onset is before age 10. Patients present with acute and rapidly progressing unilateral axial proptosis, eyelid discoloration, periocular edema, ptosis, and strabismus. There are several subtypes of rhabdomyosarcoma, varying in frequency and associated mortality (Table 25.1). The globe may be displaced inferolaterally as the tumor is frequently located superonasally.[2,53,54] Prompt imaging and biopsy, usually via anterior orbitotomy, is performed to confirm the diagnosis. Histology demonstrates striated muscle in various stages of embryogenesis, which may be more apparent on electron microscopy than traditional light microscopy. Cervical and preauricular lymph node involvement suggests regional metastases. Metastatic workup is advised, including chest x-ray, bone marrow biopsy, and lumbar puncture for cerebrospinal fluid analysis, because more distant metastases can occur.[2] Management involves radiation therapy to the orbit and systemic chemotherapy to eliminate potential microscopic metastases.[55] Recurrent cases require exenteration.

Leiomyoma and Leiomyosarcoma

Leiomyoma is a benign, slow-growing tumor of smooth muscle that may rarely involve the orbit. It typically affects children and young adults. In contrast, older adults are typically affected with the rarer, malignant form, leiomyosarcoma. Patients may present with proptosis in the case of either tumor, which is often more marked and rapidly progressive in the malignant form. CT imaging may reveal a homogenous tumor located anywhere in the orbit. Leiomyomas are encapsulated, whereas leiomyosarcomas traditionally lack a capsule and demonstrate friability. Histopathology using immunohistochemical markers is diagnostic and can be used to differentiate between benign and malignant forms. Satellite lesions are often seen with leiomyomas and can serve as a source of recurrence in the setting of incomplete excision. Hence, complete surgical excision with wide margins is the recommended treatment for both tumors.[56–58]

Orbital Cystic Lesions

Dermoid Cysts

Dermoid cysts are the most common orbital tumors of childhood. This tumor is a choristoma composed of dermal appendages, oil, and keratin. The most common location is the temporal orbit at the frontozygomatic suture. Epidermoid cysts are similar but contain only keratin and lack dermal appendages. Children usually present with a painless mass of the lateral brow that enlarges slowly. Expansion into the orbit through the frontozygomatic suture may present as a "dumbbell" cyst and clinically apparent pulsating proptosis with

TABLE 25.1 Rhabdomyosarcoma Subtypes

Type	Frequency (% of All Rhabdomyosarcomas)[71]	Histopathology[2]	Prognosis[2]	Additional Features[2,72]
Embryonal	Most common (81%)	Loose fascicles of undifferentiated spindle cells	Favorable; 94% 5-year survival rate	Superonasal location
Alveolar	12%	Compartments of fibrovascular strands with rhabdomyoblasts along connective tissue or within alveolar spaces	Poorest; 65% 5-year survival rate	Inferior orbital location
Pleomorphic	Rare	Most differentiated rhabdomyosarcoma subtype with strap-like or rounded cells with well-visualized striations	Best; 97% 5-year survival)	Occurs in adults
Botryoid	3%	Subepithelial aggregates of tumor cells	Favorable	Grape-like mass of paranasal sinuses or conjunctiva with secondary orbital spread

mastication. CT imaging reveals a round to oval well-defined mass with a hyperintense wall and hypointense center. MRI shows minimal enhancement with contrast. In chronic masses, orbital inflammation may be present as the result of leakage of cyst contents. Diagnosis is confirmed based on clinical examination findings and typical radiographic appearance. Management involves surgical excision, taking care not to rupture the cyst wall.[59–61]

Mengingocele, Encephalocele, and Meningoencephalocele

Masses composed of intracranial contents may protrude through congenital clefts in the skull or orbit. Herniated material may include meninges (meningocele), brain tissue (encephalocele), or both (meningoencephalocele). Orbital involvement typically presents anteriorly, just superior to the level of the medial canthus, with possible inferolateral globe displacement. These lesions are usually recognized in babies and often increase in size with crying or with the Valsalva maneuver. Importantly, the mass should be differentiated from nasolacrimal duct obstruction, in which the distention is inferior to the medial canthus. Multidisciplinary treatment with neurosurgery is needed for definitive management. Additionally, associated anomalies of the optic disc may be present; hence referral to an ophthalmology specialist is important.[59]

Mucocele

Mucoceles occur when communication between the paranasal sinuses and nose is obstructed, most commonly in the frontal, frontoethmoidal, and ethmoidal sinuses.[62,63] Predisposing conditions include chronic sinusitis, facial trauma, radiation to the head, and prior sinus or lacrimal apparatus surgery.[64,65] Sinus secretions form cystic structures containing desquamated respiratory epithelium that may expand and erode into the orbit. Secondary infection of these cysts can occur with purulent material, resulting in mucopyocele. Patients most commonly present with symptoms similar to that of chronic sinusitis, including headache, nasal congestion, and rhinorrhea. Dynamic proptosis, extraocular muscle restriction, ptosis, and lid ecchymoses may also occur.[63,66] Diagnosis is made with imaging. CT is best for determining the extent of bone involvement and possible infection, which demonstrates contrast enhancement. MRI is helpful for differentiating mucoceles from other soft-tissue tumors.[67] Management is surgical and most commonly performed via functional endoscopic sinus surgery, in which the mucocele is marsupialized and normal sinus drainage is reestablished.[68]

Lipomatous Tumors

Dermolipomas

Dermolipomas are solid tumors composed of adipose tissue and dense connective tissue, which typically present in the temporal subconjunctival space of the orbit. Their appearance may mimic orbital fat or lacrimal gland prolapse, but careful examination reveals small hairs on the mass surface, a unique feature of dermolipomas. Patients may report ocular irritation. Although the mass appears superficial on the globe, there is potential for deeper extension, potentially involving the extraocular muscles, orbital tissues, or lacrimal gland. These lesions can occur in isolation or as part of Goldenhar syndrome. Clinical examination is usually sufficient for diagnosis. Dermolipomas are usually observed unless the lesion is large, affects extraocular motility, or is cosmetically unacceptable to the patient. If excision is desired, only the visible portion of the mass should be removed, taking care to preserve the overlying conjunctiva, extraocular muscles, and nearby lacrimal gland ducts.[59]

TABLE 25.2 Metastatic Tumors to the Orbit Based on Patient Age

Patient age	Primary cancer by decreasing order of frequency[2,69]
Adults	Breast (females) Prostate (males) Lung Skin—melanoma Kidney Gastrointestinal tract
Children	Adrenal neuroblastoma Rarer primary cancers: Leukemia— acute lymphoblastic leukemia Ewing sarcoma Wilms tumor

Metastatic Tumors

Systemic cancer metastases to the orbit are associated with a poor systemic prognosis. The pattern of orbital metastases differs in adults and children and is overall more common in adults. Orbital metastatic disease is overwhelmingly unilateral (>90% of cases).[69] Common primary cancers are based on patient age (Table 25.2). Patients frequently present with diplopia, pain, vision loss, proptosis, and/or strabismus from early extraocular muscle involvement. Lytic CT lesions may be seen on orbital imaging.[2] Multidisciplinary treatment varies based on the primary cancer and extent of orbital involvement. Therapeutic options include radiotherapy, chemotherapy, hormone therapy, surgery, and immunotherapy.[70]

References

1. Shields, J. A., Shields, C. L., & Scartozzi, R. (2004). Survey of 1264 patients with orbital tumors and simulating lesions: The 2002 Montgomery Lecture, part 1. *Ophthalmology, 111*(5), 997–1008.
2. American Academy of Ophthalmology. (2016). Orbital neoplasms and malformations. In B. Louis, C. J. R. Cantor, & G. A. Cioffi (Eds.), *Orbit, eyelids, and lacrimal system. Basic and clinical science course* (pp. 67–114). San Francisco: American Academy of Ophthalmology.
3. Olsen, T. G., & Heegaard, S. (2019). Orbital lymphoma. *Survey of Ophthalmology, 64*(1), 45–66.
4. Demirci, H., Shields, C. L., Shields, J. A., Honavar, S. G., Mercado, G. J., & Tovilla, J. C. (2002). Orbital tumors in the older adult population. *Ophthalmology, 109*(2), 243–248.
5. Demirci, H., Shields, C. L., Karatza, E. C., & Shields, J. A. (2008). Orbital lymphoproliferative tumors: Analysis of clinical features and systemic involvement in 160 cases. *Ophthalmology, 115*(9), 1626–1631. 1631.e1621–1623.
6. Knowles, D. M., & Jakobiec, F. A. (1982). Ocular adnexal lymphoid neoplasms: Clinical, histopathologic, electron microscopic, and immunologic characteristics. *Human Pathology, 13*(2), 148–162.
7. Burkitt, D., & O'Conor, G. T. (1961). Malignant lymphoma in African children. I. A clinical syndrome. *Cancer, 14*, 258–269.
8. Templeton, A. C. (1971). Orbital tumours in African children. *British Journal of Ophthalmology, 55*(4), 254–261.

9. Brooks, H. L., Downing, J., McClure, J. A., & Engel, H. M. (1984). Orbital Burkitt's lymphoma in a homosexual man with acquired immune deficiency. *Archives of Ophthalmology, 102*(10), 1533–1537.
10. Shields, J. A., & Shields, C. L. (2016). Orbital Burkitt lymphoma. In *Eyelid, conjunctival, and orbital tumors: An atlas and textbook*. (3rd ed., p. 760). Philadelphia: Wolters Kluwer.
11. Adkins, J. W., Shields, J. A., Shields, C. L., Eagle, R. C., Flanagan, J. C., & Campanella, P. C. (1996). Plasmacytoma of the eye and orbit. *International Ophthalmology, 20*(6), 339–343.
12. Burkat, C. N., Van Buren, J. J., & Lucarelli, M. J. (2009). Characteristics of orbital multiple myeloma: A case report and literature review. *Survey of Ophthalmology, 54*(6), 697–704.
13. Thuro, B. A., Sagiv, O., Shinder, R., et al. (2018). Clinical presentation and anatomical location of orbital plasmacytomas. *Ophthalmic Plastic and Reconstructive Surgery, 34*(3), 258–261.
14. Samara, W. A., Khoo, C. T., Say, E. A., et al. (2015). Juvenile xanthogranuloma involving the eye and ocular adnexa: Tumor control, visual outcomes, and globe salvage in 30 patients. *Ophthalmology, 122*(10), 2130–2138.
15. Ortiz Salvador, J. M., Subiabre Ferrer, D., & Pérez Ferriols, A. (2017). Adult xanthogranulomatous disease of the orbit: Clinical presentations, evaluation, and management. *Actas Dermo-sifiliográficas, 108*(5), 400–406.
16. Singh, S., Kaliki, S., Reddy Palkonda, V. A., & Naik, M. N. (2018). Langerhans cell histiocytosis of the orbit: A study of eight cases. *Oman Journal of Ophthalmology, 11*(2), 134–139.
17. Betharia, S. M., Pushker, N., Sharma, V., & Sen, S. (2002). Simple dacryops: A case series and review of the literature. *Ophthalmologica, 216*(5), 372–376.
18. Chawla, B., Kashyap, S., Sen, S., et al. (2013). Clinicopathologic review of epithelial tumors of the lacrimal gland. *Ophthalmic Plastic and Reconstructive Surgery, 29*(6), 440–445.
19. Rose, G. E., & Wright, J. E. (1992). Pleomorphic adenoma of the lacrimal gland. *British Journal of Ophthalmology, 76*(7), 395–400.
20. Wolkow, N., Jakobiec, F. A., & Lee, H. (2018). Long-term outcomes of globe-preserving surgery with proton beam radiation for adenoid cystic carcinoma of lacrimal gland. *American Journal of Ophthalmology, 195*, 43–62.
21. Esmaeli, B., Yin, V. T., Hanna, E. Y., et al. (2016). Eye-sparing multidisciplinary approach for the management of lacrimal gland carcinoma. *Head and Neck, 38*(8), 1258–1262.
22. Tse, D. T., Kossler, A. L., Feuer, W. J., & Benedetto, P. W. (2013). Long-term outcomes of neoadjuvant intra-arterial cytoreductive chemotherapy for lacrimal gland adenoid cystic carcinoma. *Ophthalmology, 120*(7), 1313–1323.
23. Esmaeli, B., Golio, D., Kies, M., & DeMonte, F. (2006). Surgical management of locally advanced adenoid cystic carcinoma of the lacrimal gland. *Ophthalmic Plastic and Reconstructive Surgery, 22*(5), 366–370.
24. Andreasen, S., Esmaeli, B., Holstein, S. L., Mikkelsen, L. H., Rasmussen, P. K., & Heegaard, S. (2017). An update on tumors of the lacrimal gland. *Asia-Pacific Journal of Ophthalmology (Philadelphia, PA), 6*(2), 159–172.
25. Fathi, A. R., & Roelcke, U. (2013). Meningioma. *Current Neurology and Neuroscience Reports, 13*(4), 337.
26. Campen, C. J., & Gutmann, D. H. (2018). Optic pathway gliomas in neurofibromatosis type 1. *Journal of Child Neurology, 33*(1), 73–81.
27. Nair, A. G., Pathak, R. S., Iyer, V. R., & Gandhi, R. A. (2014). Optic nerve glioma: An update. *International Ophthalmology, 34*(4), 999–1005.
28. Falzon, K., Drimtzias, E., Picton, S., & Simmons, I. (2018). Visual outcomes after chemotherapy for optic pathway glioma in children with and without neurofibromatosis type 1: Results of the International Society of Paediatric Oncology (SIOP) Low-Grade Glioma 2004 trial UK cohort. *British Journal of Ophthalmology, 102*(10), 1367–1371.
29. Goodden, J., Pizer, B., Pettorini, B., et al. (2014). The role of surgery in optic pathway/hypothalamic gliomas in children. *Journal of Neurosurgery: Pediatrics, 13*(1), 1–12.
30. Kinori, M., Hodgson, N., & Zeid, J. L. (2018). Ophthalmic manifestations in neurofibromatosis type 1. *Survey of Ophthalmology, 63*(4), 518–533.
31. Rose, G. E., & Wright, J. E. (1991). Isolated peripheral nerve sheath tumours of the orbit. *Eye (London, England), 5*(Pt 6), 668–673.
32. Pointdujour-Lim, R., Lally, S. E., Shields, J. A., Eagle, R. C., & Shields, C. L. (2018). Orbital schwannoma: Radiographic and histopathologic correlation in 15 cases. *Ophthalmic Plastic and Reconstructive Surgery, 34*(2), 162–167.
33. Chambers, C. B., Katowitz, W. R., Katowitz, J. A., & Binenbaum, G. (2012). A controlled study of topical 0.25% timolol maleate gel for the treatment of cutaneous infantile capillary hemangiomas. *Ophthalmic Plastic and Reconstructive Surgery, 28*(2), 103–106.
34. Fridman, G., Grieser, E., Hill, R., Khuddus, N., Bersani, T., & Slonim, C. (2011). Propranolol for the treatment of orbital infantile hemangiomas. *Ophthalmic Plastic and Reconstructive Surgery, 27*(3), 190–194.
35. Rotter, A., Samorano, L. P., Rivitti-Machado, M. C., Oliveira, Z. N. P., & Gontijo, B. (2018). PHACE syndrome: Clinical manifestations, diagnostic criteria, and management. *Anais Brasileiros de Dermatologia, 93*(3), 405–411.
36. Calandriello, L., Grimaldi, G., Petrone, G., et al. (2017). Cavernous venous malformation (cavernous hemangioma) of the orbit: Current concepts and a review of the literature. *Survey of Ophthalmology, 62*(4), 393–403.
37. McNab, A. A., Selva, D., Hardy, T. G., & O'Donnell, B. (2014). The anatomical location and laterality of orbital cavernous haemangiomas. *Orbit, 33*(5), 359–362.
38. Khan, S. N., & Sepahdari, A. R. (2012). Orbital masses: CT and MRI of common vascular lesions, benign tumors, and malignancies. *Saudi Journal of Ophthalmology, 26*(4), 373–383.
39. Graeb, D. A., Rootman, J., Robertson, W. D., Lapointe, J. S., Nugent, R. A., & Hay, E. J. (1990). Orbital lymphangiomas: Clinical, radiologic, and pathologic characteristics. *Radiology, 175*(2), 417–421.
40. Hill, R. H., Shiels, W. E., Foster, J. A., et al. (2012). Percutaneous drainage and ablation as first line therapy for macrocystic and microcystic orbital lymphatic malformations. *Ophthalmic Plastic and Reconstructive Surgery, 28*(2), 119–125.
41. Mukherjee, B., Vijay, V., & Halbe, S. (2018). Combined approach to management of periocular arteriovenous malformation by interventional radiology and surgical excision. *Indian Journal of Ophthalmology, 66*(1), 151–154.
42. Barrow, D. L., Spector, R. H., Braun, I. F., Landman, J. A., Tindall, S. C., & Tindall, G. T. (1985). Classification and treatment of spontaneous carotid-cavernous sinus fistulas. *Journal of Neurosurgery, 62*(2), 248–256.
43. Meyers, P. M., Halbach, V. V., Dowd, C. F., et al. (2002). Dural carotid cavernous fistula: Definitive endovascular management and long-term follow-up. *American Journal of Ophthalmology, 134*(1), 85–92.
44. Furusato, E., Valenzuela, I. A., Fanburg-Smith, J. C., et al. (2011). Orbital solitary fibrous tumor: Encompassing terminology for hemangiopericytoma, giant cell angiofibroma, and fibrous histiocytoma of the orbit: Reappraisal of 41 cases. *Human Pathology, 42*(1), 120–128.
45. Bajaj, M. S., Sethi, A., Kashyap, S., Thanikachalam, & Pushker, N. (2004). Locally aggressive orbital fibrous histiocytoma. *Indian J Ophthalmology, 52*(1), 62–64.
46. Dorfman, D. M., To, K., Dickersin, G. R., Rosenberg, A. E., & Pilch, B. Z. (1994). Solitary fibrous tumor of the orbit. *American Journal of Surgical Pathology, 18*(3), 281–287.
47. Kim, H. J., Kim, Y. D., Yim, Y. J., et al. (2008). Solitary fibrous tumor of the orbit: CT and MR imaging findings. *American Journal of Neuroradiology, 29*(5), 857–862.
48. Ulloa, T. K., & Anderson, S. F. (1999). Orbital fibrous histiocytoma: Case report and literature review. *Journal of the American Optometric Association, 70*(4), 253–260.
49. Croxatto, J. O., & Font, R. L. (1982). Hemangiopericytoma of the orbit: A clinicopathologic study of 30 cases. *Human Pathology, 13*(3), 210–218.

50. Henderson, J. W., & Farrow, G. M. (1978). Primary orbital hemangiopericytoma. An aggressive and potentially malignant neoplasm. *Archives of Ophthalmology, 96*(4), 666–673.
51. Wang, X., Qian, J., Bi, Y., Ping, B., & Zhang, R. (2013). Malignant transformation of orbital solitary fibrous tumor. *International Ophthalmology, 33*(3), 299–303.
52. Kahana, A., Lucarelli, M. J., Grayev, A. M., Van Buren, J. J., Burkat, C. N., & Gentry, L. R. (2007). Noninvasive dynamic magnetic resonance angiography with Time-Resolved Imaging of Contrast KineticS (TRICKS) in the evaluation of orbital vascular lesions. *Archives of Ophthalmology, 125*(12), 1635–1642.
53. Shields, C. L., Shields, J. A., Honavar, S. G., & Demirci, H. (2001). Clinical spectrum of primary ophthalmic rhabdomyosarcoma. *Ophthalmology, 108*(12), 2284–2292.
54. Shields, J. A., & Shields, C. L. (2003). Rhabdomyosarcoma: Review for the ophthalmologist. *Survey of Ophthalmology, 48*(1), 39–57.
55. Raney, R. B., Walterhouse, D. O., Meza, J. L., et al. (2011). Results of the Intergroup Rhabdomyosarcoma Study Group D9602 protocol, using vincristine and dactinomycin with or without cyclophosphamide and radiation therapy, for newly diagnosed patients with low-risk embryonal rhabdomyosarcoma: A report from the Soft Tissue Sarcoma Committee of the Children's Oncology Group. *Journal of Clinical Oncology, 29*(10), 1312–1318.
56. Fernandes, B. F., Castiglione, E., Belfort, R. N., Codère, F., & Burnier, M. N. (2009). Orbital leiomyoma: Histopathologic and immunohistochemical findings of a rare tumor. *Ophthalmic Plastic and Reconstructive Surgery, 25*(1), 59–61.
57. Chaugule, S. S., Putambekar, A., Gavade, S., & Deshpande, R. (2019). Primary orbital leiomyosarcoma in an adult male. *Ophthalmic Plastic and Reconstructive Surgery, 35*(2), e27–e29.
58. Jakobiec, F. A., Howard, G. M., Rosen, M., & Wolff, M. (1975). Leiomyoma and leiomyosarcoma of the orbit. *American Journal of Ophthalmology, 80*(6), 1028–1042.
59. American Academy of Ophalmology. (2016). Congenital orbital anomalies. In L. B. Cantor, C. J. Rapuano, & G. A. Cioffi (Eds.), *Basic and clinical science course: Orbit, eyelids, and lacrimal system.* San Francisco: American Academy of Ophthalmology.
60. Ahuja, R., & Azar, N. F. (2006). Orbital dermoids in children. *Seminars in Ophthalmology, 21*(3), 207–211.
61. Shields, J. A., Kaden, I. H., Eagle, R. C., & Shields, C. L. (1997). Orbital dermoid cysts: Clinicopathologic correlations, classification, and management. The 1997 Josephine E. Schueler Lecture. *Ophthalmic Plastic and Reconstructive Surgery, 13*(4), 265–276.
62. Iliff, C. E. (1973). Mucoceles in the orbit. *Archives of Ophthalmology, 89*(5), 392–395.
63. Scangas, G. A., Gudis, D. A., & Kennedy, D. W. (2013). The natural history and clinical characteristics of paranasal sinus mucoceles: A clinical review. *International Forum of Allergy & Rhinology, 3*(9), 712–717.
64. DeParis, S. W., Goldberg, A. N., Indaram, M., Grumbine, F. L., Kersten, R. C., & Vagefi, M. R. (2017). Paranasal sinus mucocele as a late complication of dacryocystorhinostomy. *Ophthalmic Plastic and Reconstructive Surgery, 33*(3S Suppl 1), S23–S24.
65. Sheyn, A., Naylor, T., Lenes-Voit, F., & Berg, E. (2017). Maxillary sinus mucoceles and other side effects of external-beam radiation in the pediatric patient: A cautionary tale. *Ear, Nose & Throat Journal, 96*(9), E27–E28.
66. Kennedy, A., Chowdhury, H., Athwal, S., & Baddeley, P. (2015). Frontal sinus mucocoele: A rare cause of ptosis. *BMJ Case Reports, 2015.* https://doi.org/10.1136/bcr-2015-211068.
67. Van Tassel, P., Lee, Y. Y., Jing, B. S., & De Pena, C. A. (1989). Mucoceles of the paranasal sinuses: MR imaging with CT correlation. *AJR American Journal of Roentgenology, 153*(2), 407–412.
68. Tailor, R., Obi, E., Burns, J., Sampath, R., Durrani, O. M., & Ford, R. (2016). Fronto-orbital mucocele and orbital involvement in occult obstructive frontal sinus disease. *British Journal of Ophthalmology, 100*(4), 525–530.
69. Shields, J. A., Shields, C. L., Brotman, H. K., Carvalho, C., Perez, N., & Eagle, R. C. (2001). Cancer metastatic to the orbit: The 2000 Robert M. Curts Lecture. *Ophthalmic Plastic and Reconstructive Surgery, 17*(5), 346–354.
70. Valenzuela, A. A., Archibald, C. W., Fleming, B., et al. (2009). Orbital metastasis: Clinical features, management and outcome. *Orbit, 28*(2-3), 153–159.
71. Ma, X., Huang, D., Zhao, W., et al. (2015). Clinical characteristics and prognosis of childhood rhabdomyosarcoma: A ten-year retrospective multicenter study. *International Journal of Clinical and Experimental Medicine, 8*(10), 17196–17205.
72. Jurdy, L., Merks, J. H., Pieters, B. R., et al. (2013). Orbital rhabdomyosarcomas: A review. *Saudi J Ophthalmology, 27*(3), 167–175.

26 Orbital Apex Surgery and Tumor Removal

RICCARDO LENZI, MD, PhD, IACOPO DALLAN, MD, AND LUCA MUSCATELLO, MD

The orbital apex is a small, cone-shaped region located between the posterior ethmoidal foramen anteriorly and the openings of the optic canal and superior orbital fissure posteriorly. It contains many critical neurovascular structures, including the optic, oculomotor, and abducens nerves, as well as the ophthalmic branch of the trigeminal nerve. Also nearby are the cavernous sinus, carotid artery, and periarterial sympathetic plexus. At this level, the extraocular muscles attach to the annulus of Zinn, a fibrous ring that surrounds the optic canal and the inferior part of the superior orbital fissure.

Lesions in the orbital apex are rare and typically produce symptoms such as visual acuity reduction, extraocular muscle impairment with diplopia, pain, and exophthalmos. The differential diagnosis is broad and includes inflammatory, infectious, traumatic, vascular, and neoplastic causes.[1]

External surgical approaches to the orbit are well established. External orbitotomies can be performed with or without osteotomy and, in cases of more extensive tumors, the orbitozygomatic craniotomy offers a wide exposure of the orbital contents. However, medial and inferior orbital lesions are the most difficult to reach and are usually addressed via a transcutaneous or transconjunctival medial orbitotomy.[2] However, such approaches are challenging in the cases of posterior tumors, as the cone-shaped surgical field is narrow and damage to neural, muscular, or vascular structures of the orbit can have serious consequences. For intraconal lesions, a temporary section of the medial rectus muscle and retraction of the globe is sometimes necessary.

Many reports of endoscopic transnasal approaches to the orbit have been published during the past several years,[3–9] and as such, endoscopic orbital surgery is now an alternative option to traditional external approaches in the armamentarium of the surgeon for management of selected orbital lesions.

Preoperative Considerations

A complete ophthalmological evaluation is mandatory, including visual acuity, visual field, ocular mobility, and exophthalmometry. With regard to imaging, patients should have both contrast-enhanced magnetic resonance imaging and computed tomography scanning performed preoperatively. In some cases, angiography can still help to solve some clinical dilemmas. Intraoperative neuronavigation should always be available in difficult cases.

The position of the tumor is of crucial importance to determine whether or not endoscopic transnasal resection is a viable option for resection. Axial, coronal and sagittal scans must be carefully studied to determine the position of the tumor in relation to the optic nerve and other important neurovascular structures. Recently three-dimensional reconstruction has been reported as a useful tool to aid in the understanding of tumor morphology. Generally, tumors lateral to the optic nerve, but inferior to a two-dimensional plane passing from the contralateral naris and the long axis of the optic nerve, have been considered amenable to transnasal endoscopic resection.[10] Surgeons need to remember that at the orbital apex level, the possibility of manipulating and displacing structures is reduced, making this zone the most technically challenging. Although the presence of a tumor in this location may pathologically expand this zone, normally there may be less than a millimeter between the lateral border of the medial rectus muscle and the optic nerve in its greatest dimension. Additionally, the insertion of the medial rectus in the annulus of Zinn drastically limits the ability to retract the muscle medially.[11] Therefore to simplify, lesions occupying the superolateral quadrant of the orbital apex are not amenable to transnasal endoscopic resection (Fig. 26.1) and other surgical options must be considered.

Endoscopic Transnasal Approach to the Orbital Apex

After standard preparation and infiltration of the nasal cavity and lateral nasal wall, an uncinectomy is performed. The natural ostium of the maxillary sinus is identified and enlarged posteriorly to the area of the posterior fontanelle with straight-cutting forceps and the microdebrider. A large antrostomy is essential to properly visualize the posterior orbital floor and to avoid obstruction of the ostium if significant prolapse of the orbital fat occurs postoperatively.[12]

A total sphenoethmoidectomy is performed and the sphenoid anterior wall is removed, thereby allowing a wide entry into the sphenoid sinus through the posterior ethmoid. The skull base is identified and cleared and the lamina papiracea is fully exposed. The lamina papiracea can typically be fractured with a Freer elevator (Karl Storz, Tuttlingen, Germany) and flaked off. The hard palatine bone forming the posterior inferomedial orbital angle can be thinned with a small diamond burr and subsequently removed

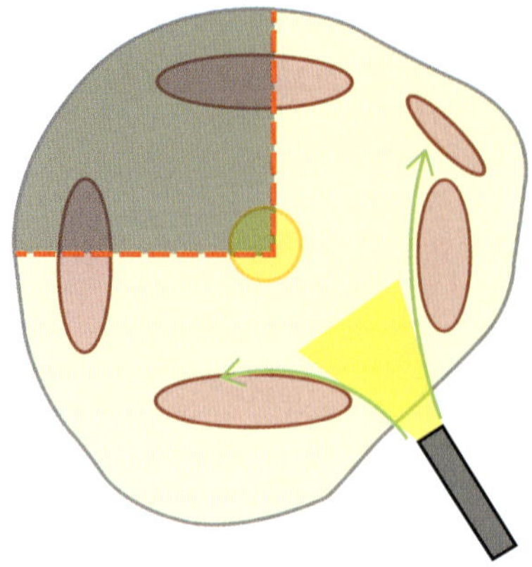

• **Fig. 26.1** Schematic Drawing Showing the Limits of the Endoscopic Transnasal Approach to the Orbit. The ideal corridor to enter the intraconal space is between the medial and inferior rectus muscle.

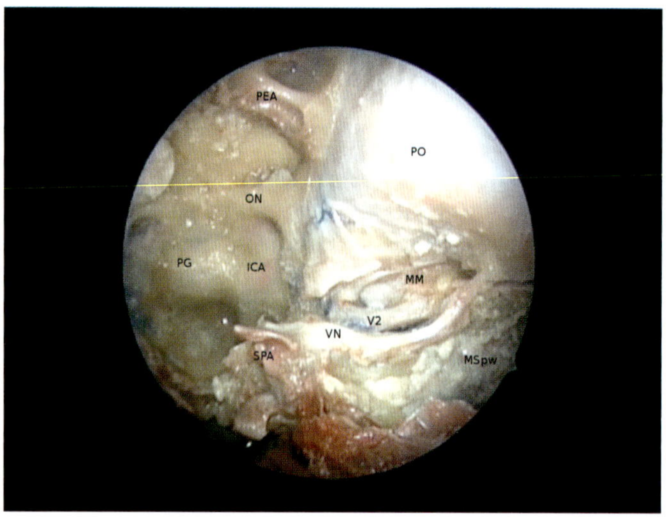

• **Fig. 26.2** Cadaver Dissection Showing the Exposition of the Orbital Apex and Pterygopalatine Fossa. The Muller muscle (*MM*) forms a fibromuscular layer that close superiorly the inferior orbital fissure. *ICA*, internal carotid artery; *MSpw*, posterior wall of the maxillary sinus; *ON*, optic nerve; *PEA*, posterior ethmoidal artery; *PG*, pituitary gland; *PO*, periorbit; *SPA*, sphenopalatine artery; *VN*, vidian nerve; *V2*, second branch of the trigeminal nerve.

safely. During the removal of the lamina papyracea it is of the utmost importance to preserve the integrity of the orbital periosteum, because herniation of fat in the surgical field can obscure the remaining bone and make its removal difficult.[13] If the pterygopalatine fossa must be entered, at this stage the posterior wall of the maxillary sinus must be removed with a Kerrison bone punch (Karl Storz, Tuttlingen, Germany) and the contents of the pterygopalatine fossa can be bluntly dissected up to the inferior orbital fissure (Fig. 26.2). Inferiorly to the optic canal, the inferomedial part of the superior orbital fissure can be skeletonized. Once the bony layer has been carefully removed, the connective tissues appear underneath. The periorbital layer presents as a continuum with the dura of the lateral sellar compartment and the fascial system covering the inferior orbital fissure and the pterygopalatine fossa[14] (Fig. 26.3). It is important to prepare an adequate bony window before proceeding with the periorbital incision. The inferomedial orbit should be fully exposed

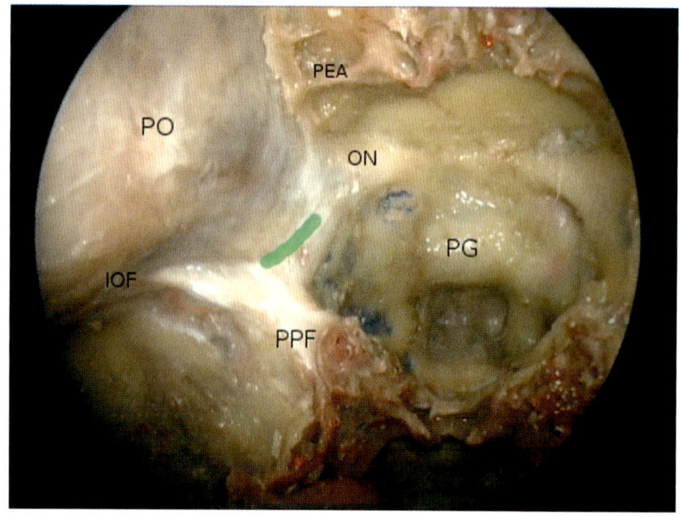

• **Fig. 26.3** Cadaver Dissection of a Right Orbit. After removing the lamina papiracea and other bone tissue surrounding the medial orbital apex, the continuity between periorbit, dura of the lateral sellar compartment, and fascial system covering the inferior orbital fissure and the pterygopalatine fossa has been shown. The *green line* represents the medial border of the superior orbital fissure. *IOF*, inferior orbital fissure; *ON*, optic nerve; *PEA*, posterior ethmoidal artery; *PG*, pituitary gland; *PO*, periorbit; *PPF*, pterygopalatine fossa.

and then entered. At this point, the pterygopalatine fossa can also be addressed as necessary if involved by the tumor or to enhance the posterior exposition of the inferomedial orbit.

When a three- or four-handed approach is planned, a posterior septectomy must be performed, wide enough to allow a second corridor for instruments from the contralateral nostril. The periorbital incision is created with a sickle knife, according to the position of the pathology.

In the case of decompressive surgery or when dealing with extraconal disease, a relatively safe blunt dissection between extraconal fat lobules is possible (Fig. 26.4). Fat lobules of the extraconal space can be carefully shrunk by bipolar electrocautery to improve visualization. In cases of tumor removal, manipulation of the diseased material can be performed with relative ease because there are no critical structures in the extraconal space (Fig. 26.5). In cadaver dissection studies, it was shown that in 83% of cases, a medial extraconal vein has been reported deep to the periorbita[14] and is known as the medial ophthalmic vein.[11]

Intraconal Dissection

The intraconal compartment is bounded medially by the muscular wall (Fig. 26.6), composed mainly of the medial rectus muscle and, to a lesser extent, the inferior rectus muscle inferiorly and the superior oblique muscle superiorly.[15] The dissection is preferably performed between the medial and inferior rectus muscles. At this point, it is necessary to retract medially or displace superiorly the medial rectus muscle. Different methods to achieve this retraction have been reported in the literature, such as double ball probe retraction, transseptal or transchoanal retraction with vessel loops, blunt dissection, or temporary detachment via a transconjunctival approach.[16] Transseptal retraction, both with suture or with a double ball probe (made by the second surgeon from the contralateral

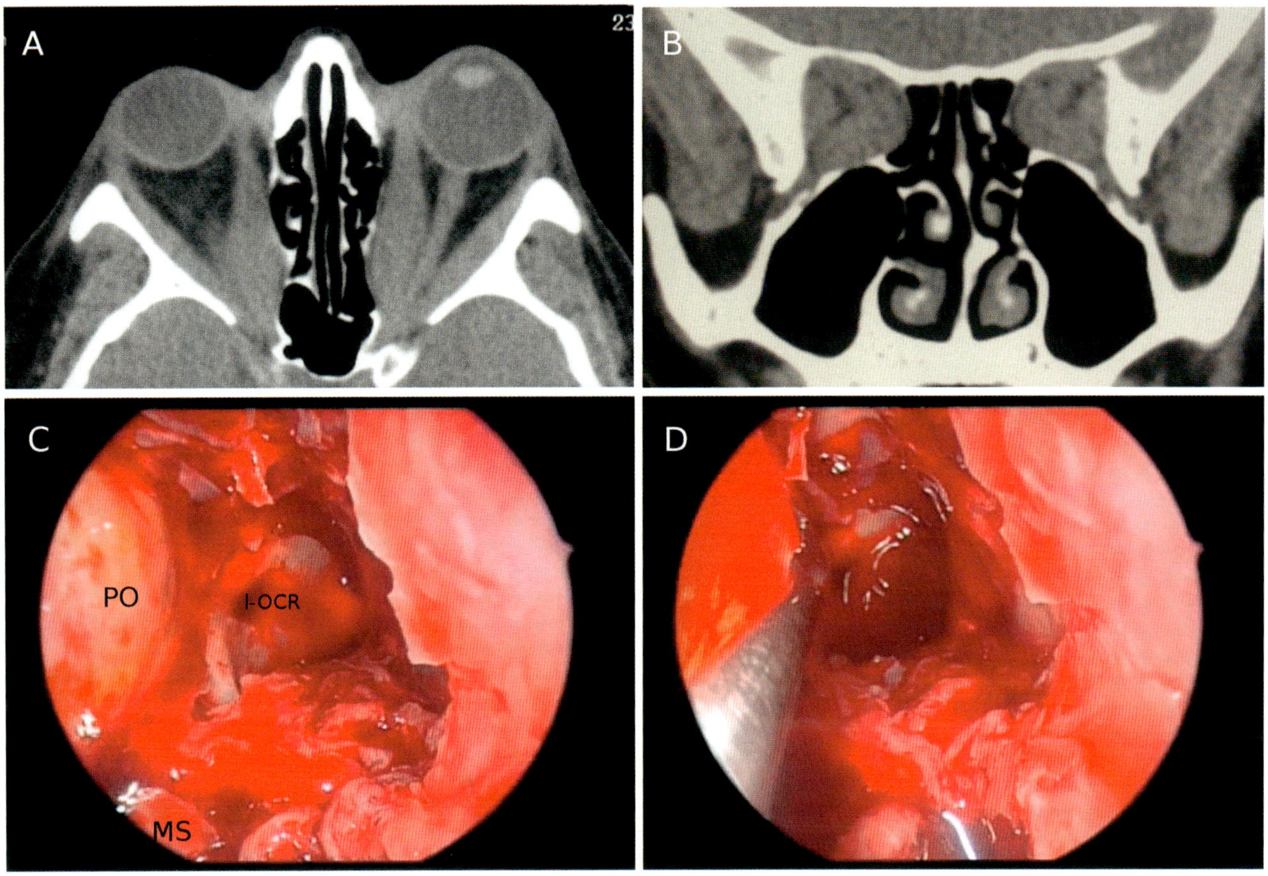

• **Fig. 26.4** Clinical Case of Endoscopic Orbital Apex Decompression. A, B, Computed tomography scan showing a bilateral "apical crowding" in a patient affected by Graves orbitopathy. C, The right medial periorbit (*PO*) is fully exposed, the maxillary (*MS*) and sphenoid sinuses are opened and the lateral optic carotid recess (*l-OCR*) is clearly visible. D, The periorbit is opened with a sickle knife in a posteroanterior direction.

nostril), showed an excellent medial displacement of the medial rectus muscle. In addition, the use of the four-handed approach may offer an advantage with respect to dynamic adjustments in retraction during the case and enhanced protection of the neurovascular inputs of the medial rectus muscle.[17] Our preference is to retract or displace the medial rectus with blunt instruments using a three- or four-handed approach if necessary.

The inferomedial muscular trunk of the ophthalmic artery passes orthogonal to the long axis of the medial intraconal space to insert on the lateral surface of the medial rectus. These arterial pedicles arise approximately 9 mm anterior to the sphenoid face, but the vascular supply to the medial rectus may be highly variable, and thus placement of a retractor less than 15 mm from the sphenoid face should be avoided[16] (Fig. 26.7). When inferior retraction of the medial rectus is needed (i.e., for access to the superomedial orbital quadrant) it must be performed with extreme caution, considering the fixed position of the anterior and posterior ethmoidal neurovascular bundles, which both pass between the medial rectus and the superior oblique muscles (Fig. 26.8). An arterial injury at this level may cause intraconal bleeding directly medial to the optic nerve.

In the superior part of the intraconal space, the nasociliary nerve runs obliquely beneath the superior rectus muscle and the superior oblique muscle where it gives rise to the anterior and posterior ethmoidal nerves. The ophthalmic artery runs anteriorly within the superomedial orbital segment, close to the nasociliary nerve. The artery usually enters the optic canal in its inferolateral portion, passes over the optic nerve, and reaches the medial wall of the orbit running beneath the inferior border of the superior oblique muscle.[15] In addition, the oculomotor nerve with its branches may be encountered when dissecting in the posterior medial intraconal space (Fig. 26.9).

Tumor Removal

The safest way to remove intraorbital lesions is by extracapsular dissection, but a large role is played by the tumor itself. Benign, well-encapsulated, and firm tumors such as cavernous hemangiomas are quite easy to dissect from the orbital fat. Consequently, they represent the ideal neoplasm to be addressed endoscopically.[18] Conversely, malignant infiltrative tumors are poor candidates for endoscopic removal; in this case endoscopic surgery may have only a diagnostic role.

Extracapsular dissection is best made with a three- or four-handed approach, allowing the first surgeon to perform the bimanual dissection. When possible, the tumor may be grasped with a Blakesley forcep (Karl Storz, Tuttlingen, Germany) on its capsule and gently pulled, paying attention to avoid excessive traction with possible damage of adjacent structures. The capsule

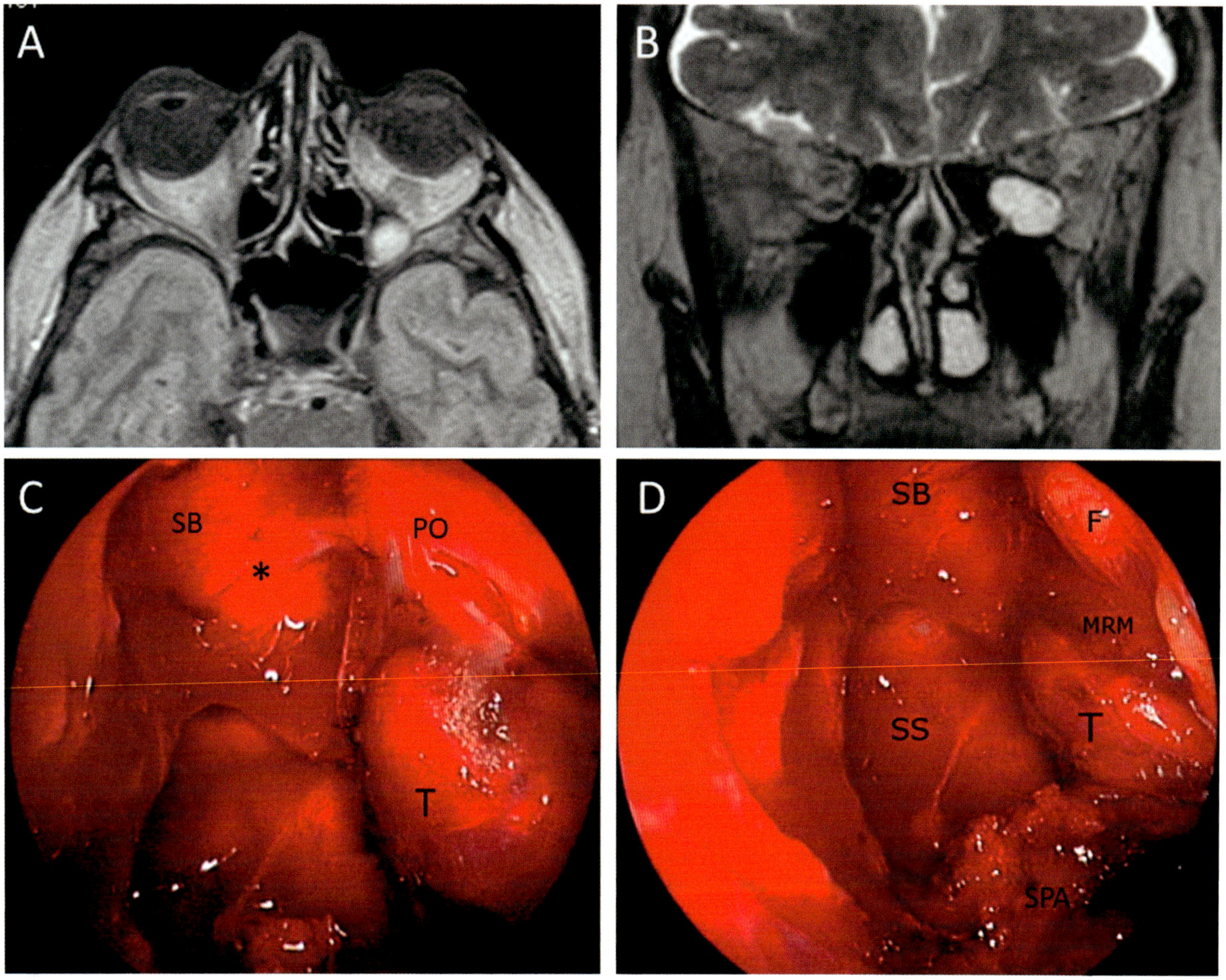

• **Fig. 26.5** A 63-year-old woman with a visual field defect in her left eye, no proptosis or dismotility on examination. A, B, Preoperative magnetic resonance imaging showing a mass in the medial quadrant of the extraconal space of the left orbit. C, Intraoperative picture; the tumor (*T*) imprinting the periorbit (*PO*) is clearly visible. The posterior ethmoidal artery (*asterisk*) along the skull base (*SB*) is also seen. D, After periorbital incision, orbital fat (*F*), medial rectus muscle (*MRM*) and the tumor (*T*) came into view. Complete resection was obtained, with recovery of visual function; no surgical complications were recorded. The lesion resulted to be a cavernous hemangioma at final histology. *SPA,* sphenopalatine artery; *SS,* sphenoid sinus.

can be dissected from the surrounding fat with a blunt elevator. When small vessels are encountered, a small endoscopic bipolar forcep can be used to coagulate the vessels, whereas for small intraoperative mucosal bleeding, warm water irrigation is an effective option to achieve hemostasis. In all cases, monopolar coagulation is to be avoided because of the high risk of thermal injury to the surrounding structures (Fig. 26.10).

With this technique it is possible to address lesions in the medial and inferior orbital apex. Lesions that extends superolaterally to the optic nerve are not amenable to endoscopic resection because the optic nerve should not typically be crossed.[8]

Reconstruction

Reconstruction of the inferomedial orbit is not always necessary, because the orbital fat can be left uncovered inside the nose without significant complications.[18] In large defects when significant manipulation of the orbital contents has been made and/or extraocular muscles are exposed, some sort of reconstruction may help to avoid complications such as diplopia, or to reduce the risk of postoperative enophhthalmos. For such reconstruction, fascia lata or a mucosal graft can be used, and a vascularized nasoseptal flap is also an appropriate option for larger defects.[9]

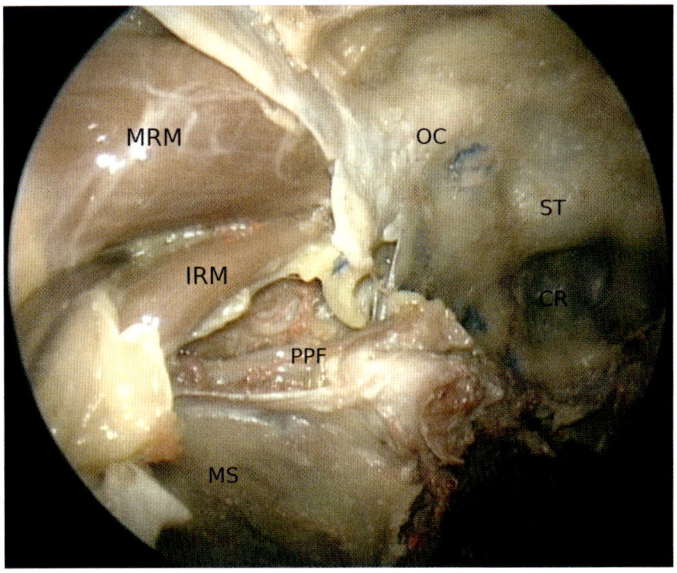

• **Fig. 26.6** Cadaver dissection of a right orbit showing the "muscular wall" that becomes evident after the extraconal orbital fat has been removed. *CR,* clival recess; *IRM,* inferior rectus muscle; *MRM,* medial rectus muscle; *MS,* maxillary sinus (posterior wall)*; OC,* optic canal; *PPF,* pterygopalatine fossa; *ST,* sella turcica; *RP,* rhinopharynx.

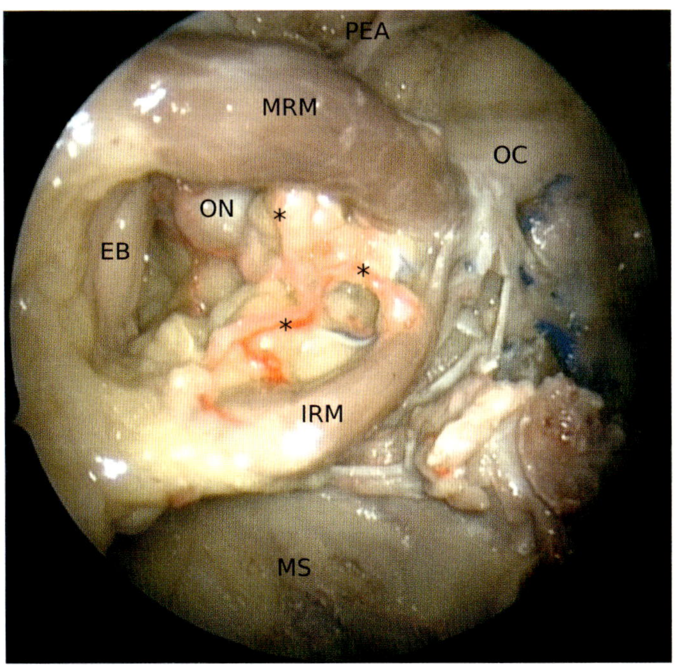

• **Fig. 26.7** A corridor between the inferior (*IRM*) and medial (*MRM*) recti muscles affords a view in the medial intraconal space. Arterial branches (*asterisk*) of the inferomedial trunk feeding the medial and inferior recti muscles are encountered. *EB,* eyeball; *MS,* maxillary sinus (posterior wall); *OC,* optic canal; *ON,* optic nerve; *PEA,* posterior ethmoidal artery.

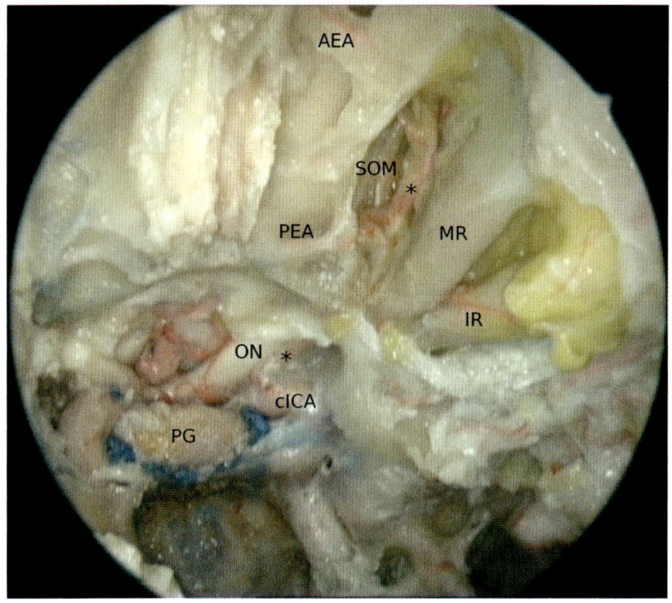

• **Fig. 26.8** Cadaver dissection of a left orbit demonstrating the course of the ophthalmic artery (*asterisk*), which rises from the cavernous internal carotid artery (*cICA*) and joins the optic nerve (*ON*) to enter the optic canal. Once in the orbit, the artery runs in the superomedial quadrant and gives two important branches: the posterior (*PEA*) and anterior (*AEA*) ethmoidal arteries, that exit from the intraconal space between the medial rectus muscle (*MR*) and the superior oblique muscle (*SOM*). *IR,* inferior rectus muscle; *PG,* pituitary gland.

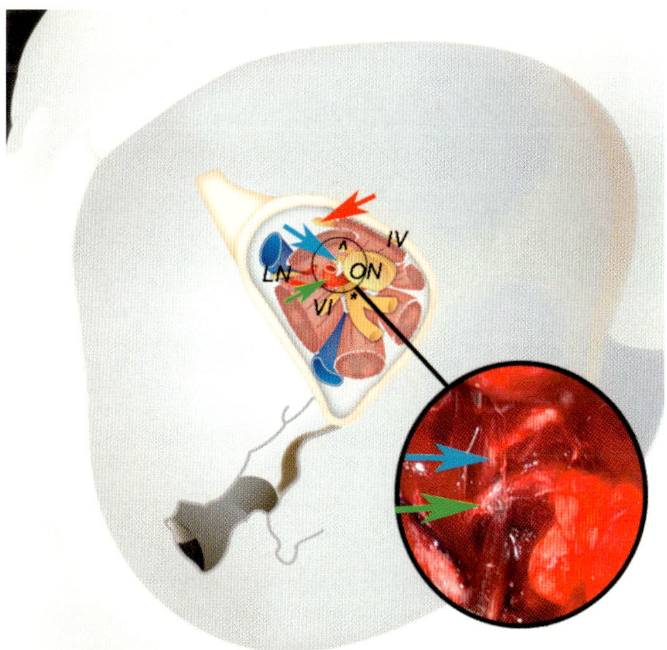

• **Fig. 26.9** Drawing and in vivo image (endoscopic transorbital view) showing the main structures of the orbital apex. Many neural structures such as the optic (*ON*), lacrimal (*LN*), throchlear (*IV*), abducens (*VI*), frontal (*red arrow*), nasociliary (^), superior (*blue arrow)* and inferior (*asterisk*) branches of the oculomotor nerve are visible. The *green arrow* indicates the ophthalmic artery.

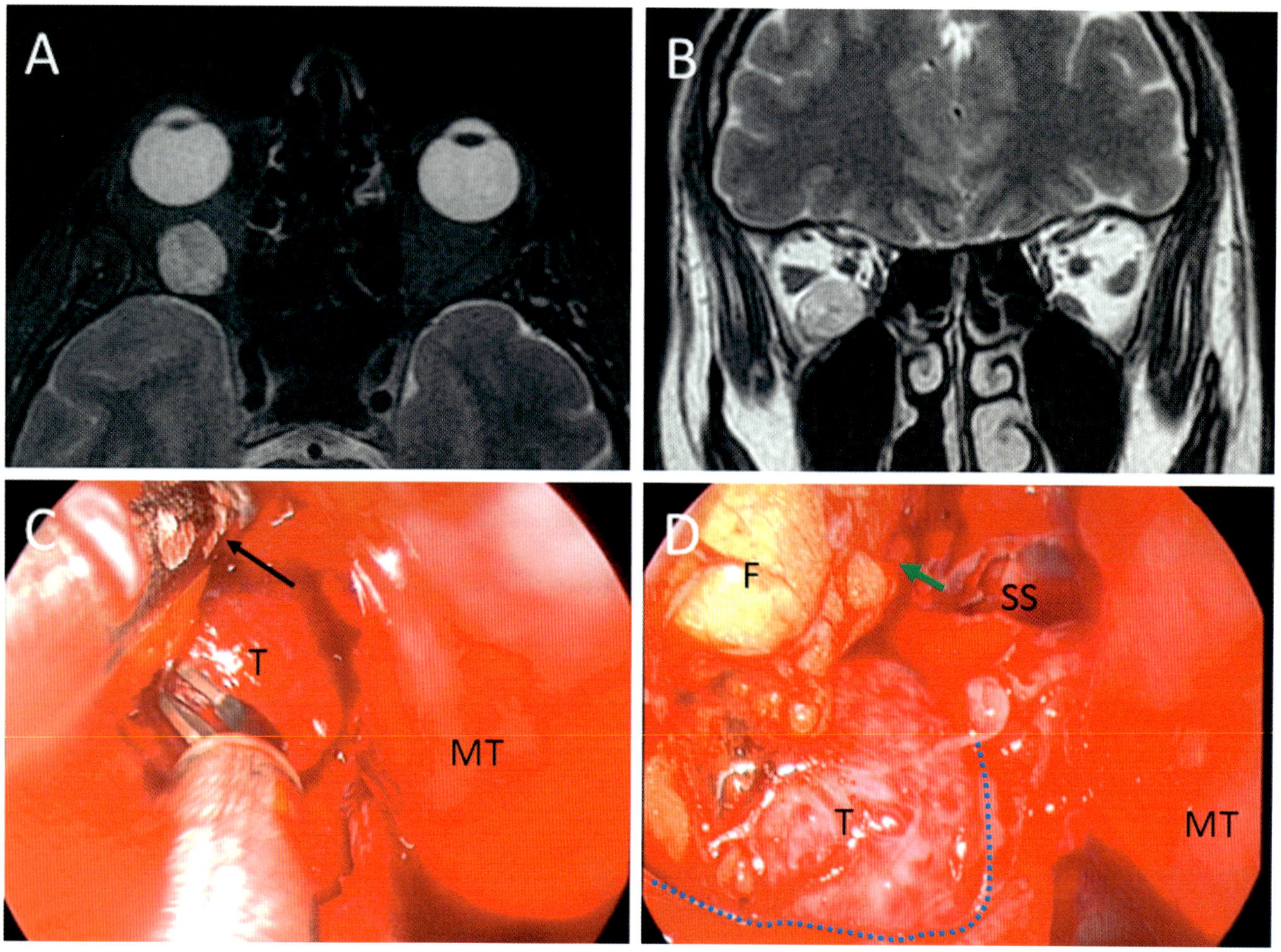

• **Fig. 26.10** A 40-year-old woman had a slight protrusion of the right eye. At the physical examination a right proptosis was observed. Ocular motility was conserved. Magnetic resonance imaging showed a mass in the inferior quadrants of the intraconal space of her right orbit (A, B). The inferior rectus muscle was dislocated medially. The lesion showed a homogeneous contrast enhancement. C, After complete sphenoethmoidectomy and middle antrostomy with middle turbinate (*MT*) sparing, the periorbita was skeletonized and incised. Inferior and medial recti muscles were identified and dislocated superiorly with a blunt instrument using a three-hand approach (*black arrow*). The tumor was identified, and small vessels around the capsule were carefully coagulated with an endoscopic bipolar forcep. D, The tumor was completely dissected from the intraconal fat and inferior rectus muscle and pulled toward the maxillary sinus (the *blue dotted line* indicates the wide right middle antrostomy) to be finally removed. Orbital fat (*F*) and the posterior part of the medial rectus muscle belly (*green arrow*) are visible. *SS*, sphenoid sinus.

Transorbital Endoscopic-Assisted Approach

In selected cases not amenable to transnasal surgery, endoscopic-assisted procedures can still be planned. In superolateral lesions of the orbital apex, external transcranial routes have classically been performed with a certain morbidity. Today the superior eyelid approach allows for the use of an endoscope via a transorbital route. An upper eyelid incision of the skin is made and the orbicolaris oculi is traversed, dividing the muscle parallel to the muscle fibers. By means of careful dissection of the preseptal space the orbital rim is reached, and the dissection proceeds in a subperiosteal plane[19] (Fig. 26.11). The increased visualization permitted by a two-surgeon procedure allows the surgeons to widely expose the superior vault of the periorbita. After the periorbital incision, a window between the superior and lateral rectus muscles can be used as a corridor to the superolateral intraconal space and the lateral aspect of the superior orbital fissure[20,21] (Figs. 26.12 and 26.13). The superior eyelid approach can be used to remove the great wing of the sphenoid bone in lateral orbital decompression or in case of lesions of the bony lateral orbital wall (Fig. 26.14), and to manage intraconal and extraconal tumors unsuitable for the transnasal approach (Fig. 26.15). In addition, this approach can be used in combination with the transnasal route to manage superomedial intraconal lesions.[22]

Complications of Endoscopic Orbital Surgery

The possible complications of endoscopic orbital surgery are numerous. However, enophthalmos and diplopia are the most frequently reported complications in various series.[16,18]

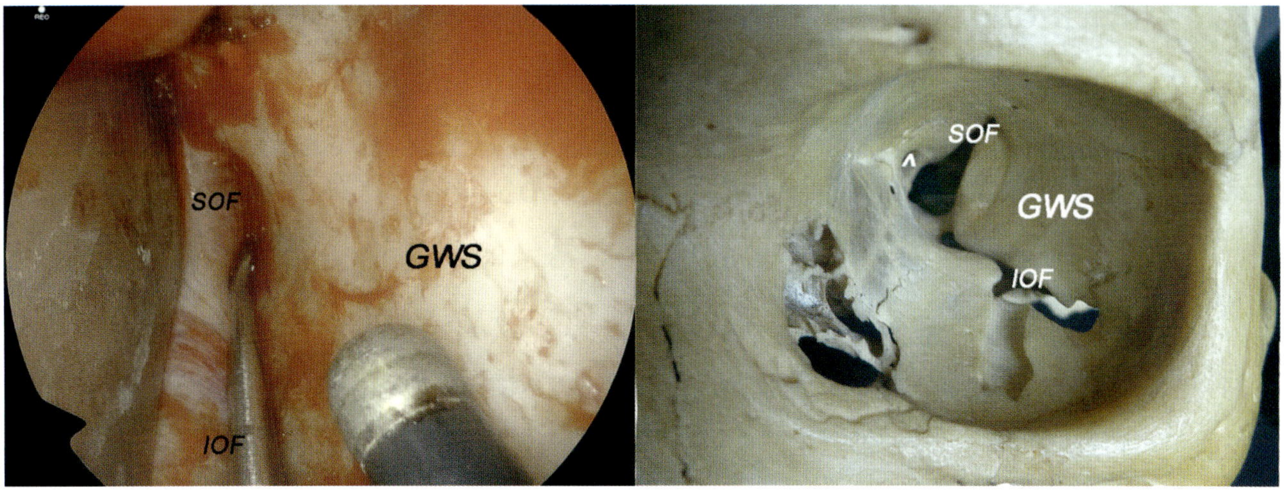

• **Fig. 26.11** Endoscopic-Assisted Transorbital Approach to the Left Superior Orbital Fissure. On the left side subperiosteal dissection of the left lateral periorbit is performed. On the right side the same landmarks are showed on a human dried skull. ^, optic canal; *GWS*, greater wing of the sphenoid; *IOF*, inferior orbital fissure; *SOF*, superior orbital fissure.

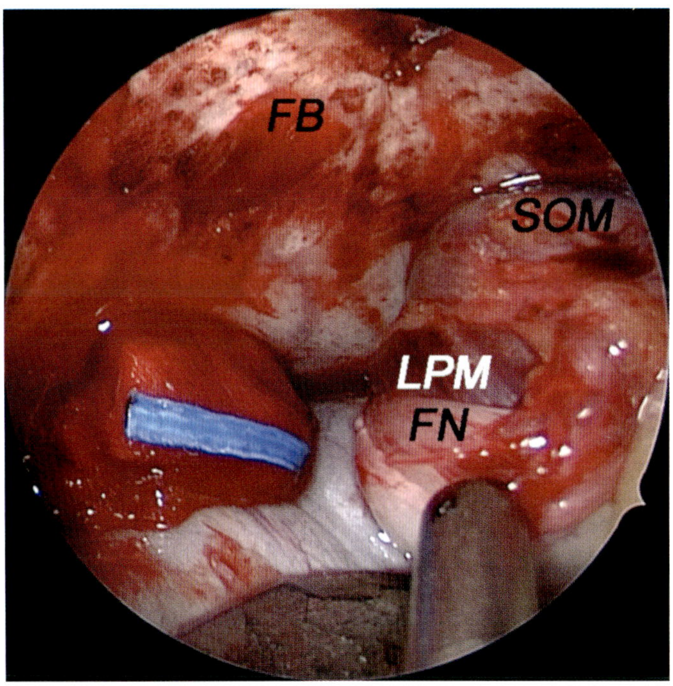

• **Fig. 26.12** Endoscopic-Assisted Transorbital Approach to the Right Supero-Lateral Orbital Quadrant. After periorbital incision the superior oblique muscle (*SOM*), the levator palpebrae muscle (*LPM*), and the frontal nerve (*FN*) are visible. *FB*, frontal bone.

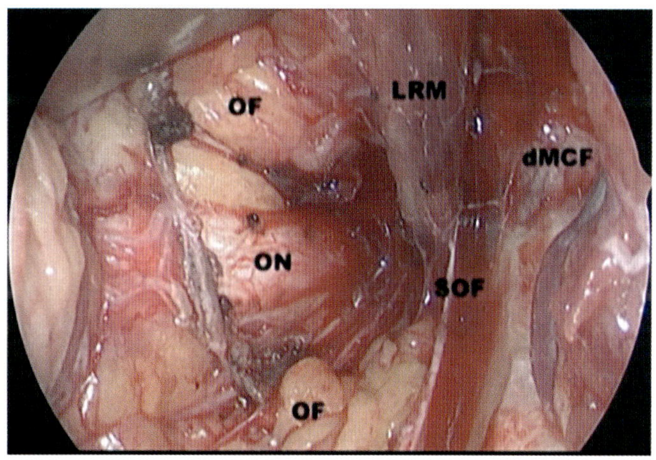

• **Fig. 26.13** Endoscopic view of the left lateral intraconal space through a transorbital superior eyelid approach, after removal of the great sphenoidal wing. *dMCF,* dura of the middle cranial fossa; *LRM,* lateral rectus muscle; *OF,* orbital fat; *ON,* optic nerve; *SOF,* superior orbital fissure.

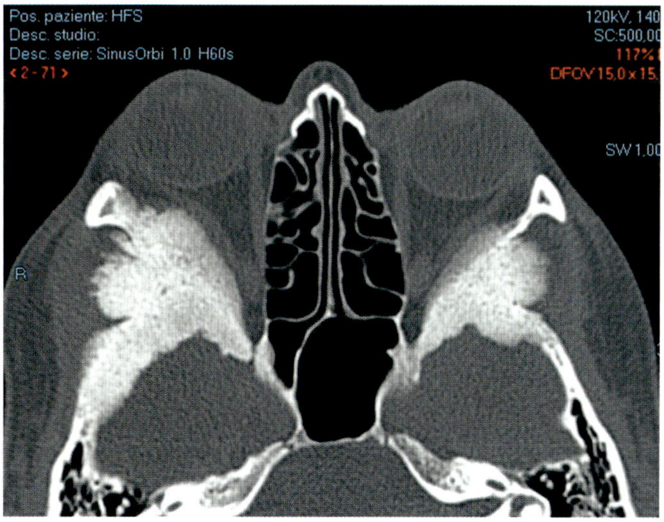

• **Fig. 26.14** A 36-year-old female with bilateral fibrous displasia of the great sphenoidal wing. Both transorbital removal of the diseased bone and endoscopic endonasal decompression of the orbital apex can be considered to manage this case.

Enophthalmos and diplopia are more common for both large approaches and in cases of extensive intraconal dissection. Diplopia can be related to eye imbalance after wide orbital wall resection or secondary to direct muscular or neural damage during intraconal surgery. Intraorbital hemorrage is a feared complication, with potential severe consequences such as blindness. Although the transnasal approach yields an orbit that is already decompressed, severe retrobulbar hemorrhages must be treated promptly with surgical revision and, if needed, with a lateral canthotomy. Identifying and controlling the bleeding vessel inside the orbit may be impossible with an endoscopic route, and the surgeon may need to resort to a Lynch incision to adequately control

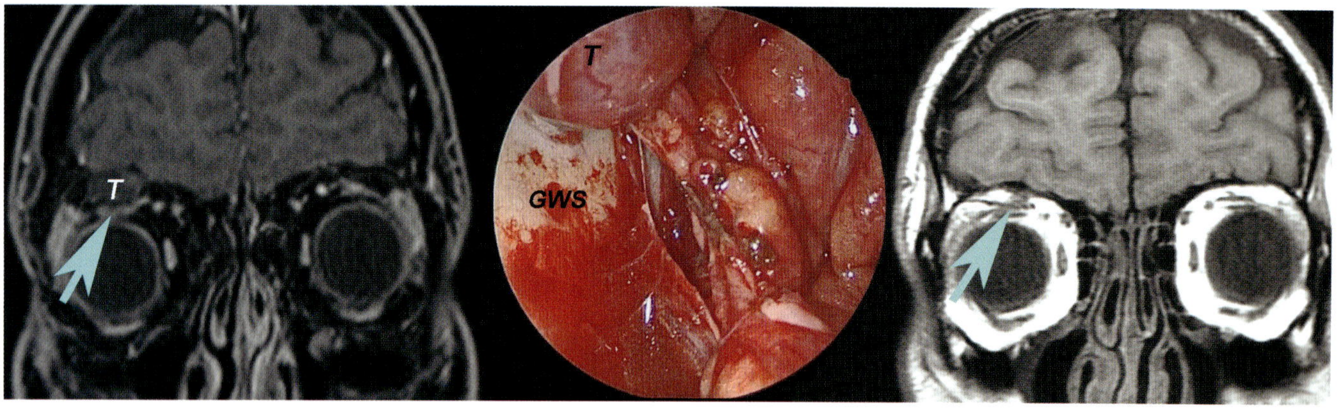

• **Fig. 26.15** Endoscopic Transorbital Removal of a Right Extraconal Tumor of the Superior Orbit. Preoperative magnetic resonance imaging (MRI) is shown on the left. The surgical approach is shown in the center. On the right the postoperative MRI shows the complete resection of the tumor (*T*). The *blue arrow* points to the levator palpebrae muscle. *GWS,* great wing of the sphenoid.

• BOX 26.1 Complications of Endoscopic Transnasal Orbital Surgery

- Enophthalmos
- Diplopia
- Intraorbital hemorrage
- Reduced visual acuity/blindness
- Visual field defects
- Infectious complications (acute orbititis)
- Hypoesthesia of the infraorbital nerve
- Nasal crusting

the hemorrhage.[23] Lesions directly involving the optic nerve may result in visual field defects, reduced visual acuity, or blindness. The optic nerve must never be crossed during surgery, as this increases the likelihood of these same complications owing to injury to the nerve. Infectious complications such as acute orbitis may occur; as such, we suggest postoperative antibiotic therapy for 7 days. When the medial orbital floor is resected, hypoesthesia of the infraorbital nerve is possible; however, it is usually temporary. Excessive nasal crusting in case of extensive endonasal resection is also possible (Box 26.1).

References

1. Yeh, S., & Foroozan, R. (2004). Orbital apex syndrome. *Current Opinion in Ophthalmology, 15,* 490–498.
2. Weisman, R. A., Kikkawa, D., Moe, K. S., & Osguthorpe, J. D. (2001). Orbital tumors. *Otolaryngologic Clinics of North America, 34,* 1157–1174.
3. Karaki, M., Kobayashi, R., & Mori, N. (2006). Removal of an orbital apex hemangioma using an endoscopic transethmoidal approach: Technical note. *Neurosurgery, 59*(1 Suppl 1). ONSE159–ONSE160; discussion ONSE160.
4. Stamm, A., & Nogueira, J. F. (2009). Orbital cavernous hemangioma: Transnasal endoscopic management. *Otolaryngology–Head and Neck Surgery, 141,* 794–795.
5. McKinney, K. A., Snyderman, C. H., Carrau, R. L., Germanwala, A. V., Prevedello, D. M., Stefko, S. T., et al. (2010). Seeing the light: Endoscopic endonasal intraconal orbital tumor surgery. *Otolaryngology–Head and Neck Surgery, 143,* 699–701.
6. Yoshimura, K., Kubo, S., Yoneda, H., Hasegawa, H., Tominaga, S., & Yoshimine, T. (2010). Removal of a cavernous hemangioma in the orbital apex via the endoscopic transnasal approach: A case report. *Minimally Invasive Neurosurgery, 53,* 77–79.
7. Murchison, A. P., Rosen, M. R., Evans, J. J., & Bilyk, J. R. (2011). Endoscopic approach to the orbital apex and periorbital skull base. *Laryngoscope, 121,* 463–467.
8. Muscatello, L., Seccia, V., Caniglia, M., Sellari-Franceschini, S., & Lenzi, R. (2013). Transnasal endoscopic surgery for selected orbital cavernous hemangiomas: Our preliminary experience. *Head and Neck, 35,* E218–E220,
9. Healy, D. Y., Jr., Lee, N. G., Freitag, S. K., & Bleier, B. S. (2014). Endoscopic bimanual approach to an intraconal cavernous hemangioma of the orbital apex with vascularized flap reconstruction. *Ophthalmic Plastic and Reconstructive Surgery, 30,* 104–106.
10. Gregorio, L. L., Busaba, N. Y., Miyake, M. M., Freitag, S. K., & Bleier, B. S. (2017). Expanding the limits of endoscopic intraorbital tumor resection using 3-dimensional reconstruction. *Brazilian Journal of Otorhinolaryngology, 85*(2), 157–161. https://doi.org/10.1016/j.bjorl.2017.11.010.
11. Bleier, B. S., Healy, D. Y., Jr., Chhabra, N., & Freitag, S. (2014). Compartmental endoscopic surgical anatomy of the medial intraconal orbital space. *International Forum of Allergy & Rhinology, 4,* 587–591.
12. Wee, D. T., Carney, A. S., Thorpe, M., & Wormald, P. J. (2002). Endoscopic orbital decompression for Graves' ophthalmopathy. *Journal of Laryngology and Otology, 116,* 6–9.
13. Sellari-Franceschini, S. (2012). Balanced orbital decompression in Graves' orbitopathy. *Operative Techniques in Otolaryngology, 23,* 219–226.
14. Dallan, I., Castelnuovo, P., de Notaris, M., Sellari-Franceschini, S., Lenzi, R., Turri-Zanoni, M., et al. (2013). Endoscopic endonasal anatomy of the superior orbital fissure and orbital apex regions: Critical considerations for clinical applications. *European Archives of Oto-Rhino-Laryngology, 270,* 1643–1649.
15. Dallan, I., Seccia, V., Lenzi, R., Castelnuovo, P., Bignami, M., Battaglia, P., et al. (2010). Transnasal approach to the medial intraconal space: Anatomic study and clinical considerations. *Minimally Invasive Neurosurgery, 53,* 164–168.
16. Bleier, B., Castelnuovo, P., Battaglia, P., Turri-Zanoni, M., Dallan, I., Metson, R., et al. (2016). Endoscopic endonasal orbital cavernous hemangioma resection: Global experience in techniques and outcomes. *International Forum of Allergy & Rhinology, 6,* 156–161.
17. Lin, G. C., Freitag, S. K., Kocharyan, A., Yoon, M. K., Lefebvre, D. R., & Bleier, B. S. (2016). Comparative techniques of medial rectus muscle retraction for endoscopic exposure of the medial intraconal space. *American Journal of Rhinology & Allergy, 30,* 226–229.

18. Lenzi, R., Bleier, B. S., Felisati, G., & Muscatello, L. (2016). Purely endoscopic trans-nasal management of orbital intraconal cavernous haemangiomas: A systematic review of the literature. *European Archives of Oto-Rhino-Laryngology, 273*, 2319–2322.
19. Sellari-Franceschini, S., Lenzi, R., Santoro, A., Muscatello, L., Rocchi, R., Altea, M. A., et al. (2010). Lateral wall orbital decompression in Graves' orbitopathy. *International Journal of Oral and Maxillofacial Surgery, 39*, 16–20.
20. Dallan, I., Locatelli, D., Turri-Zanoni, M., Battaglia, P., Lepera, D., Galante, N., et al. (2015). Transorbital endoscopic assisted resection of a superior orbital fissure cavernous hemangioma: A technical case report. *European Archives of Oto-Rhino-Laryngology, 272*, 3851–3856.
21. Dallan, I., Castelnuovo, P., Turri-Zanoni, M., Fiacchini, G., Locatelli, D., Battaglia, P., et al. (2016). Transorbital endoscopic assisted management of intraorbital lesions: Lessons learned from our first 9 cases. *Rhinology, 54*, 247–253.
22. Castelnuovo, P., Fiacchini, G., Fiorini, F. R., & Dallan, I. (2018). "Push-pull technique" for the management of a selected superomedial intraorbital lesion. *Surgery Journal (New York, NY), 4*(3), e105–e109.
23. Dallan, I., Tschabitscher, M., Castelnuovo, P., Bignami, M., Muscatello, L., Lenzi, R., et al. (2009). Management of severely bleeding ethmoidal arteries. *Journal of Craniofacial Surgery, 20*, 450–454.

27

Management of Intraconal Hemangioma: Techniques and Outcomes

CATHERINE BANKS, MD, FRACS AND BENJAMIN S. BLEIER, MD

Endoscopic orbital surgery represents a challenging arena for the endoscopic surgeon. The orbit is highly complex, with critical structures confined in a fat-filled, soft-tissue space, thereby limiting visibility, and restricting the necessary manipulation of muscles, nerves, and vessels required to resect primary orbital tumors. With the advent of increasing expertise and technology, the endoscope is now being used to transgress pneumatized sinuses and operate within the boundaries of nonpneumatized cavities. An unparalleled view of the medial orbital apex, with improved illumination, a spatial working corridor, a resection tailored to the size and location of the lesion, no external scar, and shorter hospitalization all represent advantages of the transnasal endoscopic approach to the medial orbit.

The endoscopic transnasal approach for orbital and optic nerve decompression was published almost three decades ago.[1,2] The subsequent decade provided the first report on the transnasal endoscopic removal of an intraconal orbital cavernous hemangioma (OCH).[3] This subject has lain relatively dormant for the next 20 years; however, a recent increase in publications would suggest a resurgence in this field. Despite this, the literature portrays only limited case series and case reports with only a recently evolving consensus on management strategies for intraconal lesions such as OCH.

This chapter reviews the endoscopic management of intraconal lesions and discusses the current techniques and outcomes.

Epidemiology and Etiology

The OCH is the most common primary orbital tumor of adults, with a reported incidence of 5% to 15% of all orbital tumors.[4] It is more common in women and occurs in the fourth and fifth decades of life.[5] Recent evidence regarding the immunohistochemical features of proliferative capacity, vascular differentiation, and hormone receptor status suggests that progesterone may play a role in the clinical course.[6,7] This could also explain the sudden growth of OCHs during pregnancy[8,9] and the reduction in size or stabilization in postmenopausal women.[6] However, the exact role of progesterone is yet to be fully elucidated. The natural history of OCH remains elusive. A significant number of OCHs present as asymptomatic lesions incidentally found on computed tomography (CT) or magnetic resonance imaging (MRI) performed for unrelated reasons. Previous studies have shown that asymptomatic lesions often show no progression.[10,11] In a retrospective comparative case series of OCH in 104 patients, 31 had an asymptomatic, incidental OCH on imaging. Seventy-nine patients underwent treatment and 11 of these had presented with an incidental, asymptomatic OCH that enlarged and produced symptoms or new clinical findings. In the 20 other patients, there was no or minimal change in the follow-up period of 1.2 to 20 years (mean 5.8 years, standard deviation 4.6 years). The investigators concluded that if an incidental OCH does not change over several years, it is unlikely to do so in more prolonged periods of follow-up.[12]

Anatomic Location and Characteristics

The majority of OCHs are located between the optic nerve and the extraocular muscles and are therefore considered intraconal. It is well documented that OCH have a predilection for the intraconal space. The single most common anatomic site is lateral to the optic nerve, which may reflect the relationship between the optic nerve and the distribution of the ophthalmic vasculature. This area lateral to the optic nerve, within the intraconal space, is rich in small arteries and arterioles.[13,14] However, OCHs can be found throughout the orbit, including the medial intraconal space, extraconal space, and within the optic canal.[15] Rarely they can extend beyond the confines of the orbit into the pterygopalatine fossa,[16] cavernous sinus,[17] and intracranial space.[18]

The International Society for the Study of Vascular Anomalies has classified the OCH as a slow-flow cavernous venous malformation. Histologically it is not clear if cavernous venous malformations contain exclusively venous vasculature. There is some suggestion of arterial flow on imaging studies, yet histologically there is no evidence of the elastic lamina associated with arterioles. The thicker-walled vessels are thought to be the result of thrombosis and recanalization. If any arterial component is present, it is thought to be inconsequential both histologically and clinically.[19] OCHs are characterized as lesions with mature cellular components and do not tend toward dysplasia or hypercellularity. They have a fibrous capsule that can incorporate surrounding vessels and nerves, but they do not typically infiltrate into surrounding tissue.[4] OCHs tend to be slow-growing vascular lesions with a

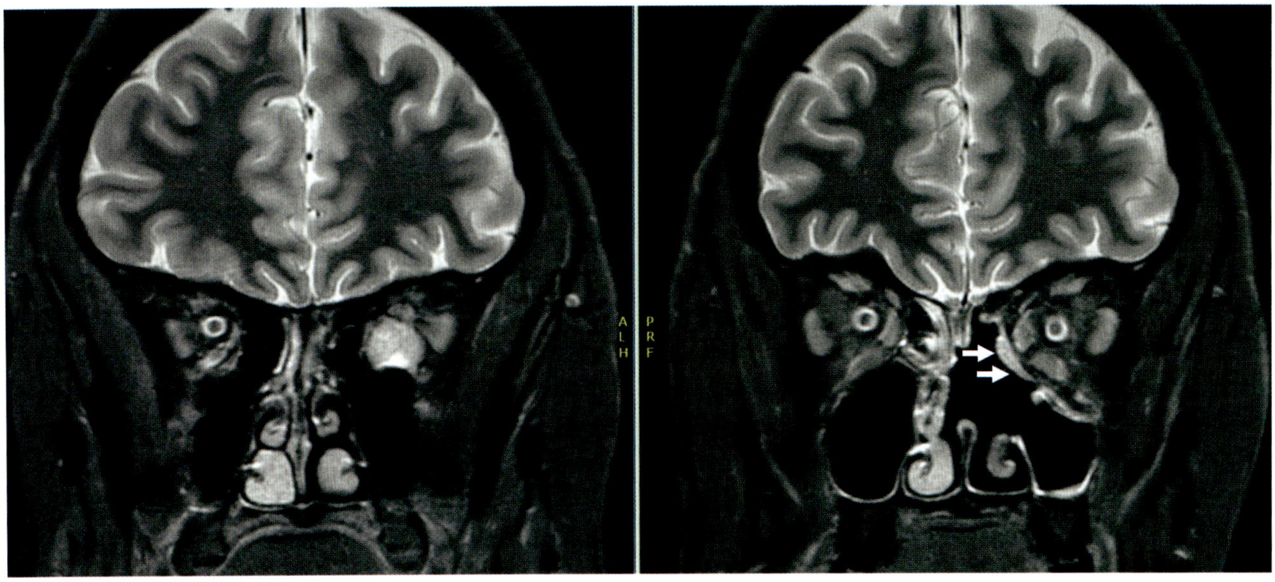

• **Fig. 27.1** *Left,* preoperative T2 coronal magnetic resonance imaging scan demonstrating the typical appearance of a left extraconal orbital cavernous hemangioma. *Right,* postoperative view demonstrating complete resection with well-healed nasoseptal flap reconstruction (*arrows*).

radiologic growth rate of 10% to 15% per year.[4] The expansion of OCH is thought to be a cycle of stasis and thrombosis with endothelial cellular proliferation and recanalization into multiple clefts and vascular channels.

Clinical Presentation and Investigations

Clinical Presentation

The presentation of intraconal OCHs is variable. Most studies reveal the most common presenting symptoms are visual impairment and proptosis, followed by pain and diplopia.[4,12,20,21] In contrast, in a series of 214 patients painless, progressive proptosis was the most frequent presenting symptom, occurring in 76.6% of patients, lasting on average 4.0 years, and ranging from 2 months to 30 years.[22] In another case series of 39 patients, 75% of whom had intraconally located OCHs, pain was the most common presenting feature in 15 patients (38.5%), followed by visual impairment in 13 (33.3%). Diplopia occurred in 4 patients (10%). The visual impairment was related to a compressive optic neuropathy in 10 patients (25.6%). Abnormal proptosis was identified in 79.5% on clinical examination, and duction deficits were seen in 20%. Papilledema, choroidal folds, and tropias were seen less commonly. A more posteriorly located lesion was associated with a relative afferent pupillary defect in 33.3%, and these individuals also had evidence of optic nerve compression on imaging.[19]

Radiologic Investigations

Radiologic imaging is a fundamental component of the preoperative workup, as a routine biopsy is not typically performed, and therefore there is a reliance on the characteristic features of OCH on imaging. Preoperative MRI and or CT are nearly universally performed. The MRI provides superior detail on the intraorbital anatomy and the relationship of the OCH to adjacent structures. OCHs are isointense or slightly hypointense on T1-weighted images and hyperintense to muscle on T2-weighted sequences[23] (Fig. 27.1). The CT scan with contrast demonstrates a well-circumscribed round or elliptical, smooth mass, rarely lobulated in shape.[24,25] OCHs appear as a soft-tissue density with contrast enhancement that varies depending on the phase of the study. Focal enhancement is seen in the early phase with a diffuse enhancement seen in the later phase. Occasionally a heterogeneous appearance can be seen, signifying irregular blood flow within the OCH. Bony erosion or demineralization is not common but has been documented.[26,27] If the OCH abuts the globe, it will tend to indent the globe rather than mold or infiltrate it. OCHs do not expand with the Valsalva maneuver, highlighting the lack of both distensible structures and arteriovenous shunting, which is characteristic of slow-flow venous malformations.[19] The MRI and CT scans have characteristic properties that secure the diagnosis in most cases; therefore although this feature can be useful to discriminate between true neoplasms and other vascular tumors,[28] it is seldom required. Angiography is also not necessary for the reasons noted earlier. Furthermore, CT scanning enables intraoperative image guidance options and visualization of the surgical trajectory, thereby assisting with preoperative planning. The use of ultrasonography to assist with the diagnosis has also been documented in the literature[22]; this would seem more of a historical investigation, made redundant by MRI and CT.

Management

Indications and Surgical Approach

Surgical resection is indicated for symptomatic lesions, whereas smaller asymptomatic lesions can be observed. The goal of surgery is definitive resection; however, given the benign nature, complete resection must be balanced against iatrogenic morbidity. Partial resections of intraconal OCHs have been reported in the literature, but long-term outcomes remain unknown.[29]

The location of the intraconal OCH within the orbit relative to the optic nerve dictates the choice of the approach. OCHs with an epicenter medial to the optic nerve or below a plane of resectability, which represents a plane subtended by the contralateral nostril and the long axis of the optic nerve, are amenable to the endoscopic approach. The feasibility and safety of this approach has been consistently demonstrated in the literature.[4,20,29-36] OCHs located lateral and superior to the plane of resectability are not candidates for a exclusively endoscopic resection.[37] The surgical team involved in these procedures varies depending on institutions; however, a multidisciplinary team approach is invaluable and should include an otolaryngologist and oculoplastic surgeon and, in some cases, a neurosurgeon.

Surgical Equipment and Techniques—Hands/Surgeons

The rigid 0-degree endoscope is most commonly used initially. Other angled scopes (30-, 45-, and 70-degree scopes) can also be of assistance.[32,34] Although image guidance is used in the majority of cases, it is not an absolute requirement as the tumor position may shift within the orbit during the approach and dissection.[20] In one report, intraoperative MRI was used when image guidance was unable to locate a small apical intraconal hemangioma.[38]

The standard single-nostril approach, using a complete uncinectomy, wide maxillary antrostomy, and sphenoethmoidectomy to create a working space and define the orbital wall and orbital axis, is a fundamental part of the surgery. The middle turbinate may be resected to increase access and visibility. A recent international multi-institutional study demonstrated the single-nostril, three-handed, two-surgeon approach or a binarial, four-handed transseptal approach is more commonly used in intraconal OCH resections, with only 31% resected using the single-nostril, two-handed approach.[4] In the binarial approach, a posterior septectomy is needed. This is associated with minimal morbidity, allows for maneuvering endoscopes and instruments, and may be incorporated into the elevation of a nasoseptal flap for medial wall reconstruction.[36] This suggests that intraconal OCH resections require consideration in the preoperative planning and operating room setup to optimize positioning and ergonomics of the second surgeon (Fig. 27.2).

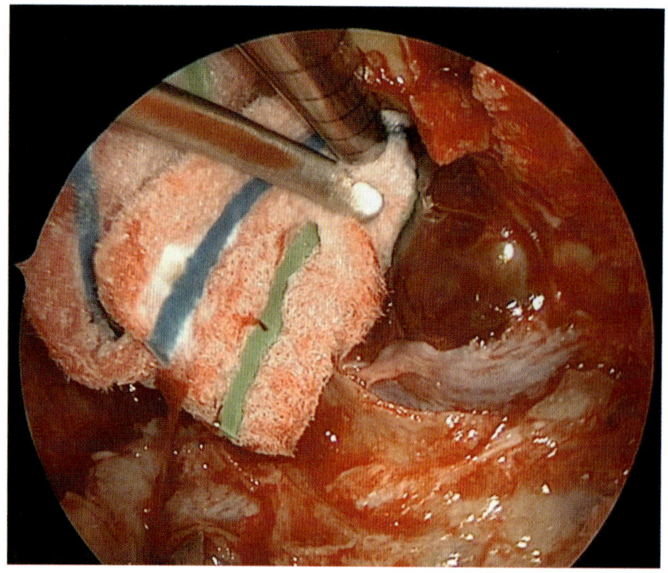

• **Fig. 27.2** Intraoperative view demonstrating three-handed binarial technique for resection of a left extracoal. orbital cavernous hemangioma. Note the use of a cottonoid pledget to retract the extraconal fat.

Surgical Management of the Medial Rectus

The intraconal dissection corridor is bounded by the medial rectus above and inferior rectus below. Creation of a periorbital window allows for identification of the muscles. The periorbita is incised in a reverse hockey-stick fashion just anterior to the tumor border to prevent unnecessary fat prolapse in the anterior field. The medial rectus serves as a landmark of the medial orbit and must be retracted to access intraconal OCHs. Numerous techniques have been described to address the retraction of the medial rectus. Transseptal sutures,[30] vessel loops,[37,39] double ball probe retraction,[4,21] blunt dissection, and detachment from the globe itself have all been reported.[37,39] The optimal method for medial rectus muscle retraction remains unknown; however, a recent international study demonstrated that immediate postoperative diplopia was evenly distributed among patients with or without medial rectus retraction. It was noted that the double-tipped ball technique was not associated with any diplopia, likely owing to avoidance of tonic traction on the neurovascular supply to the muscle.[4] This technique involves passing a right-angled double ball probe under the inferior border of the muscle and gently retracting the muscle in a superomedial direction.[4] Knowledge and appreciation of the neurovascular anatomy is crucial and directs safe placement of the ball probe on the medial rectus and the degree of retraction. The oculomotor nerve branch penetrates the medial rectus at one-third of the distance from the annulus of Zinn to its insertion onto the globe; therefore direct traction here should be avoided.[40] More studies are needed before recommendations of optimal medial rectus muscle retraction can be made.

Management of Hemostasis and Orbital Fat

Hemostasis is vital and can be achieved by a number of methods. It is widely accepted that monopolar cautery should be avoided when operating within the orbit because of a significant risk of thermal conduction to vital neural structures.[4] Judicious and precise bipolar cautery, saline solution–soaked cottonoid pledgets, and warm water irrigation have all been documented.[4]

Herniation of fat into the nasal corridor can be an issue. Although meticulous removal of extraconal fat with bipolar forceps or cutting instruments has been reported, this should be avoided by proper placement of the periorbital incision.[30,35] Preserving the extraconal fat not only helps to preserve orbital volume[32] but also minimizes the risk of medial rectus scarring and entrapment. Deliberate placement of orbital fat over the extraocular exposed muscles to prevent scarring has been described.[30,41] Keeping the intraconal corridor open is challenging, and the use of cottonoid pledgets to separate and retract the orbital fat can assist with visualization. The introduction of a small ribbon retractor has also been described to provide retraction of orbital fat.[37]

Resection Techniques for Intraconal Orbital Cavernous Hemangiomas

Resection of OCHs is facilitated by the characteristics properties of the lesion. The fibrous capsule permits dissection in the extracapsular plane with preservation of the capsule. Most case series describe a process of gentle traction, cottonoids, and blunt dissection.[27,30] Sharp cutting instruments have also been used successfully but do increase the risk of bleeding from inadvertent arteriolar injury.[30,42] An earlier study highlighted potential adherence of the OCH to surrounding structures, postulating that this may be related to the time course of the lesion.[43] Incomplete resection has been documented in cases when the lesion was adherent to the optic nerve; however, long-term follow-up remains unknown.[29]

Reconstruction of the Medial Orbital Wall

Reconstruction of the medial orbital wall should be strongly considered after removal of intraconal or large extraconal lesions with the goal of preservation of orbital volume. If reconstruction does occur, there is no clear consensus on the appropriate method of reconstruction; however, immediate rigid reconstruction does place the orbit at risk for compartment syndrome owing to edema and postoperative bleeding. Lenzi et al. performed a systematic review of 17 intraconal OCHs and noted that reconstruction was not performed in 13 cases. In the four patients who underwent reconstruction, various materials were used, including bone fragments, nasal mucosa, silicon sheet, and a pedicled nasoseptal flap.[20] The pedicled nasoseptal flap technique is preferred by the authors, as it provides the opportunity for a delayed contraction, thereby reducing the risk of diplopia and enophthalmos[41] (Fig. 27.3).

The Role of Nasal Packing

There is a lack of consensus on the use of nasal packing after surgery. Nasal packing is not recommended by some authors, citing possible exertion of pressure on the globe or optic nerve.[30,37] Alternatively, use of absorbable hemostatic packing has been reported,[44] and the use of a polyvinyl acetate sponge placed into the nasal cavity to assist with adherence and positioning of a nasoseptal flap for 7 days has been documented; however, this should not be placed in a position that could risk exerting direct pressure on the exposed orbit.[41]

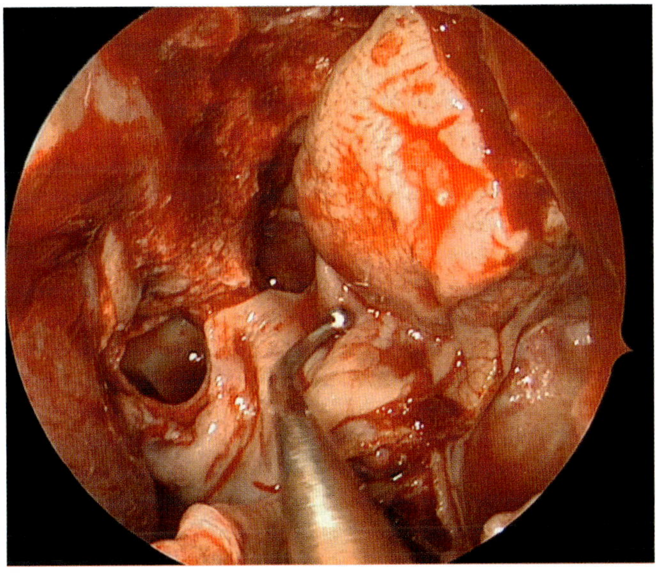

• **Fig. 27.3** Example of immediate repair of the medial orbital wall using a nasoseptal flap.

Endoscopic Orbital Cavernous Hemangioma Outcomes

The functional outcomes for the endoscopic approach to intraconal OCHs are consistent, if not better, than the current reported external approaches.[4,5,20,45] The largest systematic review to date of postoperative outcomes for purely endoscopic transnasal management of orbital intraconal cavernous hemangiomas demonstrated that vision improved or remained stable in 16 patients (one patient was not reported on). In this series of 17 patients, the complications included 3 patients with residual diplopia, 2 patients with enophthalmos, and a single case of acute orbititis.[3,20]

Conclusion

Endoscopic approaches for OCH resection have been increasing in popularity as the result of the development of improved techniques for approach, dissection, and reconstruction. This approach has been shown to be feasible, safe, and potentially superior to traditional open techniques. Further studies and wide adoption of multidisciplinary collaboration is needed for continued growth in this nascent area of endoscopic surgery.

References

1. Kennedy, D. W., Goodstein, M. L., Miller, N. R., & Zinreich, S. J. (1990). Endoscopic transnasal orbital decompression. *Archives of Otolaryngology–Head Neck Surgery*, *116*(3), 275–282.
2. Kountakis, S. E., Maillard, A. A., Urso, R., & Stiernberg, C. M. (1997). Endoscopic approach to traumatic visual loss. *Otolaryngology–Head and Neck Surgery*, *116*(6 Pt 1), 652–655.
3. Herman, P., Lot, G., Silhouette, B., Marianowski, R., Portier, F., Wassef, M., et al. (1999). Transnasal endoscopic removal of an orbital cavernoma. *Annals of Otolology, Rhinolology & Laryngology*, *108*(2), 147–150.
4. Bleier, B. S., Castelnuovo, P., Battaglia, P., Turri-Zanoni, M., Dallan, I., Metson, R., et al. (2016). Endoscopic endonasal orbital cavernous hemangioma resection: Global experience in techniques and outcomes. *International Forum of Allergy & Rhinology*, *6*(2), 156–161.
5. Calandriello, L., Grimaldi, G., Petrone, G., Rigante, M., Petroni, S., Riso, M., et al. (2017). Cavernous venous malformation (cavernous hemangioma) of the orbit: Current concepts and a review of the literature. *Survey of Ophthalmology*, *62*(4), 393–403.
6. Jayaram, A., Lissner, G. S., Cohen, L. M., & Karagianis, A. G. (2015). Potential correlation between menopausal status and the clinical course of orbital cavernous hemangiomas. *Ophthalmic Plastic and Reconstructive Surgery*, *31*(3), 187–190.
7. Gupta, A., Prabhakaran, V. C., Dodd, T., Davis, G., & Selva, D. (2012). Orbital cavernous haemangiomas: Immunohistochemical study of proliferative capacity, vascular differentiation and hormonal receptor status. *Orbit*, *31*(6), 386–389.
8. McNab, A. A., & Wright, J. E. (1989). Cavernous haemangiomas of the orbit. *Australian and New Zealand Journal of Ophthalmology*, *17*(4), 337–345.
9. Zauberman, H., & Feinsod, M. (1970). Orbital hemangioma growth during pregnancy. *Acta Ophthalmologica*, *48*(5), 929–933.
10. Scheuerle, A. F., Steiner, H. H., Kolling, G., Kunze, S., & Aschoff, A. (2004). Treatment and long-term outcome of patients with orbital cavernomas. *American Journal of Ophthalmology*, *138*(2), 237–244.
11. Harris, G. J., & Perez, N. (2002). Surgical sectors of the orbit: Using the lower fornix approach for large, medial intraconal tumors. *Ophthalmic Plastic and Reconstructive Surgery*, *18*(5), 349–354.

12. McNab, A. A., Tan, J. S., Xie, J., Selva, D., Hardy, T. G., Starte, J., et al. (2015). The natural history of orbital cavernous hemangiomas. *Ophthalmic Plastic and Reconstructive Surgery, 31*(2), 89–93.
13. McNab, A. A., Selva, D., Hardy, T. G., & O'Donnell, B. (2014). The anatomical location and laterality of orbital cavernous haemangiomas. *Orbit, 33*(5), 359–362.
14. Cheung, N., & McNab, A. A. (2003). Venous anatomy of the orbit. *Investigative Ophthalmology & Visual Science, 44*(3), 988–995.
15. Chen, Y., Tu, Y., Chen, B., Shi, J., Yu, B., & Wu, W. (2017). Endoscopic transnasal removal of cavernous hemangiomas of the optic canal. *American Journal of Ophthalmology, 173*, 1–6.
16. Yoshimura, K., Kubo, S., Yoneda, H., Hasegawa, H., Tominaga, S., & Yoshimine, T. (2010). Removal of a cavernous hemangioma in the orbital apex via the endoscopic transnasal approach: A case report. *Minimally Invasive Neurosurgery, 53*(2), 77–79.
17. Wiwatwongwana, D., & Rootman, J. (2008). Management of optic neuropathy from an apical orbital-cavernous sinus hemangioma with radiotherapy. *Orbit, 27*(3), 219–221.
18. Lee, K. Y., Fong, K. S., Loh, H. L., Heran, M. K., & Rootman, J. (2008). Giant cavernous haemangioma mimicking a fifth nerve neurofibroma involving the orbit and brain. *British Journal of Ophthalmology, 92*(3), 423–425.
19. Rootman, D. B., Heran, M. K., Rootman, J., White, V. A., Luemsamran, P., & Yucel, Y. H. (2014). Cavernous venous malformations of the orbit (so-called cavernous haemangioma), a comprehensive evaluation of their clinical, imaging and histologic nature. *British Journal of Ophthalmology, 98*(7), 880–888.
20. Lenzi, R., Bleier, B. S., Felisati, G., & Muscatello, L. (2016). Purely endoscopic trans-nasal management of orbital intraconal cavernous haemangiomas: A systematic review of the literature. *European Archives of Oto-Rhino-Laryngology, 273*(9), 2319–2322.
21. Chen, L., White, W. L., Xu, B., & Tian, X. (2010). Transnasal transsphenoid approach: A minimally invasive approach for removal of cavernous haemangiomas located at inferomedial part of orbital apex. *Clinical and Experimental Ophthalmology, 38*(5), 439–443.
22. Yan, J., & Wu, Z. (2004). Cavernous hemangioma of the orbit: Analysis of 214 cases. *Orbit, 23*(1), 33–40.
23. Dallaudiere, B., Benayoun, Y., Boncoeur-Martel, M., Robert, P., Adenis, J., & Maubon, A. (2009). Imaging features of cavernous hemangiomas of the orbit. *Journal de Radiologie, 90*(9 Pt 1), 1039–1045 (in French).
24. Mafee, M. F., Putterman, A., Valvassori, G. E., Campos, M., & Capek, V. (1987). Orbital space-occupying lesions: Role of computed tomography and magnetic resonance imaging. An analysis of 145 cases. *Radiologic Clinics of North America, 25*(3), 529–559.
25. Khan, S. N., & Sepahdari, A. R. (2012). Orbital masses: CT and MRI of common vascular lesions, benign tumors, and malignancies. *Saudi Journal of Ophthalmology, 26*(4), 373–383.
26. Yan, J., Li, Y., & Wu, Z. (2006). Orbital cavernous hemangioma with bone erosion. *Graefe's Archive for Clinical and Experimental Ophthalmology, 244*(11), 1534–1535.
27. Lee, J. Y., Ramakrishnan, V. R., Chiu, A. G., Palmer, J., & Gausas, R. E. (2012). Endoscopic endonasal surgical resection of tumors of the medial orbital apex and wall. *Clinical Neurology and Neurosurgery, 114*(1), 93–98.
28. Tanaka, A., Mihara, F., Yoshiura, T., et al. (2004). Differentiation of cavernous hemangioma from schwannoma of the orbit: A dynamic MRI study. *AJR American Journal of Roentgenology, 183*(6), 1799–1804.
29. Chhabra, N., Wu, A. W., Fay, A., & Metson, R. (2014). Endoscopic resection of orbital hemangiomas. *International Forum of Allergy & Rhinology, 4*(3), 251–255.
30. Castelnuovo, P., Dallan, I., Locatelli, D., Battaglia, P., Farneti, P., Tomazic, P. V., et al. (2012). Endoscopic transnasal intraorbital surgery: our experience with 16 cases. *European Archives of Oto-Rhino-Laryngology, 269*(8), 1929–1935.
31. Stamm, A., & Nogueira, J. F. (2009). Orbital cavernous hemangioma: Transnasal endoscopic management. *Otolaryngology–Head and Neck Surgery, 141*(6), 794–795.
32. Tomazic, P. V., Stammberger, H., Habermann, W., Gerstenberger, C., Braun, H., Gellner, V., et al. (2011). Intraoperative medialization of medial rectus muscle as a new endoscopic technique for approaching intraconal lesions. *American Journal of Rhinology & Allergy, 25*(5), 363–367.
33. Lazar, M., Rothkoff, L., & Drey, J. P. (2005). Treatment and long-term outcome of patients with orbital cavernomas. *American Journal of Ophthalmology, 139*(4), 753. author reply 753.
34. Karaki, M., Kobayashi, R., & Mori, N. (2006). Removal of an orbital apex hemangioma using an endoscopic transethmoidal approach: Technical note. *Neurosurgery, 59*(1 Suppl 1), ONSE159–160 discussion ONSE159–160.
35. Wu, W., Selva, D., Jiang, F., Jing, W., Tu, Y., Chen, B., et al. (2013). Endoscopic transethmoidal approach with or without medial rectus detachment for orbital apical cavernous hemangiomas. *American Journal of Ophthalmology, 156*(3), 593–599.
36. Murchison, A. P., Rosen, M. R., Evans, J. J., & Bilyk, J. R. (2011). Endoscopic approach to the orbital apex and periorbital skull base. *Laryngoscope, 121*(3), 463–467.
37. Paluzzi, A., Gardner, P. A., Fernandez-Miranda, J. C., Tormenti, M. J., Stefko, S. T., Snyderman, C. H., et al. (2015). "Round-the-clock" surgical access to the orbit. *Journal of Neurological Surgery Part B, Skull Base, 76*(1), 12–24.
38. Netuka, D., Masopust, V., Belsan, T., Profantova, N., & Benes, V. (2013). Endoscopic endonasal resection of medial orbital lesions with intraoperative MRI. *Acta Neurochirurgica, 155*(3), 455–461.
39. McKinney, K. A., Snyderman, C. H., Carrau, R. L., Germanwala, A. V., Prevedello, D. M., Stefko, S. T., et al. (2010). Seeing the light: Endoscopic endonasal intraconal orbital tumor surgery. *Otolaryngology–Head and Neck Surgery, 143*(5), 699–701.
40. Bleier, B. S., Healy, D. Y., Jr., Chhabra, N., & Freitag, S. (2014). Compartmental endoscopic surgical anatomy of the medial intraconal orbital space. *International Forum of Allergy & Rhinology, 4*(7), 587–591.
41. Healy, D. Y., Jr., Lee, N. G., Freitag, S. K., & Bleier, B. S. (2014). Endoscopic bimanual approach to an intraconal cavernous hemangioma of the orbital apex with vascularized flap reconstruction. *Ophthalmic Plastic and Reconstructive Surgery, 30*(4), e104–e106.
42. Stamm, A. C., Vellutini, E., Harvey, R. J., Nogeira, J. F, Jr., & Herman, D. R. (2018). Endoscopic transnasal craniotomy and the resection of craniopharyngioma. *Laryngoscope, 118*(7), 1142–1148.
43. Harris, G. J. (2010). Cavernous hemangioma of the orbital apex: Pathogenetic considerations in surgical management. *American Journal of Ophthalmology, 150*(6), 764–773.
44. Muscatello, L., Seccia, V., Caniglia, M., Sellari-Franceschini, S., & Lenzi, R. (2013). Transnasal endoscopic surgery for selected orbital cavernous hemangiomas: Our preliminary experience. *Head and Neck, 35*(7), E218–E220.
45. Jaiswal, A. K. (2017). Endonasal endoscopic approach to orbit. *Neurology India, 65*(5), 1102–1104.

28

Fibro-Osseous Lesions of the Orbit and Optic Canal

KATHLEEN M. KELLY, MD AND ASHLEIGH A. HALDERMAN, MD

Osseous tumors represent a broad range of pathologic conditions, which can be roughly categorized into fibro-osseous lesions, cartilaginous lesions, reactive bone lesions, and vascular lesions.[1] Most of these entities are extremely rare in the craniofacial skeleton, and particularly in the orbit. As such, this chapter predominantly focuses on fibro-osseous lesions, which represent a broad continuum of diseases with similar histopathologic features. Many of these lesions are slow-growing and can present with similar clinical symptoms, including proptosis, ocular displacement, and even ocular compartment syndrome when they occur in and around the orbit.[1]

Ossifying fibroma and fibrous dysplasia (FD) are similar entities consisting of collagen and fibroblasts that have replaced normal bone with a variable amount of mineralized matrix containing bone or cementum.[2] As a result, radiographic features may appear similar and can complicate diagnosis. Subtle differences between radiographic features and histopathologic features lead to an accurate diagnosis.[3] Imaging may be helpful in distinguish between these conditions and is of further value for determining the optimal surgical approach and planning the extent of surgical intervention.[4] However, despite being histopathologically benign lesions, these tumors can also cause significant orbital complications, facial deformity, and pain.[5] Additionally, as discussed later, fibrous dysplasia can give rise to osteosarcoma, a malignant fibro-osseous lesion.

Benign Fibro-Osseous Lesions

Osteoma

Osteomas are the most common benign tumor of the paranasal sinuses and show a predilection for men with a male-to-female ratio of 1.5–3:1.[6,7] The frontal (70% to 80%) and ethmoid sinuses (20% to 25%) are most commonly involved, followed by the maxillary and sphenoid sinuses, respectively.[8] Osteomas are most typically diagnosed between the third and fourth decade of life and are thought to have an incidence of up to 3% of the general population and are often discovered incidentally on imaging.[7,8] The exact underlying etiology or pathophysiology is not well understood; however prevailing theories postulate osteomas are either developmental, form secondary to trauma, or form secondary to infection.[9]

In general, osteomas are slow-growing solitary lesions with an average growth of 1.6 millimeter (mm) per year (range 0.44 to 6.0 mm per year).[10] Between 4% and 10% of osteomas produce clinical symptoms, and the symptoms are typically related to the location of the tumor, size, and growth rate.[8,11] When osteomas are symptomatic, headache localized to the area over the tumor is the most common presenting symptom.[12] Other symptoms include facial pain, swelling or deformity, nasal discharge or obstruction, and sinusitis. Orbital symptoms, including epiphora, proptosis, diplopia, and visual loss, can also be observed.[1,9,13,14]

The imaging modality of choice for osteomas is a thin-slice computed tomography (CT) scan, as it provides detail regarding the size, location, and concurrent sinonasal pathology.[11] Osteomas appear as well-circumscribed, dense masses with either a homogeneous or heterogeneous appearance (Fig. 28.1). Earwaker[8] characterized multiple types of osteomas based on CT imaging, including the following:

1. Uniformly sclerotic
2. Target-like lesion
3. Partially corticated shell with heterogeneous matrix
4. Heterogeneous matrix without a well-defined shell
5. Laminated pattern

Uniformly sclerotic lesions are the most common.[8,15] Depending on the histologic makeup of the osteoma, it may be hyperintense on T1-weighted magnetic resonance imaging (MRI), as in the case of sclerotic lesions, or it may demonstrate a signal void on all sequences, as in the case of heterogeneous lesions.[16] MRI can be used as an adjunct to evaluate for mucocele formation or intracranial and intraorbital involvement.[11,17]

Histologically osteomas are well-circumscribed lesions characterized by a variable amount of cancellous and compact, lamellar bone with haversian systems. They can be divided into ivory and mature types.

Surgical intervention is typically reserved for symptomatic patients, for cases when the osteoma is causing obstruction of the involved sinus, or if the lesion demonstrates rapid growth. In the instance of slow-growing, asymptomatic osteomas, conservative management with intermittent radiographic follow-up is recommended.[11,18] When osteomas are complicated, symptomatic, or rapidly growing, complete excision is the treatment of choice. Recurrence rates of these lesions are low with complete excision.[19] Small osteomas are often removed en bloc with curettes, whereas others require extensive drilling.[15]

In giant osteomas, which are characterized as lesions more than 30 mm in largest dimension or 110 g, dura or periorbita are often encountered during resection.[15] This has led to controversy over

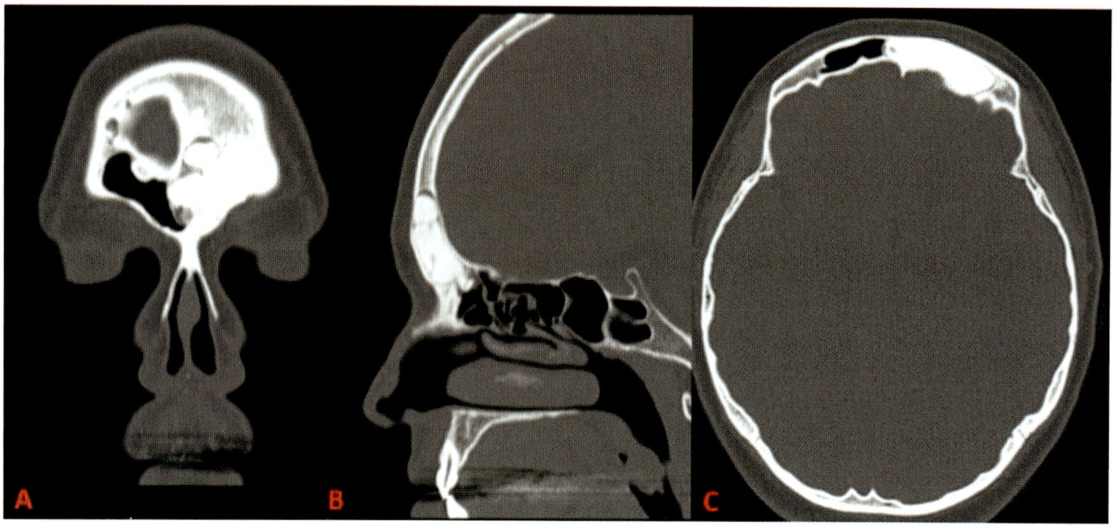

• **Fig. 28.1** Computed tomography scan demonstrating a frontal osteoma in the (A) coronal, (B) sagittal, and (C) axial planes. Note the uniform and well-circumscribed features of the tumor.

the optimal surgical approach. Overall, osteomas of the paranasal sinuses can be resected using endoscopic approaches, external approaches, or a combination of the two. Size and location typically define the approach. Endoscopic approaches have been used in all locations within the paranasal sinuses; however, traditionally open approaches have been used more frequently for frontal sinus lesions.[20] Historical approaches for these masses included a Lynch frontoethmoidectomy or osteoplastic flap to facilitate access, visualization, and treatment of possible complications such as cerebrospinal fluid leak. Cosmetic and functional concerns, in addition to the advent of improved endoscopes, instruments (such as high-speed endoscopic drills, the ultrasonic aspirator), and intraoperative navigation systems, have challenged the need for open approaches.[21] Chiu et al. identified three factors that limited endoscopic resection of osteomas from the frontal sinus: location of the base of attachment, relative size of the tumor to that of the frontal recess, and location in relation to a virtual sagittal plane through the lamina papyracea.[22] Osteomas were classified into four grades based on these characteristics, which are summarized in Table 28.1. Endoscopic resection was recommended for grades I and II disease, and open approaches were advised for grades III and IV.[22] However, there have been documented reports of successful endoscopic resections of osteomas with far lateral extent or intraorbital involvement.[23]

Purely endoscopic approaches have gained significant popularity in recent decades.[16] Although familiarity of the endoscopic modified Lothrop procedure has redefined the parameters by which frontal osteomas can be resected endoscopically, a narrow anteroposterior diameter of the frontal sinus and tumors attached to the orbital roof or anterior table of the frontal sinus significantly increase the need for open or endoscopic-assisted procedures.[16]

Osteoblastoma (Giant Osteoid Osteoma)

Osteoblastomas are rare, slow-growing benign tumors of bone that most frequently present in the long bones or vertebrae. Rarely do they occur in the paranasal sinuses. They can be locally aggressive and highly proliferative. Most often, presentation occurs between the second and fourth decades of life. Males are twice as likely to be affected.[24] Given the proliferative nature of these lesions, patients often present with pain, swelling, and tenderness over the lesion.[25]

On CT imaging, osteoblastomas often originate from the surface of the bone or within the medullary cavity (Fig. 28.2). They

TABLE 28.1 Grading System for Frontal Sinus Osteomas[22]

Grade	Base of Attachment	Location Relative to VSPLP	Anteroposterior Diameter	Recommend Approach
I	Posterior-inferior along frontal recess	Medial	AP diameter of lesion is <75% AP dimension of frontal recess	Endoscopic enodonasal
II	Posterior-inferior along frontal recess	Medial	AP diameter of lesion is >75% AP dimension of frontal recess	Endoscopic endonasal
III	Anterior or superiorly located within frontal	Lateral		External or endoscopic-assisted external
IV	Tumor fills the entire frontal sinus			External or endoscopic-assisted external

AP, anteroposterior; *VSPLP*, Virtual sagittal plane through the lamina papyracea.

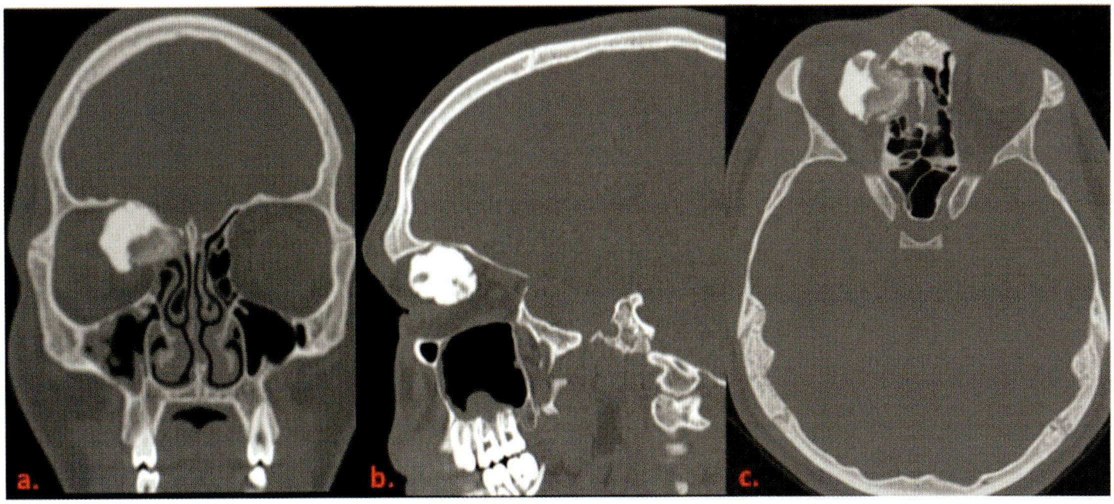

• **Fig. 28.2** Computed tomography scan demonstrating an osteoblastoma of the right superomedial orbit with inferolateral displacement of the globe shown in the (A) coronal, (B) sagittal, and (C) axial planes.

are well circumscribed with central mineralization.[26,27] The expansile tendencies of these lesions lead to destruction of cortical bone and presentation of periostitis radiographically.[28] MRI findings are nonspecific and can overestimate the size and extent of the lesion.[29] On T1- and T2-weighted imaging, osteoblastomas appear hypointense to isointense with focal areas of decreased intensity that represent calcifications. These lesions do enhance because of their vascular nature and often demonstrate enhancement of the surrounding tissue (Fig. 28.3).[29]

Histologically these lesions are similar to osteomas; however, they contain areas of woven bone trabeculae surrounded by osteoblasts, osteoclasts, and fibrovascular stroma. As a result, osteoblastomas more frequently demonstrate rapid growth, and when the lesions involve or abut the orbit, they can cause significant symptomatic effect on the eye.[30]

Complete surgical excision is recommended for these lesions, and both open and endoscopic approaches have been described.[31,32] Recurrence rates in the paranasal sinuses are difficult to determine owing to the paucity of data. However, in other sites (e.g., spine, jaw, long bones), the recurrence rate is estimated to be between 9% and 15% up to 10 years after resection.[33,34] As a result, some groups have recommended annual surveillance with CT imaging.[35] In less than 1% of cases, osteoblastomas can transform into osteosarcoma.[27]

Osteoclastoma (Giant Cell Tumor)

Osteoclastomas or giant cell tumors (GCTs) account for approximately 4% of primary bone tumors.[36] Although benign, they are known for a higher rate of recurrence compared with osteomas. GCTs are most frequently noted in patients between the ages of 20 and 45. There is a slight preponderance in women.[37] Similar to the other tumors noted in this chapter, they are more commonly found within the long bones; however, they have also been identified in the cranium.[36,38] Approximately 1% of GCTs are found in the cranium, where they occur most frequently in the sphenoid

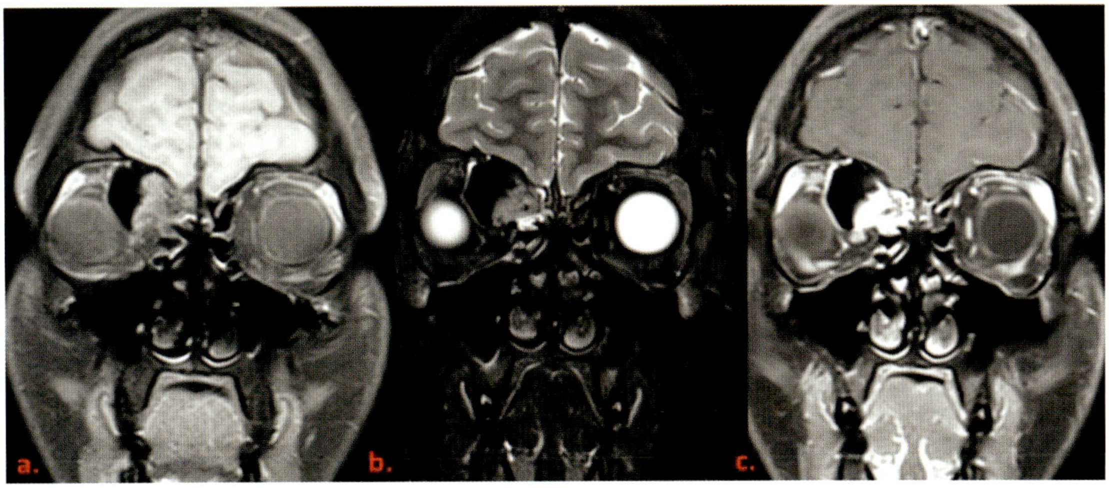

• **Fig. 28.3** A, Magnetic resonance imaging of a right orbital osteoblastoma. B, T1- and T-2 weighted imaging. C, Postcontrast images. Note the hypointense/isointense medial portion of the mass in contrast to the lateral portion where signal is dropped secondary to calcification.

and temporal bones.[36,39,40] The clinical presentation usually involves headache and dysfunction of either cranial nerve II or VIII, depending on the location of the mass.[41]

Diagnosis of GCTs based on imaging is difficult given the lack of identifiable radiologic features.[39,41] Radiographically GCTs appear as an expansive, sometimes lytic mass that may extend to other sinuses, dura, or other nearby soft tissues. Given the nonspecific radiographic features, tissue is necessary to confirm the diagnosis.

On histology, GCTs are characterized by stromal mononuclear cells and giant cells. The mononuclear cells represent the neoplastic component of the tumor, whereas the giant cells are multinucleated and have an osteoclast-like morphology. Multiple cytogenetic abnormalities have been described, with telomeric association the most frequent chromosomal aberration (75%).[39] These features separate GCTs from other osseous lesions in which multinucleated giant cells are observed, including giant cell reparative granuloma, FD, and aneurysmal bone cyst.[39]

As with osteoblastomas, complete surgical resection is recommended for GCTs, as recurrence rates are high with partial resection.[42] However, given the propensity for these tumors to develop in the sphenoid and temporal bones, aggressive surgery for complete excision must be weighed against the potential morbidity to nearby vital structures.

Ossifying Fibroma

Ossifying fibromas (OFs) are benign fibro-osseous neoplasms that involve the craniofacial bones. These tumors are divided into three variants including cement-ossifying fibroma (COF), juvenile psammomatoid ossifying fibroma (JPOF), and juvenile trabecular ossifying fibroma (JTOF). As the names imply, JPOF and JTOF are seen in juvenile patients. These tumors can be found in a fairly broad age range with some notable differences between the subtypes. JPOF and JTOF are less common than COF and typically present in the second decade of life without a gender predilection.[43] In contrast, COF is typically seen in the third to fourth decade of life and shows a 5:1 female predilection. JPOF most commonly involves the ethmoid sinuses. In contrast, JTOF is more commonly seen in the maxilla followed by the mandible.[43,44] COF occurs in the mandible most frequently, specifically in the molar and premolar regions.

Swelling is a common presenting symptom of these lesions when the maxilla and mandible are involved. Other presenting symptoms are often secondary to localized mass effect based on the location of the lesion and can include sinusitis, nasal obstruction, rhinorrhea, proptosis, diplopia, ptosis, and restriction of extraocular movements.[45] Sinonasal OFs are considered locally aggressive and may extend into adjacent structures, including the orbit, palate, optic canal, and anterior cranial fossa.[46,47] However, the lesion is bordered by a shell of bone with intact periosteum and dura mater, and thus meningitis, pneumocephalus, and neurologic deficits are rare.[46] Blindness is rare, although it has been reported.[48]

Radiographically OFs are initially predominately radiolucent and, as the tumor enlarges, begin to demonstrate a mixed density appearance.[49] A thin, radiolucent band surrounds the tumor and separates it from neighboring bone.[49] Concentric expansion of the cortical plates in keeping with a benign lesion is typically observed, and in the case of COF, the outer cortices usually remain intact (Fig. 28.4).[49,50] In contrast, the juvenile variants often show dehiscence along the expanded outer cortices (Fig. 28.5).[50] On MRI, these lesions show variable intensity on T1-weighted images and enhancement of fibrous portions after administration of contrast (Fig. 28.6).[49]

The histologic appearance depends on the specific variant. COFs demonstrate a variably hypercellular fibrous tissue with mineralized tissue that varies among tumors or even within the same tumor.[50] Mineralized tissue can consist of trabeculae of bone or osteoid with a woven and lamellar pattern or as lobulated collections of cementum-like material.[50] Another histologic feature of COFs is osteoblastic rimming.[50] Typically mitotic figures are not observed. In JTOF, however, mitotic figures can be seen within a cellular stroma with a mineralized component consisting of a cellular osteoid trabeculae focally mineralized at the center.[50] Osteoclastic giant cells can be seen and osteoblastic rimming is not

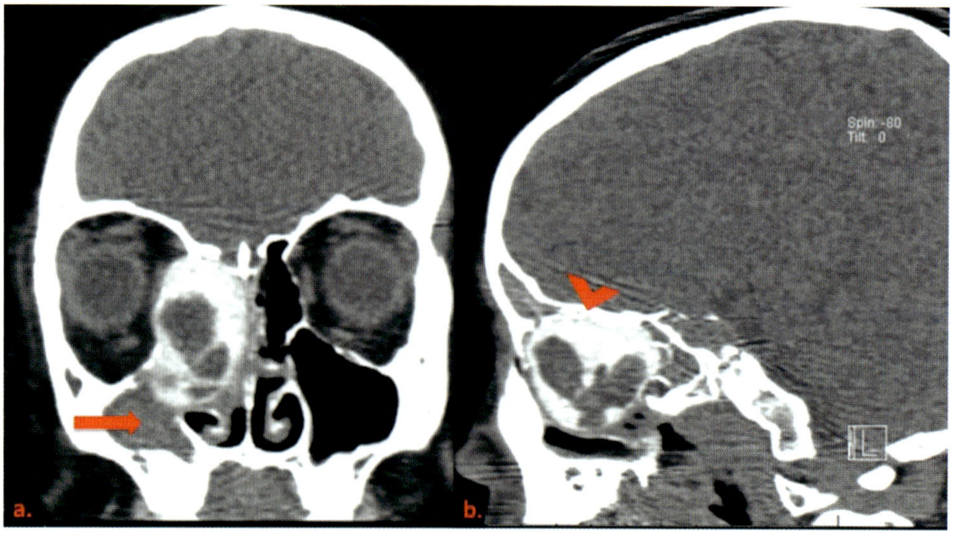

• **Fig. 28.4** Computed tomography scan of a right ethmoid cement-ossifying fibroma with involvement of the medial orbit. The coronal view is seen (A) with postobstructive maxillary sinus disease (*arrow*) and (B) the sagittal view. The tumor is abutting the skull base (*arrowhead*).

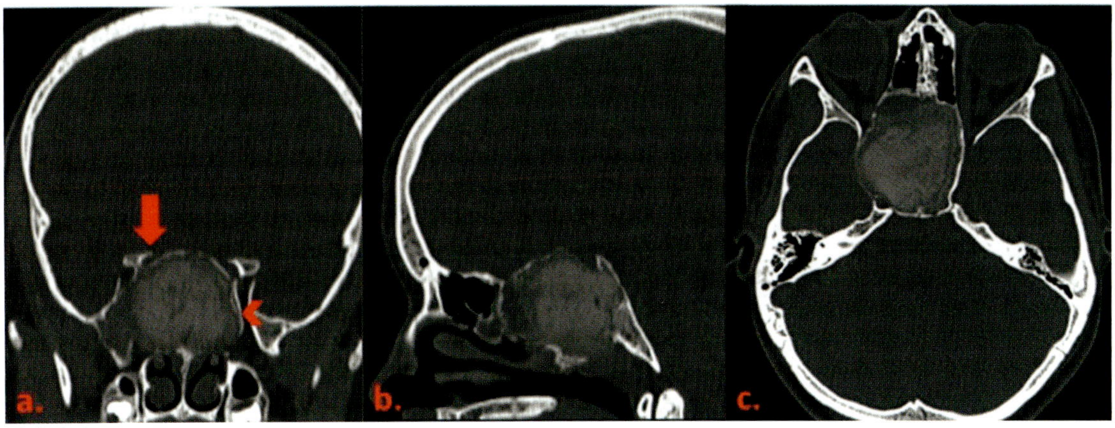

• **Fig. 28.5** Computed tomography images of a juvenile psammomatoid ossifying fibroma involving the sphenoid in the (A) coronal, (B) sagittal, and (C) axial views. The tumor was compressing the right optic canal (*arrow*). There is a thin radiolucent area of bone separating tumor from normal bone (arrowhead).

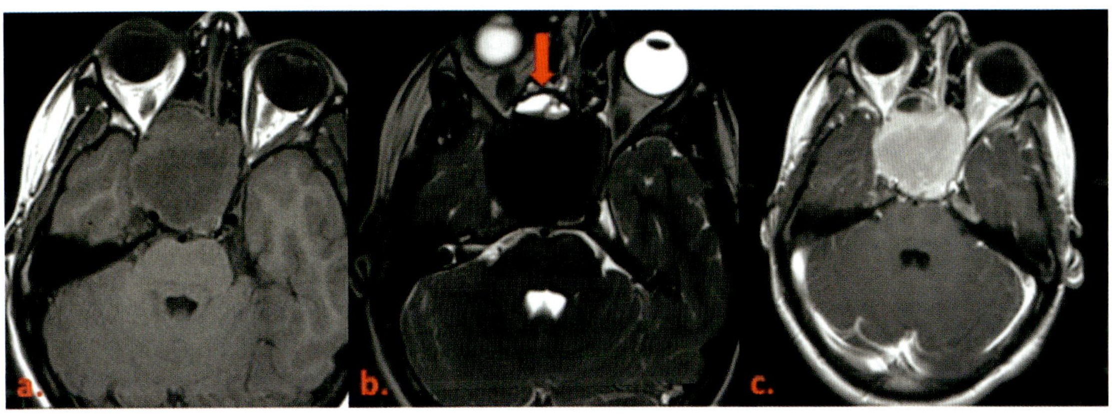

• **Fig. 28.6** Magnetic resonance imaging of a juvenile psammomatoid ossifying fibroma of the sphenoid sinus on (A) T1-weighted, (B), T2-weighted, and (C) postcontrast images. An aneurysmal bone cyst is seen arising from the juvenile psammomatoid ossifying fibroma (*arrow*).

present.[50] JPOF demonstrates numerous psammomatoid bodies that can coalesce to form large areas of mineralization.[50] On gross examination, the tumor appears white to yellow and is gritty in consistency (Figs. 28.7 and 28.8).

The treatment of choice for sinonasal OFs has typically consisted of radical resection because of the aggressive growth behavior and close proximity to both the orbit and the skull base.[51] A multidisciplinary approach with experts in radiology, neurosurgery, otolaryngology, ophthalmology, or craniofacial surgery may be required for optimal treatment planning.[52] At present, radical resection is most frequently recommended to reduce the risk of local recurrence.[44]

For many years, open surgical approaches were recommended to provide visualization of the entire lesion. Such approaches included lateral rhinotomy, sublabial approach, and craniofacial resection. However, external approaches were prone to scarring and undesirable cosmetic outcomes, as well as overresection of bone, which further placed young patients at risk for significant facial deformity. As a result, endoscopic approaches have largely replaced open approaches in an attempt to reduce scarring while achieving adequate resection.[53-55] Endoscopic approaches have the advantages of direct visualization, absence of external incisions, and reduced postoperative morbidity and length of stay. However, reports of endoscopic resection have noted significant bleeding intraoperatively as a result of removing the lesion in a piecemeal fashion.[45] These tumors are highly vascular, and with the juvenile forms are not well encapsulated, and unlike COFs, these tumors do not easily shell out. As a result, precautions, including patient positioning, optimal anesthetic, hemostatic agents, and electrocautery, should be taken to reduce intraoperative bleeding. Blood products should be readily available. Embolization of feeder vessels or ligation of branches of the external carotid artery has been reported and may be considered before surgery in some cases.[53]

Even with complete surgical excision, recurrence rates have been reported as high as 30% to 56%.[46,47] However, not all sinonasal OFs demonstrate recurrence even after a subtotal resection. Particularly in adults, there may be a role for watchful waiting with interval radiology.[45] Radiation therapy is contraindicated because of concern for malignant transformation.[56]

Lesions are most likely to recur in pediatric patients. Adjuvant systemic therapy with interferon-alfa has been explored for treatment of patients with juvenile ossifying fibroma to decrease the rate of local recurrence. In one case series, subcutaneous injections of interferon-alfa for 6 to 12 months were shown to prevent recurrence during a mean follow-up of 35 months in three patients.[57] Other chemotherapeutic agents, including cyclophosphamide, samarium, and pazopanib, have been used to try to halt progression, with mixed results.[5]

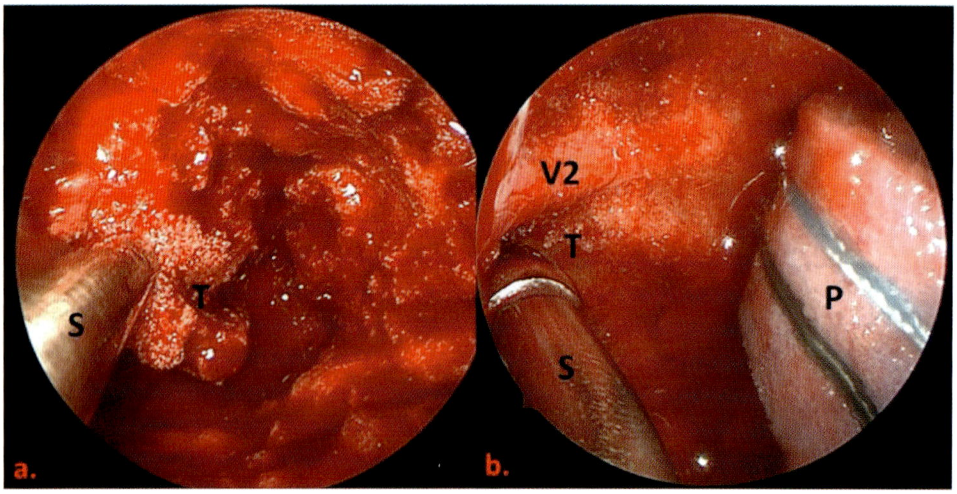

• **Fig. 28.7** Intraoperative photos from removal of a juvenile psammomatoid ossifying fibroma showing (A) the gross appearance of the tumor and (B) removal of tumor from around the maxillary division of the trigeminal nerve. *P*, pledget; *S*, suction; *T*, tumor; *V2*, maxillary division of the trigeminal nerve.

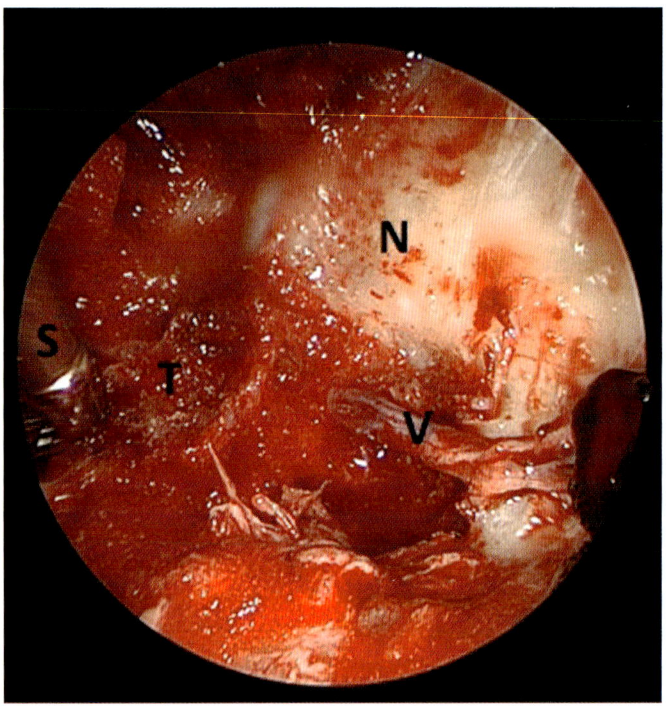

• **Fig. 28.8** Intraoperative photo from removal of a juvenile psammomatoid ossifying fibroma showing tumor within the sphenoid sinus. *N*, normal mucosa-lined bone; *S*, suction; *T*, tumor; *V*, vidian neurovascular bundle.

Fibrous Dysplasia

Fibrous dysplasia (FD) is another fibro-osseous tumor characterized by slowly progressive proliferation. Unlike ossifying fibroma, FD may be monostotic (involving a single bone) or polyostotic (involving multiple bones). The majority of cases are monostotic (75%).[58] FD is caused by missense mutations in the *GNAS* gene whose downstream effects result in changes in bone osteoprogenitor cells, leading to abnormal bone formation.[43]

FD is typically diagnosed in the first or second decade of life and does not show a gender predilection. Craniofacial bones and specifically the maxilla and mandible are some of the most common sites affected.[43] The orbital roof is often involved owing to involvement of the frontal, ethmoid, or sphenoid bones.[59] FD lesions are typically unilateral.[60] Polyostotic FD is associated with several syndromes including McCune-Albright syndrome.

Growth of FD generally slows upon completion of skeletal growth, but the disease can progress during times of hormonal change, such as pregnancy or hormone therapy. The most common presentation is painless swelling over the involved area. This can progress to significant cosmetic deformities and, in rare cases, can affect nearby vital structures. Blindness secondary to FD has been reported.[61]

The radiographic appearance of FD on CT is often characterized by a ground-glass quality of the trabecular bone (Fig. 28.9). Other descriptions include an "orange peel" or "cotton wool" appearance because of the mixed density of the lesion. Given the expansile features of the lesion, the normal morphology of nearby structures is maintained, albeit displaced.[62] The ground-glass appearance and lack of an identifiable margin are pathognomonic for FD. MRI can be misleading, as FD can appear more aggressive or even malignant. On T1-weighted images FD may have a low to intermediate signal intensity depending on the lesion's makeup of fibrous and mineralized components. On T2-weighted images, the fibrous component appears hyperintense. Because of the high vascularity of these lesions, enhancement is seen on postcontrast images.[63]

Histologically FD is characterized by trabeculae of woven bone mixed with fibrous tissue. Cancellous bone is replaced by fibrous and abnormal bone, such that there is an appearance of Chinese characters.[50,60] The bony trabeculae of FD merge with surrounding normal bone corresponding with the indistinguishable margin between tumor and normal bone seen on radiographic imaging.[50]

The treatment of choice for FD is watchful waiting and observation in the majority of cases. As mentioned previously, disease progression slows or halts with skeletal maturation. When nearby vital structures are being compromised or the disease results in significant deformity with both cosmetic and functional implications, radical resection and immediate reconstruction is the recommended approach. Partial resection is highly associated with disease recurrence.[64] However, the proximity to critical structures may

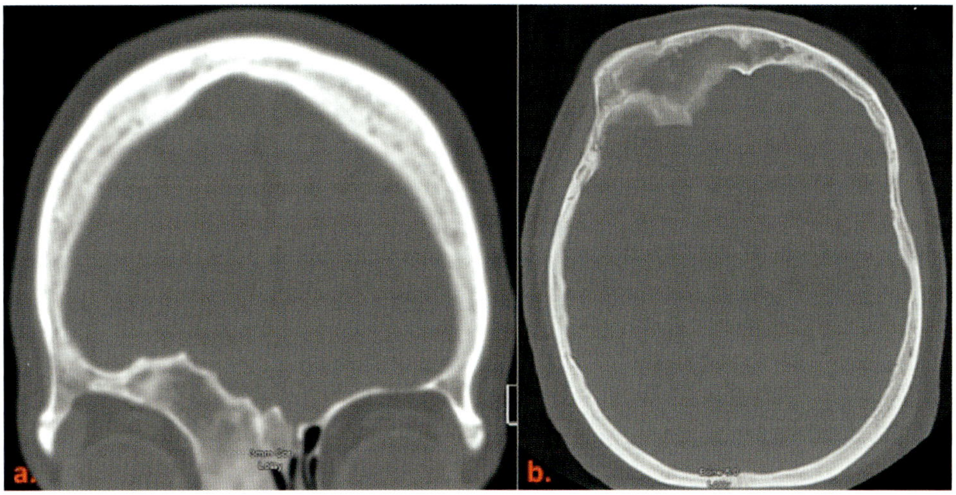

• **Fig. 28.9** Computed tomography scan showing fibrous dysplasia of the right frontal bone and orbital roof in the (A) coronal and (B) axial planes. Note the characteristic ground-glass appearance and absence of a clear margin, both of which are pathognomonic.

necessitate recontouring and delay of definitive resection until skeletal maturity has been attained and FD growth has slowed.[65]

The treatment paradigm regarding tumors invading or involving the orbital apex remains controversial. Some advocate for prophylactic decompression of the optic canal, whereas others argue against surgical intervention for these cases given the rare nature of optic neuropathy secondary to this pathology.[66-68] In support of a conservative approach, a prospective case series by Cruz et al. monitored 19 orbits with radiographic evidence of optic canal narrowing secondary to FD.[59] Of these orbits, there was only one patient who had undergone prior optic canal decompression who exhibited blindness.[59] At this time, optic canal decompression should be considered on a case-by-case basis when vision is affected, rather than prophylactically for all patients with optic canal narrowing.

Other than surgical resection, few treatment options currently exist for FD. Bisphosphonates have been used with inconsistent results.[69,70] Denosumab, a monoclonal antibody targeting RANK ligand, has shown promising results for reducing lesion growth rate and pain.[71] Historically, radiotherapy was considered a treatment option but is no longer recommended because of the risk of radiation-induced malignancies.

Although FD is a benign process, 0.4% to 6.7% of FDs can undergo malignant degeneration into osteosarcoma, fibrosarcoma, or other unspecified sarcomas even in the absence of prior radiation.[58,72] The frequency of malignant degeneration is increased in the polyostotic form and in patients with McCune-Albright and other syndromes.[58,73,74] Rapid growth, swelling, and/or pain over sites affected by FD could indicate malignant degeneration and should prompt evaluation.

Osteosarcoma

Osteosarcomas (OSs) are malignant fibro-osseous lesions. In adults, they are the second most common primary malignancy of bone with multiple myeloma being the most common.[75] OSs can occur spontaneously or can arise as a result of previous radiation, osteomyelitis, or underlying bone conditions such as FD and Paget disease.[76]

OSs in the head and neck are rare, representing 6T to 10% of all OS and less than 1% of all head and neck malignancies.[77,78] OSs of the head and neck typically present in the third and fourth decades of life, which is a later than OS of the long bones.[79-81] Men and women appear to be affected equally.[82] The most frequent site involved is the mandible followed by the maxilla and the skull.[83,84] Calvarial involvement is seen more frequently than in the skull base.[83,84] Presenting symptoms depend on the location of the tumor. Nonspecific symptoms including pain and swelling over the site are more typically seen with mandibular and maxillary involvement. Within the nasal cavity or skull base, headache, epistaxis, and nasal obstruction have been reported.[85] Involvement of the ethmoid complex or orbit can result in proptosis and varying degrees of ophthalmoplegia, whereas involvement of the sphenoid sinus or skull base can present as vision loss from optic nerve compression/involvement as well as other cranial nerve palsies.[84]

Several key characteristics of the tumor are noted on imaging. Traditional radiographs show a bony tumor with medullary and cortical destruction, a wide transition zone, and a "moth-eaten" appearance.[85] Periosteal reactions including a Codman triangle (elevation of the periosteum off the bone from underlying tumor) or a sunburst pattern (secondary to periostitis) are frequently seen.[85] Given the complex anatomy of the head and neck and overlying bony anatomy of the face, radiographs are less effective at characterizing lesions of the paranasal sinuses and skull base than other available modalities.

On CT, tumor calcification and cortical involvement are well demonstrated, and intramedullary and soft-tissue extension can also be observed (Fig. 28.10).[86] MRI provides the most detailed assessment, particularly of soft-tissue involvement and intraosseous tumor extension.[85] Mineralized components have low-intensity signals on both T1 and T2 and enhance with contrast. Soft-tissue components show an intermediate signal on T1 and a high-intensity signal on T2 (Fig. 28.11).[85] Peritumoral edema also appears bright on T2.

Histologically, OS appears as osteoid-producing spindle cells with destruction of the bony and medullary architecture and areas of necrosis.[87] Several subtypes exist and are determined by the degree of differentiation, location within bone, and histologic variants. Grade is determined by the degree of cellular atypia and

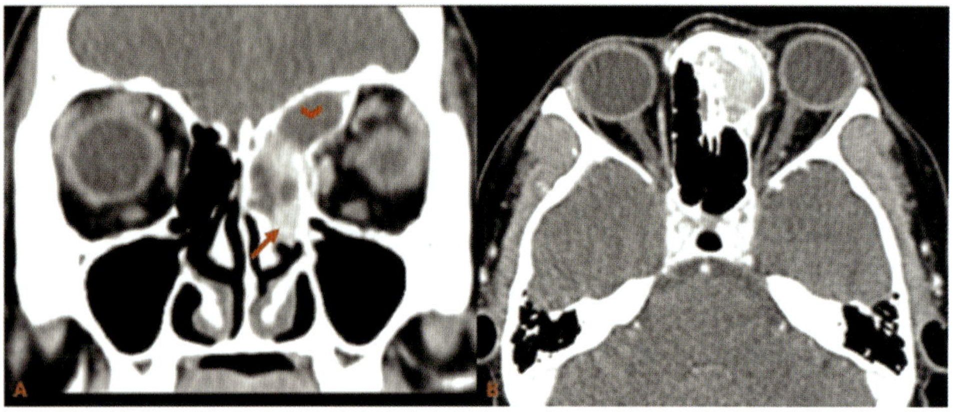

• **Fig. 28.10** Osteosarcoma of the left anterior ethmoid in the (A) coronal and (B) axial views. Note the calcifications within the tumor *(arrow)* and the intramedullary soft-tissue expansion (*arrowhead*).

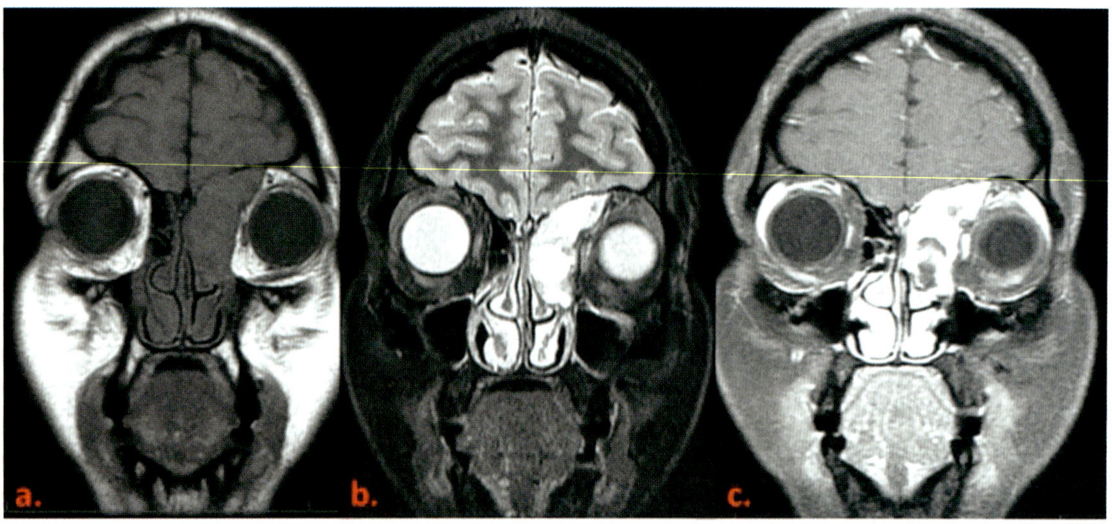

• **Fig. 28.11** Magnetic resonance imaging of an osteosarcoma of the left ethmoid sinuses and medial orbital wall showing (A) T1-weighted image, (B) T2-weighted image, and (C) postcontrast image.

architectural distortion into high, intermediate, and low grades. Of all OSs, intramedullary tumors are the most common—80%—and are divided into conventional high-grade, low-grade OSs, and telangiectatic OSs.[85] Surface or juxtacortical types account for 10% to 15% of OSs, and extraskeletal OSs represent 5% of overall tumors. Tumors are further described based on the predominate histologic differentiation as osteoblastic, chondroblastic, or fibroblastic. In one series of 14 patients with ethmoidal OS, nearly all the tumors were high grade.[88,89] High-grade tumors appear to be associated with younger age at presentation, and low-grade tumors are typically seen in older adults.[90]

In general, craniofacial OSs are less aggressive than those that occur within the long bones.[91,92] At the time of presentation, 20% or less of patients with craniofacial OSs will have distant metastases, most commonly in the lungs.[81,93] Classically OSs are clinically staged using the Enneking system, which is based on the grade, extent of primary tumor, and presence of metastases. However, use of the American Joint Commission on Cancer TNM staging system is becoming more common.

There is no consensus on the treatment approach for OSs. It has been shown that surgical resection with wide margins is associated with improved survival.[79,81,94] Furthermore, negative margins significantly predict overall and disease-specific survival.[85] Therefore complete surgical resection when possible is the mainstay of treatment. Neoadjuvant or adjuvant chemotherapy is frequently used along with surgical resection. Treatment with a number of chemotherapeutic agents has been described, including cisplatin, doxorubicin, high-dose methotrexate, ifosfamide, Adriamycin, and cyclophosphamide.[77,79,81,95] The ideal regimen for OSs has yet to be determined. Studies have shown neoadjuvant and adjuvant chemotherapy combined with surgery can decrease local recurrence and improve survival.[81] It is important to note the results mentioned previously apply to all patients with OS and not just those with craniofacial OS. Given the rarity of primary craniofacial OS, no large high-level studies have been conducted to study treatment outcomes in this specific group of patients.

The role and impact of radiation are not well defined. Some OSs appear rather radioresistant; therefore this treatment is generally reserved for specific situations. When surgical resection is incomplete or uncertain, radiation can be used for better margin control and has been shown to improve outcomes.[84] However, radiation to the head and neck is associated with a high rate of treatment-associated side effects; therefore, these possibilities must be weighed against the benefit of using radiation.[84]

In light of the above, treatment of OSs involving sites and structures around the orbit or involving the orbit itself is highly complex. Unfortunately, owing to the rarity of this disease, the literature and collective experience are sparse, consisting mainly of case reports. Therefore the treatment of OSs involving the paranasal sinuses, skull base, and/or orbit should truly be considered on a case-by-case basis. A multidisciplinary approach and involvement of a multidisciplinary tumor board is strongly recommended. It stands to reason that complete surgical resection with wide margins of a lesion involving or abutting the orbit require exenteration. In some cases, induction chemotherapy can be considered to reduce the size of the primary tumor, improve the chance of complete surgical resection, and potentially avoid orbital exenteration. Interval imaging after the start of induction chemotherapy must be done to establish if the tumor is responding. If the tumor appears to be responding, the course can be continued. If no response is observed, surgical resection should be delayed no further. If adequate surgical resection can be achieved with unilateral exenteration, this option can be offered to the patient. Bilateral orbital exenteration is not recommended. Systemic disease can be treated with chemotherapy and, in certain cases of metastatic lesions to the lungs, with pulmonary metastasectomy.

In the case of incomplete resection, postoperative radiation therapy can be considered. However, as mentioned previously, this must be weighed against the potential ocular complications associated with external beam radiation to and around the orbit. Radiation-induced cataract formation is quite common and is easily corrected with surgical treatment.[96] Unfortunately, effective treatments for late complications, such as severe keratopathy, glaucoma, and radiation retinopathy, do not yet exist. These late complications are associated with significant morbidity, including considerable pain secondary to severe keratopathy and loss of vision secondary to glaucoma and retinopathy.[96] Severe radiation keratopathy is seen with doses greater than 60 Gy, and retinopathy is seen with doses greater than 45 Gy.[96-99]

Given the complexity of the head and neck, paranasal sinuses, and skull base, complete surgical resection with wide margins is typically not feasible without substantial morbidity or risk of mortality. Therefore it is not surprising that local recurrence represents the main source of failure in craniofacial OSs.[100,101] The rate of local recurrence is reported to be between 17T and 70%.[100,101] Approximately 50% of recurrences occur within 18 months after treatment.[85] Rarely do recurrences develop after more than 5 years.[85] Overall, the prognosis for craniofacial OS involving locations other than the jaw is poor with a 5-year survival rate of approximately 20%.[81,102,103]

As stated previously, OSs can arise from prior radiation sites. In 1948, Cahan et al.[104] established four criteria for radiation-induced OS:

1. Microscopic or roentogenographic evidence of nonmalignant initial bone condition
2. Sarcoma originating in an area within the previous radiotherapeutic beam
3. A relatively long, asymptomatic latent period following irradiation before clinical appearance of a bone sarcoma
4. Histologic confirmation of sarcoma

Radiation-induced OSs (RIOS) of the craniofacial region have been described after radiotherapy for retinoblastoma, pituitary adenoma, craniopharyngioma, glioma, and other primary intracranial and head and neck pathologies.[104-106] In total, RIOS account for 3% to 5% of all OSs with an overall risk of developing the disease after radiation of 0.01% to 0.03% of all patients undergoing irradiation.[87,106] The skull ranks fourth among RIOS tumor sites, accounting for up to 13.5% of these tumor types.[87] RIOS characteristically occur at the edge of prior radiation fields when the original treatment dose exceeded 30 Gy.[86,107] In general, larger radiation doses are associated with a shorter latency period to the development of radiation-induced tumors; the mean latency period for RIOS is 9.1 years.[105,106]

The prognosis of RIOS is poorer than for primary OSs, and these tumors are associated with a high rate of local recurrence.[87,104-107] Similar to primary OSs, surgical resection and chemotherapy are the mainstays of treatment. Re-irradiation of a prior radiated field is limited by the original cumulative dose and the tolerance of nearby vital structures, such as the brain, eye, optic nerve, and so on, to further radiation.

Conclusion

A variety of fibro-osseous lesions can involve the orbit, ranging from benign to malignant. These lesions typically arise from the paranasal sinuses and therefore abut vital structures, including the orbit, optic nerve, and the skull base. For benign lesions, surgery should be considered when the lesion is symptomatic, disfiguring, or to prevent impending complications. Osteosarcoma in this area can arise as a primary tumor or develop secondary to prior radiation or underlying bone conditions. When indicated, a multidisciplinary surgical approach should be considered, and for osteosarcoma, multidisciplinary care should be standard, as surgery and chemotherapy are both indicated and, at times, radiation as well.

References

1. Selva, D., White, V. A., O'Connell, J. X., & Rootman, J. (2004). Primary bone tumors of the orbit. *Survey of Ophthalmology, 49*, 328–342.
2. Papadaki, M. E., Troulis, M. J., & Kaban, L. B. (2005). Advances in diagnosis and management of fibro-osseous lesions. *Oral and Maxillofacial Surgery Clinics of North America, 17*(4), 415–434.
3. Efune, G., Perez, C. L., Tong, L., Rihani, J., & Batra, P. S. (2012). Paranasal sinus and skull base fibro-osseous lesions, when is biopsy indicated for diagnosis? *International Forum of Allergy & Rhinology, 2*(2), 160–165.
4. Eversole, R., Su, L., & ElMofty, S. (2008). Benign fibro-osseous lesions of the craniofacial complex. A review. *Head and Neck Pathology, 2*, 177–202.
5. Merritt, H., Yin, V. T., Pfeiffer, M. L., Wang, W. L., Sniegowski, M. C., & Esmaeli, B. (2015). Treatment challenges with benign bone tumors of the orbit. *Ocular Oncology and Pathology, 1*(2), 111–120.
6. Huang, H. M., Liu, C. M., Lin, K. N., & Chen, H. T. (2001). Giant ethmoid osteoma with orbital extension, a nasoendoscopic approach using an intranasal drill. *Laryngoscope, 111*, 430–432.
7. Atallah, N., & Jay, M. (1981). Osteomas of the paranasal sinus. *Journal of Laryngology and Otology, 95*, 291–304.
8. Earwaker, J. (1993). (1993). Paranasal sinus osteomas: A review of 46 cases. *Skeletal Radiology, 22*, 417–423.
9. Menezes, C. O., & Davidson, T. M. (1994). Endoscopic resection of a sphenoethmoid osteoma: A case report. *Ear, Nose & Throat Journal, 73*, 598–600.

10. Koivunen, P., Löppönen, H., Fors, A. P., & Jokinen, K. (1990). The growth rate of osteomas of the paransal sinuses. *Clinical Otolaryngology and Allied Sciences, 15*, 397–404.
11. Georgalas, C., Goudakos, J., & Fokkens, W. J. (2011). Osteoma of the skull base and sinuses. *Otolaryngologic Clinics of North America, 44*(4), 875–890.
12. Mugliston, T. A., & Stafford, N. (1985). A cranio-facial approach to large osteomas of the fronto-ethmoidal region. *Journal of Laryngology and Otology, 99*, 979–983.
13. Cheng, K. J., Wang, S. Q., & Lin, L. (2013). Giant osteomas of the ethmoid and frontal sinuses: Clinical characteristics and review of the literature. *Oncology Letters, 5*, 1724–1730.
14. Erdogan, N., Demir, U., Songu, M., Ozenler, N. K., Uluç, E., & Dirim, B. (2009). A prospective study of paransal sinus osteomas in 1889 cases: Changing patterns of localization. *Laryngoscope, 19*, 2355–2359.
15. Lee, D. H., Jung, S. H., Yoon, T. M., Lee, J. K., Joo, Y. E., & Lim, S. C. (2015). Characteristics of paranasal sinus osteoma and treatment outcomes. *Acta Oto-Laryngologica, 135*(6), 602–607.
16. Watley, D. C., Mong, E. R., Rana, N. A., Illing, E. A., & Chaaban, M. R. (2019). Surgical approach to frontal sinus osteoma: A systematic review. *American Journal of Rhinology & Allergy, 33*(5), 462–469.
17. Castelnuovo, P., Valentini, V., Giovannetti, F., Bignami, M., Cassoni, A., & Iannetti, G. (2008). Osteomas of the maxillofacial district: Endoscopic surgery versus open surgery. *Journal of Cranio-Maxillo-Facial Surgery, 19*, 1446–1452.
18. Celenk, F., Baysal, E., Karata, Z. A., Durucu, C., Mumbuc, S., & Kanlkama, M. (2012). Paranasal sinus osteomas. *Journal of Cranio-Maxillo-Facial Surgery, 23*(5), e433–e437.
19. Badran, K., Suh, J., Namiri, N., Wrobel, B., & Ference, E. (2018). Pediatric benign paranasal sinus osteoneogenic tumors: A case series and systematic review of outcomes, techniques, and a multiportal approach. *American Journal of Rhinology & Allergy, 32*, 465–472.
20. Cokkeser, Y., Bayarogullari, H., & Kahraman, S. S. (2013). Our experience with the surgical management of paranasal sinuses osteomas. *European Archives of Oto-Rhino-Laryngology, 270*, 123–128.
21. Sciarretta, V., Pasquini, E., Frank, G., Modugno, G. C., Cantaroni, C., Mazzatenta, D., et al. (2006). Endoscopic treatment of benign tumors of the nose and paranasal sinuses: A report of 33 cases. *American Journal of Rhinology, 20*, 64–71.
22. Chiu, A. G., Schipor, I., Cohen, N. A., Kennedy, D. W., & Palmer, J. N. (2019). Surgical decisions in the management of frontal sinus osteomas. *American Journal of Rhinology, 19*, 191–197.
23. Turri-Zanoni, M., Dallan, I., Terranova, P., Battaglia, P., Karligkiotis, A., Bignami, M., et al. (2012). Frontoethmoidal and intraorbital osteomas. *Archives of Otolaryngology–Head Neck Surgery, 138*, 498–504.
24. Caltabiano, R., Serra, A., Bonfiglio, M., Platania, N., Albanese, V., Lanzafame, S., et al. (2012). A rare location of benign osteoblastoma: Case study and a review of the literature. *European Review for Medical and Pharmacological Sciences, 16*(13), 1891–1894.
25. Atesok, K. I., Alman, B. A., Schemitsch, E. H., Peyser, A., & Mankin, H. (2011). Osteoid osteoma and osteoblastoma. *Journal of the American Academy of Orthopaedic Surgeons, 19*, 678–689.
26. Lucas, D. R. (2010). Osteoblastoma. *Archives of Pathology & Laboratory Medicine, 134*, 1460–1466.
27. Nielsen, G. P., & Rosenberg, A. E. (2007). Update on bone forming tumors of the head and neck. *Head and Neck Pathology, 1*, 87–93.
28. Greer, R. O., Marx, R. E., Greer, R. O., Marx, R. E., Said, S., & Prok, L. D. (2016). Neoplasms of bone and fibro-osseous lesions of the craniofacial skeleton. In *Pediatric head and neck pathology* (pp. 391–440). Cambridge: Cambridge University Press.
29. Shaikh, M. I., Saifuddin, A., Pringle, J., Natali, C., & Sherazi, Z. (1999). Spinal osteoblastoma: CT and MRI imaging with pathological correlation. *Skeletal Radiology, 28*(1), 33–40.
30. McHugh, J. B., Mukherji, S. K., & Lucas, D. R. (2009). Sino-orbital osteoma: A clinicopathologic study of 45 surgically treated cases with emphasis on tumors with osteoblastoma-like features. *Archives of Pathology & Laboratory Medicine, 33*(10), 1587–1593.
31. Patel, A. A., Friedel, M. E., Liu, J. K., & Eloy, J. A. (2012). Endoscopic endonasal resection of extensive anterior skull base sinonasal osteoblastoma. *Otolaryngology–Head and Neck Surgery, 147*, 594–596.
32. Sidani, C. A., Karam, A. R., Bruce, J. H., & Sklar, E. (2010). Osteoblastoma of the frontal sinuses presenting with headache and blurred vision: Case report and review of the literature. *Journal of Radiology Case Reports, 4*(6), 1–7.
33. Choque-Velasquez, J., Colasanti, R., Piippo, A., & Niemela, M. (2017). Suboccipital osteoblastoma: Microsurgical resection of a rare entity. *Surgical Neurology International, 8*, 33. https://doi.org/10.4103/sni.sni_444_16.
34. Zileli, M., Cagli, S., Basdemir, G., & Ersahin, Y. (2003). Osteoid osteomas and osteoblastomas of the spine. *Neurosurgery Focus, 15* (5), E5.
35. Hicks, K., Moe, K., & Humphreys, I. (2018). Bilateral transorbital and transnasal endoscopic resection of a frontal sinus osteoblastoma and orbital mucocele, a case report and review of the literature. *Annals of Otolology, Rhinolology & Laryngology, 127*, 864–869.
36. Glasscock, M. E., 3rd, & Hunt, W. E. (1974). Giant-cell tumor of the sphenoid and temporal bones. *Laryngoscope, 84*, 1181–1187.
37. Zelig, S., Eilon, A., Deutsch, E., & Ariel, I. (1982). Giant cell tumor of the temporal bone: A case report. *ORL Journal for Oto-rhino-laryngology and Its Related Specialties, 44*, 318–322.
38. Bertoni, F., Unni, K. K., Beabout, J. W., & Ebersold, M. J. (1992). Giant cell tumor of the skull. *Cancer, 70*(5), 1124–1132.
39. Tsai, Y.-F., Chen, L.-K., Su, C.-T., Lee, C.-C., Wai, C.-P., & Chen, S.-Y. (2000). Giant cell tumor of the skull base: A case report. *Chinese Journal of Radiology, 25*, 223–227.
40. Chatterjee, D., Gupta, K., Singla, N., & Kapoor, A. (2016). Sphenoid bone, a rare site for giant cell tumor—case report with literature review. *Clinical Neuropathology, 35*, 385–388.
41. Wolfe, J. T., Cheithauer, B. W., & Dahlin, D. C. Giant-cell tumor of the sphenoid bone, review of 10 cases. *Journal of Neurosurgery, 59* (2), 322–327.
42. Company, M. M., & Ramos, R. (2009). Giant cell tumor of the sphenoid. *Archives of Neurology, 66*(1), 134–135.
43. Mofty, E. (2017). Odontogenic and maxillofacial bone tumours. In A. K. El-Naggar, J. K. C. Chan, J. R. Grandis, T. Takata, & P. J. Slootweg (Eds.), *WHO classification of head and neck tumors* (4th ed., Vol. 9, pp. 251–255). Lyon, France: International Agency for Research on Cancer.
44. Brannon, R. B., & Fowler, C. B. (2001). Benign fibro-osseous lesions: A review of current concepts. *Advances in Anatomic Pathology, 8*(3), 126–143.
45. Wang, H., Sun, X., Liu, Q., Wang, J., & Wang, D. (2014). Endoscopic resection of sinonasal ossifying fibroma, 31 cases report at an institution. *European Archives of Oto-Rhino-Laryngology, 271*, 2975–2982.
46. Johnson, L. C., Yousefi, M., Vinh, T. N., Heffner, D. K., Hyams, V. J., & Hartman, K. S. (1991). Juvenile active ossifying fibroma: Its nature, dynamics and origin. *Acta Oto-Laryngologica Supplementum, 488*, 1–40.
47. Eversole, L. R., Leider, A. S., & Nelson, K. (1985). Ossifying fibroma, a clinicopathologic study of sixty-four cases. *Oral Surgery, Oral Medicine, and Oral Pathology, 60*, 505–511.
48. Hasturk, A., Tun, K., Guvenc, Y., & Kaptanoglu, E. (2010). Cranial ossifying fibroma causing visual disorder. *Journal of Craniofacial Surgery, 21*, 768–770.
49. Ahmad, M., & Gaalaas, L. (2018). Fibro-osseous and other lesions of bone in the jaws. *Radiologic Clinics of North America, 56*, 91–104.
50. Nelson, B. L., & Phillips, B. L. (2019). Benign fibro-osseous lesions of the head and neck. *Head and Neck Pathology, 13*(3), 466–475.
51. Marvel, J. B., Marsh, M. A., & Catlin, F. I. (1991). Ossifying fibroma of the mid-face and paranasal sinuses: Diagnostic and therapeutic considerations. *Otolaryngology–Head and Neck Surgery, 104* (6), 803–808.

52. Hartstein, M. E., Grove, A. S., Jr., Woog, J. J., Shore, J. W., & Joseph, M. P. (1998). The multidisciplinary management of psammomatoid ossifying fibroma of the orbit. *Ophthalmology, 105*, 591–595.
53. Donnellan, K. A., & Carron, J. D. (2010). Endoscopic resection of an aggressive juvenile ossifying fibroma. *Laryngoscope, 120*(Suppl 4), S223.
54. Post, G., & Kountakis, S. E. (2005). Endoscopic resection of large sinonasal ossifying fibroma. *American Journal of Otolaryngology, 26*(1), 54–56.
55. Cansiz, H., Tuskan, K., Karaman, E., & Dervisoglu, S. (2004). Endoscope assisted removal of cementoossifying fibroma in the paranasal sinuses in a five-year-old girl. *International Journal of Pediatric Otorhinolaryngology, 68*(4), 489–493.
56. Vaidya, A. M., Chow, J. M., Goldberg, K., & Stankiewicz, J. A. (1998). Juvenile aggressive ossifying fibroma presenting as an ethmoid sinus mucocele. *Otolaryngology–Head and Neck Surgery, 119*(6), 665–668.
57. Kelly, P. R. (2008). Poster 014: Interferon alpha therapy for aggressive juvenile ossifying fibroma. *Journal of Oral and Maxillofacical Surgery, 66*(8 Suppl), 76–77.
58. Riddle, N. D., & Bui, M. M. (2013). Fibrous dysplasia. *Archives of Pathology & Laboratory Medicine, 137*, 134–138.
59. Cruz, A. A., Constanzi, M., de Castro, F. A., & dos Santos, A. C. (2007). Apical involvement with fibrous dysplasia, implications for vision. *Ophthalmic Plastic and Reconstructive Surgery, 23*, 450–454.
60. Ozek, C., Gundogan, H., Bilkay, U., Tokat, C., Gurler, T., & Songur, E. (2002). Craniomaxillofacial fibrous dysplasia. *Journal of Craniofacial Surgery*, (*3*), 382–389.
61. Gupta, D., Garg, P., & Mittal, A. (2017). Computed tomography in craniofacial fibrous dysplasia: A case series with review of the literature and classification update. *Open Dentistry Journal, 11*, 384–403.
62. MacDonald-Jankowski, D. S., Yeung, R., Li, T. K., & Lee, K. M. (2004). Computed tomography of fibrous dysplasia. *Dentomaxillofacial Radiology, 33*(2), 114–118.
63. Larheim, T. A., & Westesson, P. L. (2006). Maxillofacial *imaging*. New York: Springer.
64. Goisis, M., Biglioli, F., Guareschi, M., Frigerio, A., & Mortini, P. (2006). Fibrous dysplasia of the orbital region: Current clinical perspectives in ophthalmology and cranio-maxillofacial surgery. *Ophthalmic Plastic and Reconstructive Surgery, 22*, 383–387.
65. El-Mofty, S. K. (2014). Fibro-osseous lesions of the craniofacial skeleton: An update. *Head and Neck Pathology, 8*(4), 432–444.
66. Chen, Y. R., Breidahl, A., & Chang, C. N. (1997). Optic nerve decompression in fibrous dysplasia: Indications, efficacy, and safety. *Plastic and Reconstructive Surgery, 99*, 22–30; discussion 31–33.
67. Papay, F. A., Morales, L., Jr., Flaharty, P., Smith, S. J., Anderson, R., Walker, J. M., et al. (1995). Optic nerve decompression in cranial base fibrous dysplasia. *Journal of Craniofacial Surgery, 6*, 5–10.
68. Michael, C. B., Lee, A. G., Patrinely, J. R., Stal, S., & Blacklock, J. B. (2000). Visual loss associated with fibrous dysplasia of the anterior skull base: Case report and review of the literature. *Journal of Neurosurgery, 92*, 350–354.
69. Lee, J. S., Fitzgibbon, E. J., Chen, Y. R., Kim, H. J., Lustig, L. R., Akintoye, S. O., et al. (2012). Clinical guidelines for the management of craniofacial fibrous dysplasia. *Orphanet J Rare Dis, 7* (suppl 1), S2.
70. Boyce, A. M., Kelly, M. H., Brillante, B. A., Kushner, H., Wientroub, S., Riminucci, M., et al. (2014). A randomized, double blind, placebo-controlled trial of alendronate treatment for fibrous dysplasia of bone. *Journal of Clinical Endocrinology and Metabolism, 99*(11), 4133–4140.
71. Boyce, A. M., Chong, W. H., Yao, J., Gafni, R. I., Kelly, M. H., Chamberlain, C. E., et al. (2012). Denosumab treatment for fibrous dysplasia. *Journal of Bone and Mineral Research, 27*, 1462–1470.
72. Ruggieri, P., Sim, F. H., Bond, J. R., & Unni, K. K. (1994). Malignancies in fibrous dysplasia. *Cancer, 73*, 1411–1424.
73. Schwartz, D. T., & Alpert, M. (1964). The malignant transformation of fibrous dysplasia. *American Journal of the Medical Sciences, 247*, 1–20.
74. Jhala, D. N., Eltoum, I., Carroll, A. J., Lopez-Ben, R., Lopez-Terrada, D., Rao, P. H., et al. (2003). Osteosarcoma in a patient with McCune-Albright syndromes and Mazabraud's syndrome: A case report emphasizing the cytological and cytogenetic findings. *Human Pathology, 34*, 1354–1357.
75. Anil, S., Krishnan, A. P., & Rajendran, R. (2012). Osteosarcoma of the mandible masquerading as a dental abscess: Report of a case. *Case Reports in Dentistry, 2012*. 635062.
76. Erdem, E., Angtuaco, E. C., Van Hemert, R., Park, J. S., & Al-Mefty, O. (2003). Comprehensive review of intracranial chordoma. *Radiographics, 23*, 995–1009.
77. Chennupati, S., Norris, R., Dunham, B., & Kazahaya, K. (2008). Osteosarcoma of the skull base, a case report and review of the literature. *International Journal of Pediatric Otorhinolaryngology, 72*, 115–119.
78. Krishnamurthy, A., & Palaniappan, R. (2018). Osteosarcomas of the head and neck region: A case series with a review of the literature. *Journal of Maxillofacial and Oral Surgery, 17*(1), 38–43.
79. Gadwal, S. R., Gannon, F. H., Fanburg-Smith, J. C., Becoskie, E. M., & Thompson, L. D. (2001). Primary osteosarcoma of the head and neck in pediatric patients: A clinicopathologic study of 33 cases with a review of the literature. *Cancer, 91*, 598–605.
80. Potter, B. O., & Sturgis, E. M. (2003). Sarcomas of the head and neck. *Surgical Oncology Clinics of North America, 39*, 521–530.
81. Ha, P. K., Eisele, D. W., Frassica, F. J., Zahurak, M. L., & McCarthy, E. F. (1999). Osteosarcoma of the head and neck: A review of the of the Johns Hopkins experience. *Laryngoscope, 109*, 964–969.
82. Daw, N. C., Mahmoud, H. H., Meyer, W. H., Jenkins, J. J., Kaste, S. C., Poquette, C. A., et al. (2000). Bone sarcomas of the head and neck in children: The St Jude Children's Research Hospital experience. *Cancer, 88*, 2172–2180.
83. Malalis, J. F., Lee, J. M., & Jay, W. M. (2013). Primary osteosarcoma of the skull base in a pregnant patient. *Neuro-Ophthalmology, 37*(1), 38–40.
84. Mathkour, M., Garces, J., Beard, B., Bartholomew, A., Sulaiman, O. A., & Ware, M. L. (2016). Primary high-grade osteosarcoma of the clivus: A case report and literature review. *World Neurosurgery, 89*, 730e9–730e13.
85. Gonzalez, M. E., Raghavan, P., Cho, B., Muttikkal, T. J., & Rehm, P. K. (2016). Primary osteogenic osteosarcoma of the ethmoid sinus in an adolescent: Case report. *Journal of Radiology Case Reports, 10*(2), 1–9.
86. Lee, Y. Y., Tassel, P. V., Nauert, C., Raymond, A. K., & Edeiken, J. (1988). Craniofacial osteosarcomas: Plain film, CT, and MRI findings in 46 cases. *AJR American Journal of Roentgenology, 150*, 1397–1402.
87. Huvos, A. G. (1981). *Bone tumors: Diagnosis, treatment and prognosis* (2nd ed., pp. 85–252). Philadelphia: Saunders.
88. Park, H. R., Min, S. K., Cho, H. D., & Cho, S. (2004). Osteosarcoma of the ethmoid sinus. *Skeletal Radiology, 33*(5), 291–294.
89. Vlychou, M., Ostlere, S. J., Kerr, R., & Athanasou, N. A. (2007). Low-grade osteosarcoma of the ethmoid sinus. *Skeletal Radiology, 36*(5), 459–462.
90. Park, Y. K., Yang, M. H., Choi, W. S., & Lim, Y. J. (1995). Well-differentiated, low-grade osteosarcoma of the clivus. *Skeletal Radiology, 24*, 386–388.
91. Smeele, L. E., Kostense, P. J., van der Waal, I., & Snow, G. B. (1997). Effect of chemotherapy on survival of craniofacial osteosarcoma: A systematic review of 201 patients. *Journal of Clinical Oncology, 15*, 363–367.
92. Uysal, K. M., Koyuncuoğlu, M., Akman, F., Güneri, A., Sarialioğlu, F., Kargi, A., et al. (2001). A rare tumor of craniofacial bones in children: A pediatric chondroblastic osteosarcoma case with diagnostic and therapeutic problems. *Pediatric Hematology and Oncology, 18*, 147–152.

93. Mark, R. J., Sercarz, J. A., Tran, L., Dodd, L. G., Seich, M., & Calcaterra, T. C. (1991). Osteogenic sarcoma of the head and neck: The UCLA experience. *Archives of Otolaryngology–Head Neck Surgery, 117*, 761–766.
94. Oda, D., Bavisotto, L. M., Schmidt, R. A., McNutt, M., Bruckner, J. D., Conrad, E. U., 3rd, et al. (1997). Head and neck osteosarcoma at the University of Washington. *Head & Neck, 19*, 513–523.
95. O'Neill, J. P., Bilsky, M. H., & Kraus, D. (2013). Head and neck sarcomas: Epidemiology, pathology, and management. *Neurosurgery Clinics of North America, 24*, 67–78.
96. Takeda, A., Shigematsu, N., Suzuki, S., Fujii, M., Kawata, T., Kawaguchi, O., et al. (1999). Late retinal complications of radiation therapy for nasal and paranasal malignancies: Relationship between irradiated-dose area and severity. *International Journal of Radiation Oncology, Biology, Physics, 44*(3), 599–605.
97. Kwok, S. K., Ho, P. C., Leung, S. F., Gandhi, S., Lee, V. W., Lam, D. S., et al. (1998). An analysis of the incidence and risk factors of developing severe keratopathy in eyes after megavoltage external beam irradiation. *Ophthalmology, 105*(11), 2051–2055.
98. Emami, B., Lyman, J., Brown, A., Coia, L., Goitein, M., Munzenrider, J. E., et al. (1991). Tolerance of normal tissue to therapeutic irradiation. *International Journal of Radiation Oncology, Biology, Physics, 1991, 21*, 109–122.
99. Jiang, G. L., Tucker, S. L., Guttenberger, R., Peters, L. J., Morrison, W. H., Garden, A. S., et al. (1994). Radiation-induced injury to the visual pathway. *Radiotherapy and Oncology, 30*, 17–25.
100. Guadagnolo, B. A., Zagars, G. K., Raymond, A. K., Benjamin, R. S., & Sturgis, E. M. (2009). Osteosarcoma of the jaw/craniofacial region. *Cancer, 115*, 3262–3270.
101. Canadian Society of Otolaryngology-Head and Neck Surgery Oncologic Study Group. (2004). Osteogenic sarcoma of the mandible and maxilla: A Canadian review (1980-2000). *Journal of Otolaryngology, 33*, 139–144.
102. Durnali, A., Alkis, N., Yukruk, F. A., Dikmen, A. U., Akman, T., Seker, M. M., et al. (2004). Osteosarcoma of the jaws in adult patients: A clinicopathological study of 15 patients. *Sarcoma Research International, 1*, 4.
103. Lim, S., Lee, S., Rha, S. Y., & Rho, J. K. (2016). Craniofacial osteosarcoma: Single institutional experience in Korea. *Asia-Pacific Journal of Clinical Oncology, 12*(1), e149–e153.
104. Cahan, W. G., Woodard, H. Q., Higinbotham, N. L., Stewart, F. W., & Coley, B. L. (1948). Sarcoma arising in irradiated bone: Report of 11 cases. *Cancer, 1948, 1*(1), 3–29.
105. Ito, T., Ozaki, Y., Sato, K., Oikawa, M., Tanino, M., Nakamura, H., et al. (2010). Radiation-induced osteosarcomas after treatment for frontal gliomas: A report of two cases. *Brain Tumor Pathology, 27*, 103–109.
106. Salvati, M., Cervoni, L., Ciappetta, P., & Raco, A. (1994). Radiation-induced osteosarcoma of the skull: Report of two cases and review of the literature. *Clinical Neurology and Neurosurgery, 96*, 226–229.
107. Arlen, M., Higgenbotham, N. L., Huvos, A. G., Marcove, R. C., Miller, T., & Shah, I. C. (1971). Radiation induced sarcoma of bone. *Cancer, 28*, 1087–1099.

29

Endoscopic Orbital Exenteration

DONALD CHARLES LANZA, MD, MS AND LUISAM TARRATS, MD, JD

Endoscopic-Assisted Orbital Exenteration

Malignant diseases involving the orbit can result in an incalculable amount of human suffering, as their natural course can progress to include bleeding, pain, disfigurement, blindness, and premature death (Fig. 29.1). Orbital exenteration to treat such a malady, whether performed by open surgery or endoscopically, is challenging and is best accomplished through a multidisciplinary approach. The recommendation to exenterate the orbital content is typically based on two critical considerations: (1) will it lengthen life? and/or (2) will it maintain or improve quality of life? The recommendation to exenterate is made more difficult by the lack of controlled studies or even consensus as to when it is absolutely indicated. Regardless of whether orbital exenteration is best performed through a traditional approach or is endoscopically assisted is based on the disease being treated and the experience of the surgeon. Open orbital exenteration is most commonly performed for malignancy arising from within the orbit and its adnexa. Endoscopic-assisted orbital exenteration (EAOE) is typically used for orbital disease arising within the nasal and sinus passages.[1,2]

Traditionally orbital exenteration describes removal of all orbital contents, including the globe, eyelids, conjunctiva, and periorbital structures.[3] However, based on the nature, extent, and location of the disease being treated, the exenteration may be subtotal (eyelids left intact) or extended (removal of adjacent bony structures).[4] At the conclusion of the traditional exenteration, substantial frontal, sphenoid, and/or zygomatic bone is typically left exposed within the exenteration cavity. The average length of time for an exenteration cavity to heal by secondary intention is estimated to be 5 months.[3,4] In the case of cancer, without immediate reconstruction with split-thickness skin graft, regional tissue transfer, or myocutaneous free flaps, there will be an unacceptable delay in the initiation of postoperative radiation. EAOE, however, represents an alternative approach that permits preservation of the superior and lateral periosteum/periorbita that can greatly facilitate wound healing.

EAOE, introduced by Batra and Lanza in 2005,[1,2] evolved from experiences with endoscopic dacryocystorhinostomy and endoscopic decompressions of the orbit and the optic nerve. The endoscopic approach offers improvements in visualization and facilitates a more natural transition from the sinonasal portion of the procedure to the orbital exenteration. It allows for better assessment of tissues at the sino-orbital interface if the final decision to exenterate is made intraoperatively. This approach can facilitate postresection mapping to obtain clean margins. EAOE expedites the removal of orbital adnexa, such as the fat, extraocular muscles, lacrimal gland, sac, duct, vessels, and nerves, by using a soft-tissue shaver (microdebrider). Endoscopic resection readily permits eyelid and brow preservation. It is important to note that during EAOE, the globe and distal optic nerve are removed intact, anteriorly through the palpebral fissure. This precludes any risk of contralateral blindness secondary to sympathetic ophthalmia. Despite its advantages, the place of EAOE in our surgical armamentarium is yet to be clearly delineated.

Examining Indications for Endoscopic-Assisted Orbital Exenteration

The indications for EAOE resemble those for traditional exenteration and can include cancer, infections, trauma, inflammatory disorders, and even massive expanding benign tumors. Yet, in most circumstances, there are immediate alternatives to exenteration. However, once the extraocular muscles, intraconal fat (Fig. 29.2A), and/or the globe are involved by destructive disease arising within the paranasal sinuses, aggressive therapy is warranted.[5,6] However, involvement of the lamina papryacea, lacrimal bone, maxillary bone, or even the periorbita is no longer considered by many treating physicians as absolute indications for orbital exenteration. Accurately determining which of these tissues are directly involved by malignancy can be difficult to ascertain by preoperative imaging even with magnetic resonance imaging (MRI).[7] Surrounding tissue edema secondary to the cancer may be mistaken on imaging for extraocular muscle invasion[7] (Fig. 29.2B). Therefore the final determination on critical orbital involvement may be delayed based on intraoperative tissue sampling/pathology results.

In the case of acute invasive fungal sinusitis, orbital exenteration might be delayed until antifungal therapy, reversal of immune dysfunction, and endoscopic sinus surgery can be given a chance to be effective. Topical or injected intraorbital amphotericin B might also be used.[8] Limited treatment without exenteration is more likely to be effective in those patients whose immune deficit can be reversed and/or when mucormycosis is not the infection invading tissue. However, in the case of severe immunosuppression with fulminant mucormycosis tissue invasion, EAOE performed with early signs of involvement is known to be lifesaving.

In the case of sinus malignancy, it is widely accepted that invasion of orbital contents through the periorbita heralds a poorer prognosis for overall and disease-free survival.[9,10] The standard

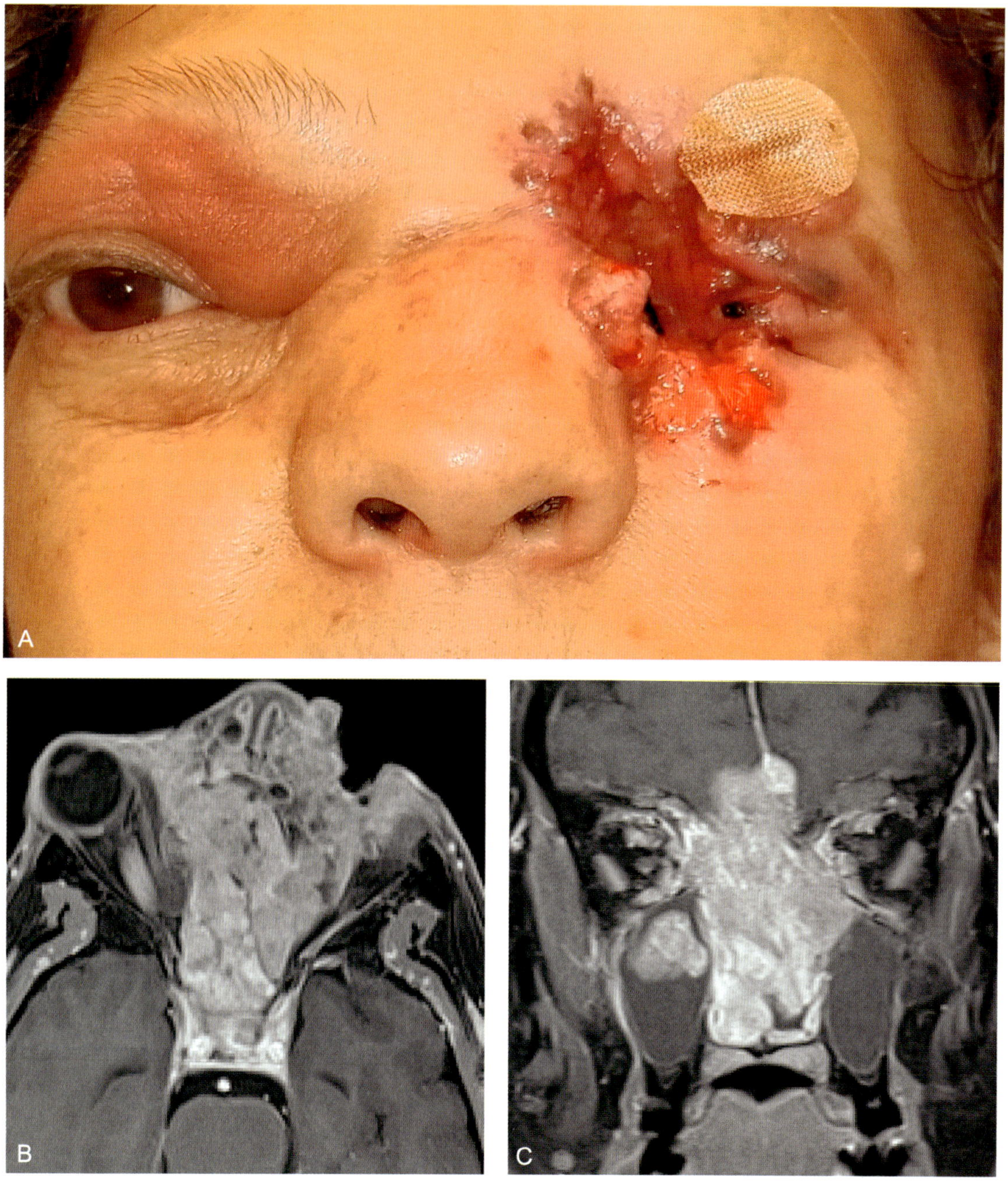

• **Fig. 29.1** A, 61-year-old woman showing the 6-year course of an insufficiently treated collision tumor with basal cell of the eyelid and squamous cell carcinoma of the paranasal sinuses. B, Postcontrast axial and magnetic resonance imaging scan. C, Postcontrast coronal and magnetic resonance imaging scan. (Image courtesy the Sinus & Nasal Institute of Florida Foundation.)

of care is a combination of surgery with adjuvant radiation therapy with or without chemotherapy.[11-14] However, whether orbital exenteration improves disease-free survival or overall survival is unclear.[13] This lack of clarity makes the choice to exenterate an orbit for sinus malignancy especially difficult.[13,15] Moreover, the existing data for sinus malignancy examine traditional orbital exenteration, but similar data are not available for EAOE. Yet early results for endoscopic management of sinus malignancy yield comparable results to open surgery.[14] Endoscopic resection of sinus malignancy alone or in combination with EAOE may be delayed or avoided depending on the malignancy type, extent of involvement, the patient's choice for neoadjuvant chemotherapy and/or radiation, and patient motivation to preserve the eye.

In one study, induction chemotherapy was successful in downstaging sinus cancer, leading to orbital preservation in 82% of patients.[13] However, nearly 20% did not respond adequately to therapy, potentially jeopardizing those lives to preserve an orbit.[13,16] In another study, treatment of basal cell carcinoma invading the orbit with an oral hedgehog pathway inhibitor called vismodegib (Erivedge) has prevented blindness and preserved the orbit in select cases.[17] Adding to the controversy is an international collaborative report of 334 patients with ethmoid malignancies

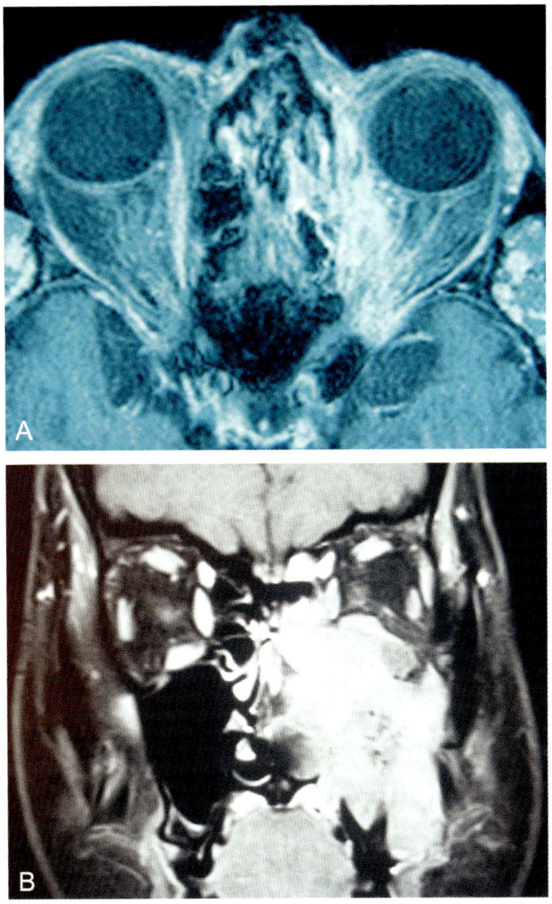

• **Fig. 29.2** A, Postcontrast axial magnetic resonance imaging (MRI) showing recurrent/persistent squamous cell carcinoma of the septum, despite surgery and radiation at an outside facility. Note the involvement of the right orbital apex. B, Postcontrast MRI of stage T4B squamous cell carcinoma of the left maxilla when frozen histopathology did not reveal orbital involvement. (Image courtesy the Sinus & Nasal Institute of Florida Foundation.)

who underwent craniofacial resection with and without radiation/chemotherapy.[9] This report indicates that orbital involvement reduces 5 year disease-specific survival from 78.0% to 44.4%.[9] Unfortunately, there is insufficient evidence from even this large study to determine whether orbital exenteration yields a better 5-year survival rate. The survival impact of orbital exenteration, from a series with the most promising results, is 93.4% at 1 year and 53.1% at 5 years.[18] Lastly, orbital invasion by cancer is associated with inferior outcomes even from salvage surgery.[19]

Preoperative Assessment

Preoperative surgical planning requires careful review of computed tomography and MRI to assess the extent of sinonasal and orbital pathology.[7] All patients undergo nasal endoscopy, typically with tissue sampling and preoperative ophthalmologic evaluation. Consultation with oncology, radiation oncology, the reconstructive team, neurosurgery, and/or maxillofacial prosthetic specialists is obtained when appropriate. Informed consent for orbital exenteration is obtained after frank discussion about limitations, risks, benefits, and alternatives. The patient's psychological status is taken into consideration, as orbital exenteration surgery may have significant emotional repercussions.

Endoscopic-Assisted Orbital Exenteration: Surgical Technique

The operative suite is set up for computer-aided endoscopic sinus surgery, and the patient is prepared for general anesthesia with appropriate intravenous access, should blood transfusion be necessary. The face is prepped and draped with special protections afforded to the contralateral eye with corneal shield, lubricant, and/or temporary tarsorrhaphy suture. The ipsilateral eye may be similarly protected until the intraoperative decision to exenterate is finalized based on pathology findings. The intraoperative navigation system is properly positioned, registered, and its accuracy verified. Nasal decongestion is obtained with 0.05% oxymetazoline hydrochloride on cotton pledgets. Transnasal sphenopalatine and lateral nasal wall injections are performed with 1% lidocaine with 1:200,000 of epinephrine. Large sinonasal neoplasms may preclude sufficient intranasal injections; transoral greater palatine foramen block may be used in these circumstances. Bleeding is controlled with topical vasoconstrictors applied on $^1/_2 \times$ 3-inch pledgets and unipolar suction cautery. Topical adrenaline, 1:1000 colored with fluorescein to prevent drug confusion (with injected medications), can be helpful when safely administered. Three 1 × 36-inch petroleum jelly–impregnated gauze packs are opened on the field should they be needed for brisk bleeding. The transnasal segment of the procedure is initiated first.

After endoscopic complete sphenoethmoidectomy, maxillary anstrostomy. and frontal sinusotomy are performed, disease extending beyond the sinuses, into the clivus, pterygoid plates, pterygomaxillary space, or infratemporal fossa is resected endoscopically. A wide sphenoidotomy and maxillary antrosomy facilitates the exposure of the orbital apex. The region of the medial orbit, inferior orbit, lacrimal sac, and optic nerve are exposed. Residual lamina papryacea is removed with a curette, Cottle elevator (Karl Storz, Germany), and/or drilled away with a concurrently irrigating diamond burr. Bone at the orbital apex is removed with the diamond burr to expose the annulus of Zinn. The involved portions of the lacrimal sac are removed endoscopically. Tissue sampling for pathology are sent for mapping of the disease. The periorbita is incised with 6700 and/or bent 7200 Beaver blade (BVI [Beaver-Visitec] International, Waltham, MA) to expose the orbital fat and muscles.

Angled instruments typically used in frontal sinus surgery as well as 30-degree and 70-degree telescopes are needed for this approach. Soft-tissue shavers (microdebriders) facilitate expeditious removal of the periorbital contents while the suction constantly clears blood from the surgical field. Extraocular muscles, orbital fat, lacrimal gland and pathology are very amenable to soft-tissue debridement with straight, 40-degree, 60-degree, 90-degree, and even 120-degree shaver tips (Medtronic Xomed, Jacksonville, FL). The orbit is skeletonized as the debulking proceeds from medial to lateral and inferior to superior. Removal of the lacrimal gland and inferior oblique muscle at its lateral attachment is typically performed with 70-degree endoscope and either a 90-degree or 120-degree soft-tissue shaver tip. Properly grounded unipolar suction cautery is used for bleeding control during soft tissue resection. Unipolar cautery is avoided at the orbital apex and on tissues adjacent to the dura. Again, with careful resection, the lateral and superior orbital periosteum can typically be preserved. Once the orbital adnexa are removed, the globe and optic nerve remain intact. The tough collagen of the episclera renders the globe somewhat impervious to inadvertent damage by the soft-tissue shaver. The cauterized extraocular muscle stumps with the origins at the annulus of Zinn remain visible. The optic nerve and ophthalmic artery are cross-clamped at the orbital apex using a long thin right-angle hemostat placed transnasally.

Exteriorly, using overhead lighting and magnified direct visualization, the globe is released by making relaxing incisions in the conjunctiva at the surgical limbus. The conjunctiva is elevated and preserved back toward the conjunctival fornix. The globe is mobilized medially and laterally by sharp release of the medial and lateral canthal tendons. A Wells enucleation spoon (Novo Surgical, Oak Brook, IL) (Fig. 29.3) is placed behind the globe to provide traction during the endonasal transection of the optic nerve. Incision is made endoscopically proximal to the right angle hemostat at the orbital apex with a 7200 Beaver blade. The globe and optic nerve trunk are withdrawn with the Wells enucleation spoon through the palpebral fissure. While protecting the eyelids, the optic nerve /ophthalmic artery stump is tied with two 2-0 silk suture ligatures through the palpebral fissure into the exenteration cavity. Frozen sections can be obtained from the orbital apex and optic nerve to ensure adequate removal of disease. Bipolar cautery is used to control residual bleeding.

Although reconstruction can be delayed or immediate, typically dissolvable and removable bacteriostatic packing is applied to fill the sino-orbital defect and exposed areas of bone. First, a "microfibrillar collagen slurry" is applied to all areas of exposed bone. This is prepared by mixing 1 gm of Avitene microfibrillar collagen hemostat flour BD Bard, Warwick, RI) with 6 to 7 mL of

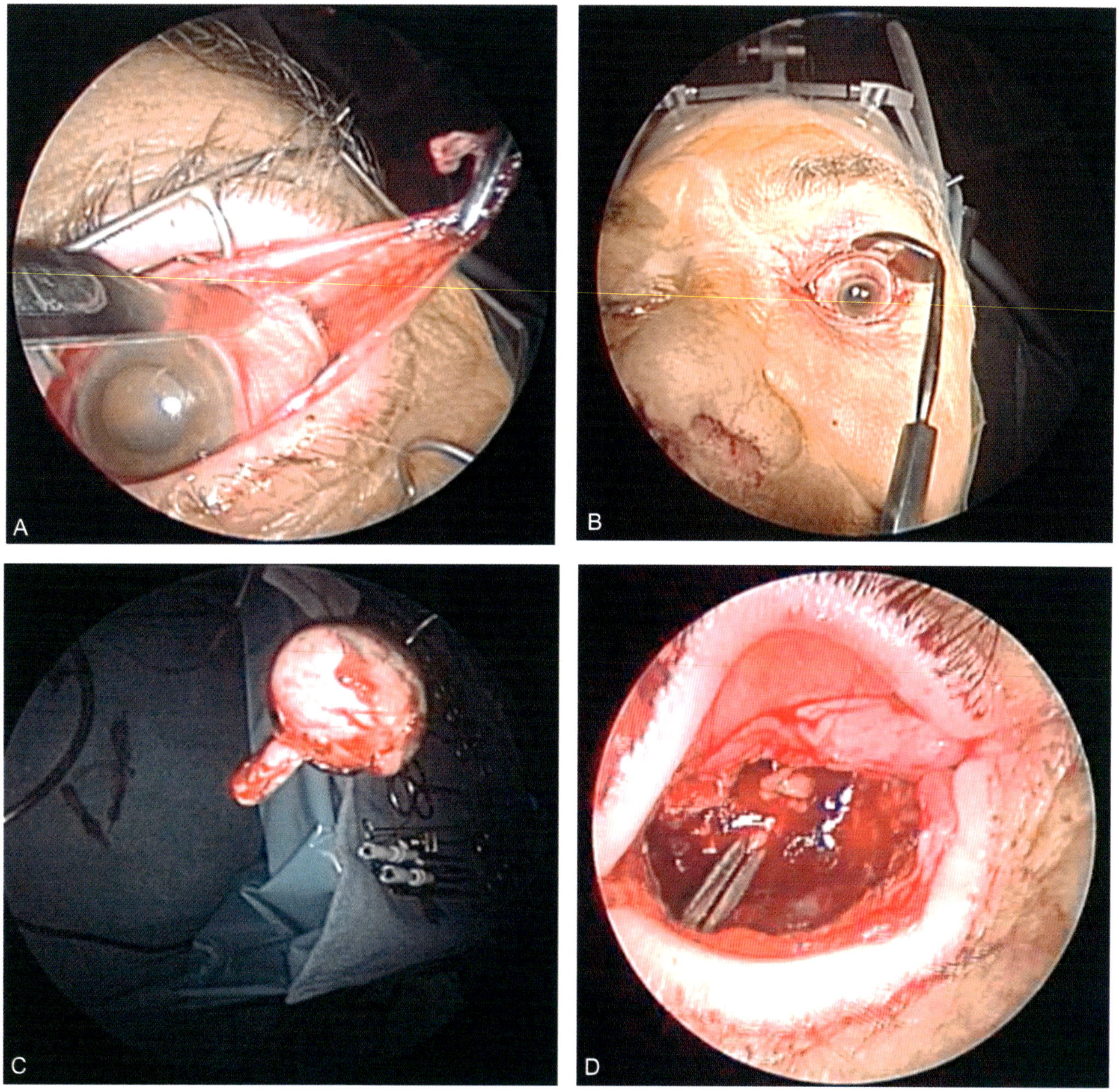

• **Fig. 29.3** External steps for endoscopic-assisted orbital exenteration. A, Freeing up the globe from the conjunctiva. B, Insertion of the Wells enucleation spoon. C, removal of the globe and optic, D, Right-angle clamp seen through palpebral fissure for suture ligature of the ophthalmic artery and the optic nerve. (Image courtesy the Sinus & Nasal Institute of Florida Foundation.)

gentamicin-saline (160 mg/L). The barrel of a 3-mL Luer-lock syringe is filled with the slurry with its plunger removed. Once filled, the plunger is reinserted and a 10-gauge angiocath (without its needle) is attached to the Luer lock tip. The microfibrillar collagen paste is now readily applied to the optic nerve stump and exposed bony surfaces of the sino-orbital cavity. The sinonasal cavity is then transnasally packed with a combination of 2% mupirocin ointment–coated Merocel sponges (Medtronic Xomed, Jacksonville, FL). The Merocel packing configuration (3.5 cm and 8 cm) varies based on the geometry of the defect. Drawstrings from the Merocel packing are secured to the nasal dorsum with $^1/_2$ × 4-inch Steri-strips (3M, St. Paul, MN) after preparing the skin with 3M Steri-Strip Compound Benzoin Tincture. The uninvolved eye is carefully protected while applying this skin prep. Before preparing the skin for the Steri-strips application, the orbital cavity is packed with bacteriostatic Xeroform petrolatum gauze (Covidien Medtronic, Mansfield, MA) strips and/or dry $^1/_2$ inch × 5 yards cotton gauze packing that is coated with 2% mupirocin ointment. All packing is sized and placed to facilitate transnasal endoscopic removal 1 week after surgery.

The posterior aspects of the conjunctiva of the upper and lower lids are approximated to one another and sewn with 4-0 Vicryl sutures on an atraumatic needle. Gentamicin ophthalmic ointment is applied to the conjunctiva. The eyelids are then managed by lateral permanent tarsorrhaphy.[20] The orbit is then patched. The corneal shield is removed from the contralateral eye. Through forces of contracture, the lids will eventually retract into the orbital cavity; the orbital prosthesis can later be fitted directly over the lids (Fig. 29.4).

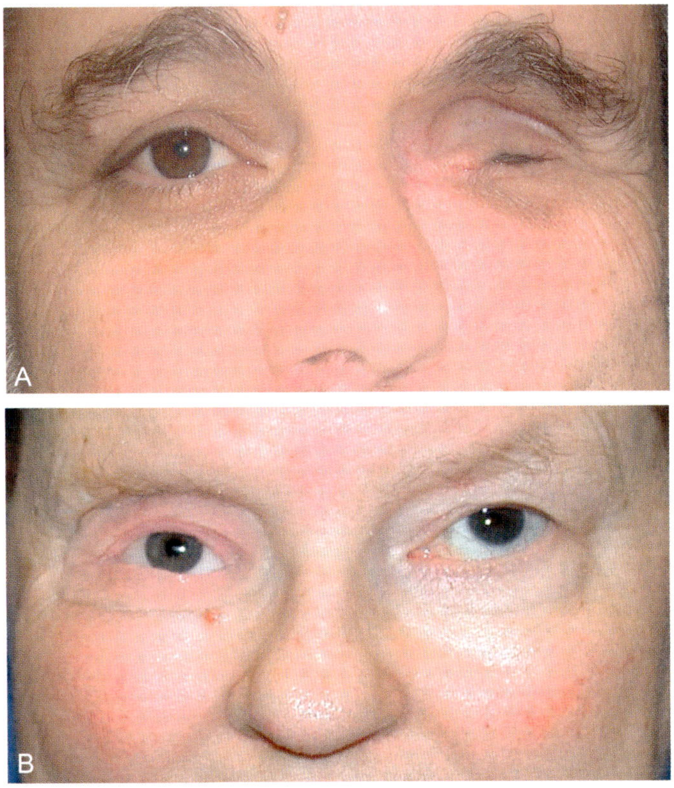

• **Fig. 29.4** A, Postoperative appearance of left eyelids after endoscopic-assisted orbital exenteration. B, Right eye orbital prosthesis. (Image courtesy the Sinus & Nasal Institute Florida Foundation.)

EAOE has found a place in our surgical armamentarium in select patients to treat sinus malignancy invading the orbit and acute fungal infection, but it may also evolve to be useful in other disorders affecting the orbit. Four advantages of EAOE are as follows:

1. It renders a superb view of the orbital contents.
2. It facilitates direct control of the ophthalmic artery,
3. It permits preservation of the superior and lateral periosteum, which facilitates wound healing.
4. It permits sparing of uninvolved tissues thereby improving the fitting of external orbital/facial prosthesis.

Caution is advised, especially for less-experienced surgeons, in managing bulky tumors or highly vascular neoplasms with EAOE. Diffuse bleeding in these cases may be more difficult to control endoscopically. Regardless of the approach, patients should be counseled on the risks of monocular vision. With the consequent loss of depth perception, there is an increased risk of subsequent trauma that requires strategies and patient education.[21] Whenever orbital exenteration is used, assembly of a multidisciplinary team is strongly advised to serve the individual needs of each patient.

References

1. Batra, P. S., & Lanza, D. C. (2005). Endoscopic power-assisted orbital exenteration. *American Journal of Rhinology, 19*, 297–301.
2. Batra, P. S., & Lanza, D. C. (2008). Endoscopic power-assisted orbital exenteration: A novel technique. *Operative Techniques in Otolaryngology, 19*, 202–204.
3. Nemet, A. Y., Martin, P., Benger, R., Kourt, G., Sharma, V., Ghabrial, R., et al. (2007). Orbital exenteration: A 15-year study of 38 cases. *Ophthalmic Plastic and Reconstructive Surgery*, (6), 468–472.
4. Ben Simon, G. J., Schwarcz, R. M., Douglas, R., Fiashetti, D., McCann, J. D., & Goldberg, R. A. (2005). Orbital exenteration: One size does not fit all. *American Journal of Ophthalmology, 139*, 11–17.
5. Iannetti, G., Valentini, V., Rinna, C., Ventucci, E., & Marianetti, T. M. (2005). Ethmoido-orbital tumors: Our experience. *Journal of Craniofacial Surgery, 16*(6), 1085–1091.
6. Neel, G. S., Nagel, T. H., Hoxworth, J. M., & Lal, D. (2017). Management of orbital involvement in sinonasal and ventral skull base malignancies. *Otolaryngologic Clinics of North America, 50*(2), 347–364.
7. Eisen, M. D., Yousem, D. M., Loevner, L. A., Thaler, E. R., Bilker, W. B., & Goldberg, A. N. (2000). Preoperative imaging to predict orbital invasion by tumor. *Head and Neck, 22*, 456–462.
8. Kalin-Hajdu, E., Hirabayashi, K. E., Vagefi, M. R., & Kersten, R. C. (2017). Invasive fungal sinusitis: Treatment of the orbit. *Current Opinion in Ophthalmology, 28*(5), 522–533.
9. Ganly, I., Patel, S. G., Singh, B., Kraus, D. H., Bridger, P. G., Cantu, G., et al. (2005). Craniofacial resection for malignant paranasal sinus tumors: Report of an International Collaborative Study. *Head and Neck, 27*, 575–584.
10. Suarez, C., Llorente, J. L., Fernandez De Leon, R., Maseda, E., & Lopez, A. (2004). Prognostic factors in sinonasal tumors involving the anterior skull base. *Head and Neck, 26*, 136–144.
11. McCary, W. S., Levine, P. A., & Cantrell, R. W. (1996). Preservation of the eye in the treatment of sinonasal malignant neoplasms with orbital involvement: A confirmation of the original treatise. *Archives of Otolaryngology–Head Neck Surgery, 122*(6), 657–659.
12. Lisan, Q., Kolb, F., Temam, S., Tao, Y., Janot, F., & Moya-Plana, A. (2016). Management of orbital invasion in sinonasal malignancies. *Head and Neck, 38*(11), 1650–1656.
13. Khoury, T., Jang, D., Carrau, R., Ready, N., Barak, I., & Hachem, R. A. (2019). Role of induction chemotherapy in sinonasal malignancies:

A systematic review. *International Forum of Allergy & Rhinology*, *9*(2), 212–219.

14. Lund, V. J., Stammberger, H., Nicolai, P., Castelnuovo, P., Beal, T., Beham, A., et al. (2010). European position paper on endoscopic management of tumours of the nose, paranasal sinuses and skull base. *Rhinology Supplement*, *22*, 1–143.
15. Reyes, C., Mason, E., Solares, C. A., Bush, C., & Carrau, R. (2015). To preserve or not to preserve the orbit in paranasal sinus neoplasms: A meta-analysis. *Journal of Neurological Surgery Part B, Skull Base*, *6*(2), 122–128.
16. Ock, C. Y., Keam, B., Kim, T. M., Han, D. H., Won, T. B., Lee, S. H., & al, et. (2016). Induction chemotherapy in head and neck squamous cell carcinoma of the paranasal sinus and nasal cavity: A role in organ preservation. *Korean Journal of Internal Medicine*, *31*(3), 570–578.
17. Mathis, J., Doerr, T., Lin, E., & Ibrahim, S. F. (2019). Oral hedgehog pathway inhibition as a means for ocular salvage in locally advanced intraorbital basal cell carcinoma. *Dermatologic Surgery*, *45*(1), 17–25.
18. Hoffman, G. R., Jefferson, N. D., Reid, C. B., & Eisenberg, R. L. (2016). Orbital exenteration to manage infiltrative sinonasal, orbital adnexal, and cutaneous malignancies provides acceptable survival outcomes: An institutional review, literature review, and meta-analysis. *Journal of Oral and Maxillofacical Surgery*, *74*(3), 631–643.
19. Kaplan, D. J., Kim, J. H., Wang, E., & Snyderman, C. (2016). Prognostic indicators for salvage surgery of recurrent sinonasal malignancy. *Otolaryngology–Head and Neck Surgery*, *154*(1), 104–112.
20. University of Iowa Health Care, Opthalmology and Visual Services (2015). *Lateral tarsorrhaphy.* Available from https://webeye.ophth.uiowa.edu/eyeforum/video/plastics/2/Lateral-tarsorrhaphy.htm. Accessed 3 March 2019.
21. Neimkin, M. G., & Custer, P. L. (2017). Compliance with protective lens wear in anophthalmic patients. *Ophthalmic Plastic and Reconstructive Surgery*, *33*(1), 61–64.

PART 6

Transorbital Techniques

30

Endoscopic Subperiosteal Abscess Drainage

CHARLES SAADEH, MD, JACKSON DEERE, BS, GOPI SHAH, MD, AND RON MITCHELL, MD

Right Orbital Subperiosteal Abscess Drainage

Acute rhinosinusitis (ARS) accounts for one-fifth of all adult and pediatric antibiotic prescriptions.[1,2] Bacterial ARS can lead to orbital or intracranial infections by direct or hematogenous spread. If left untreated, this can result in permanent vision loss, meningitis, intracranial abscess, sepsis, and death. The incidence of serious complications from ARS has been estimated to be 1:12,000 in children and 1:32,000 in adults.[3] Orbital complications are more common than intracranial complications and most commonly occur in male children.[4,5]

Orbital complications have historically been categorized by Chandler's classification, as shown in Table 30.1.[6] Most orbital complications occur from an infected ethmoid sinus, whereas the other paranasal sinuses are less frequently the source of the infection.[7] Theories for explaining orbital spread include congenital dehiscence of the lamina papyracea, direct spread via ethmoid artery foramina, and the presence of valveless venous anastomoses draining the ethmoid and maxillary sinuses.[8]

Subperiosteal abscesses (SPAs) of the orbit most commonly affect the medial wall but can also involve the inferior and superior orbital walls. In the past, surgical approaches for abscess drainage involved open orbitotomies and external approaches to the sinuses. More recently, endoscopic sinus surgery has largely replaced open techniques, as this obviates the need for a facial incision. However, visualization can be difficult owing to bleeding from the inflamed mucosa.[9] This chapter illustrates the surgical management of SPAs that are amenable to transnasal endoscopic drainage.

Clinical Presentation

Children are frequently seen in clinics with symptoms of fever, nasal congestion, nasal drainage, and facial pain consistent with ARS. Those with orbital complications are distinguished by ophthalmologic symptoms including eye swelling, blurry vision, pain, and limited ocular movements. Examination can demonstrate upper and lower eyelid swelling, decreased visual acuity, ophthalmoplegia, chemosis, and/or proptosis. SPAs may be difficult to distinguish from orbital cellulitis by clinical examination, but lateral or inferior displacement of the globe is suggestive of abscess formation. Nasal endoscopy may show swollen turbinates and purulent nasal drainage.

The initial workup includes a full ophthalmologic evaluation including assessment of the pupil, retina, intraocular pressure (IOP), extent of proptosis, and presence of chemosis. Laboratory tests, including complete blood count, basic metabolic panel, and inflammatory markers, are useful to establish baseline values and trends in cases that are observed or do not quickly resolve. If there is a concern for an orbital complication beyond preseptal cellulitis, computed tomography (CT) of the sinuses, preferably with contrast, is the investigation of choice. It is useful for preoperative planning to determine the extent of infection and specifically to exclude involvement of the cavernous sinus.[10-12] A CT scan is quick and readily available, does not normally require sedation, and defines the bony and soft-tissue anatomy well. Many authors advocate broad-spectrum intravenous antibiotics for 24 to 48 hours and a CT scan only if there is worsening or no improvement.[13] If there is concern for intracranial complications or invasive fungal sinusitis, magnetic resonance imaging (MRI) should be performed. However, MRI is not indicated for routine workup for orbital complications of ARS.[4] Figs. 30.1 and 30.2 illustrate examples of SPAs.

Management

Medical management should be initiated in all children with SPAs and includes antibiotics and nasal hygiene, including high-volume saline rinses and a short course of decongestants (i.e., oxymetazoline). Initial antibiotic therapy may be empiric and cover the most common responsible organisms. Coudert et al. reviewed 48 children with SPAs and found that 60% of cultured abscesses grew *Streptococcus*, 12% *Staphylococcus*, and 12% anaerobic species.[14] We recommend starting a regimen of a single-agent antibiotic such as ampicillin-sulbactam or a third-generation cephalosporin such as ceftriaxone in children 9 years or younger, in whom polymicrobial infections is less common.[15] If the child has a penicillin allergy, clindamycin is used instead. Liao et al. reported a 6.5% (3/46) rate of methicillin-resistant *Staphylococcus aureus* (MRSA) on culture and recommended that the initial broad-spectrum antibiotic regimen should include MRSA coverage.[16] Based on our hospital antibiogram, we do not need to use empiric antibiotic therapy that includes MRSA coverage, but the need to do so may differ in other regions. Conversely, in a child 10 to 15 years or older in whom the infection has a higher chance of being polymicrobial or odontogenic in origin, broader anaerobic and MRSA coverage is part of

TABLE 30.1 Chandler Classification of Orbital Complications of Sinusitis

Grade	Symptoms
1	Preseptal cellulitis
2	Orbital cellulitis
3	Subperiosteal abscess
4	Orbital abscess
5	Cavernous sinus thrombosis

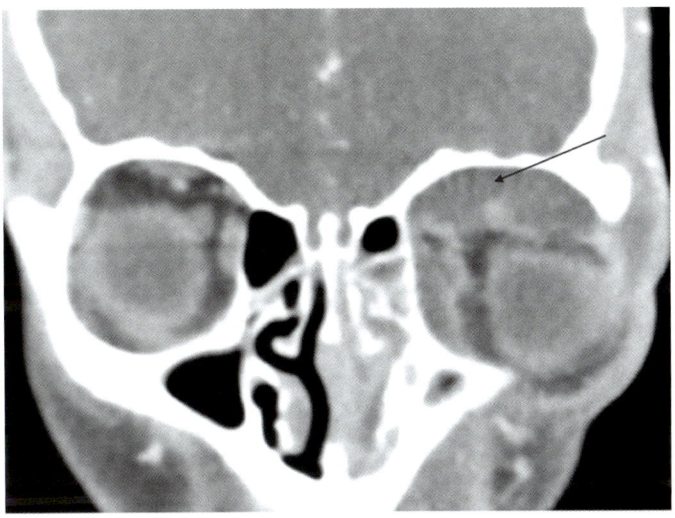

• **Fig. 30.1** Computed tomography scan of sinus with contrast, coronal cut showing left subperiosteal medial and superior abscesses (*arrow*).

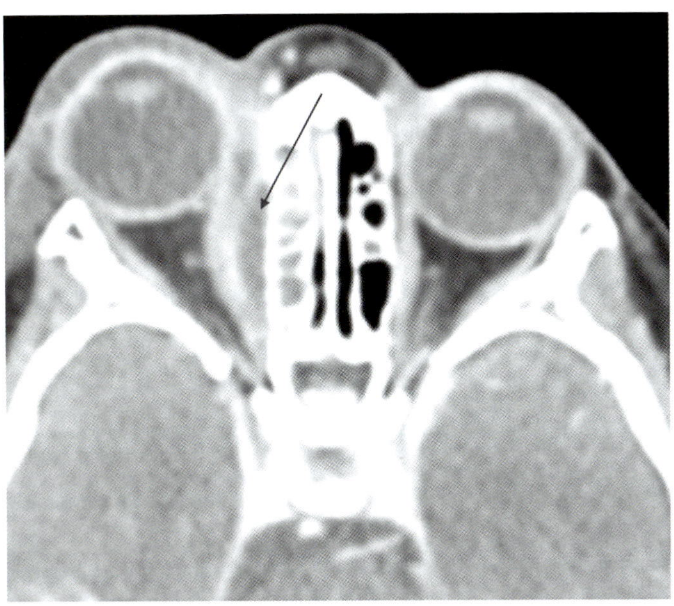

• **Fig. 30.2** Computed tomography of sinus with contrast, axial cut showing a right medial subperiosteal abscess (*arrow*).

initial antibiotic therapy.[17-19] If there is concern for meningeal involvement or associated intracranial complications, double coverage with a third-generation cephalosporin and metronidazole is indicated at a dose appropriate to pass through the blood–brain barrier[14]

The decision to start medical treatment and observe versus drainage of a SPA is a critical part of the decision making. A neurologic and ophthalmologic examination is crucial. Patients with a normal visual acuity, pupil, and retina and with no ophthalmoplegia, with an IOP less than 20 mm Hg and proptosis less than 5 mm, may be treated with medical management and close observation.[20] Patients with compromised vision or rapid progression to intracranial complication need immediate drainage. "Immediate drainage" is not well defined, but in our institution it is within 12 to 24 hours of presentation.

Age plays a determining factor in the decision making to drain a SPA. Children older than the first decade of life tend to have more aggressive bacteria by culture with a higher likelihood of anaerobes. Older children and adults are more prone to intracranial complications of sinusitis. In any older child or adult who presents with an orbital complication of sinusitis, there should be no hesitation to proceed with surgical decompression.[18]

Several studies have investigated abscess width and volume on CT as factors considered for initial medical versus surgical management. Abscess width of less than 10 mm with normal findings on ophthalmologic examination may be medically treated initially.[20,21] Abscess volume greater than 500 mm^3 usually requires surgical intervention.[22,23] These measurements may be difficult to determine consistently, as there is no standard way to measure width or volume on a CT scan.

Thus in children younger than 10 years without visual compromise, normal IOPs, smaller abscess size, and no neurologic involvement, we recommend medical management with close observation. It is worth noting that children with a large-volume SPA (volume >500 mm^3) may have a longer hospital stay and duration of antibiotic therapy and a higher incidence of peripherally inserted central catheters.[8] Patients whose conditions do no improve after 48 to 72 hours or in whom worsening occurs in 48 hours should be considered for surgical management; decision making requires close communication between the otolaryngology and ophthalmology services. We do not recommend routine repeat imaging before surgery, but studies on this subject are lacking.

Surgical Management

The location of the SPA directs the approach. Most medial and inferior abscesses are amenable to endoscopic drainage. Superior and lateral abscesses are less common and less accessible endonasally and are more likely to require an external orbitotomy.[24] Endoscopic sinus surgery for acute SPAs is challenging, primarily owing to the inflamed and hyperemic mucosa that can lead to increased blood loss and poor visualization (see Video). The setup is similar to functional endoscopic sinus surgery, and intraoperative image-guided navigation is recommended.[25] The efficacy of reconstructed non–image-guided CT scans used for endoscopic surgery is unknown, although we would rarely recommend a repeat scan for the purpose of using image-guided surgery.

Noninvasive measures for hemostasis should be used, including bed elevation, keeping the blood pressure low, and topical vasoconstriction with oxymetazoline pledgets. The nasal mucosa is injected with 1% lidocaine with 1:100,000 epinephrine. Fakhri describes injections of the lateral nasal wall, using as few injections as possible to minimize bleeding from these sites.[9] We recommend injecting the head and axilla of the middle turbinate, and, if able to visualize, the region adjacent to the sphenopalatine artery posterior to the maxillary sinus along the lateral nasal wall.

Traditionally a 4-mm endoscope is used; however, in small children, a 2.7-mm endoscope may be necessary. A smaller-diameter scope does compromise visualization but may be the best option in a small swollen nasal cavity. The middle turbinate is medialized, and an uncinectomy is performed and the maxillary sinus ostium identified. Using a 30-degree endoscope, a maxillary antrostomy is performed to drain the maxillary sinus and to provide a surgical landmark for the orbital floor. Purulence should be collected for culture when encountered. The ethmoid bulla is then entered and an anterior ethmoidectomy is performed, exposing the middle turbinate lateral to the lamina papyracea. Based on the size and posterior extent of the abscess, the basal lamella of the middle turbinate is entered and a posterior ethmoidectomy is performed to provide posterior access to the medial orbit. A posterior-to-anterior total ethmoidectomy can then be performed along the skull base, taking care to fully expose the lamina laterally. Froehlich et al. report good results with a limited anterior ethmoidectomy with dissection immediately lateral to the lamina in a small number of children with SPAs.[26] However, the authors continue to recommend a more extensive dissection because we feel it is less likely to lead to incomplete drainage.

The lamina is inspected for dehiscences and spontaneous purulent drainage. If no areas of purulence are noted, the lamina is entered sharply with either a curette or a periosteal elevator and the abscess is drained with assistance of external pressure on the orbit.[24] The lamina does not need to be completely removed after the abscess is drained. Good hemostasis is achieved and nasal packing is avoided, maximizing decompression. If intraoperative bleeding obscures safe access to the orbit, an external approach should be used (see Video).

Further research is indicated for management of the uninvolved side, as well as the utility of concurrent adenoidectomy in younger patients. Although most medially based abscesses along the lamina papyracea are amenable to endonasal endoscopic drainage, the presence of a superolateral component may require a combined procedure with an ophthalmologist for an orbitotomy (Fig. 30.3). The presence of an intraconal abscess requires intraoperative ophthalmologic input and may require serial measurements of IOP.[9]

If there is clinical improvement after 24 to 48 hours of surgical drainage, patients are usually transitioned to 14 days of oral antibiotics directed by culture results. However, if there is no improvement or worsening of eye swelling, proptosis, IOP, and/or visual acuity, a repeat CT scan is recommended to evaluate for abscess recurrence or progression. Early surgical intervention within 24 hours of presentation has been shown to decrease abscess recurrence by a small amount (12%), but this is of doubtful clinical significance.[27] In cases of recurrence or lack of complete drainage, repeat endoscopic drainage or external ethmoidectomy may be needed with or without an orbitotomy. The emergence of neurologic signs may require MRI to evaluate for intracranial complications, such as epidural empyema or subdural abscess. Prolonged intravenous antibiotic therapy and close evaluation by ophthalmology and infectious disease specialists are essential in recalcitrant cases that require multiple procedures.

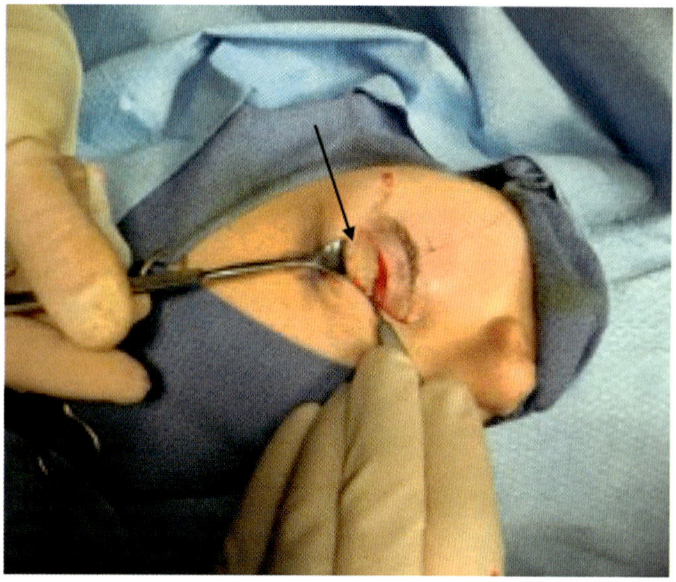

• **Fig. 30.3** Intraoperative photo of superior orbitotomy for superior subperiosteal abscess in conjunction with ophthalmology (*arrow*).

Conclusion

Management of SPAs with endonasal endoscopic techniques has decreased the morbidity of surgery. Younger patients with smaller abscesses may be treated initially with medical therapy and close observation, but any patient whose condition does not improve after 48 to 72 hours requires operative drainage. Surgeons should be prepared for increased blood loss and inflamed mucosa that can make the approach challenging. Management of SPAs requires a multidisciplinary team with close communication with ophthalmology and infectious disease specialists.

References

1. Antimicrobial treatment guidelines for acute bacterial rhinosinusitis. (2000). *Otolaryngology–Head and Neck Surgery, 123*, S1–S32.
2. Oxford, L. E., & McClay, J. (2005). Complications of acute sinusitis in children. *Otolaryngology–Head and Neck Surgery, 133*, 32–37.
3. Hansen, F. S., Hoffmans, R., Georgalas, C., & Fokkens, W. J. (2012). Complications of acute rhinosinusitis in The Netherlands. *Family Practice, 29*, 147–153.
4. Segal, N., Nissani, R., Kordeluk, S., Holcberg, M., Hertz, S., Kassem, F., et al. (2016). Orbital complications associated with paranasal sinus infections—a 10-year experience in Israel. *International Journal of Pediatric Otorhinolaryngology, 86*, 60–62.
5. Huang, S. F., Lee, T. J., Lee, Y. S., Chen, C. C., Chin, S. C., & Wang, N. C. (2011). Acute rhinosinusitis-related orbital infection in pediatric patients: A retrospective analysis. *Annals of Otolology, Rhinolology & Laryngology, 120*, 185–190.
6. Chandler, J. R., Langenbrunner, D. J., & Stevens, E. R. (2009). The pathogenesis of orbital complications in acute sinusitis. *Laryngoscope, 80*, 1414–1428.
7. Sciarretta, V., Demattè, M., Farnetti, P., Fornaciari, M., Corsini, I., Piccin, O., et al. (2017). Management of orbital cellulitis and subperiosteal orbital abscess in pediatric patients: A ten-year review. *International Journal of Pediatric Otorhinolaryngology, 96*, 72–76.
8. Nation, J., Lopez, A., Grover, N., Carvalho, D., Vinocur, D., & Jiang, W. (2017). Management of large-volume subperiosteal

abscesses of the orbit: Medical vs surgical outcomes. *Otolaryngology–Head and Neck Surgery, 157*, 891–897.
9. Fakhri, S. (2008). Endoscopic drainage of subperiosteal orbital abscesses. *Operative Techniques in Otolaryngology, 19*, 195–198.
10. DeMuri, G., & Wald, E. R. (2013). Acute bacterial sinusitis in children. *Pediatrics in Review, 34*, 429–437.
11. Slavin, M. L., & Glaser, J. S. (1987). Acute severe irreversible visual loss with sphenoethmoiditis-"posterior" orbital cellulitis. *Archives of Ophthalmology (Chicago, Ill., 1960), 105*, 345–348.
12. Anderson, R. L., & Edwards, J. J. (1980). Bilateral visual loss after blepharoplasty. *Annals of Plastic Surgery, 5*, 288–292.
13. Nathoo, N., Nadvi, S. S., van Dellen, J. R., & Gouws, E. (1999). Intracranial subdural empyemas in the era of computed tomography: A review of 699 cases. *Neurosurgery, 44*, 529–535.
14. Coudert, A., Ayari-Khalfallah, S., Suy, P., & Truy, E. (2018). Microbiology and antibiotic therapy of subperiosteal orbital abscess in children with acute ethmoiditis. *International Journal of Pediatric Otorhinolaryngology, 106*, 91–95.
15. Liao, J. C., & Harris, G. J. (2015). Subperiosteal abscess of the orbit. *Ophthalmology, 122, 639–647.*
16. Liao, S., Durand, M. L., & Cunningham, M. J. (2010). Sinogenic orbital and subperiosteal abscesses: Microbiology and methicillin-resistant *Staphylococcus aureus* incidence. *Otolaryngology–Head and Neck Surgery, 143*, 392–396.
17. Ketenci, I., Unlü, Y., Vural, A., Doğan, H., Sahin, M. I., & Tuncer, E. (2013). Approaches to subperiosteal orbital abscesses. *European Archives of Oto-Rhino-Laryngology, 270*, 1317–1327.
18. Harris, G. (2001). Subperiosteal abscess of the orbit: Older children and adults require aggressive treatment. *Ophthalmic Plastic and Reconstructive Surgery, 17*, 395–397.
19. Brook, I. (2006). The role of anaerobic bacteria in sinusitis. *Anaerobe, 12*(1), 5–12.
20. Oxford, L. E., & McClay, J. (2006). Medical and surgical management of subperiosteal orbital abscess secondary to acute sinusitis in children. *International Journal of Pediatric Otorhinolaryngology, 70*, 1853–1861.
21. Ryan, J. T., Preciado, D. A., Bauman, N., Pena, M., Bose, S., Zaizal, G. H., et al. (2009). Management of pediatric orbital cellulitis in patients with radiographic findings of subperiosteal abscess. *Otolaryngology–Head and Neck Surgery, 140*, 907–911.
22. Tabarino, F., Elmaleh-Bergès, M., Quesnel, S., Lorrot, M., Van Den Abbeele, T., & Teissier, N. (2015). Subperiosteal orbital abscess: Volumetric criteria for surgical drainage. *International Journal of Pediatric Otorhinolaryngology, 79*, 131–135.
23. Gavriel, H., Yeheskeli, E., Aviram, E., Yehoshua, L., & Eviatar, E. (2011). Dimension of subperiosteal orbital abscess as an indication for surgical management in children. *Otolaryngology–Head and Neck Surgery, 145*, 823–827.
24. Campbell, A. P., Bergmark, R. W., & Metson, R. (2017). Orbital complications of acute sinusitis. Oper. Tech. *Otolaryngology–Head and Neck Surgery, 28*, 213–219.
25. White, J., & Parikh, S. (2005). Early experience with image guidance in endoscopic transnasal drainage of periorbital abscesses. *Journal of Otolaryngology, 34*, 63–65.
26. Froehlich, P., Pransky, S. M., Fontaine, P., Stearns, G., & Morgon, A. (1997). Minimal endoscopic approach to subperiosteal orbital abscess. *Archives of Otolaryngology–Head Neck Surgery, 123*, 280–282.
27. Teinzer, F., Stammberger, H., & Tomazic, P. V. (2014). Transnasal endoscopic treatment of orbital complications of acute sinusitis: The Graz concept. *Annals of Otolology, Rhinolology & Laryngology, 124*, 368–373.

31

Transorbital Techniques to Frontal Sinus Diseases

KOFI BOAHENE, MD

The frontal sinus is commonly affected by inflammatory diseases, traumatic fractures, benign tumors, and malignant neoplasms. Because of its proximity to the brain, eye, and nose, disease processes originating from these anatomic sites can extend to involve the frontal sinuses. Transnasal endoscopic surgery is presently the principal approach for managing frontal sinus pathologies, with open external approaches mostly limited to the repair of frontal sinus fractures. The trend away from classic external frontal sinus approaches to contemporary endonasal techniques exploded over the past two decades with the introduction of specialized instruments, the development of high-powered endoscopes, and image-guided surgical navigation systems. A major limitation of transnasal endoscopic frontal sinus surgery is access to the lateral and most anterior aspects of the frontal sinus. Access to the lateral and anterior sections of the frontal sinus is feasible through expanded transnasal techniques, such as the Draf procedures, but the working angles are somewhat less favorable and disruption of healthy paranasal sinus system is often necessary.[1,2] Nonetheless, the anterior and lateral segments of the frontal sinus are easily accessible through the classic bicoronal cranial exposure with osteoplastic bone flaps.[3] However, the bicoronal approach involves a broad field surgery far beyond the outlines of the frontal sinus. An approach to the frontal sinus that allows access to all aspects of the frontal sinus that combines the minimally invasive advantages endoscopic and the exposure of open access surgery is desirable.

Transorbital approaches to frontal sinus diseases offer an alternative to pure endonasal approaches, combining the desirable aspects of classic external approaches and the more contemporary endonasal approaches. Because the thin superior and medial walls of the orbit are intimately associated with the frontal sinus, osteotomy windows in the fronto-orbital complex offer a direct surgical corridor to frontal sinus pathologies. Lim et al. and Boahene et al. have contributed extensively to the popularity of transorbital anterior skull base approaches with a series of publications over the past decade.[4-7]

Surgical Technique

There are four main technical aspects to transorbital frontal sinus surgery: soft-tissue exposure of the fronto-orbital bone complex, creation of a mini-orbitofrontal bone window, management of the targeted pathology, and reconstruction. These four technical components are performed in a minimally invasive manner over short working distances with bimanual dissection in a coplanar fashion augmented or enhanced with endoscopes or surgical microscopes.

Soft-Tissue Exposure of the Frontoorbital Bone Complex

Exposure of the orbitofrontal bone complex for the transorbital approach is through an upper eyelid supratarsal crease or conjunctival incision. The access incision—supratarsal versus conjunctival—is selected depending on the targeted subsite of the frontal sinus.

The supratarsal crease incision is the workhorse approach through which the entire fronto-orbital bar can be exposed (Fig. 31.1). The supratarsal crease is a distinct skin fold above the upper eyelid margin that results from insertion of the levator aponeurosis into the eyelid skin. Incisions placed in this crease are routinely used for upper eyelid blepharoplasty and camouflage well. An extension of the incision into a lateral orbital wrinkle expands the soft-tissue exposure and heals acceptably well provided the scar does not extend past the bony orbital rim.

The supratarsal crease should be outlined preoperatively with the patient sitting upright. The incision extends from the inner canthal region to the lateral canthal area following the natural upper eyelid crease. At least 3 mm of skin is left intact over the medial canthus to prevent webbing. The lateral extension of the incision is planned in a natural wrinkle line. When appropriately planned, the marked line should not be visible when the eyelids are open (see Fig. 31.1).

To protect the cornea, a temporary Frost suture or cornea shield is placed. The forehead and upper eyelid are infiltrated with local anesthetic with vasoconstrictive agents. The infiltration also hydrodissects the tissue planes to facilitate dissection. The incision is carried through the skin and orbicularis oculi muscle. The orbital septum deep to the orbicularis oculi muscle is kept intact, preventing fat herniation. Dissection is carried over the orbital septum to the superior orbital rim. The periosteum along the superior orbital rim is sharply incised and released along the superior and lateral orbital rim. Subperiosteal dissection is widely performed to expose the entire anterior frontal sinus wall and the superior orbital rim (see Fig. 31.1). Releasing the periosteal attachments at the

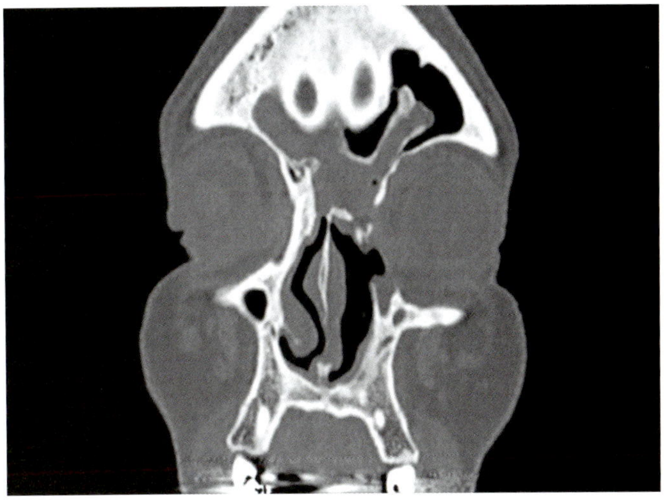

• **Fig. 31.1** Supratarsal approach.

temporal line broadens the exposure. The supraorbital neurovascular bundle should be carefully released from its foramen or notch and protected. An orbitofrontal minicraniotomy can now be performed to provide access to the frontal sinus. To protect the eyelid skin, pledgets are placed along the skin edge as a protective cushion when retracting.

The orbital walls can also be accessed via conjunctival incisions. The transconjunctival approach may be used to expose all quadrants of the orbit. A precaruncular medial conjunctival incision with extensions into the upper and lower eyelids is ideal for exposing lesions along the medial aspects of the frontal sinus floor (Fig. 31.2). The upper and lower lacrimal puncta are identified and preserved. They can be cannulated to prevent inadvertent injury. The conjunctiva behind the caruncle is infiltrated with local anesthetic. A precaruncular conjunctival incision down to bone is made with a guarded needle-tip cautery. Through this access the periorbital along the medial and superior orbital wall is elevated as extensively as needed. The anterior and posterior ethmoid arteries become visible, bridging the gap between the periorbital and orbital bone at the level of the cribiform plate. They should be ligated and divided to provide more working space. The ethmoid arteries are important landmarks in this surgical approach, as they mark a level above which intracranial access can then be gained after removal of a thin orbital bone. The working surgical cavity is maintained by gentle distraction with a malleable retractor, which can be held in place with a clamp holder.

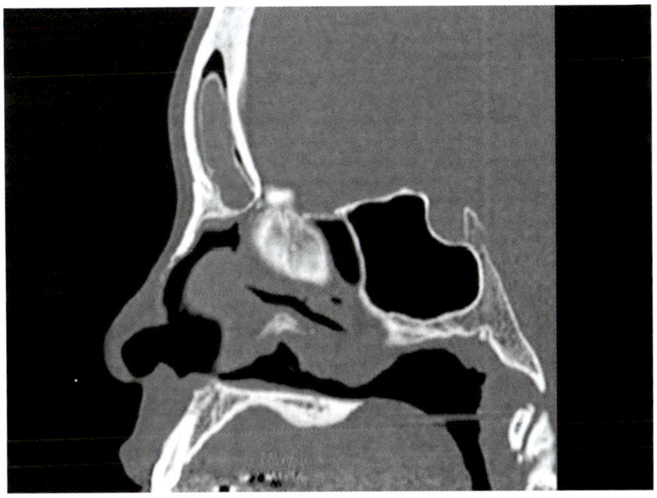

• **Fig. 31.2** Transconjunctival approach.

Orbitofrontal Bone Window

A computed tomography–guided image mapping of the outline of the frontal sinus is essential in planning and opening an optimal orbitofrontal bone window. The bone window can be variably positioned based on the location of the target pathology to provide the most direct exposure for instrumentation (see Fig. 31.1). To access the frontal sinus recess, intersinus septum, and contralateral sinus, the bone window should be positioned close to the frontonasal suture line. A laterally centered bone window is necessary for exposing the lateral frontal sinus recesses. The planned ostectomy may be limited only to the anterior frontal sinus wall and superior orbital ridge or extended to include the orbital roof and frontal sinus floor depending on the targeted pathology. Once the planned osteotomy is designed, the osteotomy site may be preplated to facilitate an anatomic reconstruction after the procedure. Low-profile 1.0 titanium plates are adequate. The minicraniotomy is then performed using an oscillating saw or ultrasonic bone scalpel and osteotomes. Beveling the bone cuts inward allows the bone flap to be replaced on a supported lip at the end of the case. A 1.5- to 2.5-cm orbitocranial window is usually adequate for direct visualization and bimanual instrumentation. Illumination and a detailed view of the frontal sinus are greatly enhanced by endoscopic magnification.

Management of Selected Targeted Disease

Inverting Papilloma

Inverting papilloma is a rare, benign, sinonasal tumor that is locally aggressive and has a tendency to recur.[8,9] Complete resection is critical because up to 9% of inverting papillomas can progress to squamous cell carcinoma.[10] Complete resection of the tumor and adjoining predisposed mucosa after fully outlining the disease extent within the frontal sinus decreases the likelihood of recurrence.

A trabsorbital approach through a supratarsal crease incision is a versatile approach for thorough resection of inverting papilloma with extensive involvement of the frontal sinus (Fig. 31.3). The transorbital approach is combined with a transnasal endoscopic approach to comprehensively address disease in the nose and sinuses.[11,12]

The procedure usually begins with the endonasal portion. The extent of endonasal resection is determined by the extent of the disease. A medial maxillectomy, total ethmoidectomy, and resection of any involved turbinate are performed in the standard fashion as needed. Extension of disease into the frontal sinus is typically addressed with a Draf IIb or Draf III procedure.

A Draf IIb procedure involves removal of the frontal sinus floor between the nasal septum and the lamina papyracea. This exposure provides access for introduction of angled instruments to address disease involving the walls of the frontal sinus. For disease involving both frontal sinuses, a Draf III procedure is performed. With a Draf III procedure, a Draf IIb procedure is carried out on both sides and communicated across the midline, resulting in a common frontal sinus floor opening. When performed in combination with a transorbital approach, we find drilling the frontal sinus floor

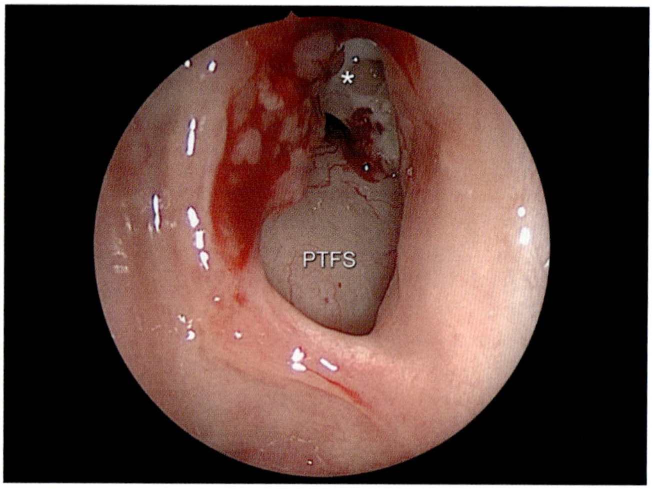

• **Fig. 31.3** Inverting papilloma.

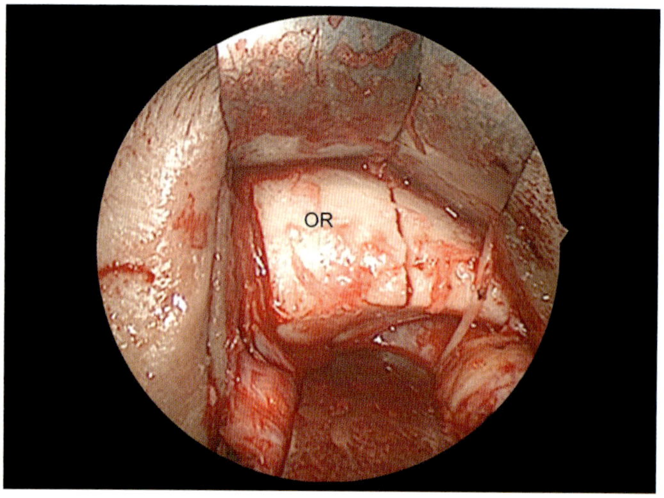

• **Fig. 31.4** Meningocele repair.

much easier and faster when performed through the transorbital exposure (see Fig. 31.3).

Through the endonasal approach, a portion of the superior nasal septum is removed at the junction of the quadrangular cartilage and the perpendicular plate of the ethmoid. After communication between the nasal cavities is achieved, the mini-orbitofrontal craniotomy is performed through the eyelid approach. The access incision for the orbitofrontal craniotomy is through the supratarsal crease as described. The size of the orbitofrontal craniotomy is tailored to allow the use of two to three instruments at a time to effectively address the entire frontal sinus. This is usually guided by stereotactic navigation and may be as little as 1.5 cm × 1.5 cm. Extending the craniotomy window medially toward the midline provides exposure and access to both frontal sinuses if desired. Tumor dissection within the frontal sinus is performed under direct or endoscopic visualization. Tumor dissection is carried out by submucosal elevation off the underlying bone. The exposed bone is drilled down with an ultrasonic bone drill or a coarse diamond burr.

Intrasinus bony septations are removed to create a single open cavity. The floor of the frontal sinus can now be drilled out as in a Draf procedure. Simultaneous visualization and dissection through the orbitocranial and endonasal corridors can be performed to ensure continuity of diseased tissue removal from the sinus to the nose. Periorbital and bone defects into the orbit may be repaired with collagen regeneration matrix or fascia grafts to provide a barrier against fat herniation into the sinus. After complete tumor resection, the bone flap is replaced and fixated. The upper eyelid incision is closed in a layered fashion.

Meningocele With Cerebrospinal Fluid Leaks

Meningoceles of the frontal lobe commonly expand through the anterior cranial base to involve the frontal and ethmoid sinuses. The transorbital approach is an efficient technique for managing frontoethmoid meningoceles and cerebrospinal fluid (CSF) leaks.[13]

Transpalpebral Repair of Meningoceles and Cerebrospinal Fluid Leaks

The supratarsal crease provides an ideal access for transorbital exposure of meningoceles and CSF leaks of the frontal sinus. With image guidance, a fronto-orbital bone window is designed for a direct working trajectory to the cranial base defect and the neck of the meningocele. Once the bone flap is removed, the meningocele is first encountered and is usually covered by sinus mucosa. The meningocele is carefully amputated as it exits the bony defect. Care should be taken to control any incorporated vessels to prevent intracranial bleeding from retracted vessels. With the meningocele removed, the outline of the bony skull base defect becomes clearer (Fig. 31.4). The exposed dura can then be carefully elevated circumferentially around the bone defect for placement of a fascia or collagen matrix barrier to seal off any CSF leak. Similarly, frontal sinus mucosa can be elevated around the skull base defect to allow placement of a second layer of barrier. The barrier may be immobilized with fibrin glue. The frontal sinus outflow track should be left undisturbed. The bone flap is repositioned and the eyelid incision closed as described.

Transconjunctival Repair of Cerebrospinal Fluid Leaks

Smaller skull base defects with CSF leaks isolated to the frontoethmoid region may be accessed through a transconjunctival transorbital approach.[14] The primary advantage of this approach is the ability to isolate the defect over a short working distance and placement of sealing materials on top of the skull base while preserving the paranasal sinus system (Fig. 31.5). As described earlier, a precaruncular incision is made with an electrocautery and periorbtal elevation carried out to

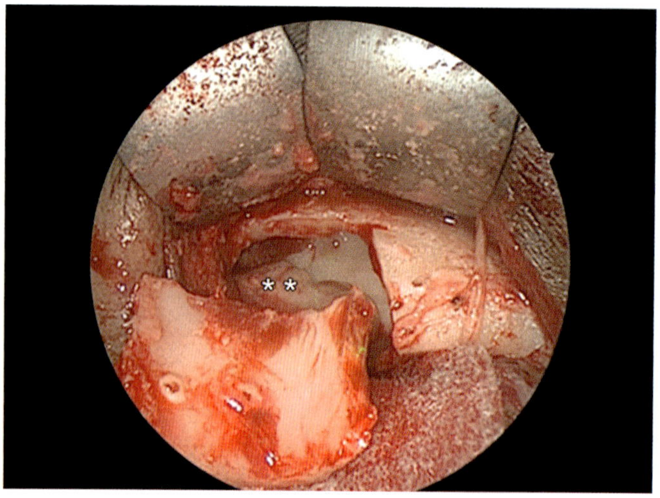

• **Fig. 31.5** Transconjuctival cerebrospinal fluid repair.

expose the superomedial orbital wall (see Fig. 31.2). The anterior and posterior ethmoid arteries are identified, ligated, and divided. Above the level of the ethmoid arteries, guided by stereotactic navigation, an orbitotomy window is drilled out adjacent to the skull base defect. The bone window is first made in a small confined area to expose the underlying dura and is gradually expanded with a Kerrison punch to a size adequate for exposure and instrumentation. The dura is then carefully elevated until the defect site is exposed. The precise location of the defect can be found aided by stereotactic navigation or intrathecal fluorescein dye. Once identified, the defect is repaired by placing a layer of fat, fascia, or collagen matrix immobilized and sealed with fibrin glue. Because of the approach and exposure, a sealing graft much larger than the dural and bone defect can be applied on a base of stable cranial base bone.

Frontal Sinus Fractures

Frontal sinus fractures may involve the anterior or posterior walls with or without extension into the frontal recess. Minimally displaced anterior or posterior frontal sinus fractures can be observed because they heal well without intervention. Severely displaced or comminuted frontal sinus fractures require intervention to address associated CSF leaks, minimize secondary infections or mucocele formation, and manage forehead contour changes. The transorbital approach may be used to address simple to complex frontal sinus fractures.[15,16] This approach avoids the need for an extensive bicoronal scalp incision and exposure. The transpalpebral exposure of the frontorbital bone complex through a supratarsal crease incision provides adequate exposure for reducing and fixating anterior wall fractures with titanium plates (Fig. 31.6). When the posterior wall is involved, a severely comminuted anterior wall fracture is usually present. The fractured anterior wall bone is removed to gain access to the posterior wall. The posterior wall defect is carefully reduced and sealed with underlay grafts as needed to address any CSF leaks. Rarely is there the need for cranialization if the frontal recess is functional. We avoid obliteration of the frontal sinus in these situations to minimize chances of delayed mucocele formation.

Postoperative Management

After surgery, patients are typically prescribed oral antibiotics. To minimize periorbital swelling, the patient's head is inclined at 30 degrees. Artificial eye tears and ice packs are applied over a period of 2 days. The patient is instructed to clean the eyelid incision daily and apply ophthalmic antibiotic ointment. The most common complication we have encountered with the transorbital approach to the frontal sinus is upper eyelid swelling. This is minimized by ensuring absolute hemostasis in the eyelid dissection field before closure and early application of ice packs around the eye. Perioperative steroids may also be used to minimize swelling. Retraction of upper eyelid may cause epidermolysis of the skin edges. This can be avoided by placing pledgets along the eyelid incision before placing skin retractors. Temporary numbness over the forehead is expected but resolves over several weeks.

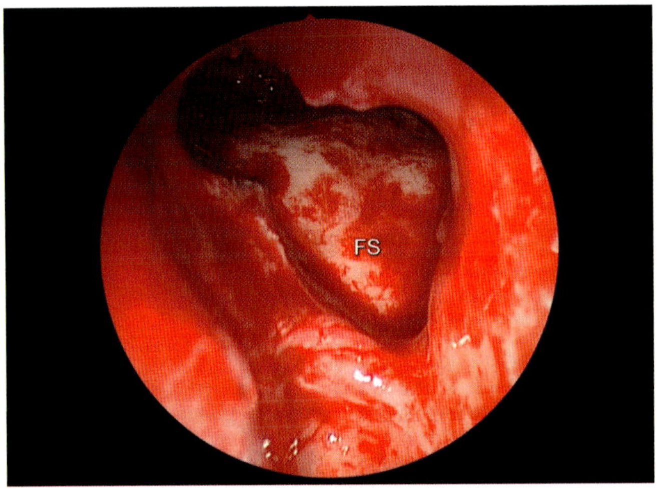

• **Fig. 31.6** Frontal sinus fracture repair.

References

1. Conger, B. T., Jr., Illing, E., Bush, B., & Woodworth, B. A. (2014). Management of lateral frontal sinus pathology in the endoscopic era. *Otolaryngology–Head and Neck Surgery*, *151*(1), 159–163.
2. Weber, R., Draf, W., Kratzsch, B., Hosemann, W., & Schaefer, S. D. (2001). Modern concepts of frontal sinus surgery. *Laryngoscope*, *111*, 137–146.
3. Hardy, J. M., & Montgomery, W. W. (1976). Osteoplastic frontal sinusotomy: An analysis of 250 operations. *Ann Otol Rhinol Laryngol*, *85*(Pt 1), 523–532.
4. Lim, J. H., Sardesai, M. G., Ferreira, M., Jr., & Moe, K. S. (2012). Transorbital neuroendoscopic management of sinogenic complications involving the frontal sinus, orbit, and anterior cranial fossa. *Journal of Neurological Surgery Part B, Skull Base*, *73*, 394–400.
5. Moe, K. S., Bergeron, C. M., & Ellenbogen, R. G. (2010). Transorbital neuroendoscopic surgery. *Neurosurgery*, *67*(3 Suppl Operative), ons16–ons28.
6. Raza, S. M., Boahene, K. D., & Quiñones-Hinojosa, A. (2010). The transpalpebral incision: Its use in keyhole approaches to cranial base brain tumors. *Expert Rev Neurother*, *10*(11), 1629–1632.
7. Owusu Boahene, K. D., Lim, M., Chu, E., & Quiñones-Hinojosa, A. (2010). Transpalpebral orbitofrontal craniotomy: A minimally invasive approach to anterior cranial vault lesions. *Skull Base*, *20*, 237–244.
8. Melroy, C. T., & Senior, B. A. (2006). Benign sinonasal neoplasms: A focus on inverting papilloma. *Otolaryngologic Clinics of North America*, *39*(3), 601–617.
9. Sham, C. L., Woo, J. K., van Hasselt, C. A., & Tong, M. C. (2009). Treatment results of sinonasal inverted papilloma: An 18-year study. *American Journal of Rhinology & Allergy*, *23*(2), 203–211.
10. Krouse, J. H. (2001). Endoscopic treatment of inverted papilloma: Safety and efficacy. *American Journal of Otolaryngology*, *22*, 87–99.
11. Albathi, M., Ramanathan, M., Jr., Lane, A. P., & Boahene, K. D. O. (2018). Combined endonasal and eyelid approach for management of extensive frontal sinus inverting papilloma. *Laryngoscope*, *128*(1), 3–9.
12. Dubin, M. G., Sonnenburg, R. E., Melroy, C. T., Ebert, C. S., Coffey, C. S., & Senior, B. A. (2005). Staged endoscopic and combined open/endoscopic approach in the management of inverted papilloma of the frontal sinus. *American Journal of Rhinology*, *19*, 442–445.
13. Moe, K. S., Kim, L. J., & Bergeron, C. M. (2011). Transorbital endoscopic repair of cerebrospinal fluid leaks. *Laryngoscope*, *121*, 13–30.
14. Raza, S. M., Boahene, K. D., & Quiñones-Hinojosa, A. (2010). The transpalpebral incision: Its use in keyhole approaches to cranial base brain tumors. *Expert Review of Neurotherapeutics*, *10*(11), 1629–1632.
15. Gassner, H., Schwan, F., & Schebesch, K. M. (2016). Transorbital approaches: Minimally invasive access to the anterior skull base. In K. Boahene & A. Quiñones-Hinojosa (Eds.), *Minimal access skull base surgery: Open and endoscopic approaches* (pp. 62–72). New Delhi: Jaypee Brothers Medical Publishing.
16. Guy, W. M., & Brissett, A. E. (2013). Contemporary management of traumatic fractures of the frontal sinus. *Otolaryngologic Clinics of North America*, *46*, 733–748.

32

Endoscopic Management of Mucoceles With Significant Orbital Involvement

GRIFFIN D. SANTARELLI, MD, STEPHEN C. HERNANDEZ, MD, CHARLES S. EBERT, JR., MD, MPH, ADAM J. KIMPLE, MD, PHD, ADAM M. ZANATION, MD, AND BRIAN D. THORP, MD

Patient Demographics, Clinical Presentation, and Preoperative Workup

Sinonasal mucoceles are benign lesions arising from progressive expansion of respiratory epithelium. Obstruction of the natural ostia of the corresponding sinus leads to noted expansion of the sinus epithelium with mucoid secretions.[1] The mucocele can expand and exert mass effect on surrounding nasal, orbital, and intracranial structures. The inciting factor for mucocele development can range and include chronic infection, trauma, postoperative scarring, and systemic disease states.[1-3]

Sinonasal mucoceles represent approximately 8% of all sinus masses. The most common site of occurrence is the frontal sinus followed by the ethmoid cavity. Approximately 70% to 90% of mucoceles occur in the frontoethmoidal region.[4] The globe is therefore at risk owing to associated mass effects and potential infectious progression to a mucopyocele. In addition, there is a cytokine cascade with local upregulation of osteolytic cytokines such as interleukin 1 potentiating bony erosion of the orbit with mucocele propagation.[5]

The onset of symptoms is typically insidious, and the spectrum of presentation of orbital mucoceles is variable. In a retrospective study of 102 patients with mucoceles who underwent operative intervention, the most common presenting symptoms were headache (42%), facial pressure (28%), and congestion (26%). Although patients traditionally present with accompanying symptoms of rhinosinusitis, a heightened index of suspicion should be included for patients with proptosis, diplopia, ophthalmoplegia, orbital cellulitis, or facial asymmetry. Retrospective studies of mucoceles with significant intraorbital extension have shown the most common presenting symptoms to include ptosis (33%) and periorbital swelling (29%).[6]

Patients present to a wide spectrum of providers before diagnosis because of the interplay between the sinuses and the orbit. Diagnosing patients appropriately is dependent on clinical history, physical examination including endoscopic examination, and radiographic findings. Patients typically present with a long-standing history of rhinosinusitis symptoms, a history of sinus surgery, or facial trauma. Mucocele development is not an acute process, and the clinical history needs to include chronic conditions as there is a delay between sinonasal insult and mucocele development. One study noted patients presented on average 5.3 years after functional endoscopic sinus surgery (FESS), 17 years after maxillofacial trauma, and 18 years after open surgery.[7]

In addition to the clinical history, a thorough physical examination can help identify sequelae of mucocele expansion. Providers should perform a comprehensive head and neck examination including a focus on the orbit. Visual acuity, visual field testing, and extraocular movements should all be included in the ophthalmologic test battery. Identifying vision loss is key, especially in the acute setting. A systematic review of patients with orbital mucoceles presenting with vision loss concluded that vision loss is potentially reversible in most cases. In a review of 207 patients, those who presented with vision equal to 20/650 or worse and had operative management within 6 days were those that were most likely to have a visual acuity improvement with an improvement comparable to progressing from 20/200 to 20/20.[8] Therefore early identification and intervention are critical for any vision loss associated with orbital mucoceles.

Although a clinical index of suspicion can help identify patients with potential orbital mucoceles, maxillofacial/sinus imaging is critical to identify intracranial and intraorbital extension of mucoceles. Computed tomography helps delineate sinonasal structures and the extent of bony erosion. Magnetic resonance imaging is useful for the evaluation of the orbital, soft-tissue, and intracranial contents. Computed tomography and magnetic resonance imaging have a complementary role in identifying intracranial and intraorbital disease. At a tertiary referral center that surgically addressed 133 mucoceles, intracranial and intraorbital extension was identified preoperatively in 14% and 20% of cases, respectively.[7] Intraorbital extension was most commonly associated with frontoethmoidal mucoceles.

Management of mucoceles requires surgical extirpation and long-term follow-up. Surgical approaches include open approaches, endoscopic approaches, or combined techniques. The varying techniques for surgically addressing sinonasal mucoceles with orbital involvement are discussed further in this chapter.

Approaches

Transnasal Endoscopic Approaches

Historically, expansile mucoceles involving the orbit and anterior cranial fossa were managed with open techniques.[9] Original thought processes revolved around complete mucocele resection with implementation of obliterative techniques to prevent further recurrence.[9,10] Although descriptions and outcomes of these operations demonstrated some initial success, the associated morbidity of open procedures to achieve the desired goal remained. Howarth became the first to champion the idea of preservation of mucosal lining and simple marsupialization, which he described in 1921.[10] This slowly gained acceptance during the early 20th century, but for extensive mucoceles, open surgical techniques remained the mainstay of definitive management.

Transnasal techniques progressively gained popularity and were used with increasing frequency,[11] demonstrating acceptable outcomes with limited morbidity. Ultimately, with the technological advancement of endoscopes and the early descriptions of FESS, endoscopic endonasal techniques became the primary operation for management of mucoceles involving the paranasal sinuses.[12] Morbidity was certainly decreased, and the frequency of recurrence was comparable to those of open procedures. It would be later demonstrated that the epithelial lining of mucoceles maintained the normal respiratory epithelium with its associated physiologic properties of mucociliary clearance. Postoperative imaging also showed bony remodeling and neo-osteogenesis of suspected areas of erosion after adequate marsupialization.[13] As otolaryngologists gained experience with endoscopic sinus surgery, outcomes of endoscopic endonasal marsupialization were published. Woodworth et al. reported a 92% success rate (34 of 37 patients) over a mean follow-up interval of 32.6 months with endoscopic management of mucoceles involving erosion of the anterior table of the frontal sinus.[14] Similarly, Sautter et al. described outcomes of 57 patients treated endoscopically for mucoceles with anterior skull base and/or orbital erosion. Fifty-six patients (98.2%) were found to have a patent cavity with no evidence of recurrence at a mean follow-up of 15 months, with no major complications reported.[15] Other case series and meta-analyses have demonstrated similar efficacy and complication rates similar to those previously reported.[16,17]

Endoscopic techniques for management of frontoethmoid mucoceles follow the same principles as those described for endoscopic sinus surgery. With the frontal and ethmoid sinuses being the most common location for mucoceles to develop, the pseudocyst is often present in the middle meatus (Figs. 32.1 and 32.2). The floor of the mucocele is removed, and the contents can subsequently be expressed. Palpation of the orbit often allows for visualization of any site of bony dehiscence, while simultaneously assisting in evacuation of the mucocele contents. After this has been completed, the cavity is then widely marsupialized. Mucosal-sparing sphenoethmoidectomy is often completed with the approach given the expansile nature of the mucocele. This maneuver also improves visualization and postoperative clinical surveillance.

Transorbital Endoscopic Approaches

Although transnasal endoscopic approaches remain the mainstay of surgical management of paranasal sinus mucoceles, there are times when adjunct procedures may be required. Frontoethmoid mucoceles at the least require endonasal management to restore an appropriate outflow tract and address any underlying sinonasal pathology, but access can sometimes be limited secondary to individual patient anatomy. In particular, lateral access in a well-pneumatized frontal sinus can be difficult to reach via the endonasal corridor. This was demonstrated by Timperley et al., who showed that only 10% of orbital roofs could be accessed beyond the midorbital point in a cadaveric dissection in which a modified endoscopic Lothrop procedure was performed.[18]

Transorbital approaches to skull base pathology have gained increasing favor, particularly over the past 10 years. Initially introduced by Moe et al. to address a variety of pathologies, including skull base fractures, cerebrospinal fluid (CSF) leaks, and tumors, among other indications.[19] The superior lid crease and the precaruncular approaches permit access to the paranasal sinuses and anterior skull base. Advantages include a direct approach, access to the lateral frontal sinus and orbit, and preclusion of angled endoscopes and instrumentation. Incisions are well disguised and cosmesis is excellent. With respect to frontoethmoid mucoceles involving the orbit, the transorbital approach can be adjunctive in access to the lateral aspect of the frontal sinus and orbit that cannot be reached with traditional endoscopic endonasal techniques. The transorbital approach also provides direct access where there may be dural exposure or even CSF leaks that would need to be concurrently addressed. Lim et al. demonstrated how the transorbital approaches could be used for those patients with sinogenic complications involving the orbit.[20] In this series of 13 patients, 5 presented with mucoceles or mucopyoceles that involved the orbit. Along with traditional transnasal techniques, they successfully accessed the lateral frontal sinus and superolateral orbit when inaccessible through the transnasal route alone.

As physicians continue to gain experience with these transorbital techniques, expanded indications may be seen for these approaches used for lateral access in extensive mucoceles. However, transnasal approaches remain the definitive procedure, as it permits direct access, addresses any underlying sinonasal pathology, and reestablishes a normal outflow tract.

External Approaches

As previously discussed, open approaches were the traditional approach for extensive mucoceles involving the anterior cranial fossa and orbit. This largely consisted of a frontal osteoplastic flap with removal of the mucosal lining and subsequent frontal sinus obliteration. This has largely grown out of favor given the evolution of endoscopic sinus surgery and advanced endoscopic techniques, but there are still instances for open approaches or combined approaches. Herndon et al. described 13 patients with extensive frontoethmoid mucoceles involving the orbit and anterior cranial base.[21] Eight patients underwent open procedures with frontal sinus obliteration, but it is important to note that four of these patients had previously undergone frontal sinus obliteration and the remainder had significant erosion of the anterior table of the frontal sinus. A systematic review was also performed evaluating large frontal sinus mucoceles, revealing that 65.9% of patients underwent external approaches.[22] Indications included associated subdural empyema, intracranial complication, and extensive anterior table erosion. Although a role for open or combined approaches still remains, it often involves an attempt at obliteration of the frontal sinus. This necessitates removal of all mucosa, and in those instances when the posterior table of the frontal sinus or roof of the orbit are dehiscent, the mucosa needs to be lifted from the dural surface or periorbita. This can be extremely difficult to achieve and certainly lends itself to a greater degree of complications. With the success rates of endoscopic marsupialization and ease of clinical surveillance, transnasal approaches should continue to be first-line treatment with open or combined approaches reserved for select cases.

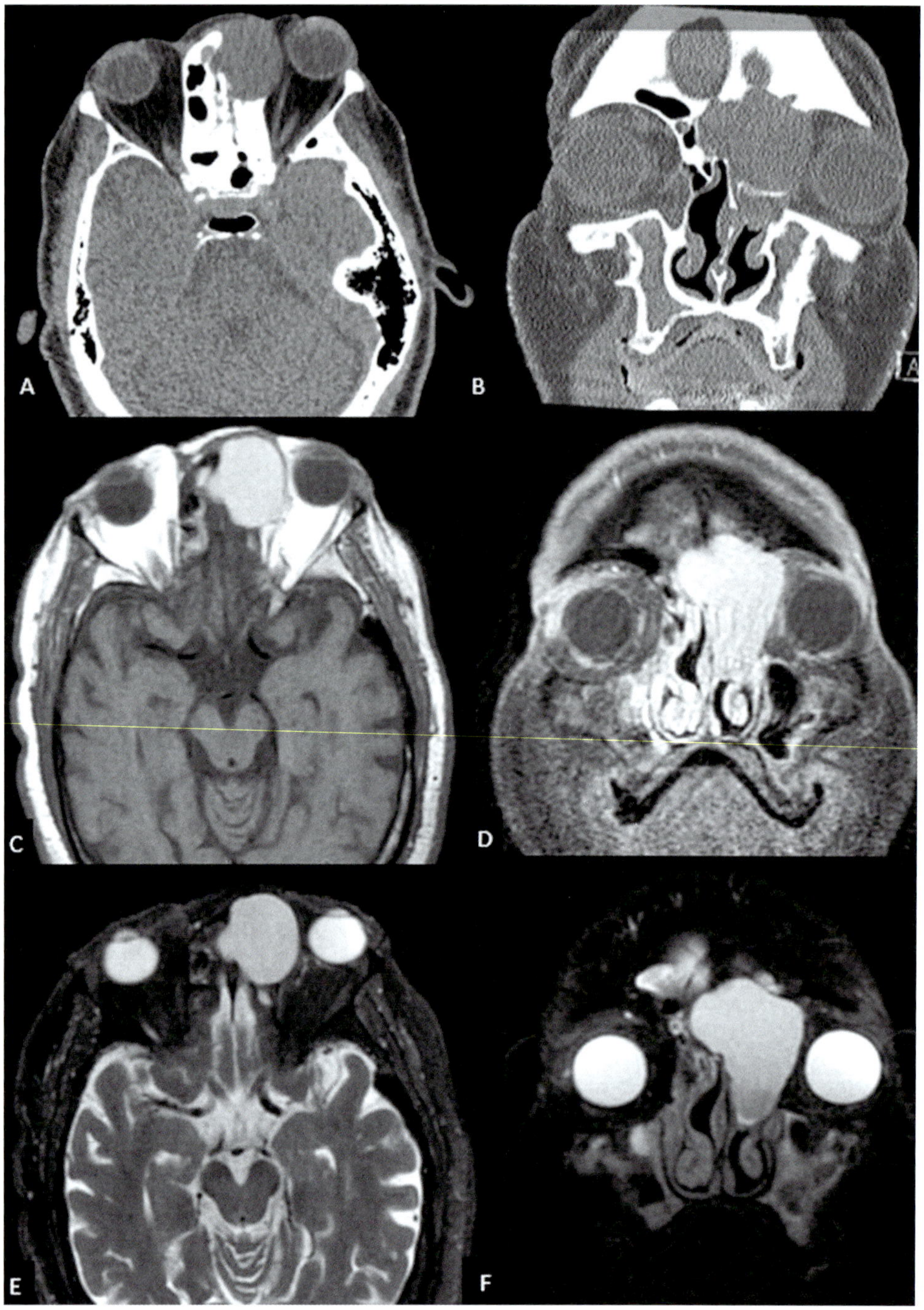

• **Fig. 32.1** Computed tomography demonstrating erosion anteriorly and laterally through the medial orbital wall (A, B). T1-weighted (C, D) and T2-weighted (E, F) magnetic resonance imaging demonstrating classic radiographic features of a frontoethmoid mucocele.

Complications and Pitfalls

Endoscopic management of orbital mucoceles is the mainstay of therapy. Endoscopic transnasal approaches represent the most common approach; however, transorbital endoscopic techniques are also an emerging technique. Regardless of the technique used, the complication profile is similar. In addressing mucoceles, there can be a large polyposis or sinusitis burden that distorts anatomy or increases the complexity of the case. Addressing the accompanying disease is critical to minimize recurrence. Despite appropriate surgery, recurrence of mucoceles is common and occurs in approximately 25% of cases.[1] Major complications such as postoperative epistaxis, diplopia, and CSF leaks secondary to surgery are possible.[23] It is therefore critical to understand the anatomy and be prepared for more extensive surgery. It is also key to creating a surgical cavity that can provide long-term endoscopic surveillance.

Orbital mucoceles can also cause proptosis, diplopia, or notable shifts in eye position. Patients accommodate to those changes because of the insidious nature of disease. However, surgical management/marsupialization of the mucocele can lead to rapid orbital

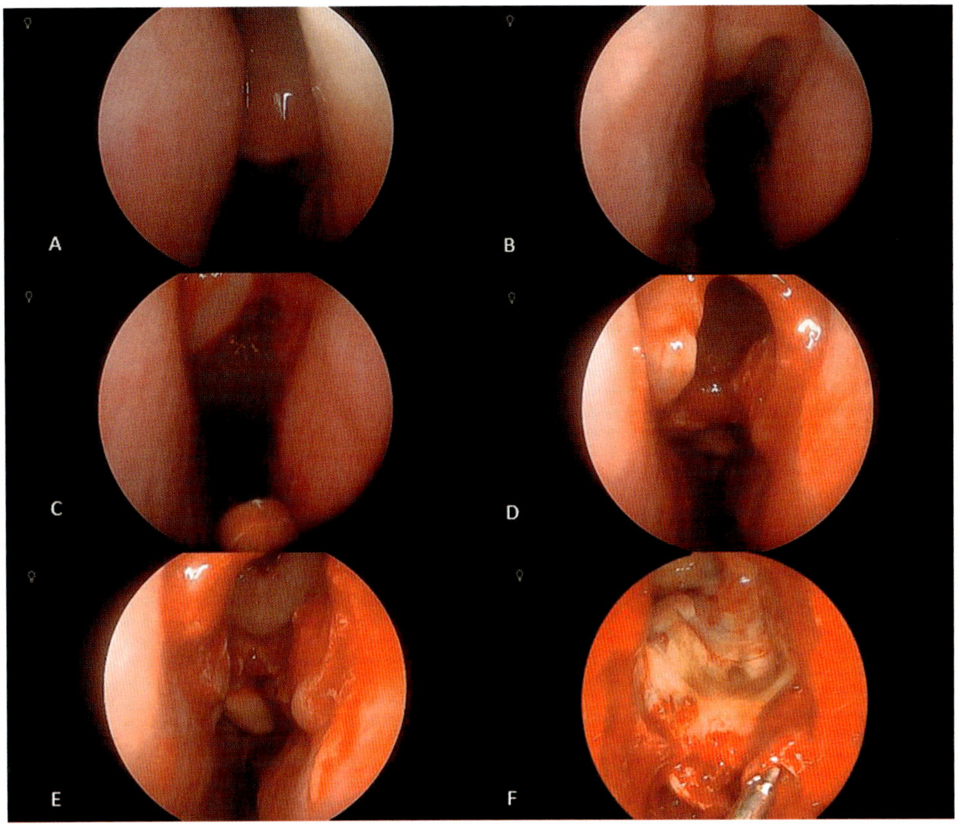

• **Fig. 32.2** Intraoperative photos of a left frontoethmoid mucocele. The mucocele is seen in the left middle meatus (A), and the floor of the mucocele is removed to expose the pseudocyst lining (B). The inspissated secretions of the mucocele are then expressed (C) and the cavity is opened (D). Zero-degree (E) and 45-degree (F) endoscopic views of the widely marsupialized mucocele cavity.

volume and positioning changes. Patients should be counseled regarding possible postoperative diplopia that can ensue secondary to the rapid orbital volume changes. Patients tend to adjust with time, but it is a possible surgical sequela that requires adequate counseling.

Bony changes secondary to the expansile effects of mucoceles are common, with complete resorption of the orbital bones possible. Traditionally the bony defect does not need to be reconstructed because the mucoperiosteum tends to be preserved. In a study of 116 patients who underwent operative intervention and had complete bone resorption, 12 patients had postoperative imaging and were noted to have bone regeneration. Reconstruction was avoided and enophthalmos, meningoceles, or facial deformities did not develop. The preservation of the mucoperiosteum is thought to serve as a strong enough impetus for bone regeneration.[24]

Conclusion

Sinonasal mucoceles with orbital extension are a common rhinologic pathology. Endoscopic management of mucoceles is a safe and effective modality of treatment. Open obliterative procedures are less common, and endoscopic approaches allow the sinuses to regain normal mucociliary function. Intracranial and intraorbital involvement are common, and an understanding of the complex interplay among sinonasal, cranial, and orbital anatomy is key to surgically addressing the mucoceles and for long-term follow-up.

References

1. Devars du Mayne, M., Moya-Plana, A., Malinvaud, D., Laccourreye, O., & Bonfils, P. (2012). Sinus mucocele: Natural history and longterm recurrence rate. *European Annals of Otorhinolaryngology, Head and Neck Diseases*, *129*, 125–130.
2. Obeso, S., Llorente, J. L., Rodrigo, J. P., Sanchez, R., Mancebo, G., & Suarez, C. (2009). Paranasal sinuses mucoceles: Our experience in 72 patients. *Acta Otorrinolaringológica Española*, *60*(5), 332–339 (in Spanish).
3. Palmer-Hall, A. M., & Anderson, S. F. (1997). Paraocular sinus mucoceles. *Journal of the American Optometric Association*, *68*, 725–733.
4. Natvig, K., & Larsen, T. E. (1978). Mucocele of the paranasal sinuses: A retrospective clinical and histologic study. *Journal of Laryngology and Otology*, *92*, 1075–1082.
5. Lund, V. J., Henderson, B., & Song, Y. (1993). Involvement of cytokines and vascular adhesion receptors in the pathology of frontoethmoidal mucocoeles. *Acta Oto-Laryngologica*, *113*, 540–546.
6. Lee, T. J., Li, S. P., Fu, C. H., Huang, C. C., Chang, P. H., Chen, Y. W., et al. (2009). Extensive paranasal sinus mucoceles: A 15-year review of 82 cases. *American Journal of Otolaryngology*, *30*, 234–238.
7. Scangas, G. A., Gudis, D. A., & Kennedy, D. W. (2013). Natural history and clinical characteristics of paranasal sinus mucoceles: A clinical review. *International Forum of Allergy & Rhinology*, *3*, 712–717.
8. Zukin, L. M., Hink, E. M., Liao, S., Getz, A. E., Kingdom, T. T., & Ramakrishnan, V. R. (2017). Endoscopic management of paranasal sinus mucoceles: Meta-analysis of visual outcomes. *Otolaryngology–Head and Neck Surgery*, *157*, 760–766.
9. Lynch, R. C. (1921). The technique of a radical frontal sinus operation which has given me the best results. *Laryngoscope*, *31*, 1–5.

10. Howarth, W. G. (1921). Mucocele and pyocele of the nasal accessory sinuses. *Lancet*, *2*, 744–746.
11. Wolfowitz, B. L., & Solomon, A. (1972). Mucoceles of the frontal and ethmoidal sinuses. *Journal of Laryngology and Otology*, *86*, 79–82.
12. Kennedy, D. W., Josephson, J. S., Zinreich, S. J., Mattox, D. E., & Goldsmith, M. M. (1989). Endoscopic sinus surgery for mucoceles: A viable alternative. *Laryngoscope*, *99*, 885–895.
13. Serrano, E., Klossek, J. M., Percodani, J., Yardeni, E., & Dufour, X. (2004). Surgical management of paranasal sinus mucoceles: A long-term study of 60 cases. *Otolaryngology–Head and Neck Surgery*, *131*, 133–140.
14. Woodworth, B. A., Harvey, R. J., Neal, J. G., Palmer, J. N., & Schlosser, R. J. (2008). Endoscopic management of frontal sinus mucoceles with anterior table erosion. *Rhinology*, *46*, 231–237.
15. Sautter, N. B., Citardi, M. J., Perry, J., & Batra, P. S. (2008). Paranasal sinus mucoceles with skull-base and/or orbital erosion: Is the endoscopic approach sufficient? *Otolaryngology–Head and Neck Surgery*, *139*, 570–574.
16. Dhepnorrarat, R. C., Subramanium, S., & Sethi, D. S. (2012). Endoscopic surgery for front-ethmoidal mucoceles: A 15-year experience. *Otolaryngology–Head and Neck Surgery*, *147*, 345–350.
17. Courson, A. M., Stankiewicz, J. A., & Lal, D. (2014). Contemporary management of frontal sinus mucoceles: A meta-analysis. *Laryngoscope*, *124*, 378–386.
18. Timperley, D. G., Banks, C., Robinson, D., Roth, J., Sacks, R., & Harvey, R. J. (2011). Lateral frontal sinus access in endoscopic skull-base surgery. *International Forum of Allergy & Rhinology*, *1*, 290–295.
19. Moe, K. S., Bergeron, C. M., & Ellenbogen, R. G. (2010). Transorbital neuroendoscopic surgery. *Neurosurgery*, *67*, 16–28.
20. Lim, J. H., Sardesai, M. G., Ferreira, M. Jr., & Moe, K. S. (2012). Transorbital neuroendoscopic management of sinogenic complications involving the frontal sinus, orbit, and anterior cranial fossa. *Journal of Neurological Surgery Part B, Skull Base*, *73*, 394–400.
21. Herndon, M., McMains, K. C., & Kountakis, S. E. (2007). Presentation and management of extensive front-orbital-ethmoid mucoceles. *American Journal of Neuroradiology*, *28*, 145–147.
22. Stokken, J., Wali, E., Woodard, T., Recinos, P. F., & Sindwani, R. (2016). Considerations in the management of giant frontal mucoceles with significant intracranial extension: A systematic review. *American Journal of Rhinology & Allergy*, *30*, 301–305.
23. Har-El, G. (2001). Endoscopic management of 108 sinus mucoceles. *Laryngoscope*, *111*, 2131–2134.
24. Terranova, P., Karligkiotis, A., Digilio, E., Basilico, F., Bernardini, E., Pistochini, A., et al. (2015). Bone regeneration after sinonasal mucocele marsupialization: What really happens over time? *Laryngoscope*, *125*, 1568–1572.

33

Endoscopic Orbital Fracture Repair

GIOVANNI FELISATI, MD, ALBERTO MARIA SAIBENE, MD, MA, FEDERICO BIGLIOLI, MD, AND GIACOMO COLLETTI, MD

Endoscopic Repair of a Medial Orbital Wall Facture With the "Milan Technique"

Endoscopic Medial Orbital Wall Reconstruction After Removal of an Orbital Mass Via a Transnasal Approach

Among the seven bones composing the orbit, the maxillary bone and the ethmoid bone represent the thinnest boundaries. Therefore blunt trauma to the orbit most often results in inferior and/or medial wall fractures rather than lateral wall and orbital roof injuries.[1] More specifically, the lamina papyracea of the ethmoid bone, aptly named because of its extreme frailty, composes most of the medial orbital wall, which makes medial wall fractures very common.[2]

Medial and inferior orbital wall fractures do not necessarily have absolute surgical indications (small, isolated blow-out medial wall fractures generally might not require treatment, although late enophthalmos can become an aesthetic concern for such patients[3]). However, complications are very likely to occur with fractures exceeding 1 cm^2 or 50% of the wall.[4] Furthermore, extrinsic orbital muscle impinging in the fracture margins, thereby inducing ophthalmoplegia and subsequent diplopia, represents another general indication for medial and inferior orbital wall fractures repair.[1]

There is an intrinsic technical challenge associated with orbital fracture surgery, as well as some risk of complications in restoring the orbital rim and in functionally reconstructing the globe, the extraocular muscles, the lacrimal system, and other structures. The optic nerve, the extrinsic muscles, and the lacrimal system can be hindered by even minor mistakes, with predictable dire consequences. Furthermore, the complex anatomy and a constrained surgical filed sometimes make exposing the structures and correcting defects with implants a significant challenge.[5]

Several traditional open surgical accesses to the orbit have been proposed over the course of many years to provide the best exposition of tissues coupled with minimal invasiveness and optimal aesthetic outcomes.[6,7] The anterior half of the orbit is managed through a group of incision collectively designated as anterior orbitotomy, with the incision located according to the orbital quadrant requiring intervention. Access to the orbit is gained either subperiosteally (via the orbital rim) or orbitally (via the orbital septum) approach. The orbital rim can be reached with incisions, including direct brow, subbrow, Lynch, inferior rim, Kronlein, subciliary, subtarsal, and transconjunctival, with or without lateral canthotomy. None of these approaches is risk free, and poor cosmetic or functional outcomes have led to abandoning some of these procedures. The historic (and still valid from a tissue exposition standpoint) Lynch incision, for example, provides excellent exposure to the medial orbit at the cost of medial canthal web formation, a visible scar, and potential medial canthal malpositioning, whereas subciliary approaches allow broad access to the orbital floor but can cause lower lid retraction and malposition.[8] The latter approaches grant only limited access to the medial wall. Transconjunctival incision might allow lower morbidity than cutaneous incisions (although this was not scientifically proven) and was originally described in 1924; it is mostly used to access the orbital floor.[9]

Although the anterior, inferior, and medial orbit are easily managed with these accesses, the lateral and posterior orbit, as well as the orbital roof, require more complex strategies, such as lateral orbitotomy to access the lateral orbit and the retrobulbar space,[10] with lateral canthotomy or extended eyelid crease skin incision as the most common procedures, with possible implementation of neurosurgical approaches, such as coronal incision or fronto-orbito-zygomatic cranio-orbitotomy.[11] These complex approaches entail significant operative and recovery time and neurosurgical-related morbidity.

Endoscopy in orbital surgery presents, as in other surgical fields, the opportunity to couple extensive surgical field vision with minimally invasive approaches. The first attempt in endoscopically accessing the orbit dates back to the early 1980s with the work of Norris and Cleasby,[12] furthered by Braunstein and colleagues research in the mid-1990s.[13] These techniques initially failed to allow a safe and expandable cavity for surgery. With the wide diffusion of endoscopic surgery in otolaryngology in the late 1990s, transnasal and transantral endoscopic orbital surgery gradually became a surgical tool for maxillofacial surgeons, otolaryngologists, and ophthalmologists.[14] Currently the application of endoscopic techniques to orbital fracture repair allows complete exposition of fractures, regardless of depth, and incarcerates tissues, encouraging accurate implant placement and reducing injuries to noble orbital structures with marginal invasiveness.[5]

This chapter focuses on the treatment of medial orbital wall fractures, with special emphasis on transnasal endoscopic approaches, which allow for excellent functional and esthetic results while completely avoiding problems related to external approaches. The last section of the chapter provides useful information on managing complex fractures with the aid of endoscopy and on using endoscopy as a tool for addressing the management of complex orbital fractures.

Medial Orbital Wall Fractures

The medial orbital wall, as the locus minoris resistentiae, is the second most frequently injured orbital boundary after blunt trauma. As covered further in the chapter, medial orbital wall fractures can also present concomitant orbital floor fractures in a more complex scenario.[1]

Two different etiopathogenic theories have been suggested as an explanation for medial orbital blow-out fractures: the hydraulic theory and the buckling theory.[15] According to the first paradigm, intraorbital pressure becomes elevated owing to retropulsion of the orbit; such elevated pressure leads to fracturing the medial orbital wall in the point of lowest resistance. The latter paradigm links medial orbital wall breaches to a direct trauma involving the medial orbital rim. Independent of the physiopathogenic mechanism, any blunt trauma involving the eyeball and/or the medial orbital rim can lead to a fracture of the lamina papyracea, causing herniation of the medial orbital content into the nasal cavity. This means that not only the fatty orbital content, but also the muscles can enter the nasal cavity with a non-negligible chance of muscular entrapment; again, enophthalmos and/or diplopia may follow.

From an anatomic standpoint, it is worth remembering that the medial orbital wall is formed not only by the lamina papyracea (which almost inevitably is fractured), but also by the lacrimal bone anteriorly, the maxillary bone inferiorly, and the lesser wing of the sphenoid posteriorly. A suture runs at the border between the ethmoid and the frontal bone, in close proximity to the anterior and posterior ethmoidal arteries. This suture represents the closest point to the dura and thus should be approached with the utmost attention to avoid cerebrospinal fluid leaks. Ethmoidal arteries can allow for an average estimate of the anteroposterior orbital depth, given that the anterior ethmoidal artery runs 24 mm from the lacrimal crest, whereas the posterior ethmoidal artery lies 12 mm posterior to this and the orbital apex 6 mm further posteriorly.

As mentioned earlier, both fat and muscle (more specifically, the medial rectus muscle) can herniate toward the nasal cavity; therefore, indications for medial orbital wall repair are diplopia and significant enophthalmos. Although evaluating gaze in all position is always recommended because the medial rectus muscle is usually affected, the horizontal gaze should be given the maximum attention during evaluation to identify the slightest restrictions. Although clinically relevant enophthalmos, as well as diplopia, are generally appreciable with a careful clinical examination, a CT scan is mandatory to provide information on the fracture site, the number of fragments, and anatomic relationships. This is especially relevant if a pure transnasal endoscopic access is planned, which must rely on the usual landmarks of endoscopic sinus surgery to avoid damage to noble structures. Furthermore, the CT scan provides information on the size of the fracture, allowing for proper planning. Mirrored CT images coupled with neuronavigation enable also more precise orbital reconstructions.[16]

Medial wall fractures have been approached historically in countless ways. The first reliable proposal was the Lynch incision, ultimately abandoned because of poor overall aesthetic results.[17] Currently the approaches to medial wall usually rely on transconjunctival accesses, including the transcaruncular, precaruncular, and retrocaruncular routes.[18] All these accesses usually couple swift direct access to the fracture site with an acceptable surgical field. Nevertheless, these approaches are hampered by very limited visibility of the posterior and superior areas of the medial wall and by potential injuries to the lacrimal sac and to the lower oblique muscle. The need for eyeball manipulation is another disadvantage, though minor, in these approaches. To overcome these disadvantages, many authors have relied on endoscopy, which has been used as an aid to traditional approaches or in completely new ways through the transnasal route.[19,20]

Many recently introduced techniques saw a tight collaboration among ophthalmologists, maxillofacial surgeons, and otolaryngologists. Most of these techniques have been developed to address both tumors and orbital fractures, with a specific focus on the posteriormost areas—the orbital apex and the periorbital skull base—which are the areas least easily exposed through external approaches. Excellent case series have been published (e.g., Murchison et al.[21]). In this series a multidisciplinary team (neurosurgeon, otolaryngologist, and orbital surgeon) performed ethmoidectomy, sphenoidotomy, and posterior lamina papyracea removal to enter the orbit in 18 patients with a range of pathologies including cavernous hemangiomas, juvenile angiofibromas, and invasive cutaneous squamous cell carcinoma. Approaching these lesions somehow led the way to approaching with a higher degree of safety, smaller, localized lesions, such as medial wall fractures. In these regards, it may be worth noting that in these case series, complications were relatively common (22% of the patients) and included decreased postoperative visual acuity and cerebrospinal fluid leak. Although the extent of exposition for approaching medial wall fractures is considerably more limited, the orbital surgeon should never forget that the orbit should always be regarded as a high-risk location.

Other interesting case series on endoscopic approaches were published by Chhabra et al.[22] and Bleier et al.[23] These two articles report a detailed experience in treating orbital venous malformations (commonly misnamed as cavernous hemangiomas[24]), a condition that frequently requires extensive dissection, removal of the papyracea, and extrinsic orbital muscle dissection. The experience with these patients not only strengthened the anatomic knowledge of the medial orbital wall from an endoscopic perspective but also added information on an important feature common to medial orbital wall—that is, the enophthalmos caused by the herniation of orbital content toward the nasal cavity. Although modern views on these techniques state that minimally invasive accesses do not tend to induce enophthalmos,[25] the same approach we describe in detail for medial orbital wall fractures could be adopted to reconstruct the medial orbital wall after endoscopic orbital mass removal.[26]

Restricting once again the focus on endoscopic reconstruction of medial orbital wall fractures, it is worth noting that the transnasal-transethmoidal and transcaruncular approaches and conjunctival incisions are the most commonly used approaches and both grant the avoidance skin incisions and optimization of cosmesis. Among the first notable case series was the one from Hinohira et al.,[27] who performed a transnasal endoscopic medial wall reconstruction on 23 patients with isolated medial blowout fractures with a 95.5% success rate. When using the transnasal approach, nevertheless, most authors usually rely on supporting the medial wall with a silicone sheet[28] and/or using additional long-term nasal packing to contain the herniated orbital content,[29] with obvious patient discomfort and a theoretical increased risk of infection. Conversely, the use of other materials such as high-density porous polyethylene[30] with an endoscopic transcaruncular approach (which means an external approach aided by the endoscope, not a pure endoscopic approach) showed excellent results with minimal discomfort.

The Milan Approach to Medial Wall Orbital Fractures

Our group developed the so-called Milan technique for medial orbital walls fracture repairs. The technique combines the expositional advantages offered by the transnasal endoscopic approach and the effectiveness of reconstruction with stable porous polyethylene implants. This endoscopic transnasal technique has an excellent success rate, requires no packing or prolonged hospital stays, and has proved its efficacy—even in the long term—in a considerably sized patient group.[31,32]

This technique can be applied to any patient with medial wall fractures dating back no more than 15 days who have enophthalmos and/or extrinsic orbital muscle movement impairment. A preoperative CT scan is required to measure the expected lamina papyracea defect and to identify the anatomic landmarks. The CT scan further allows quantification of the enophthalmos and identifies whether fat tissue alone or fat and muscle are herniating into the nasal cavity. We do not rely on any intraoperative navigation for fracture repair purposes.

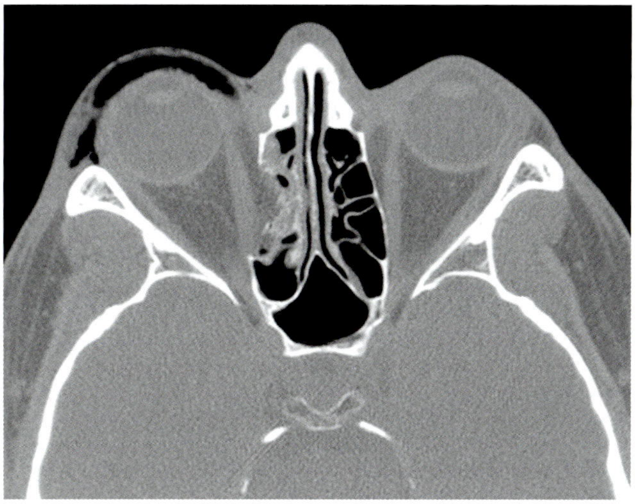

• **Fig. 33.1** Axial plain computed tomography image of the head showing right medial orbital wall fracture. The orbital soft tissues are herniating toward the ethmoid with an appreciable degree of enophthalmos.

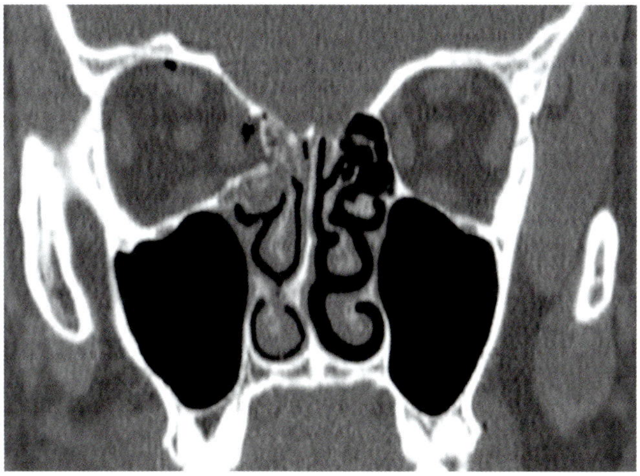

• **Fig. 33.2** Coronal plain computed tomography image of the head showing right medial orbital wall fracture.

Technique

With the Milan technique, surgery begins by placing the patient in the standard position for endoscopic sinus surgery; both eyes must be visible in the operating field. After nasal mucosa decongestion, the procedure is started with a 0-degree scope; uncinectomy, middle antrostomy, and radical ethmoidectomy are performed in the affected side to approach the lamina papyracea and expose the orbital floor. Although the use of powered instruments (debriders and such) can be considered, we prefer to exert extreme care while approaching the fractured lamina papyracea, removing the ethmoid bone with cutting forceps and grasping forceps, avoiding powered instruments. Because such patients usually do not have a nasal inflammatory condition, bleeding is most often minimal. The swollen mucosa must be distinguished from the herniated orbital content and removed carefully to minimize the risk for postoperative mucoceles. All the fractured fragments of the lamina papyracea must then be removed to avoid pushing them back in the orbit at the time of positioning the reconstructive sheet. After removing all mucosa and fractured bone fragments, constant landmarks can be identified; anteriorly, superiorly, and inferiorly it must be possible to identify the healthy, solid margins of the medial wall. In this maneuver a 45-degree scope can assist the surgeon in visualizing the margins. The posterior aspect of the fracture is typically shaped as an acute angle connecting the upper and lower margins. With the aid of a ruler (usually a flexible disposable ruler), the anteroposterior size of the defect is measured and a 0.8-mm thick porous high-density polyethylene sheet is shaped accordingly, exceeding the measured defect by few millimeters both in length and height.

The shape of the prosthesis should be shaped as a guitar pick, with a medial concavity, going toward the orbit. The polyethylene prosthesis is placed over the herniated content and gently pushed laterally into the orbit until entering the fracture margins. A curved instrument (suction tip or such) can be used to aid positioning the sheet inside the fracture margins. After it is placed inside the fractured margins, the sheet becomes then self-containing, impinging on the fracture margins (this requires a precise shaping of the implant itself by the surgeon). No stenting, packing, or prosthesis covering is required. We advise intraoperative antibiotic prophylaxis and obtaining a postoperative CT scan 24 to 48 hours after the procedure to confirm the correct reconstruction. Figs. 33.1 to 33.4 show a typical case of medial orbital wall fracture addressed with this technique.

Endoscopic Assistance for Complex Fractures or Management of Complications of Previous Conventional Fracture Treatment

As emphasized previously, one of the major drawbacks of traditional external approaches to the inferior and medial orbital wall—just slightly less when endoscopically assisted (i.e., using the endoscope through an external approach)—is the dismal performance in visualizing the uppermost and deepest parts of the orbit. Similarly, we have already noted how these problems are addressed swiftly by relying on an endoscopic endonasal approach.

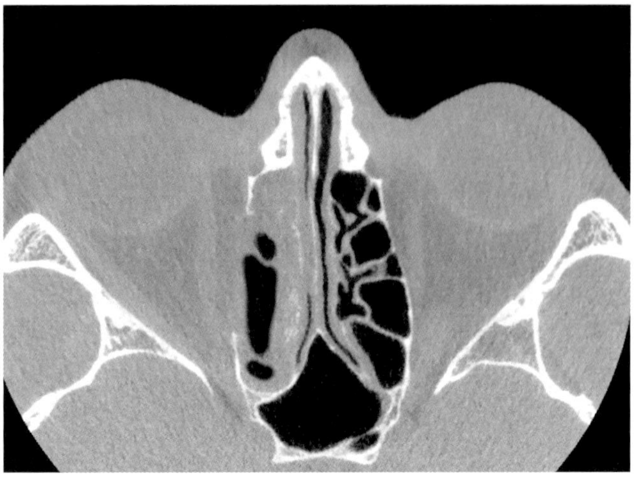

• **Fig. 33.3** Postoperative axial plain computed tomography image of the head. The right orbital content herniation is completely corrected by the polyethylene sheet and the enophthalmos is no longer appreciable.

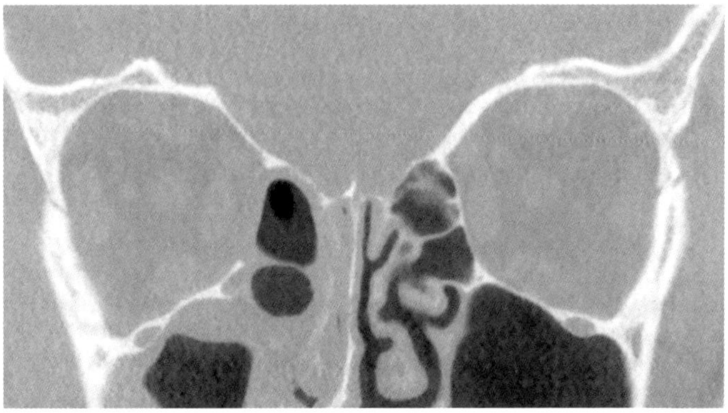

• **Fig. 33.4** Postoperative coronal plain computed tomography image of the head. After complete correction, the orbits are symmetric.

When managing "normal" fractures, the endoscopic endonasal approach allows for better aesthetic outcomes, less discomfort, the use of hassle-free reconstruction materials such as polyethylene, optimal fracture reduction, and overall reduced hospital stays. However, the endoscopic endonasal approach proves also useful in another unusual setting: managing fractures that are deemed complex for a number of reasons or fractures for which the standard reconstruction methods have failed, with displacement of meshes or other support structures or poor aesthetic outcomes.

A first criterion of complexity is represented by the size of the fracture and its anteroposterior position. In cases of wider fractures ($\geq$3 cm) or posterior fractures, transnasal endoscopy allows isolation of the entire fracture margins, even when their position is close to the orbital apex. Furthermore, the gentle movements required for placing endoscopic reconstruction prosthesis reduce the stress imposed on the optical nerve and the chance of tearing the ethmoidal blood vessels. This is especially true for the medial orbital wall.

Another group of complex fractures is characterized by the herniation of orbital content into the sinonasal cavities. The surgeon might face a massive herniation of fat and muscular tissue (most often in case of wider fractures) or a less massive herniation but presenting with muscular impingement. The latter can be a result of fractured bone fragments blocking the muscle or an unusual position of the fracture, with the muscle(s) falling into a small fracture and thus becoming functionally impotent. In either case, the transnasal approach allows removal of all the fragmented bone, thereby reducing the risk of small spiculae penetrating the muscle even secondarily and allows a better—and less traumatic—manipulation of the muscle, for which we encourage the use of cotton paddies. This maneuver is in no way different from the gentle dissection used to free endo-orbital masses during endoscopic dissection.

A third and final group of difficult-to-treat group orbital fractures in which endoscopic aid is helpful consists of fractures extending to other nearby noble structures—that is, the anterior skull base, the lacrimal system, and the optic nerve.[33-35] Fractures extending to these nearby areas are not commonplace and most often occur in dire settings of polytrauma with central nervous system involvement when the surgeons' effort is focused on other life-threatening injuries. In these cases, it is appropriate to consider endoscopy as a helping tool. Endoscopic procedures for cerebrospinal fluid leak repair (monolayered or multilayered, with autologous or synthetic materials) are at present routinely employed by almost any nasal endoscopist and can be employed transnasally after correcting the orbital fractures. In these cases, adequate nasal packing and antibiotic prophylaxis should be employed as required by the surgical setting. More technically demanding, but just as rewarding and safe as simple fracture treatment, is the use of optic nerve decompression in cases of traumatic neuropathy. Such types of decompression can follow the removal of the lamina papyracea fracture fragments and require the removal of all the posterior part of the lamina papyracea toward the orbital apex. Gentle dissection of the orbital content, following the periorbital plane whenever possible to reduce risk for vessels, extrinsic muscles, and nerves, must be performed posteriorly to remove all the bone composing the orbital nerve canal. A wide sphenoidotomy can help the surgeon visualize the optic nerve itself in the context of other important landmarks such as the internal carotid artery. Less risky, but still extremely useful, is the possible use of dacryocystorhinostomy, with or without lacrimal stent placement, to warrant the patency of the lacrimal system when the blunt force causing the trauma induces a tearing of the lacrimal sac or a compression/closure of the nasolacrimal duct, primarily preventing the development of epiphora or recurrent dacryocystitis.

As introduced at the beginning of this section, transnasal endoscopic orbital approaches can also be a useful tool in secondary treatment of patients with an unsatisfying correction of combined medioinferior wall orbital fractures, either from an aesthetic or functional end point. Previously discussed in this chapter are how traditional external techniques may lack the chance to correctly explore the deepest part of the orbit; this situation may in turn lead to mispositioning of the reconstructive meshes that can impinge muscles or prolapse into the sinonasal cavities. Patients with postoperative impairment in eyeball movement or persisting enophthalmos should undergo a CT study to identify reconstructive problems. Most often these problems can be solved by using endoscopic aid in a second surgical procedure. After the already explored exposition of the bony boundaries of the orbit, endoscopic vision and blunt dissection instruments usually allow for correct repositioning of the meshes and freeing the extrinsic muscle wherever needed. Should repositioning be impossible, the meshes can obviously be substituted with more appropriate ones or extended with other more pliable materials to provide the correct degree of correction.

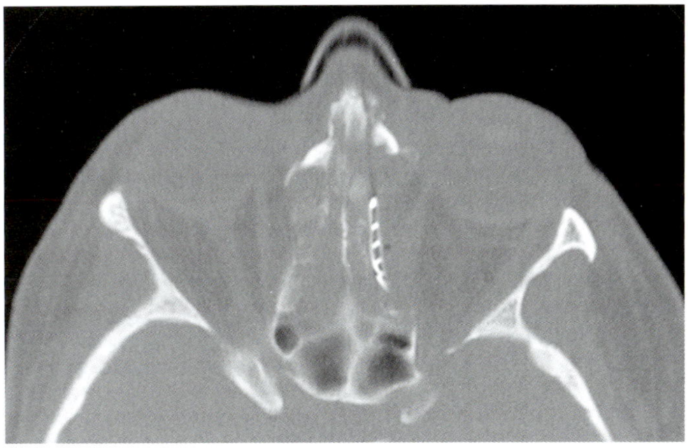

• **Fig. 33.5** Axial plain computed tomography image of the head showing a left inferior and medial orbital wall fracture treated by an external approach with a titanium mesh. The mesh is protruding toward the midline, leaning on the nasal septum, owing to a misplacement during the approach.

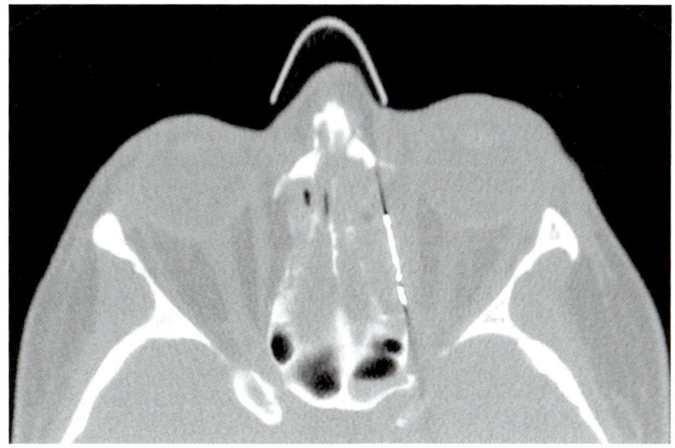

• **Fig. 33.7** Postoperative axial computed tomography image of the head showing the results of the transnasal endoscopic correction of the mesh displacement. The medial orbital wall is symmetrized without substituting the mesh.

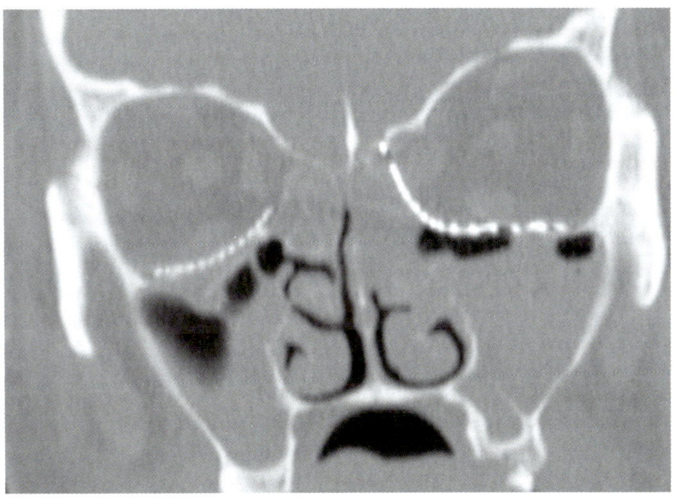

• **Fig. 33.6** Coronal plain computed tomography image of the head showing a left inferior and medial orbital wall fracture treated by an external approach with a titanium mesh. The mesh displacement determines a patent asymmetry of the orbits.

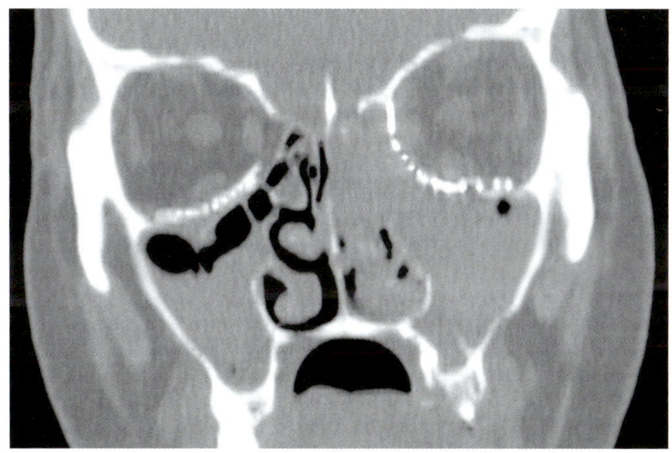

• **Fig. 33.8** Postoperative coronal plain computed tomography image of the head showing the results of the transnasal endoscopic correction of the mesh displacement. The mesh is secured to the intact inferior and medial orbital wall with good symmetrization.

In our experience with cases of improperly positioned preformed two-wall reconstructive meshes, we were able to reposition them through a transnasal approach in a precise manner made possible by the simple identification of the upper and posterior border of the fracture that must have been impossible to repair in the first traditional surgical setting. Figs. 33.5 to 33.8 show a typical case of improper mesh positioning corrected by a transnasal endoscopic approach.

References

1. Grob, S., Tao, J., & Yonkers, M. (2017). Orbital fracture repair. *Seminars in Plastic Surgery*, *31*, 31–39.
2. Choi, K.-E., Lee, J., Lee, H., Chang, M., Park, M., & Baek, S. (2015). The paradoxical predominance of medial wall injuries in blowout fracture. *Journal of Craniofacial Surgery*, *26*, e752–e755.
3. Fan, X., Li, J., Zhu, J., Li, H., & Zhang, D. (2003). Computer-assisted orbital volume measurement in the surgical correction of late enophthalmos caused by blowout fractures. *Ophthalmic Plastic and Reconstructive Surgery*, *19*, 207–211.
4. Burnstine, M. A. (2002). Clinical recommendations for repair of isolated orbital floor fractures: An evidence-based analysis. *Ophthalmology*, *109*, 1207–1210.
5. Zhang, S., Li, Y., & Fan, X. (2013). Application of endoscopic techniques in orbital blowout fractures. *Frontiers of Medicine*, *7*, 328–332.
6. Yoon, M., Campbell, A., & Grob, S. (2015). Novel surgical approaches to the orbit. *Middle East African Journal of Ophthalmology*, *22*, 435–441.
7. Schick, U. T. A., & Unterberg (2012). Surgical approaches to the orbit. In *Schmidek and Sweet operative neurosurgical techniques: Indications, methods, and results* (6th ed.) (pp. 603–612). Philadelphia: Elsevier Saunders.
8. Kang, S. J., & Kim, J. W. (2012). Surgical treatment of enophthalmos using an endoscope and T-shaped porous polyethylene fabricated with a mirror image. *International Journal of Oral and Maxillofacial Surgery*, *41*, 1186–1191.

9. Lorenz, H. P., Longaker, M. T., & Kawamoto, H. K. Jr. (1999). Primary and secondary orbit surgery: The transconjunctival approach. *Plastic and Reconstructive Surgery*, *103*, 1124–1128.
10. Kim, J. W., Yates, B. S., & Goldberg, R. A. (2009). Total lateral orbitotomy. *Orbit*, *28*, 320–327.
11. Lew, H., Rootman, D. B., Nassiri, N., Goh, A., & Goldberg, R. A. (2014). Transorbital approach without craniotomy to orbital tumors with extradural intracranial extension. *Orbit*, *33*, 343–351.
12. Norris, J. L., & Cleasby, G. W. (1981). Endoscopic orbital surgery. *American Journal of Otolaryngology*, *91*, 249–252.
13. Braunstein, R. E., Kazim, M., & Schubert, H. D. (1995). Endoscopy and biopsy of the orbit. *Ophthalmic Plastic and Reconstructive Surgery*, *11*, 269–272.
14. Rose, G. E. (2002). Endoscopic removal of periorbital lesions—where next? *Orbit*, *21*, 261–262.
15. Bullock, J. D., Warwar, R. E., Ballal, D. R., & Ballal, R. D. Mechanisms of orbital floor fractures: A clinical, experimental, and theoretical study. *Transactions of the American Ophthalmological Society*, *97*, 87–110.
16. Ho, S., & Lee, G. (2016). Orbital adherence syndrome following the use of titanium precontoured orbital mesh for the reconstruction of posttraumatic orbital floor defects. *Craniomaxillofac Trauma & Reconstruction*, *10*, 77–83.
17. Damgaard, O. E., Larsen, C. G., Felding, U. A., Toft, P. B., & von Buchwald, C. (2016). Surgical timing of the orbital "blowout" fracture: A systematic review and meta-analysis. *Otolaryngology–Head and Neck Surgery*, *155*, 387–390.
18. Kempton, S. J., Cho, D. C., Thimmappa, B., & Martin, M. C. (2016). Benefits of the retrocaruncular approach to the medial orbit: A clinical and anatomic study. *Annals of Plastic Surgery*, *76*, 295–300.
19. Copelli, C., Manfuso, A., d'Ecclesia, A., Catanzaro, S., Cassano, L., Pederneschi, N., et al. (2015). Endoscopic transnasal approach and intraoperative navigation for the treatment of isolated blowout fractures of the medial orbital wall. *Journal of Cranio-Maxillo-Facial Surgery*, *43*, 1974–1978.
20. Jin, H.-R., Yeon, J.-Y., Shin, S.-O., Choi, Y.-S., & Lee, D.-W. (2007). Endoscopic versus external repair of orbital blowout fractures. *Otolaryngology–Head and Neck Surgery*, *136*, 38–44.
21. Murchison, A. P., Rosen, M. R., Evans, J. J., & Bilyk, J. R. (2011). Endoscopic approach to the orbital apex and periorbital skull base. *Laryngoscope*, *121*, 463–467.
22. Chhabra, N., Wu, A. W., Fay, A., & Metson, R. (2014). Endoscopic resection of orbital hemangiomas. *International Forum of Allergy & Rhinology*, *4*, 251–255.
23. Bleier, B. S., Castelnuovo, P., Battaglia, P., Turri-Zanoni, M., Dallan, I., Metson, R., et al. (2016). Endoscopic endonasal orbital cavernous hemangioma resection: Global experience in techniques and outcomes. *International Forum of Allergy & Rhinology*, *6*, 156–161.
24. Colletti, G., & Deganello, A. (2017). Cavernous hemangioma: A term to be canceled. *European Archives of Oto-Rhino-Laryngology*, *274*, 2069–2070.
25. Castelnuovo, P., Fiacchini, G., Fiorini, F. R., & Dallan, I. (2018). "Push-pull technique" for the management of a selected superomedial intraorbital lesion. *Surgery Journal (New York, NY)*, *4*, e105–e109.
26. Colletti, G., Saibene, A. M., Pessina, F., Duvina, M., Allevi, F., Felisati, G., et al. A shift in the orbit. *Journal of Cranio-Maxillo-Facial Surgery*, *28*, 2027–2029.
27. Hinohira, Y., Takahashi, H., Komori, M., & Shiraishi, A. (2009). Endoscopic endonasal management of medial orbital blowout fractures. *Facial Plastic Surgery*, *25*, 17–22.
28. Park, C. H., Choi, D. J., Lee, J. H., Hong, S. M., Kwon, T. K., Joung, H. H., et al. (2009). Endoscopic reduction of medial orbital wall fractures using the rolled silastic sheet technique. *Journal of Trauma*, *66*, 1421–1424.
29. Kim, K., Song, K., Choi, S., Bae, Y., Choi, C., Oh, H., et al. (2012). Endoscopic transnasal approach for the treatment of isolated medial orbital blow-out fractures. *Annals of Plastic Surgery*, *68*, 161–165.
30. Wu, W., Jing, W., Selva, D., Cannon, P. S., Tu, Y., & Chen, B. (2013). Endoscopic transcaruncular repair of large medial orbital wall fractures near the orbital apex. *Ophthalmology*, *120*, 404–409.
31. Colletti, G., Pipolo, C., Lozza, P., Felisati, G., Allevi, F., Biglioli, F., et al. (2018). Orbital medial wall fractures: Purely endoscopic endonasal repair with polyethylene implants. *Clinical Otolaryngology*, *43*, 396–398.
32. Colletti, G., Saibene, A. M., Giannini, L., Dessy, M., Deganello, A., Pipolo, C., et al. (2018). Endoscopic endonasal repair with polyethylene implants in medial orbital wall fractures: A prospective study on 25 cases. *Journal of Cranio-Maxillo-Facial Surgery*, *46*, 274–282.
33. Hasheminia, D., Kalantar Motamedi, M. R., Hashemzehi, H., Nazeri, R., & Movahedian, B. (2015). A 7-year study of 1,278 patients with maxillofacial trauma and cerebrospinal fluid leak. *Journal of Cranio-Maxillo-Facial Surgery*, *14*, 258–262.
34. Urolagin, S. B., Kotrashetti, S. M., Kale, T. P., & Balihallimath, L. J. (2012). Traumatic optic neuropathy after maxillofacial trauma: A review of 8 cases. *Journal of Cranio-Maxillo-Facial Surgery*, *70*, 1123–1130.
35. Uzun, F., Karaca, E. E., & Konuk, O. (2016). Surgical management of traumatic nasolacrimal duct obstruction. *European Journal of Ophthalmology*, *26*, 517–519.

PART 7

Intracranial/Skull Base Surgery and the Optic Apparatus

34

Surgical Anatomy of the Optic Nerves and Chiasm

OMAR H. AHMED, MD, EZEQUIEL GOLDSCHMIDT, MD, PhD,
JUAN C. FERNANDEZ-MIRANDA, MD, AND ERIC W. WANG, MD

The optic nerve and chiasm can be involved with pathology affecting the orbit, orbital apex, and skull base. When surgically addressing these structures, it is critical to maintain not only their neural integrity but also their vascular supply, as this will allow for superior visual outcomes. Even relatively common procedures such as endoscopic endonasal transsellar resections of pituitary adenomas require a robust surgical knowledge of the optic apparatus.

Surgical decompression of the optic nerve and chiasm may be indicated for either decompression or tumor resection. Perhaps the most common indication for isolated decompression of the optic nerve is traumatic optic neuropathy; however, this may also be performed for nontraumatic optic neuropathy related to compressive pathologies such as Graves ophthalmopathy, fibrous dysplasia, or mucocele.[1,2] Anterior skull base tumors involving the optic canals or chiasm are particularly characteristic of tuberculum sellae and planum sphenoidale meningiomas, with the incidence of optic canal invasion reported to be approximately 27% to 77%[3-8] and as high as 97%[9] in one series. These tumors necessitate surgical access to the optic apparatus for curative resection, improvement of visual deficits, or exploration to delineate tumor extent.[9] Access can be achieved by either open or endonasal endoscopic approaches and is influenced by the compartment of the optic canal that needs to be addressed (e.g., medial or lateral), tumor size and location, and the goals of surgery.[10] Lateral approaches include transorbital or craniotomy approaches. The endoscopic endonasal approach (EEA) ideally addresses medial lesions; allows for direct access to the orbital apex, optic nerve, and suprasellar cistern; and provides enhanced visualization of the subchiasmatic space. EEA approaches also potentially confer the advantages of less morbidity, less brain or orbital retraction, and superior cosmesis, as there are typically no external incisions.[11]

Surgical Anatomy

The optic nerve should be considered an extension of the brain, as it contains meninges including a cerebrospinal fluid–containing subarachnoid space. There are four segments of the optic nerve distal to the optic chiasm: intracranial, intracanalicular, intraorbital, and intraocular. The optic chiasm and nerve are covered in this chapter proximally to distally.

Anatomy of the Optic Chiasm

The optic chiasm lies within the suprasellar cistern. The bony chiasmatic groove or sulcus, a bony depression bordered anteriorly by the limbus sphenoidale and posteriorly by the tuberculum sellae, is a consistent anatomic landmark for the level of the optic chiasm. The optic chiasm usually lies above the diaphragm and pituitary gland in 70% of cases, but in the remaining 30%, the optic chiasm can overlie the tuberculum sella in a "prefixed" configuration or the dorsum sellae in a "postfixed" configuration.[12] Superior to the optic chiasm are the anterior cerebral and anterior communicating arteries (Fig. 34.1). Immediately posterior to the optic chiasm is the pituitary infundibulum. Laterally, the optic chiasm is abutted by the supraclinoid internal carotid arteries (ICAs).

As the optic chiasm traverses the circle of Willis, it receives blood supply from it via the anterior cerebral and communicating arteries, posterior cerebral and communicating arteries, and the basilar artery.[13] The optic chiasm also receives significant blood supply from the superior hypophyseal artery (SHA). The SHA is typically composed of two arteries (one proximal and the other distal) that arise from each ICA. The proximal artery typically has three main branches: infundibular (supplies the pituitary stalk and optic chiasm), optic (supplies the ventral and anterior optic chiasm as well as the proximal optic nerves), and descending (supplies the sellar diaphragm, stalk, and adenohypophysis) (Fig. 34.2). Unilateral injury to or sacrifice of the SHA is unlikely to cause endocrine or chiasmal deficits owing to redundant blood supply but may pose significant risk to the proximal optic nerves as they have minimal collateral blood supply.[14]

Anatomy of the Intracranial Segment of the Optic Nerve

The intracranial segment is the portion of the optic nerve between the optic chiasm and intracanalicular segment, and is approximately 12 to 16 mm in length and 4.5 mm in caliber.[15] This segment is perfused by the ophthalmic, anterior cerebral, anterior communicating, and SHAs.[16] Lateral to the optic nerve in this segment is the supraclinoid ICA (Fig. 34.3). The ophthalmic artery originates from the supraclinoid ICA and generally courses inferolaterally to the nerve within its meninges as they both enter the optic canal. However, in approximately 15% of cases, the ophthalmic artery lies

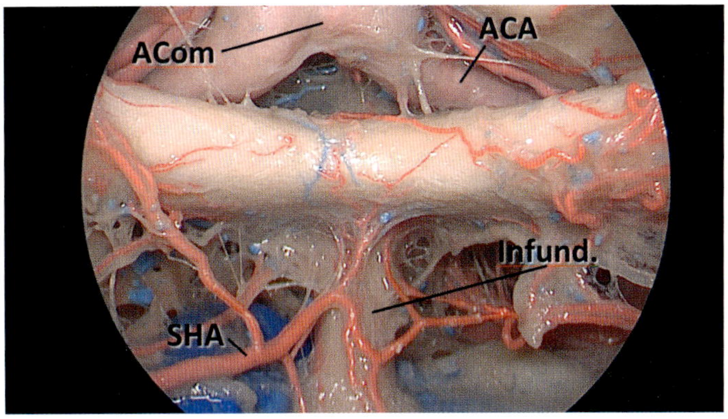

• **Fig. 34.1** Optic chiasm. *ACA,* anterior cerebral artery; *ACom,* anterior communicating artery; *SHA,* superior hypophyseal artery; *Infund,* pituitary infundibulum.

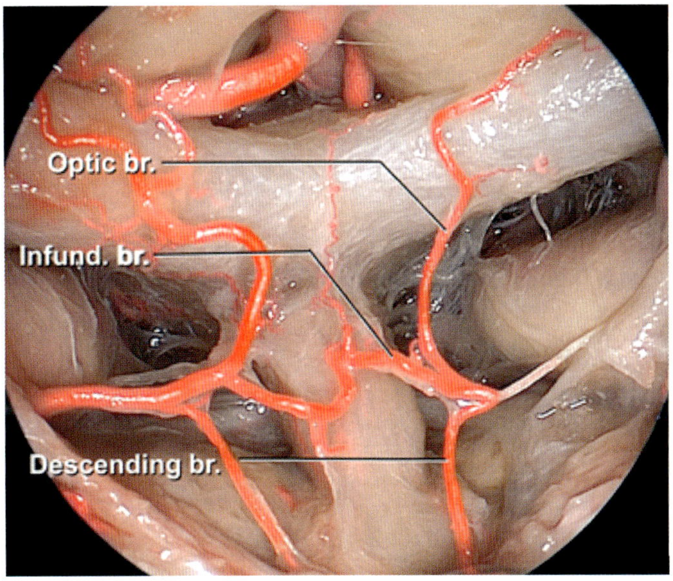

• **Fig. 34.2** Branches of the superior hypophyseal artery. (From Truong, H. Q., Najera, E., Zanabria-Ortiz, R., Celtikci. E., Sun, X., Borghei-Razavi. H., et al. [2018]. Surgical anatomy of the superior hypophyseal artery and its relevance for endoscopic endonasal surgery. *Journal of Neurosurgery, 13,* 1–9. Used with permission.)

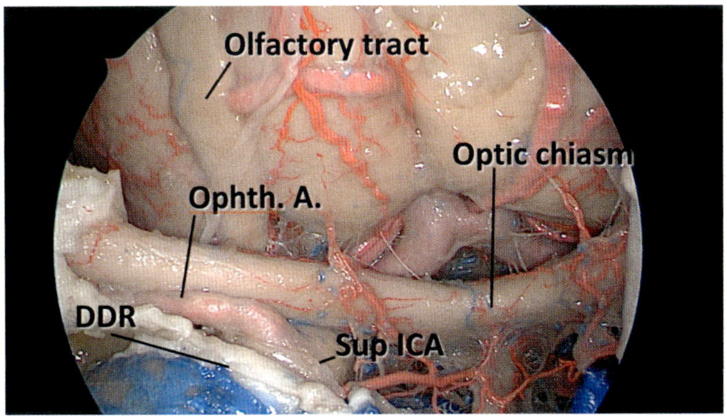

• **Fig. 34.3** Intracranial optic nerve. *Ophth A,* ophthalmic artery; *Sup ICA,* supraclinoid internal carotid artery; *DDR,* distal dural ring.

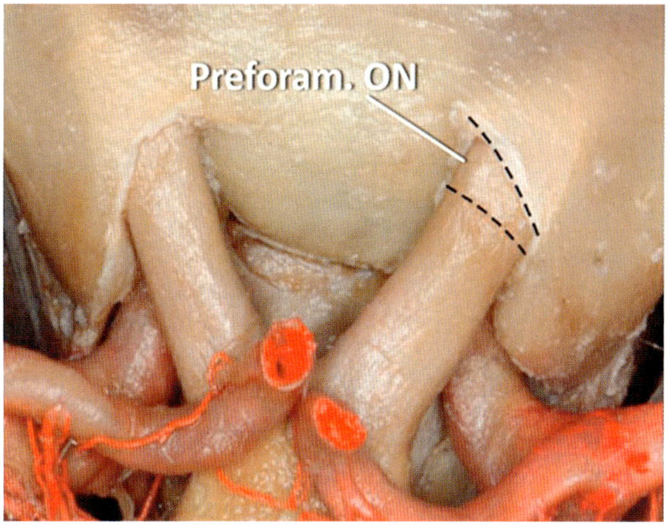

• **Fig. 34.4** Falciform ligament and the intracranial optic nerve. The falciform ligament overlying the intracranial optic nerves has been removed bilaterally in this cadaveric photo. The area demarcated between the *dashed black lines* is where the falciform ligament spanned, marking the preforaminal intracranial segment of the optic nerve before its entry into the osseous optic canal. (From Abhinav, K., Acosta, Y., Wang, W. H., Bonilla, L. R., Koutourousiou, M., Wang, E., et al. [2015]. Endoscopic endonasal approach to the optic canal: Anatomic considerations and surgical relevance. *Neurosurgery, 11*[suppl]), 431–445. Used with permission.)

inferomedial to the nerve, potentially posing risk during EEA approaches that require the optic canals to be drilled.[17] The ophthalmic artery gives off many small emissary vessels that supply the surrounding meninges and underlying optic nerve. Above the optic nerve in the intracranial segment are the gyri recti of the frontal lobes. Just proximal to where the intracranial optic nerve enters into its osseous canal, a fibrous band termed the *falciform ligament* (Fig. 34.4) runs anteromedially from the anterior clinoid to the limbus sphenoidale, forming the roof of this preforaminal portion of the intracranial optic nerve. The falciform ligament covers the nerve superiorly for approximately 3 mm in length.[18]

Anatomy of the Intracanalicular Segment of the Optic Nerve

The intracanalicular segment of the optic nerve bridges the intracranial and intraorbital segments and spans approximately 9 mm in length (Fig. 34.5).[17,18] This segment is supplied by the plial arterial network from the ophthalmic artery.[16] The intracanalicular portion lies within an oblong cylinder of bone formed by the confluence of the optic strut and anterior clinoid process. As the nerve courses through the canal and transitions into its intraorbital segment, this bony exit is known as the optic foramen. The diameter of the intracanalicular portion is greater mediolaterally than superoinferiorly, and the anteroposterior distance is greater laterally than medially. However, as the nerve courses toward the optic foramen to exit into the orbit, the dimensions of the optic foramen are wider superoinferiorly than mediolaterally.[15,18,19] The roof of the optic canal is the anterior root of the lesser sphenoid wing, which is continuous laterally with the anterior clinoid process and medially with the limbus sphenoidale (Fig. 34.6). The optic strut is the bony floor of the optic canal that connects the anterior clinoid process to the lateral sphenoid sinus and separates the optic canal from

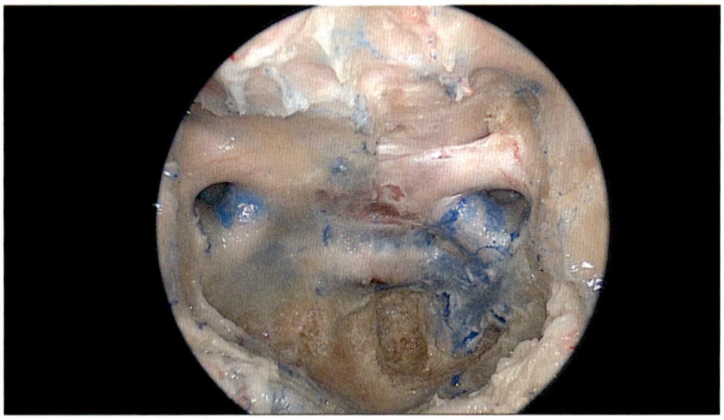

• **Fig. 34.5** Intracanalicular optic nerve. In this photo, the medial aspect of the intracanalicular canal has been drilled to expose the intracanalicular optic nerve and its dural sheath from the orbital apex to the intracranial optic nerve.

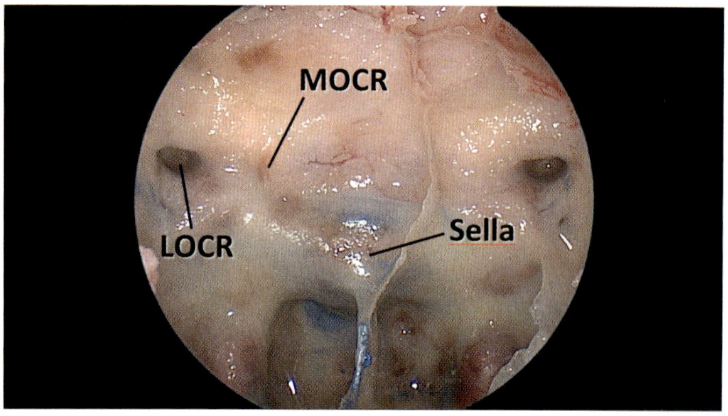

• **Fig. 34.7** Opticocarotid recess. A well-pneumatized lateral opticocarotid recess (*LOCR*) is shown. The medial opticocarotid recess (*MOCR*) and sella are also labeled.

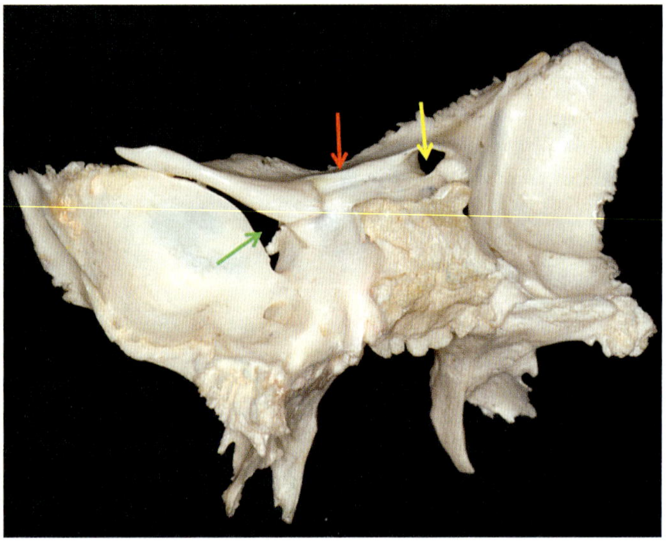

• **Fig. 34.6** Optic canal. The *yellow arrow* denotes the oblong optic canal. The *red arrow* denotes the limbus sphenoidale. The *green arrow* denotes the superior orbital fissure. The roof of the optic canal is the anterior root of the lesser sphenoid wing and its floor is the optic strut.

the superior orbital fissure inferiorly. The medial wall is formed by the body of the sphenoid and is often thin (78%) or even dehiscent in up to 28% of cases.[19,20] Distally, the intracanalicular optic canal is narrower and the bone composing it is thicker. The thickness of the medial bony wall at this point, where the optic canal courses near the orbit, is 0.57 mm on average, in contrast to the medial wall proximally toward the chiasm, where it is markedly thinner, measuring approximately 0.21 mm.[18] The distal aspect of the canal as it terminates at the optic foramen contains particularly thick bone medially and is termed the optic tubercle. The optic tubercle is typically too hardy to be fractured off with instruments and instead requires a high-speed drill. The optic tubercle can be visualized to varying degrees and may lie within the sphenoid sinus or at the sphenoethmoidal junction, depending on the pneumatization pattern of the sphenoid and posterior ethmoid sinuses.[21]

The intracanalicular optic canal can usually be seen within the sphenoid sinus superolateral to the parasellar ICA as its medial wall forms a noticeable convexity. However, in approximately 25% of cases, the prominence of the optic canal is not apparent.[20] The parasellar ICA lies inferomedial to the optic prominence, and the bone overlying this segment is typically less than 0.5 mm, with the vessel covered only by mucosa in up to 8% of cases.[20] The opticocarotid recess is an imprint on the lateral sphenoid wall outlining the parasellar carotid and optic nerve (Fig. 34.7). It has both medial and lateral components. The lateral opticocarotid recess (LOCR) is a pneumatization of the optic strut, whereas the medial opticocarotid recess represents a pneumatization of the middle clinoid process.[19,22] The middle clinoid process is a bony projection that extends from the superolateral sella at approximately the junction of the intracavernous and paraclinoidal internal carotid artery segments to cover the anteromedial aspect of the cavernous sinus and partially encase the anterior genu of the intracavernous carotid artery.[23] The middle clinoid process is not always present, estimated to be identifiable in approximately 36% to 74% of the population.[24,25] Even more uncommonly, but important to recognize to avoid inadvertent injury to the cavernous carotid artery, is an osseous bridge or "caroticoclinoid ring" that connects the anterior clinoid process to the middle clinoid process. The pattern of pneumatization of the LOCR can be quite variable; thus the endoscopic surgeon should consider it as just one among many other landmarks that can be used to identify the optic canal. The LOCR is typically more pronounced than the medial opticocarotid recess.[19]

Anatomic variants with respect to approaching the optic canal must be recognized preoperatively on computed tomography imaging. The presence of Onodi cells, posterior ethmoid cells that extend above the sphenoid sinus laterally and/or posteriorly, distorts the typical compartmentalization between the ethmoid and sphenoid sinuses. This anatomic variant can predispose the optic canal to iatrogenic injury because the bone overlying the intracanalicular optic nerve is typically thin and may course within the Onodi cell itself. Also, the degree of sphenoid sinus pneumatization is an important factor in the endonasal identification of this segment of the optic nerve. The three classic types of sphenoid sinus pneumatization patterns described are conchal, presellar, and sellar. The conchal pattern is characterized by solid bone underlying the sella. The presellar pattern is characterized by pneumatization of the sphenoid sinus only anterior to the coronal plane of the sellar wall. In the sellar type, which is the most common (76% of subjects), pneumatization is present anterior to and below the sella, from the sphenoid rostrum to the clivus posteriorly.[20] In conchal and presellar sphenoid sinuses, landmarks typically identifiable after sphenoidotomy (such as the sella, carotid canal, optic canal, and opticocarotid recess) are obscured and are thus at risk of iatrogenic injury.

The bony optic canal can be endoscopically decompressed up to 270 degrees, from chiasm to orbital apex, after meticulous removal of the roof, floor, medial walls, and detachment of the falciform ligament.[19] The lateral wall of the optic canal is difficult to safely drill out without posing significant risk of injury to the nerve through an endonasal approach. Open approaches also allow for 270 degrees of decompression but are limited in accessing the inferomedial aspect, which is the aspect of the optic canal most frequently involved by tumors such as tuberculum sellae meningiomas.

Anatomy of the Intraorbital Segment of the Optic Nerve

The intraorbital optic nerve is the segment between the optic foramen and the nerve's entry into the globe (Fig. 34.8). It is primarily supplied by the plial circulation derived from the ophthalmic artery.[16] As the ophthalmic artery courses into the orbit, it later penetrates the optic nerve sheath to run within the nerve into the optic disc. It is at this point, on average 10 mm proximal to the globe, that the vessel is known as the central retinal artery.

The intraorbital optic nerve is approximately 25 mm in length, with redundancy of several millimeters relative to the anteroposterior distance from the globe to the optic foramen, conferring protection from eye movements or proptosis from conditions such as Graves ophthalmopathy.[16] The intraorbital optic nerve continues to be surrounded by its meninges as it courses into the orbit from the optic foramen. The outer layer of the dura enveloping the intracanalicular optic nerve runs contiguously with the periorbita. This area just distal to the optic foramen is known as the orbital apex. It is here that the annulus of Zinn, a fibrous ring surrounding the contents of the optic foramen and central aspect of the superior orbital fissure, emanates from the merging of the pia and arachnoid. The annulus of Zinn also forms the common origin for four of the six extraocular muscles that define the boundaries of the intraconal space. The intraorbital optic nerve transitions into the intraocular segment or optic nerve head, which is approximately 1 mm in length.

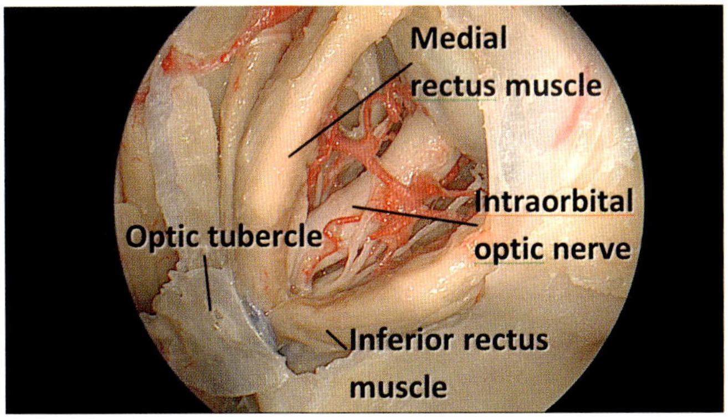

• **Fig. 34.8** Intraorbital optic nerve. The medial orbital wall, periorbita, and orbital fat have been removed to expose the intraorbital optic nerve from the orbital apex and annulus of Zinn to the intraocular segment (optic disc). (Photo credit: Huy Q. Truong, MD.)

Conclusion

Understanding the anatomy of the optic chiasm and nerves is imperative for safe surgery. From the optic chiasm to its terminus into the globe, there are four segments: intracranial, intracanalicular, intraorbital, and intraocular (optic disc). Each segment has distinct anatomic nuances and vascular supply.

References

1. Tandon, D., Thakar, A., Mahapatra, A., & Ghosh, P. (1993). Transethmoidal optic nerve decompression. *Clinical Otolaryngology, 19*, 98–104.
2. DeKlotz, T. R., Stefko, S. T., Fernandez-Miranda, J. C., Gardner, P. A., Snyderman, C. H., & Wang, E. W. (2017). Endoscopic endonasal optic nerve decompression for fibrous dysplasia. *Journal of Neurological Surgery Part B, Skull Base, 78*(1), 24–29.
3. Liu, J. K., Christiano, L. D., Patel, S. K., Tubbs, R. S., & Eloy, J. A. (2011). Surgical nuances for removal of tuberculum sellae meningiomas with optic canal involvement using the endoscopic endonasal extended transsphenoidal transplanum transtuberculum approach. *Neurosurgical Focus, 30*(5), E2.
4. Mahmoud, M., Nader, R., & Al-Mefty, O. (2010). Optic canal involvement in tuberculum sellae meningiomas: Influence on approach, recurrence, and visual recovery. *Neurosurgery, 67*(3 Suppl Operative), ons108–ons118. 2010.
5. Margalit, N. S., Lesser, J. B., Moche, J., & Sen, C. (2003). Meningiomas involving the optic nerve: Technical aspects and outcomes for a series of 50 patients. *Neurosurgery, 53*(3), 523–532.
6. Sade, B., & Lee, J. H. (2009). High incidence of optic canal involvement in tuberculum sellae meningiomas: Rationale for aggressive skull base approach. *Surgical Neurology, 72*(2), 118–123.
7. Nozaki, K., Kikuta, K., Takagi, Y., Mineharu, Y., Takahashi, J. A., & Hashimoto, N. (2008). Effect of early optic canal unroofing on the outcome of visual functions in surgery for meningiomas of the tuberculum sellae and planum sphenoidale. *Neurosurgery, 62*(4), 839–844.
8. Koutourousiou, M., Fernandez-Miranda, J. C., Stefko, S. T., Wang, E. W., Snyderman, C. H., & Gardner, P. A. (2014). Endoscopic endonasal surgery for suprasellar meningiomas: Experience with 75 patients. *Journal of Neurosurgery, 120*(6), 1326–1339.
9. Nimmannitya, P., Goto, T., Terakawa, Y., Sato, H., Kawashima, T., Morisako, H., et al. (2016). Characteristic of optic canal invasion in 31 consecutive cases with tuberculum sellae meningioma. *Neurosurgical Review, 39*(4), 691–697.
10. Attia, M., Kandasamy, J., Jakimovski, D., Bedrosian, J., Alimi, M., Lee, D. L., et al. (2012). The importance and timing of optic canal exploration and decompression during endoscopic endonasal resection of tuberculum sella and planum sphenoidale meningiomas. *Neurosurgery, 71*, 58–67.
11. Kong, D. S., Hong, C. K., Hong, S. D., Nam, D. H., Lee, J. I., Seol, H. J., et al. (2018). Selection of endoscopic or transcranial surgery for tuberculum sellae meningiomas according to specific anatomical features: A retrospective multicenter analysis (KOSEN-002). *Journal of Neurosurgery, 18*, 1–10.
12. Renn, W. H., & Rhoton, A. L. (1975). Microsurgical anatomy of the sellar region. *Journal of Neurosurgery, 43*, 288–298.
13. Rubin, R. M., Sadun, A. A., & Piva, A. P. (2014). Optic chiasm, parasellar region, and pituitary fossa. In M. Yanoff & J. S. Duker (Eds.), *Ophthalmology* (4th ed., pp. 900–908). Oxford: Elsevier.
14. Truong, H. Q., Najera, E., Zanabria-Ortiz, R., et al. (2018). Surgical anatomy of the superior hypophyseal artery and its relevance for endoscopic endonasal surgery. *Journal of Neurosurgery, 13*, 1–9.
15. Sadun, A. A. (2014). Anatomy and physiology. In M. Yanoff & J. S. Duker (Eds.), *Ophthalmology* (4th ed., pp. 866–868). Oxford: Elsevier.

16. Goldberg, J. L. (2011). Optic nerve. In L. A. Levin, S. Nilsson, J. Ver HoeveJ, S. M. Wu, P. L. Kaufman, & A. Alm (Eds.), *Adler's physiology of the eye* (11th ed., pp. 550–573). Philadelphia: Elsevier.
17. Barham, H. P., Ramakrishnan, V. R., & Kingdom, T. T. (2019). Optic nerve decompression. In A. G. Chiu, J. N. Palmer, & N. D. Adappa (Eds.), *Atlas of endoscopic sinus and skull base surgery* (11th ed., pp. 550–573). Philadelphia: Elsevier.
18. Maniscalco, J. E., & Habal, M. B. (1978). Microanatomy of the optic canal. *Journal of Neurosurgery*, *48*(3), 402–406.
19. Abhinav, K., Acosta, Y., Wang, W. H., Bonilla, L. R., Koutourousiou, M., Wang, E., et al. (2015). Endoscopic endonasal approach to the optic canal: Anatomic considerations and surgical relevance. *Neurosurgery*, *11*(suppl 3), 431–445.
20. Fujii, K., Chambers, S. M., & Rhoton, A. L. Jr. (1979). Neurovascular relationships of the sphenoid sinus: A microsurgical study. *Journal of Neurosurgery*, *50*(1), 31–39.
21. Stammberger, H. R., Kennedy, D. W., & Anatomic Terminology Group. (1995). Paranasal sinuses: Anatomic terminology and nomenclature. *Annals of Otology. Rhinology & Laryngology Supplement*, *167*(Part 2), 7–16.
22. Gardner, P. A., Kassam, A. B., Thomas, A., Snyderman, C. H., Carrau, R. L., Mintz, A. H., et al. (2008). Endoscopic endonasal resection of anterior cranial base meningiomas. *Neurosurgery*, *63*(1), 36–52.
23. Fernandez-Miranda, J. C., Tormenti, M., Latorre, F., Gardner, P., & Snyderman, C. (2012). Endoscopic endonasal middle clindoiectomy: Anatomic, radiological, and technical note. *Neurosurgery*, *71*(2 Suppl Operative), ons233–ons239.
24. Erturk, M., Kayalioglu, G., & Govsa, F. (2004). Anatomy of the clinoidal region with special emphasis on the caroticoclinoid foramen and the interclinoid osseous bridge in a recent Turkish population. *Neurosurgical Review*, *27*(1), 22–26.
25. Efthymiou, E., Thanopoulou, V., Kozompoli, D., Kanellopoulou, V., Fratzoglou, M., Mytilinaios, D., et al. (2018). Incidence and morphometry of caoticoclinoid foramina in Greek dry human skulls. *Acta Neurochirurgica*, *160*(10), 1979–1987.

35

Transcranial Approaches to the Optic Apparatus

SHAHERYAR F. ANSARI, MD, GARNI BARKHOUDARIAN, MD, PhD, HOWARD KRAUS, MD, AND DANIEL F. KELLY, MD

Transcranial approaches to the optic apparatus include both traditional approaches, such as frontotemporal (pterional) and bifrontal craniotomies, as well as more recent minimally invasive keyhole approaches, including the supraorbital eyebrow approach and minipterional approach.[1-5] Given advances in understanding anatomy, instrumentation, and, perhaps most importantly, the addition of high-definition endoscopy, the use of these smaller, minimally invasive approaches is becoming increasingly incorporated into routine neurosurgical practice at many centers for pathology involving the optic apparatus and parasellar area.[6-11]

This chapter focuses on the use and limitations of the supraorbital and minipterional transcranial approaches for tumors affecting the optic apparatus, with minimal attention to the traditional larger approaches. Because it is addressed in other chapters, we do not discuss the use of the transorbital approach, which is being increasingly applied to skull base pathology. Attention is directed to the most common tumors approachable by these two keyhole routes, including meningiomas, craniopharyngiomas, intrinsic lesions of the optic apparatus and lamina terminalis, and metastatic tumors.[3,12-24] Because the optic apparatus is located centrally in the skull base, in close proximity to the circle of Willis, cavernous sinus, hypothalamus, infundibulum, and pituitary gland, many patients with tumors in this region may present with nonvisual symptoms, such as diplopia, endocrinopathy, personality changes and/or headache. In such patients, the goal of surgery is maximal safe tumor removal while preserving the integrity of the optic apparatus.

The keyhole supraorbital and minipterional transcranial approaches, when used and executed appropriately and with ideal neuroanesthetic techniques, low-profile instrumentation, and endoscopic assistance, offer excellent exposure to the optic apparatus.[7, 9,11,22-30] These two approaches have proven quite versatile and effective even for many large tumors that affect the optic nerves, chiasm, and optic tracts, although in some cases of very large tumors, a conventional large pterional or bifrontal craniotomy may be preferred.[11]

The advantage of these smaller keyhole approaches is that they provide access to the parasellar area, anterior, and middle cranial fossae with minimal exposure of the cerebral surface, without the need for brain retraction.[a] As such, these approaches allow access to the critical neurovascular structures of the skull base while reducing approach-related morbidity. Although the window to the area of interest is limited, the use of endoscopy as an adjunct to the microscope allows the surgeon to gain high-definition visualization, illumination, and access into the deep cisternal spaces.[b]

Choice of Approach: Supraorbital Versus Minipterional Versus Endonasal Versus Conventional Craniotomy

Several keyhole and conventional approaches allow surgeons to reach tumors affecting the optic apparatus. From a purely anatomic standpoint, given the midline location of the optic chiasm and optic nerves, most lesions that affect the optic apparatus can be approached from the supraorbital or endonasal routes. For tumors affecting the optic chiasm from below (predominantly pituitary adenomas, Rathke cleft cysts, and retrochiasmal craniopharyngiomas), the preferred approach is endonasal. For tumors impacting the optic apparatus from above, laterally, or those that push the optic chiasm posteriorly (predominantly meningiomas), the supraorbital approach is often preferred. For tumors that in part encircle an optic nerve or the chiasm, either an approach from above or below may be reasonable depending on the pathology and the goals of the surgery. For tumors with a significant extension or origin lateral to the optic nerves and tracts that grow into the middle fossa and the lateral orbit, a minipterional approach may be optimal. Finally, for very large, extensive tumors that involve both the middle and frontal fossae, orbit and that may impinge into the suprasellar cistern, a conventional frontotemporal (pterional) craniotomy may be preferred. We discuss some of the nuances in choosing the optimal approach for specific tumors with an emphasis on the use of the supraorbital and minipterional routes.

Use of Supraorbital and Minipterional Approaches

Indications and Choice of Approach

Intra-axial and extra-axial tumors of the anterior cranial fossa, anterior aspect of the middle fossa, and frontal lobe can be accessed

[a]References 6, 9, 10, 16,22, 24, 27, 31.

[b]References 16, 17, 21, 24, 25, 32, 33.

TABLE 35.1 Most Common Pathologies Approached by Supraorbital Craniotomy

Extra-Axial Tumors	Intra-Axial Tumors
Meningioma	Germinoma
Craniopharyngioma	Glioma
Pituitary adenoma	Metastatic carcinoma
Rathke cleft cyst	Lymphoma
Arachnoid cyst	

through the supraorbital and minipterional keyhole approaches. As detailed in Table 35.1, the most common tumors affecting the optic apparatus (including the intracranial optic nerves, chiasm, and optic tracts) and that are appropriate for the supraorbital or minipterional craniotomy are parasellar meningiomas, craniopharyngiomas, some gliomas, pituitary adenomas, and metastatic brain tumors.

Meningiomas arising from the tuberculum sellae and posterior planum region, anterior clinoid process, and in some instances, the medial sphenoid wing are ideally approached from the supraorbital route.[13] Some invasive parasellar meningiomas that have extensive sellar, cavernous sinus, and/or Meckel cave growth may need to be approached from the supraorbital route for optic apparatus decompression; however, many if not most of these can also be effectively debulked from the endonasal route. Regarding tuberculum sellae meningiomas, for which both endonasal and transcranial approaches are feasible, the three key factors in choosing the approach are tumor size, sellar depth, and lateral tumor extension. As we have previously described, ideal meningiomas for the endonasal route include those less than 3 cm without lateral extension beyond the optic nerves and supraclinoid carotid arteries and a deepened sella.[13] The remainder of tuberculum sella and anterior clinoidal meningiomas, including those that in part involve the medial sphenoid wing, can often be removed by a supraorbital or conventional frontotemporal craniotomy.

The supraorbital approach, which places the ipsilateral optic nerve directly in line with the route, creates a relative surgical blind spot along the undersurface of the ipsilateral optic nerve (Fig. 35.1). Meningiomas of the tuberculum sella elevate the nerve and chiasm and can often grow into the optic canal. Compression of the chiasm can cause a bitemporal hemianopsia, and stenosis of the optic canal by tumor can cause loss of visual acuity as well as variable visual field loss. This poses a challenge to the surgeon, as decompression of the optic canal may be required. Although the supraorbital approach does allow for bony decompression of the optic canal roof, the area inferior to the optic nerve ipsilateral to the approach is not visible in the line of sight of the microscope. Leaving this tumor behind risks continued visual disturbance and increases the likelihood of recurrence. Angled endoscopes and instruments allow the surgeon to visualize and reach under the ipsilateral nerve and remove tumors in this location.

Craniopharyngiomas pose a particular challenge as they can have a variable relationship with the optic nerves and chiasm. Given that most craniopharyngiomas are retrochiasmal in location, resulting in a prefixed chiasm (Fig. 35.2), they are best approached from an endonasal route to minimize manipulation of the optic apparatus. This approach also typically puts the surgical trajectory along the long-axis of the tumor. Craniopharyngiomas that arise

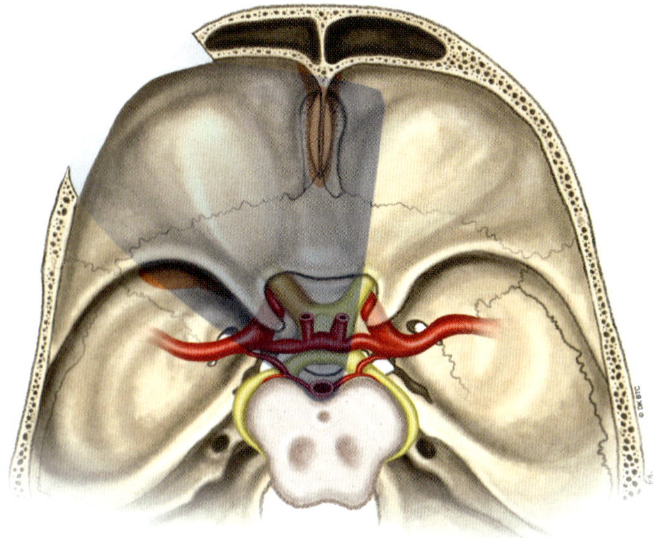

• **Fig. 35.1** Drawing of supraorbital craniotomy showing range of exposure (*blue shading*) and three potential blind spots (highlighted in *orange*), including the anterior cribiform plate area, the inferior to the ipsilateral optic nerve, and the ipsilateral sphenoid wing area. Notably, all of these areas can typically be well visualized and accessed with the aid of angled endoscopy.

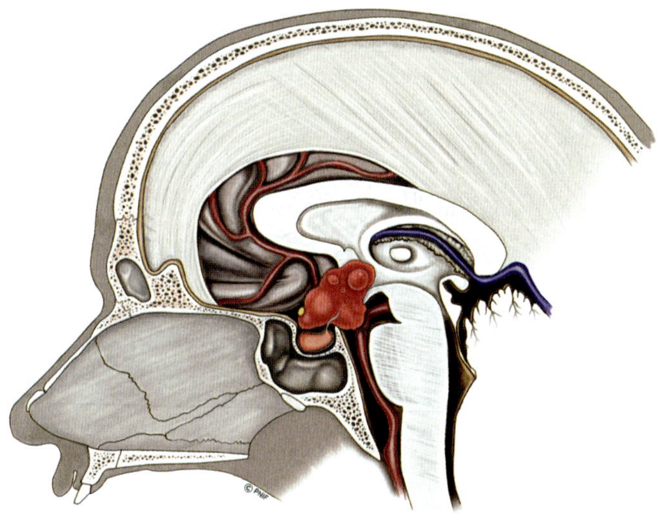

• **Fig. 35.2** Drawing of a retrochiasmal craniopharyngioma causing a prefixed chiasm (*yellow*).

anterior to the optic chiasm (postfixed chiasm), or elevate it superiorly (Fig. 35.3), or which have suprachiasmatic anterolateral extensions into the frontal and middle fossae, can often be approached transcranially (in most cases via the supraorbital approach rather than the minipterional approach). Pituitary adenomas with exophytic supradiaphragmatic extensions can similarly be removed from the supraorbital approach, whereas the minipterional route is rarely needed.

Gliomas, lymphomas, germinomas, and metastatic lesions affecting or intrinsic to the optic apparatus are often ideally approached via the supraorbital or minipterional route given that these tumor types are typically above the plane of the optic apparatus (and in the case of gliomas and metastases are intra-axial). As shown in the case example later in this chapter, germinomas often

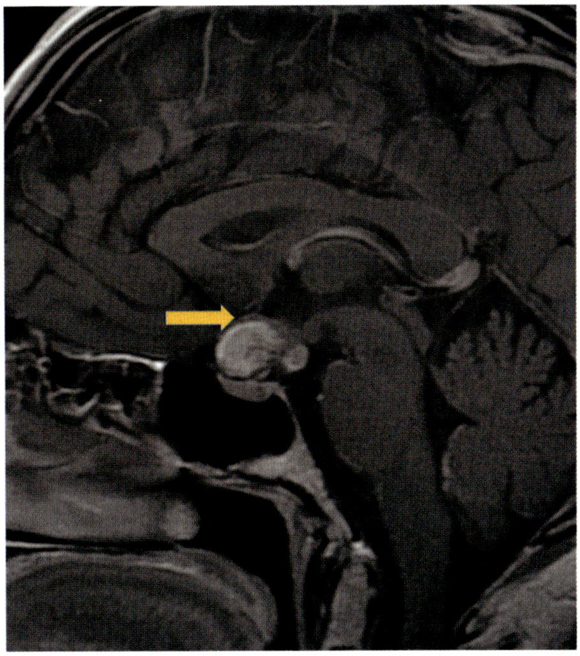

• **Fig. 35.3** Sagittal postcontrast magnetic resonance imaging scan showing an elevated chiasm displaced by a suprasellar craniopharyngioma.

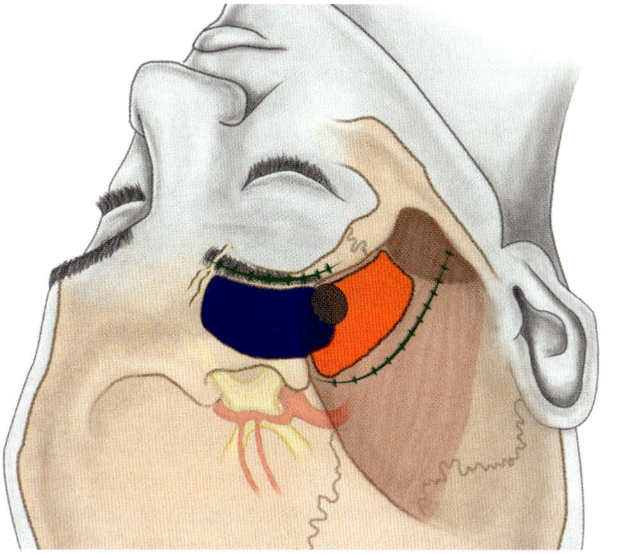

• **Fig. 35.4** Drawing showing the relative positions and overlap of the supraorbital (*blue*) and minipterional (*orange*) incisions and craniotomies, as well as relevant landmarks including the superior temporal line and supraorbital nerve.

extend up along the infundibulum and may invade the lamina terminalis; as such, the supraorbital route with endoscopic assistance is ideal for accessing this area. In our practice, the supraorbital route, relative to the minipterional route, is favored for accessing anterior cranial fossa and parasellar lesions, as well those extending into the proximal sylvian fissure and medial temporal lobe, and is used almost five times as often as the minipterional route.

The traditional pterional craniotomy is a workhorse approach in neurosurgery, allowing access to the entire circle of Willis, sylvian fissure, optic apparatus, pituitary gland and infundibulum, and the base of the skull in the anterior and middle cranial fossae. The minimally invasive variant of this approach allows similar access to all of these structures, with the only limitation access to the distal sylvian fissure. As detailed in Table 35-2, the minipterional approach is particularly well suited for lesions that are predominantly in the middle fossa with extension to the ipsilateral optic nerve and chiasm, as well as tumors that extend into the orbit or traverse the superior orbital fissure. Meningiomas are by far the most common tumor approached via the minipterional route, which is particularly effective for sphenoid wing meningiomas that invade the orbital apex and/or optic canal. Bony decompression of the optic canal, orbital apex, and orbit can be accomplished via the minipterional route. Sphenoid wing meningiomas are relatively easy to access with this approach, as the lateral aspect of the wing is drilled and the tumors present themselves close to the surface, as seen in the later example. An anterior clinoidectomy can also be performed extradurally or intradurally. The limitation of the minipterional approach, as with most keyhole approaches, is the difficulty getting light to the deep structures. This is overcome by introducing the endoscope to look up close at the neurovascular structures of the skull base, as well as around corners and into blind spots. This can aid the surgeon in finding small remnants of tumors and improve the likelihood of a complete resection. Fig. 35.4 indicates the overlap and the difference between minipterional and supraorbital approaches. The minipterional approach is better suited for lateral orbital apex and optic canal lesions, whereas the subraorbital approach is ideal for lesions involving the entire optic apparatus.

TABLE 35.2 Most Common Pathologies Approached by Minipterional Craniotomy

Extra-Axial Tumors	Intra-Axial Tumors
Meningioma	Glioma
Optic nerve sheath tumor	Metastatic carcinoma
Orbital tumors	Lymphoma

Nuances of Endoscopy and Endoscope-Assisted Transcranial Tumor Removal

For most tumor resection with either endoscopy or endoscope-assisted approaches, the microscope provides excellent visualization and illumination, and in some instances, the endoscope is of little value. However, for certain anatomic regions and to better understand key neurovascular-tumor relationships, the endoscope is invaluable. The most common utility for the panoramic angled visualization provided by the endoscope is visualization of the region behind or under the optic nerve or chiasm or overlying brain without retraction. Provided a potential intracranial space has been created, the endoscope can be brought into this space and illuminate what cannot be seen by the microscope. In most instances, this means that most of the tumor has already been debulked, the brain is relaxed, and there is sufficient space to maneuver effectively and safely to determine if additional tumor can be safely removed. Using the endoscope at this stage of the surgery in most instances allows one to see these spaces without directly retracting the optic apparatus or the brain, which is otherwise necessitated if one is using only the line-of-sight visualization of the microscope. For an already compromised optic nerve or chiasm, even minimal manipulation may lead to permanent vision damage.

The endoscope thus allows visualization of parts of the skull base around the optic apparatus that are otherwise too risky to clearly visualize with the microscope alone. This up-close endoscopic view, however, comes with several of its own risks. First, given the small opening, there is the potential for instrument conflict and poor maneuverability. Second, the actual heat of the endoscope light must be appreciated and proximity to the optic apparatus and associated vasculature must be respected. Decreasing the light intensity and frequent irrigation can help mitigate this effect. Third, the surgical team must continually be cognizant of the passage of instruments in and out of the field. In laparoscopic or thoracoscopic surgeries, a port is placed that enables safe passage of instruments without traumatizing superficial tissues. This is not possible in cranial surgery, as the instruments and the endoscope are advanced through the same opening. This requires extra caution and coordination on the part of the surgical team to maintain a coaxial view of the instruments upon entry through the craniotomy. This maneuvering is complicated by the need to maintain a two-handed surgical technique. Although various endoscope holding arms are available, the authors recommend that a skilled assistant should drive the endoscope, as this allows for dynamic focus to be maintained over the entire surgical field both superficially and in the deep parts of the field, using synchronized movements of the endoscope, as instruments are inserted and removed throughout the procedure.

Surgical Technique: General Room Setup and Essential Instrumentation for Keyhole Surgery in the Optic Apparatus Region

Given that the endoscope will be used for at least part of the procedure, the room monitor should be set up with this need in mind (Fig. 35.5 A, B) so that it can be swung into position easily when the endoscopes are used. Rigid-4 mm 0-, 30-, and 45-degree rod-lens endoscopes are ideal. Additionally, given the relatively restricted opening of the supraorbital and minipterional approaches, keyhole low-profile bayoneted or pistol-grip instrumentation should be used. Other essential equipment include the Doppler probe for vessel localization, two-dimensional ultrasonography for assessing completeness of tumor removal, with aneurysm clips and appliers readily available. Consideration should also be given to evoked potential monitoring, including somatosensory evoked potentials and motor evoked potentials depending upon the pathology. If it is anticipated that the frontal sinus will be entered, the right or left lower quadrant of the abdomen should be prepared to harvest a fat graft.

Surgical Technique: Supraorbital Craniotomy

The supraorbital craniotomy was first described by Fedor Kraus in 1908[34] and was subsequently modified with a decrease in the size of the bony opening while preserving access to the skull base as described by Reisch et al. in 2003.[6] The supraorbital craniotomy is now considered a workhorse approach to access the anterior cranial fossa and optic apparatus. Fig. 35.1 shows the broad access to the base of the skull allowed by this approach. The patient is placed supine on the operating table with the head in a Mayfield clamp. The head is turned to the contralateral side, typically 20 to 45 degrees depending on the pathology, and extended so that the malar eminence is the most prominent part of the head (Fig. 35.6 A, B). The degree of turning is dependent on the location of the pathology; more medial pathology requires more of a head turn. For a typical tuberculum sella meningioma, a 30-degree head turn with the malar eminence prominent is ideal. Intraoperative navigation is used as an adjunct to localize the lateral border of the frontal sinus as well as intermittently throughout the procedure to localize relevant anatomy.

The incision is made within the eyebrow to minimize a visible scar (Fig. 35.7A), starting from just medial to the

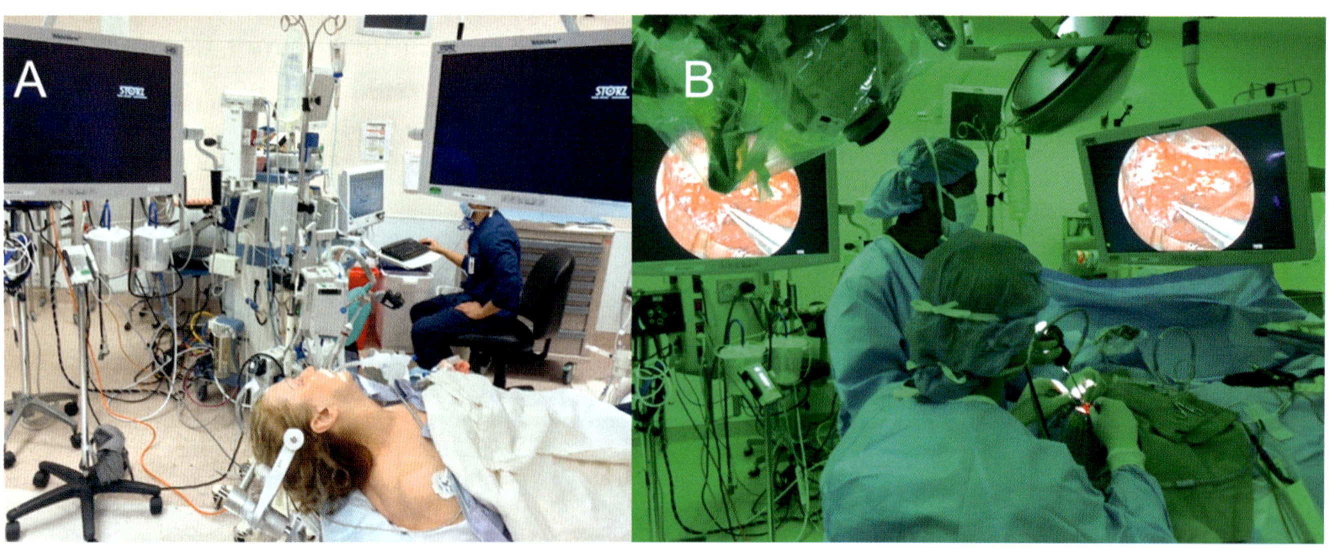

• **Fig. 35.5** Room setup for intracranial endoscopy. A, Positioning of a patient and room setup for right supraorbital craniotomy for both microscope and endoscope-assisted surgery with the monitors positioned to easily swing into position for endoscopy. B, Endoscopic portion of the operation with microscope swung out of position, surgeon sitting, and endoscope being driven by assistant.

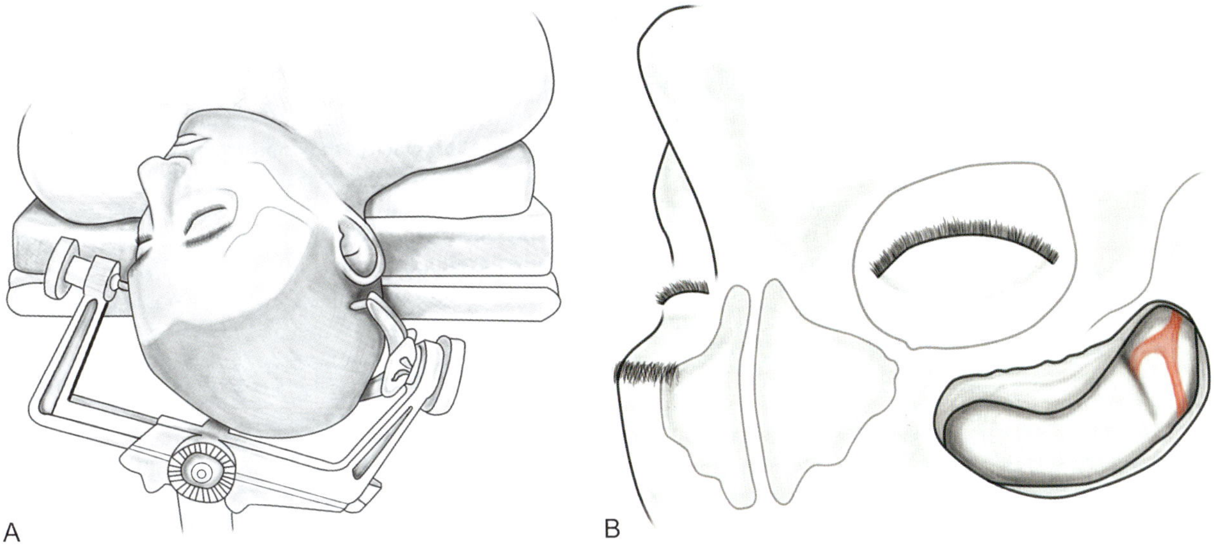

• **Fig. 35.6** A, Head positioning for supraorbital approach. B, Position of the craniotomy relative to the frontal sinus and exposure of the skull base.

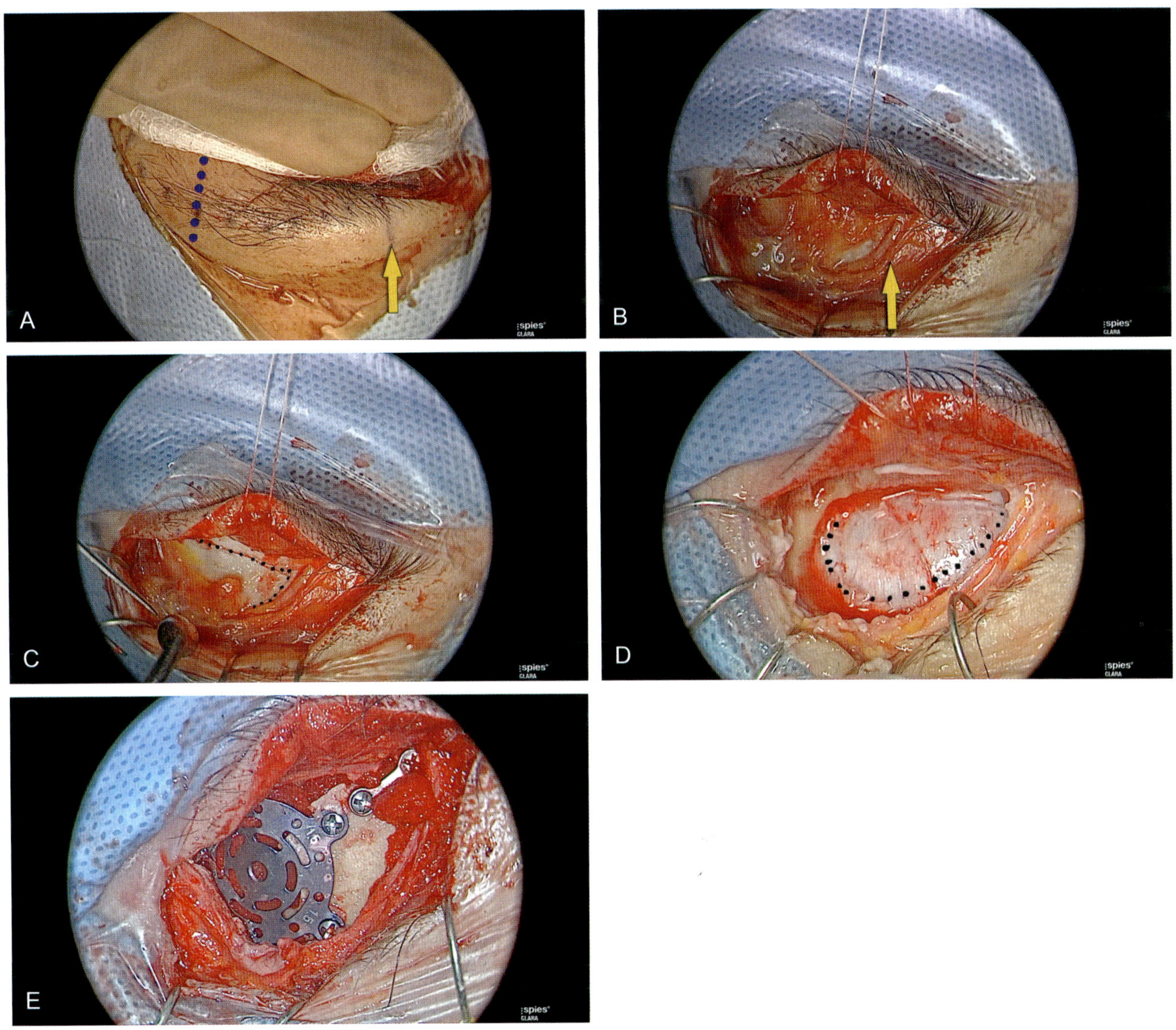

• **Fig. 35.7** A, Incision of supraorbital approach, intraoperative photo. Supraorbital notch (*black arrow).* Temporal line (*dotted line*). B, Exposure of pericranium (*black arrow,* supraorbital nerve). C, Pericranial incision (*dotted line*). D, Supraorbital exposure after skull base drilling. Dural incision (*dotted line*). E, Plated bone flap.

supraorbital notch to just beyond the superior temporal line. The lateral termination may need to extend a few millimeters beyond the termination of the eyebrow for adequate incision length. The subcutaneous tissues are opened sharply until the pericranium is reached. A stitch is placed through the skin and subcutaneous tissues of the inferior aspect of the incision for gentle retraction. The supraorbital nerve is then dissected out bluntly with scissors and carefully preserved (Fig. 35.7B). The pericranium is incised just above the supraorbital rim from the supraorbital nerve medially, to the superior temporal line, continuing along the temporalis fascia and muscle down to bone (Fig. 35.7C). An intersecting cut is made parallel and immediately lateral to the supraorbital nerve, and the pericranium directly over the site of the craniotomy is elevated superiorly. Multiple fish hooks are placed for gentle but effective superior retraction. Achieving adequate superior exposure is critical to the success of the eyebrow craniotomy. A bone flap that is less than 2 cm in height will be very restricting for the procedure and potentially unsafe to adequately maneuver and perform microneurosurgery. The high-speed drill with matchstick bit is used to create a burr hole at the keyhole just behind the frontozygomatic process. The dura is carefully stripped away from the inner table and the craniotome is used to fashion a craniotomy that is approximately 2.5 cm width and 2.0 cm high. If the frontal sinus is entered, a piece of Gelfoam (Pfizer, Groton, NY) or collagen soaked in betadine is placed inside for the duration of the procedure. Small openings can be sealed off with bone wax, but larger openings need to be obliterated and reinforced with an abdominal fat graft. The dura is dissected off the floor of the anterior cranial fossa, and the matchstick bit is again used to thin down the inner table of the frontal bone and the roof of the orbit, making a flat plane (Fig. 35.7D).

The dura is opened in a curvilinear fashion based on the floor and tacked back with a stitch. The first intradural maneuver should attain brain relaxation by opening the subarachnoid cisterns; the opticocarotid, prechiasmatic, and carotid-oculomotor cisterns are accessible, and whichever of these is not obstructed by the pathology should be opened and drained of cerebrospinal fluid (CSF). This allows the frontal lobe to fall away from the frontal fossa floor and create space to work. For large tumors with obstruction of these cisterns, the surgeon should be prepared for brain herniation and inform the anesthesiologist accordingly to perform the required maneuvers of head elevation, hyperventilation, and osmotic diuresis. When there is no access to CSF spaces, rapid debulking of the tumor is required to relieve the pressure on the brain. In extreme cases, pial violation and resection of inferior frontal gyri or gyrus rectus may be required to obtain adequate brain relaxation. The brain should be covered by telfa or collagen for protection; no fixed retractor is necessary. The subsequent dissection and removal of pathology depends on the individual lesion. The falciform ligament can be sectioned to aid in decompression of the optic canal. The reconstruction is performed by reapproximating the dura and closing off the frontal sinus with an abdominal fat graft, if it was entered with the craniotomy. The entire opening is then covered with collagen sponge (Helistat, Integra LifeSciences, Plainsboro, NJ). Fibrin glue is optional. The bone flap is plated with a low-profile plating system using a burr hole cover and a short straight plate medially (Fig. 35.7E), which is secured so that there is no gap on the superior aspect of the exposure to prevent a cosmetically unappealing dent in the forehead. The inferior bone gap that is directly under the eyebrow is then filled in with bone cement, which helps prevent CSF egress into the subdural space and enhances cosmesis. Once hemostasis is obtained, closure is performed in layers by first approximating the pericranium and then closing the subcutaneous tissue and dermis with absorbable stitches. No skin glue is used in the eyebrow, and a gentle compressive ace head wrap is applied for 24 to 48 hours.

Case Examples

Case 1

A 29-year-old woman presented with progressive right-sided headaches that ultimately prompted magnetic resonance imaging (MRI) revealing a large ($5 \times 5 \times 6$ cm), homogeneously enhancing mass extending superiorly from the medial sphenoid wing with hyperostosis of the right sphenoid bone (Fig. 35.8), consistent with a clinoidal and sphenoid wing meningioma, causing significant distortion of the right optic nerve and chiasm. She had a nonfocal neurologic examination including normal visual acuity and fields. Given the large tumor size, she underwent attempted tumor embolization of the external carotid arterial supply, but the angiogram showed vascularity primarily derived from the ophthalmic artery (Fig. 35.9 A,B), resulting in termination of the procedure.

The patient was subsequently taken to the operating room for a right supraorbital eyebrow craniotomy for tumor resection. The exposure was performed as described earlier and the brain was found to be quite full upon dural opening. As the tumor obstructed the pathway to the parasellar cisterns, the tumor was entered and debulked until the top of the tumor was separated from the base. This technique eventually allowed access to the carotid-oculomotor cistern, which relaxed the brain considerably. This maneuver allowed arachnoidal dissection to proceed along the dome of the tumor to separate it from the brain, alternating with debulking using ultrasonic aspiration. There were discrete regions of pial invasion with vascularity from the brain. As the most posterior extent of the tumor was removed, the right frontal horn was entered and sealed with collagen and fibrin glue. The tumor base along the clinoid and anterior cranial fossa was then carefully dissected free. Doppler ultrasonography was used periodically to identify and attempt to map the course of the supraclinoid carotid artery, and somatosensory evoked potentials were monitored throughout the operation. As the resection proceeded, significant bleeding was encountered along the clinoid portion of the tumor. This was further evaluated and found to be a dural arterial supply to the tumor, which was controlled with standard hemostatic measures. Endoscopy was used to look over the edge of the sphenoid wing and ensure no tumor remained in the middle fossa, as well as to look under the ipsilateral optic nerve to confirm this was clear of tumor. The reconstruction was performed as described earlier. The patient awoke with no postoperative deficit except an expected right frontalis paresis. The postoperative MRI (Fig. 35.10) showed a greater than 98% resection with a small residual, which has been stable over 3 years since surgery (Fig. 35.11). The pathology indicated a World Health Organization (WHO) I meningioma with a slightly increased proliferation index of 10% with positive estrogen receptor staining. Her frontalis weakness normalized by 3 months after surgery.

Case 2

A 20-year-old male presented with a 3-month history of vision loss in the right eye. The vision loss worsened and progressed

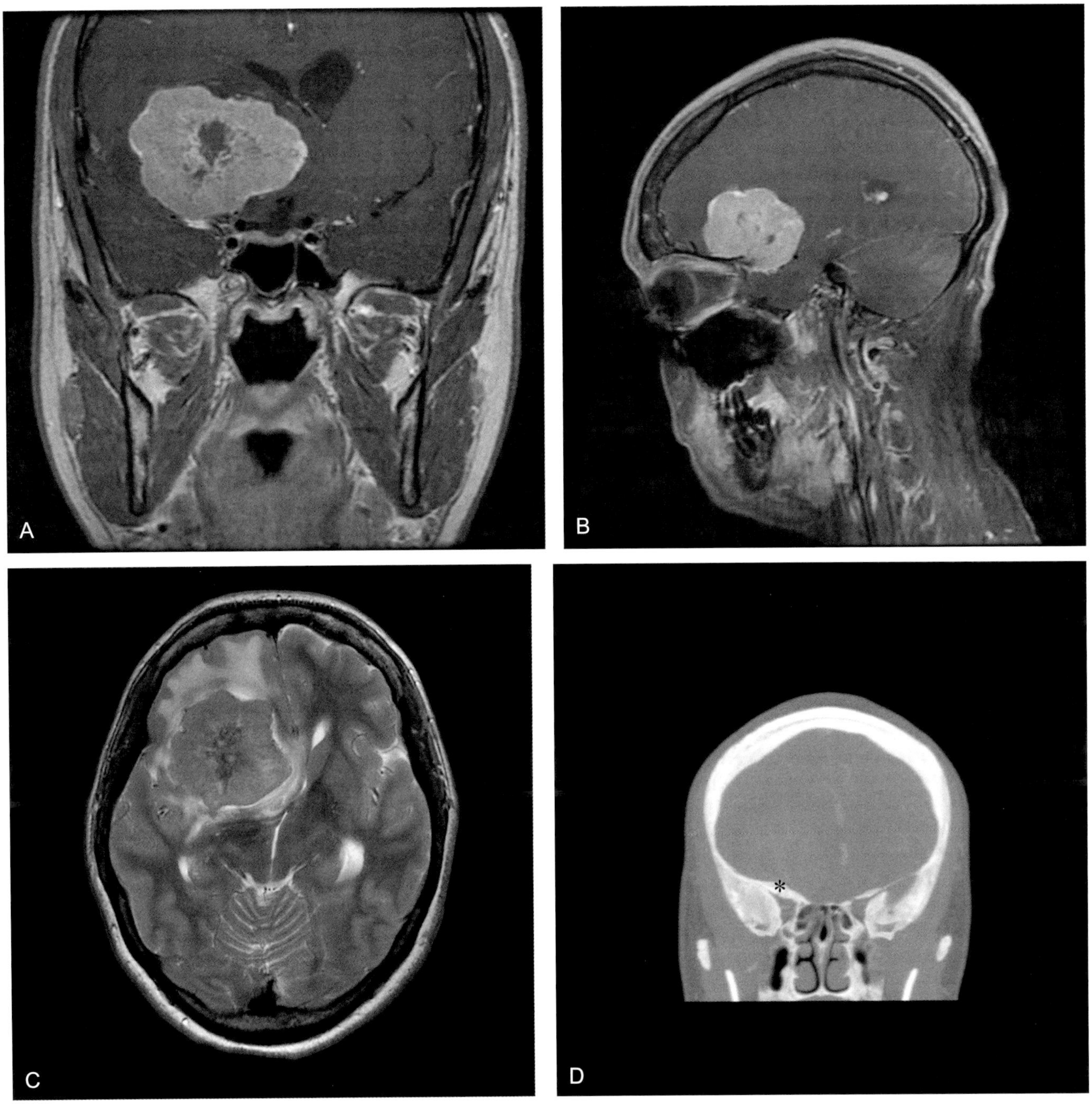

• **Fig. 35.8** A, Preoperative magnetic resonance imaging (MRI) scan for patient in Case 1 (coronal postcontrast T1). B, Preoperative MRI scan for patient in Case 1 (sagittal postcontrast T1). C, Preoperative MRI scan for patient in Case 1 (axial T2 showing significant vasogenic edema). D, Computed tomography angiography scan of patient in Case 1 showing hyperostosis (*asterisk*).

to include the left eye, and the patient began having difficulty reading road signs. An initial MRI scan was interpreted as normal. He then presented with polydipsia and polyuria and was admitted to the hospital with a sodium level of 160 mg/dL. He was treated for presumed diabetes insipidus. A repeat MRI scan at this time showed a thickened optic chiasm and lamina terminalis with abnormal enhancement extending up along the infundibulum almost to the hypothalamus (Fig. 35.12). Upon examination, the patient had 20/100 vision in his left eye and a bitemporal superior quadrantanopsia. The patient underwent a lumbar puncture for CSF tumor markers, which revealed a normal cytologic profile and no diagnostic tumor markers. Given the uncertain diagnosis and his progressive visual decline and diabetes insipidus, he was taken to the operating room for a left supraorbital craniotomy for biopsy of the chiasmal–lamina terminalis lesion. The exposure was undertaken in the fashion described earlier and there was entry into the frontal sinus, which was filled with betadine-soaked Gelfoam sponge. Under microscopic vision, the left opticocarotid cistern was opened for brain relaxation. The ipsilateral optic nerve was identified and followed to the

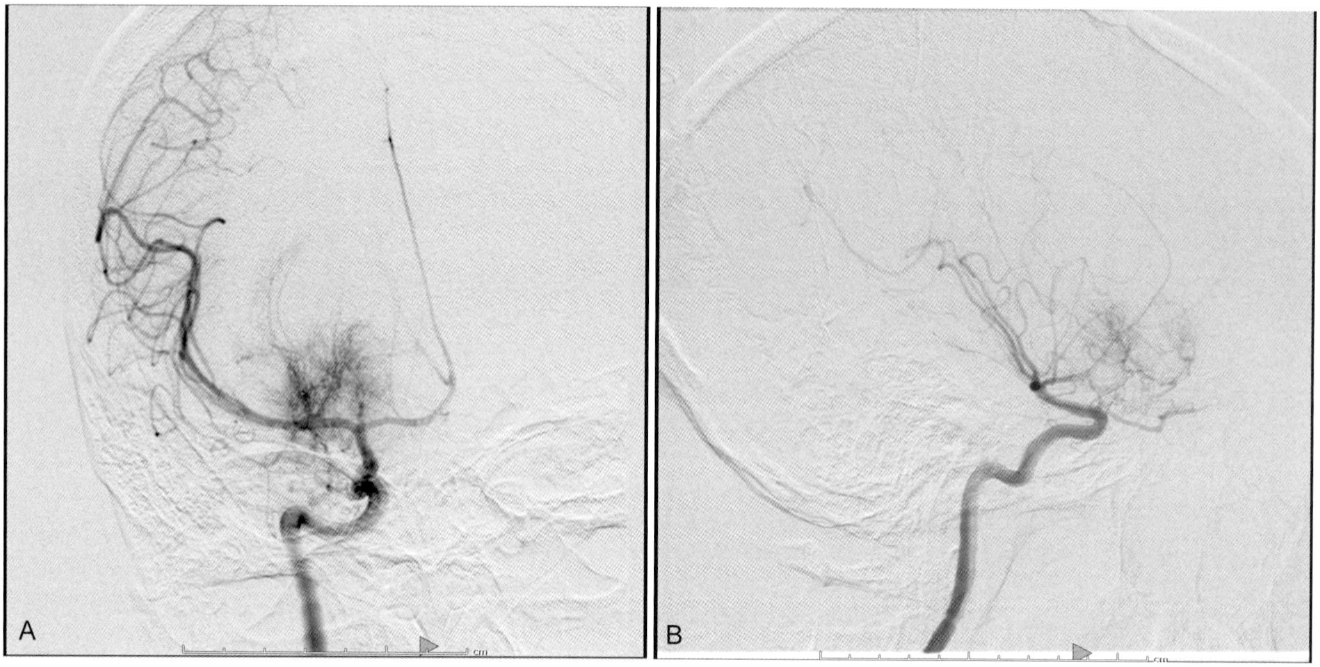

• **Fig. 35.9** A, Preoperative anteroposterior cerebral angiogram of patient in Case 1. B, Lateral view of angiogram.

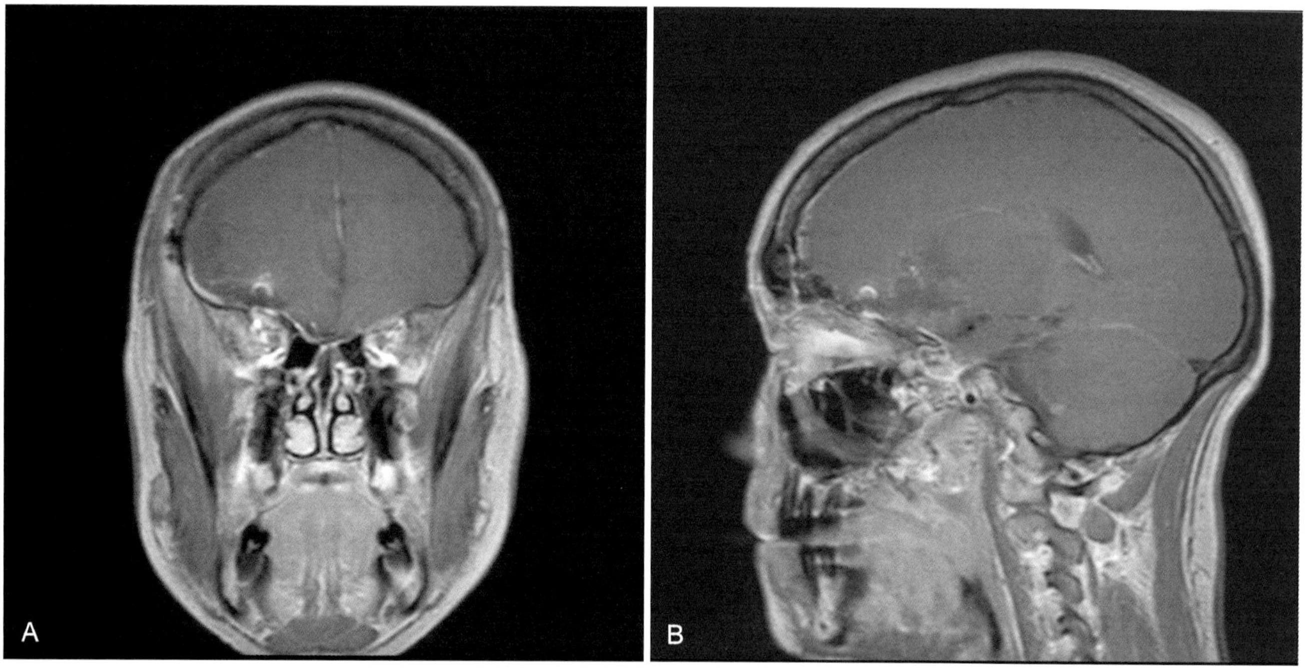

• **Fig. 35.10** A, Immediate postoperative magnetic resonance imaging scan for patient in Case 1 (postcontrast coronal T1). B, Sagittal postcontrast T1 image.

optic chiasm. The arachnoid was opened sharply at the interface of the left optic nerve and chiasm with the overlying frontal lobe, allowing exposure posterior to the chiasm and lamina terminalis region, all of which was clearly abnormally expanded by tumor (Fig. 35.13). At this point, the 30-degree endoscope was used for ideal visualization of the lamina terminalis and anterior cerebral arteries, without the need for brain retractors. Once the navigation probe confirmed the enhancing lesion in this location, the abnormal-appearing area of the lamina terminalis was biopsied, confirming a diagnosis of germinoma. After hemostasis, the dura was closed, the frontal sinus breach was repaired with an abdominal fat graft, and a layered collagen reconstruction was performed. The remainder of the closure proceeded in the usual fashion. The patient had an uneventful postoperative recovery with no further deterioration in his vision and persistent hypopituitarism. His transient left frontalis palsy resolved after 6 months and he went into remission of his germinoma with chemotherapy and stereotactic radiotherapy.

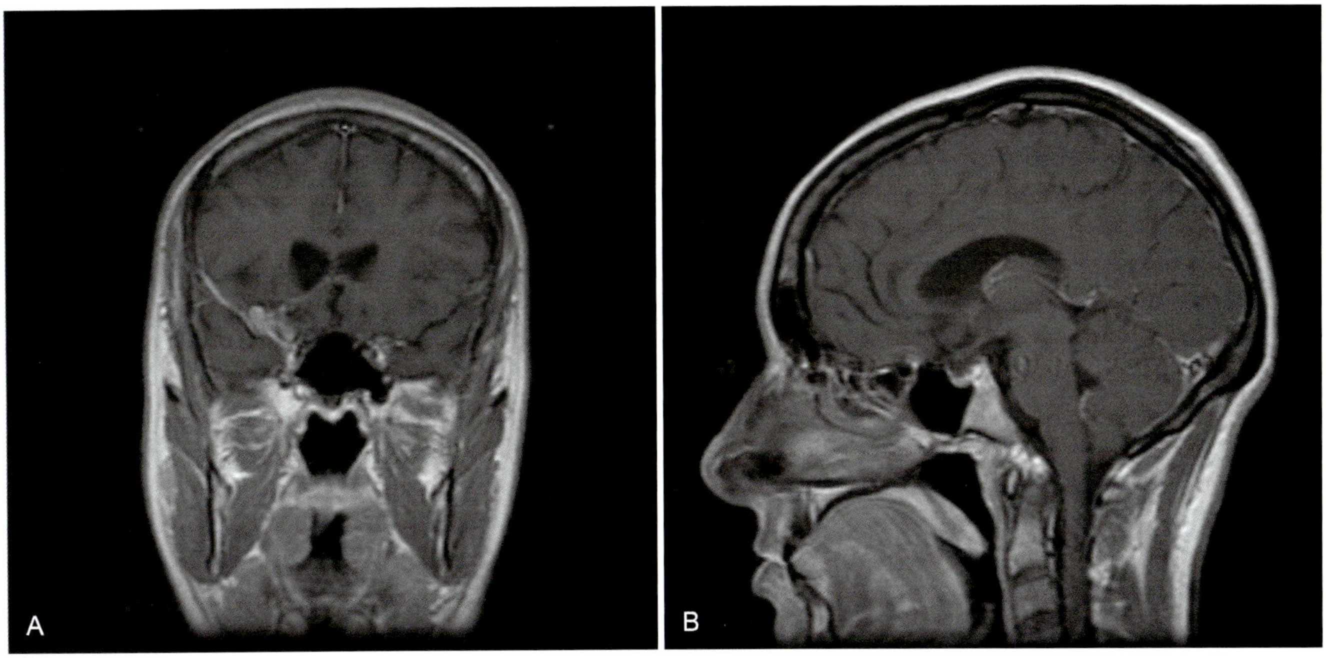

• **Fig. 35.11** A, One-year postoperative magnetic resonance imaging scan (coronal postcontrast T1) showing no recurrence. B, Sagittal T1 image after contrast.

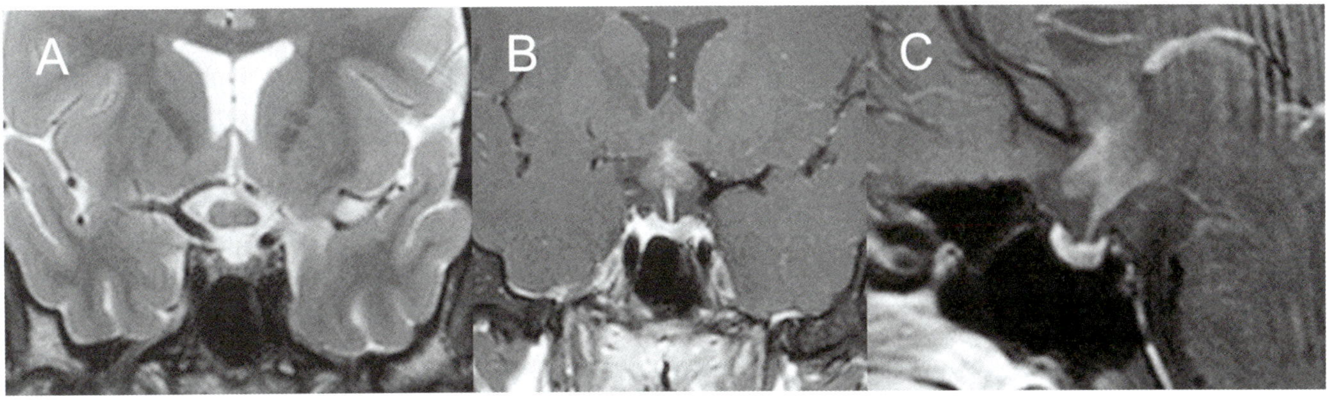

• **Fig. 35.12** Preoperative magnetic resonance imaging scan for patient in Case 2 of chiasmal and lamina terminals germinoma. A, Coronal T2; B, coronal T1 postgadolinium; and C, sagittal T1 postgadolinium scans showing enlarged and enhancing infundibulum, chiasm, and lamina terminalis.

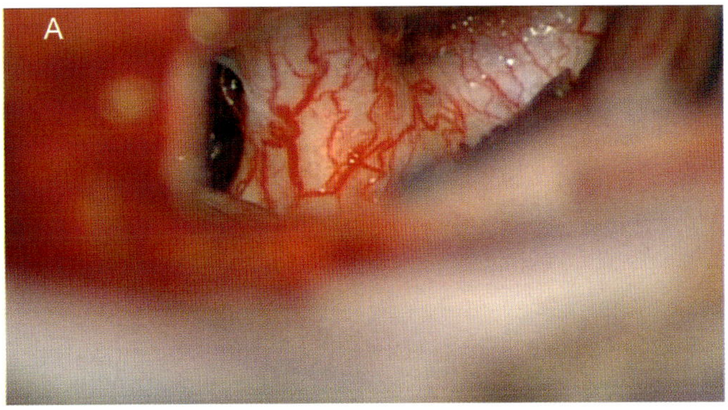

• **Fig. 35.13** A, Intraoperative microscopic view of patient in Case 2 via left supraorbital craniotomy showing a partial view of the left optic nerve, chiasm, and right optic nerve.

Continued

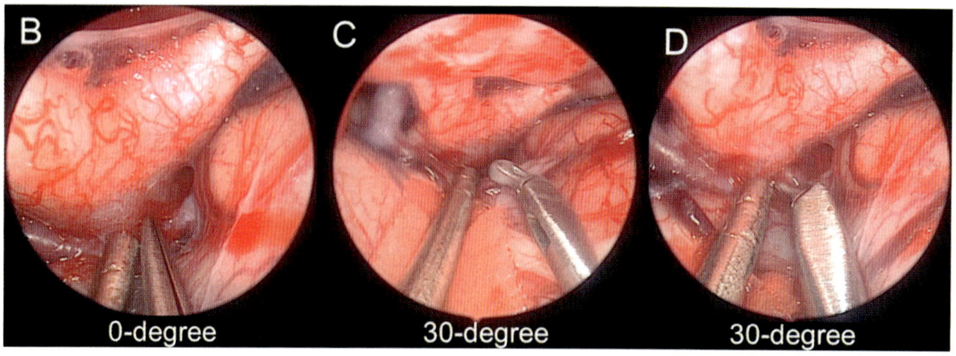

• **Fig. 35.13, cont'd** Intraoperative endoscopic view in Case 2 via left supraorbital craniotomy showing a more complete view with (B) 0-degree and (C, D) 30-degree endoscope facilitating lamina terminalis biopsy without a retractor.

Case 3

A 70-year-old woman presented with a 20-year history of vision loss of the left eye for which she underwent cataract surgery. Her left eye vision remained diminished after surgery but then progressively worsened several years later. She was evaluated by various ophthalmologists until an MRI scan of her brain was ordered and revealed a left planum and clinoidal mass with displacement of the optic nerve, consistent with a meningioma. She was found to have 20/200 vision in her left eye with an inferior altitudinal defect. Her MRI (Fig. 35.14) scan showed a 13 × 15 mm homogeneously enhancing, extra-axial mass based on the clinoid with severe lateral compression of the left optic nerve and contact with the optic chiasm. She underwent a left supraorbital craniotomy for tumor resection. At surgery, the prechiasmatic cistern and proximal sylvian fissure were easily opened for excellent brain relaxation. The tumor separated well from the carotid, and as it was debulked, the mass effect on the optic chiasm was also reduced. Ultimately, the entire optic nerve was able to be exposed from the chiasm to the optic canal. The 30-degree endoscope was then introduced to evaluate the inferior and medial portions of the optic nerve (Fig. 35.15). A fibrous remnant remained densely adhered to the proximal carotid and optic nerve, and this small remnant was left behind. The patient awoke from surgery with improved vision. Her mild left frontalis paresis (Fig. 35.16) resolved within 3 months. Pathology studies confirmed a typical WHO grade I meningioma. Her postoperative MRI scans have shown a small (Fig. 35.17) 6 × 5 mm tumor remnant along the left optic nerve and clinoid that has remained stable at 1 year after surgery.

Surgical Approach: Minipterional Craniotomy

The minipterional craniotomy was first described by Figueiredo et al. in 2007[35] and is a modification of the traditional pterional craniotomy described by Yasargil and Fox in 1975.[5] As shown in Fig. 35.18, the key structure to expose is the pterion (sphenoid wing), the removal of which allows access to the cisterns, circle of Willis, and optic apparatus.[14,35] The minipterional approach demonstrates that it is not strictly necessary to expose large surfaces of the frontal and temporal lobes to accomplish the goals of surgery around the base of the skull.[30] As in the supraorbital approach,

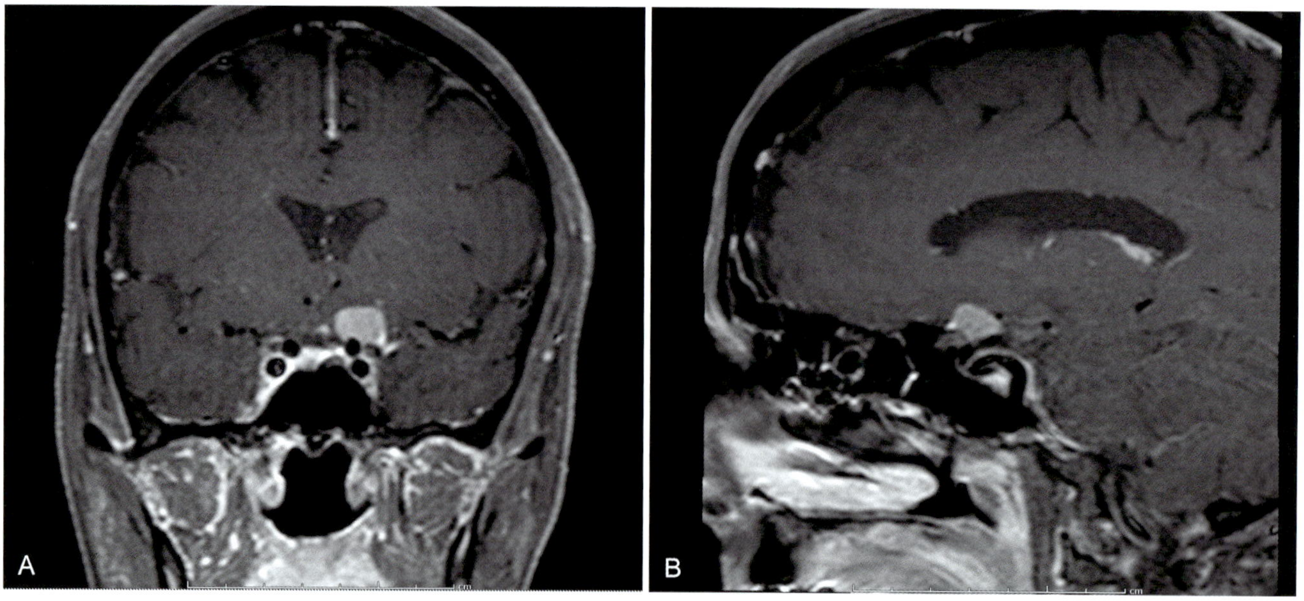

• **Fig. 35.14** A, Preoperative magnetic resonance imaging scan of patient in Case 3 (coronal T1 postcontrast) showing clinoidal enhancing lesion. B, Sagittal postcontrast T1 image.

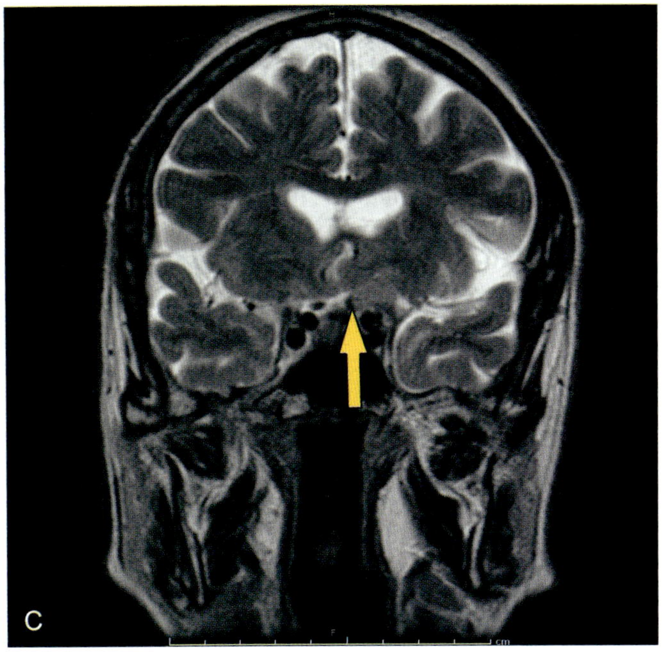

• **Fig. 35.14, cont'd** C, Coronal T2 image showing displacement of the optic nerve (*yellow arrow*).

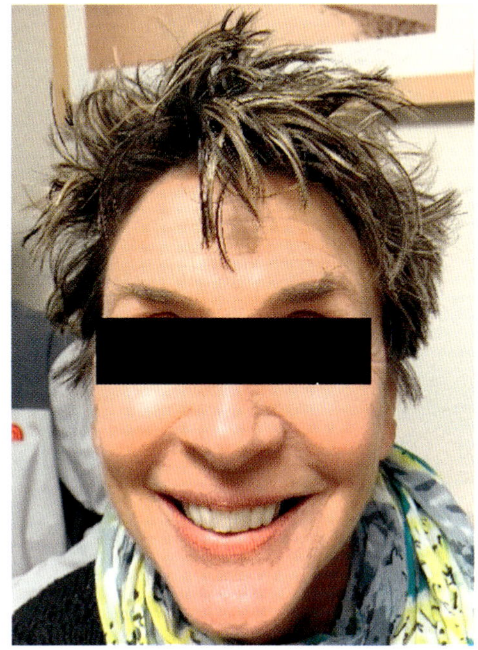

• **Fig. 35.16** Photo of patient in Case 3 at 3 months with resolution of scar and frontalis palsy.

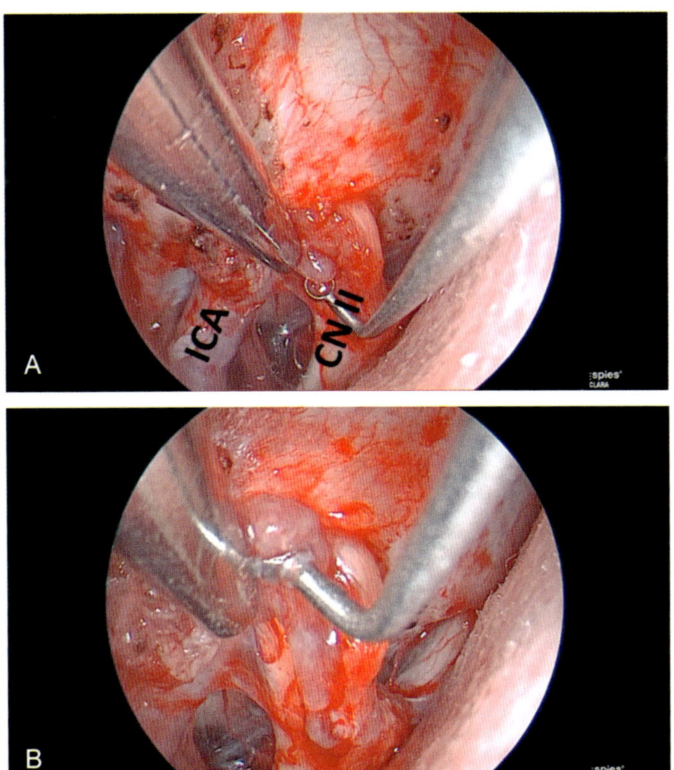

• **Fig. 35.15** A, B, Intraoperative photos showing a 30-degree endoscopic view of removing additional tumor along the superolateral aspect of the left optic nerve. A small remnant of densely adherent tumor was left attached to optic nerve.

endoscopy is a useful and important adjunct to improve visualization in the region. The patient's head is placed in a similar fashion as for a standard pterional craniotomy, with the neck extended and the head turned based on the pathology.

A 3- to 4-cm, curvilinear incision is made starting at the zygoma and curving anteriorly toward the orbital rim.[8,9,35,36] The incision is placed more anterior than the traditional pterional incision but remains at or behind the hairline for cosmesis[11] (Fig. 35.18, large image). It is imperative that the incision not be placed anterior to the midpoint of the zygoma to avoid injury to the frontalis branch of the facial nerve. Additionally, the temporalis muscle and fascia are elevated in a myocutaneous fashion, again to protect the frontalis branch.[37] For most optic apparatus lesions, particularly pathology in the optic canal or lateral orbital apex, dissecting the temporalis muscle inferoposteriorly allows optimum access to these structures.

The burr hole is made as usual at the keyhole. The dura is carefully stripped from the inner table and the floor of the anterior cranial fossa is identified. A craniotome is then used to complete the opening. Using a matchstick or diamond bit, the pterion is drilled to flatten the roof of the orbit and sphenoid wing (Fig. 35.18A). The meningo-orbital band is identified, coagulated, and sectioned, allowing the dura to be elevated as far medially as the cavernous sinus, if necessary. For dural-based lesions, this allows early devascularization of the tumor before dural opening.[8] The dura is opened in a curvilinear fashion based on the pterion and retracted back with tacking sutures (Fig. 35.18B). As with the supraorbital approach, the first maneuver should relax the brain by releasing CSF. This is most easily performed by opening the opticocarotid cistern (Fig. 35.18C). This allows the frontal lobe to fall away from the floor of the anterior cranial fossa and exposes the optic nerve and chiasm. The pathology can then be addressed. The opening can be modified in a superior or inferior direction as needed based on the pathology and can reach as low as the floor of the middle cranial fossa if needed. As with the supraorbital approach, the falciform ligament can be sectioned to help decompress the optic canal. The more lateral approach afforded by the minipterional also allows drilling of the optic strut for inferolateral optic canal decompression if needed. This approach can nicely access the orbital apex and the entire length of the orbit. Reconstruction entails

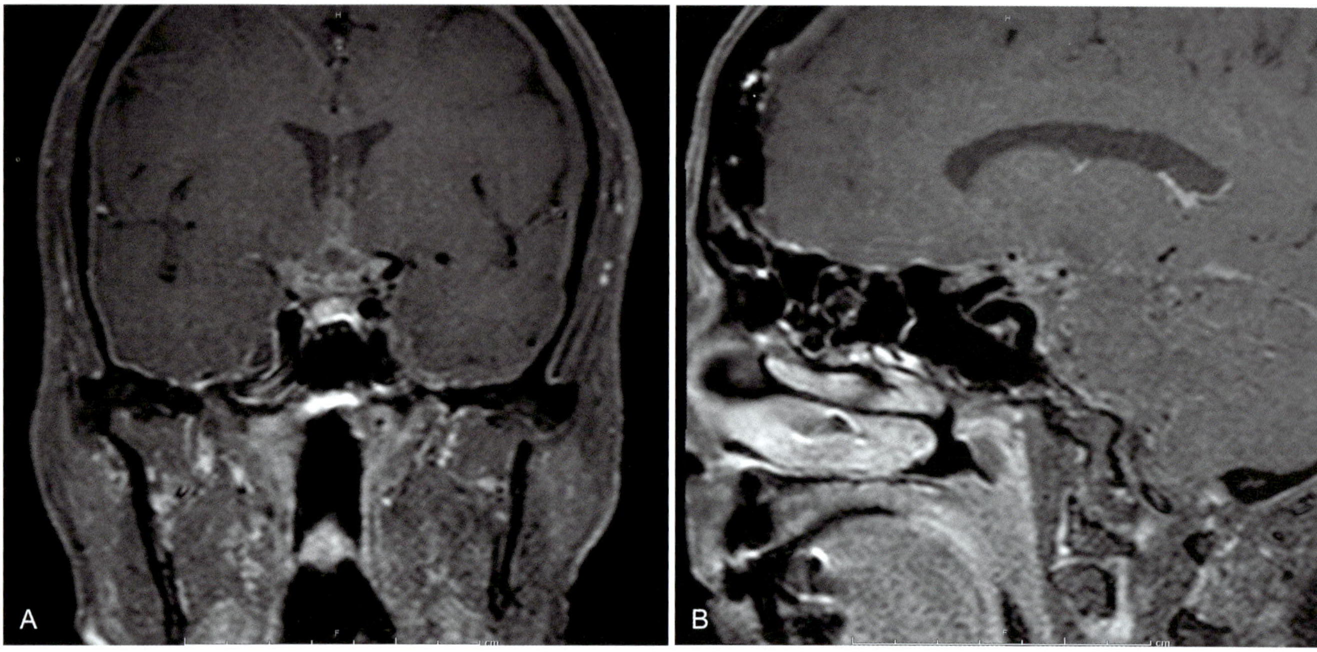

• **Fig. 35.17** A, Postoperative magnetic resonance imaging (MRI) scan of patient in Case 3 (coronal T1 postcontrast). B, Postoperative MRI of patient in Case 3 (sagittal T1 postcontrast).

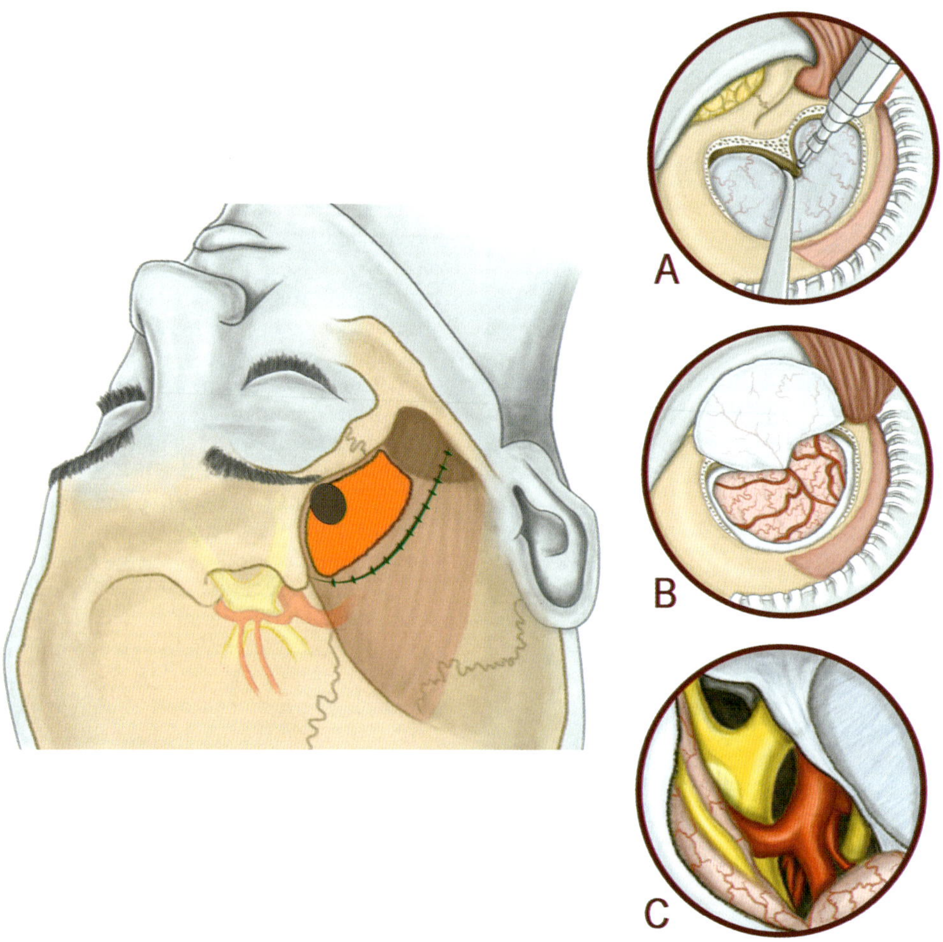

• **Fig. 35.18** Large image: incision of minipterional approach. A, Initial exposure with bony drilling. B, Initial intradural exposure. C, Cisternal exposure after opening the arachnoid of the opticocarotid cistern.

reapproximation of the dura and replacement of the bone flap with titanium plates. The epidural space is filled with collagen (Helistat). The bony defect at the pterion may optionally be filled with bone cement. The temporalis muscle and fascia are reapproximated and the subcutaneous tissues and skin are closed in a cosmetic fashion with absorbable subcutaneous stitches.

Case Example

A 36-year-old, previously healthy woman became aware of a progressive bulging of her left eye for approximately 18 months. She was initially thought to have Graves disease, but laboratory analysis did not bear this out. A subsequent MRI scan revealed an enhancing skull base tumor involving the left sphenoid wing and partially filling the orbit and extending into the sphenoid sinus, measuring 5.4 × 3.1 cm (Fig. 35.19), suggestive of a spheno-orbital meningioma. She had a nonfocal neurologic examination except for limited abduction of the left eye and proptosis. Visual acuity and fields were normal.

Given the lateral extent of the tumor, a minipterional approach was undertaken for a planned subtotal removal. The approach was performed as described earlier with extension to the middle fossa floor, and upon bone removal extradural tumor was visible. Removal of this tumor exposed the dura of the anterior and middle fossae. The very soft tumor was removed piecemeal until the floor of the middle fossa, temporal lobe, and sylvian fissure were visualized. The tumor was quite adherent to the temporal lobe. Doppler ultrasonography was used to localize the cavernous carotid artery. The bony opening was extended back to the orbital apex using the drill and rongeurs. The tumor itself did not extend to the cisternal portion of the optic nerve. The tumor extending into the orbit was removed by the neuro-ophthalmology team. The intraorbital resection was halted once the lateral rectus muscle was visualized (Fig. 35.20). Endoscopy was used to visualize the anterolateral orbit, and angled instruments were used to remove some additional tumor. Along the base of the skull, tumor was removed down to the foramen ovale region. An abdominal fat graft was harvested owing to proximity to the air sinuses and invasion of tumor into them. Reconstruction and closure were then performed in the usual fashion. The patient awoke without deficit.

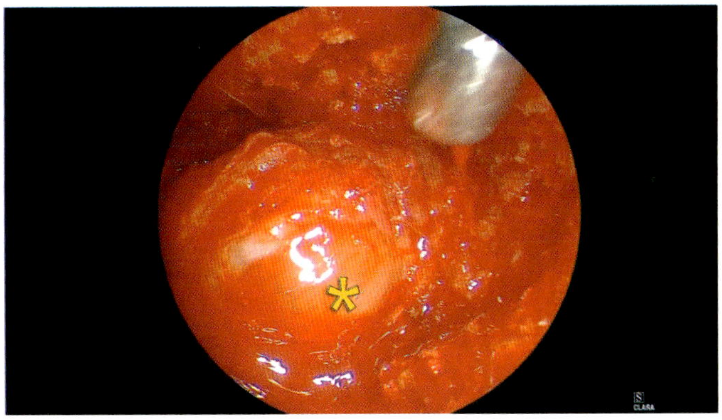

• **Fig. 35.20** Intraoperative photo showing a bulge of the lateral rectus muscle (*asterisk*).

Unfortunately, her postoperative MRI can the following day showed significant residual tumor medial to the lateral rectus muscle that was not evident intraoperatively (Fig. 35.21). As such, the patient was returned to the operating room for additional tumor removal because of concern that failure to remove this tumor would not alleviate the patient's proptosis. Intraoperatively, the stereotactic navigation indicated that the patient's residual tumor was most significant between the lateral and inferior rectus muscles. After careful dissection of the lateral rectus muscle, piecemeal debulking of the tumor was performed. Most of the tumor within the muscle cone was thus removed. Following this, the lateral rectus muscle continued to appear to bulge laterally. The area just under the muscle was opened sharply and tumor tissue was found and debulked. Once again, the angled endoscope allowed visualization of the area behind the globe and out of site of the microscope (Fig. 35.22). Additional fat was harvested to fill the larger defect, and the reconstruction and closure were performed in the usual fashion. The patient's postoperative MRI scan showed resection of the intraorbital contents of the tumor (Fig. 35.23). The patient awoke with a mild lateral rectus palsy. Three months postoperatively, the palsy had resolved, and her eye bulge had improved to almost normal. The pathologic analysis revealed a WHO II meningioma with focal brain invasion with positive progesterone receptor and proliferation index of 3% to 4%.

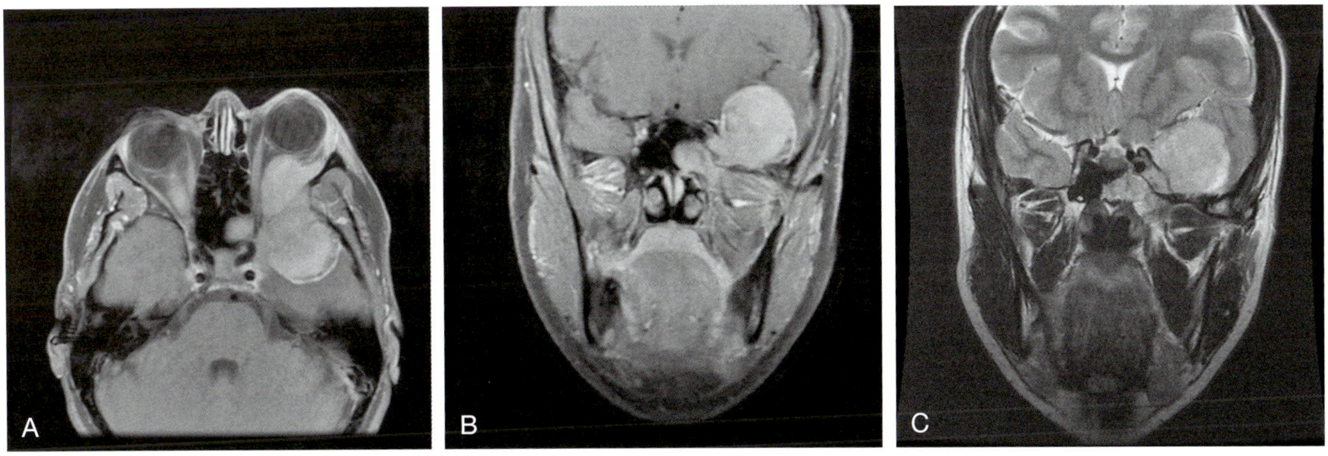

• **Fig. 35.19** A, Preoperative magnetic resonance imaging scan of patient in case description (axial T1 postcontrast). B, Coronal T1 (postcontrast). C, Coronal T2 (postcontrast).

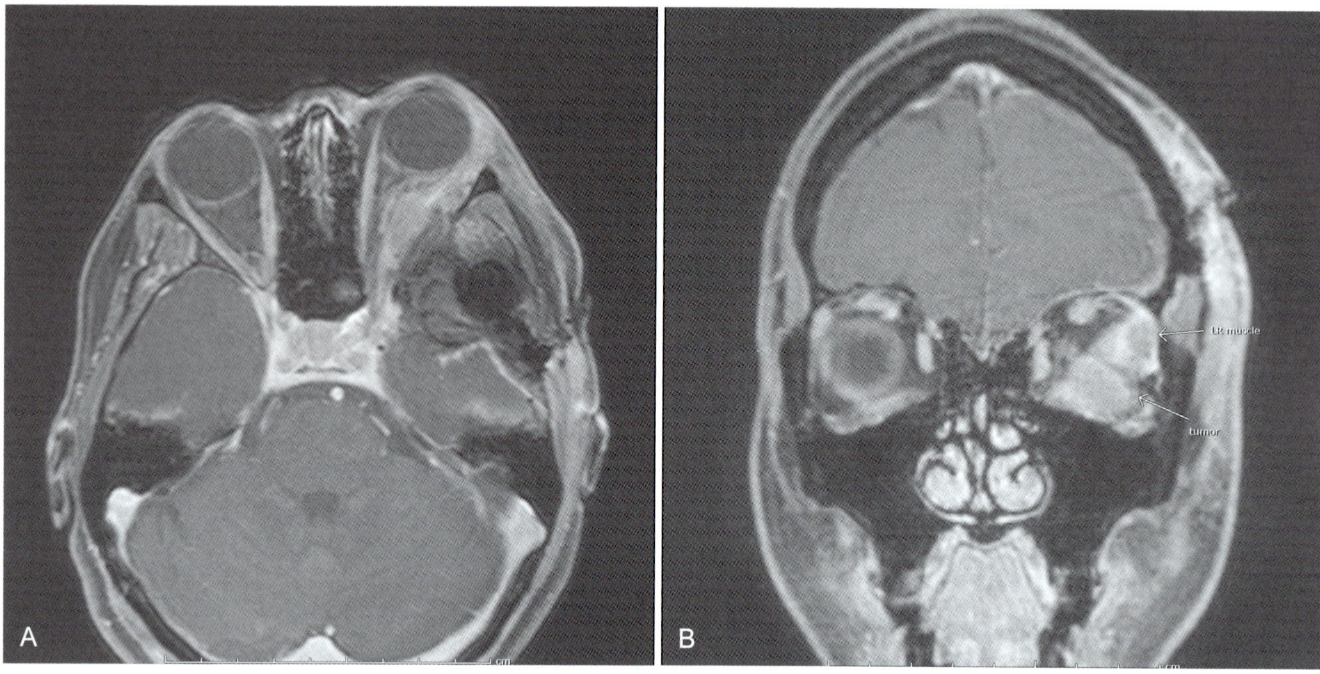

• **Fig. 35.21** A), Initial postoperative magnetic resonance imaging scan (axial T1 postcontrast). B, Coronal T1 postcontrast imaging showing residual tumor in the orbit, medial to the lateral rectus muscle.

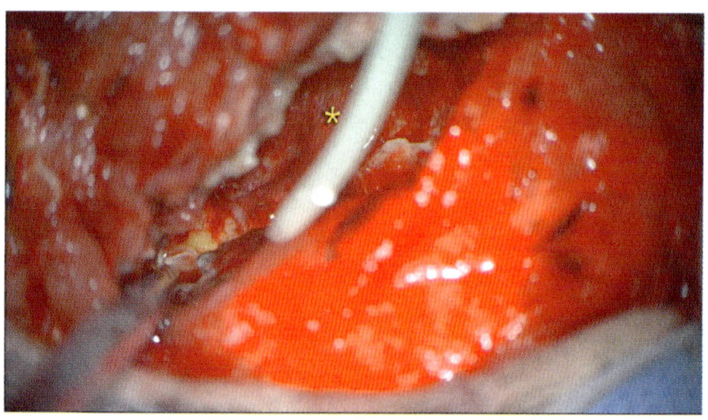

• **Fig. 35.22** Intraoperative photograph showing complete resection with visible orbital fat and decompressed lateral rectus muscle (asterisk).

Authors' Experience

We have performed 122 operations in 118 patients with the supraorbital approach and 24 operations in 22 patients with the minipterional approach. We have found that the supraorbital approach is generally versatile and offers a very similar exposure with an improved cosmetic outcome relative to the minipterional approach. The only situation in which the supraorbital approach is limited is in tumors that extend deep into the middle fossa or into the orbit. In these situations we elect to use the minipterional approach. The supraorbital approach provides a broad exposure to the optic apparatus anteromedially and allows access to lesions lateral to the chiasm and nerve as well. There are many cases of tumors (namely meningiomas) situated near the optic apparatus

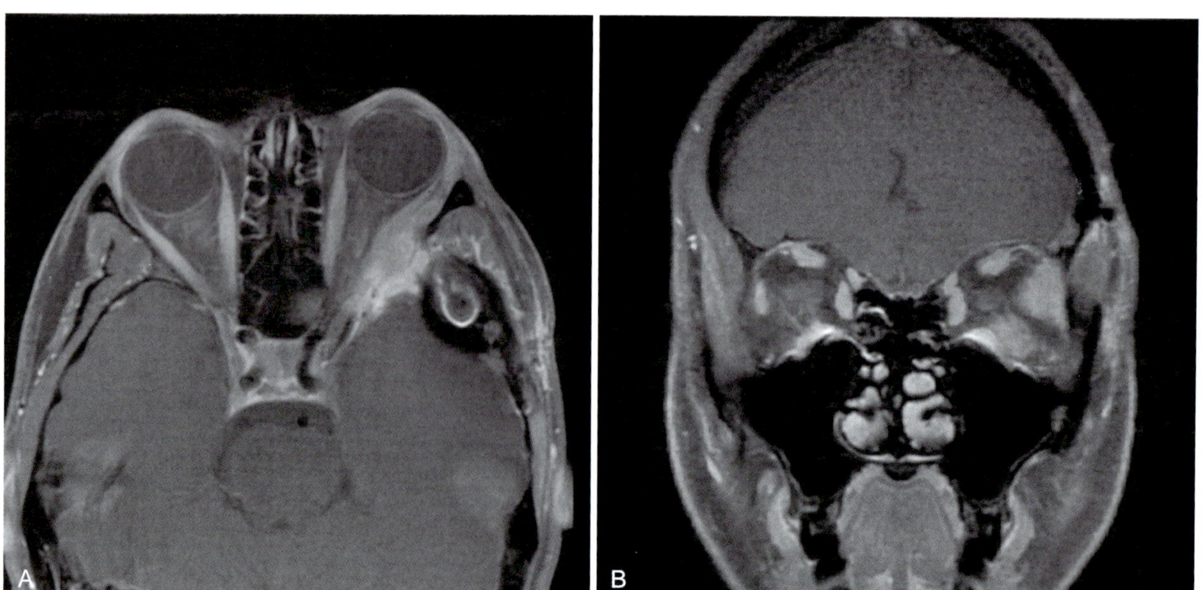

• **Fig. 35.23** A, Second postoperative magnetic resonance imaging scan (axial T1 postcontrast). B, Coronal T1 postcontrast scan showing removal of the intraorbital tumor and decompression of the orbital contents.

but with presenting symptoms other than visual loss. In 23 of our 122 cases, parasellar tumors, including meningiomas, pituitary adenomas, and dural-based metastatic tumors, presented without visual dysfunction. Patients with such tumors most commonly presented with headaches (11), neurologic or endocrine deficit (6), cognitive decline (3), and incidental discovery (3). We found that the average maximal tumor diameter of the lesions in patients who presented with visual loss was smaller than that of the patients who did not present with visual loss (average maximum diameter 3.19 cm vs. 1.93 cm). This implies that the likelihood of a tumor to cause visual loss is related more to its location than its size, and that larger tumors are more likely to cause headaches from edema and increased intracranial pressure before they cause visual decline. This is exemplified in the contrast between Cases 1 and 3 earlier, in which a patient with a smaller tumor had visual loss, whereas a patient with a very large tumor did not.

Conclusion

The supraorbital and minipterional approaches are minimally invasive approaches with limited cortical and soft-tissue retraction that provide excellent access to the anterior and middle cranial fossae and bilateral access to the optic nerves and chiasm. Combined with the endonasal endoscopic approach, they allow 360-degree access to the optic apparatus. Endoscopy is a powerful adjunct that greatly augments the visualization provided by the microscope and allows the surgeon to obtain a greater extent of resection while aiding the safety of the operation by eliminating blind spots.

References

1. Delashaw, J. B., Jr., Tedeschi, H., & Rhoton, A. L. (1992). Modified supraorbital craniotomy: Technical note. *Neurosurgery, 30*, 954–956.
2. Jane, J. A., Park, T. S., Pobereskin, L. H., Winn, H. R., & Butler, A. B. (1982). The supraorbital approach: Technical note. *Neurosurgery, 11*, 537–542.
3. Noguchi, A., Balasingam, V., McMenomey, S. O., & Delashaw, J. B., Jr. (2005). Supraorbital craniotomy for parasellar lesions: Technical note. *Journal of Neurosurgery, 102*, 951–955.
4. Sanchez-Vazquez, M. A., Barrera-Calatayud, P., Mejia-Villela, M., Palma-Silva, J. F., Juan-Carachure, I., Gomez-Aguilar, J. M., et al. (1999). Transciliary subfrontal craniotomy for anterior skull base lesions: Technical note. *Journal of Neurosurgery, 91*, 892–896.
5. Yasargil, M. G., & Fox, J. L. (1975). The microsurgical approach to intracranial aneurysms. *Surgical Neurology, 3*, 7–14.
6. Reisch, R., Perneczky, A., & Filippi, R. (2003). Surgical technique of the supraorbital key-hole craniotomy. *Surgical Neurology, 59*, 223–227.
7. Thaher, F., Hopf, N., Hickmann, A. K., Kurucz, P., Bittl, M., Henkes, H., et al. (2015). Supraorbital keyhole approach to the skull base: Evaluation of complications related to csf fistulas and opened frontal sinus. *Journal of Neurological Surgery Part A, Central European Neurosurgery, 76*, 433–437.
8. Tra, H., Huynh, T., & Nguyen, B. (2018). Minipterional and supraorbital keyhole craniotomies for ruptured anterior circulation aneurysms: Experience at single center. *World Neurosurgery, 109*, 36–39.
9. Tullos, H. J., Conner, A. K., Baker, C. M., Briggs, R. G., Burks, J. D., Glenn, C. A., et al. (2018). Mini-pterional craniotomy for resection of parasellar meningiomas. *World Neurosurgery, 117*, e637–e644.
10. van Lindert, E., Perneczky, A., Fries, G., & Pierangeli, E. (1998). The supraorbital keyhole approach to supratentorial aneurysms: Concept and technique. *Surgical Neurology, 49*, 481–489.
11. Welling, L. C., Figueiredo, E. G., Wen, H. T., Gomes, M. Q., Bor-Seng-Shu, E., Casarolli, C., et al. (2015). Prospective randomized study comparing clinical, functional, and aesthetic results of minipterional and classic pterional craniotomies. *Journal of Neurosurgery, 122*, 1012–1019.
12. Ditzel Filho, L. F., McLaughlin, N., Bresson, D., Solari, D., Kassam, A. B., & Kelly, D. F. (2014). Supraorbital eyebrow craniotomy for removal of intraaxial frontal brain tumors: A technical note. *World Neurosurgery, 81*, 348–356.
13. Fatemi, N., Dusick, J. R., de Paiva Neto, M. A., Malkasian, D., & Kelly, D. F. (2009). Endonasal versus supraorbital keyhole removal of craniopharyngiomas and tuberculum sellae meningiomas. *Neurosurgery, 64*, 269–284.
14. Figueiredo, E. G., Welling, L. C., Preul, M. C., Sakaya, G. R., Neville, I., Spetzler, R. F., et al. (2016). Surgical experience of minipterional craniotomy with 102 ruptured and unruptured anterior circulation aneurysms. *Journal of Clinical Neuroscience, 27*, 34–39.
15. Gandhi, S., Cavallo, C., Zhao, X., Belykh, E., Lee, M., Yoon, S., et al. (2018). Minimally invasive approaches to aneurysms of the anterior circulation: Selection criteria and clinical outcomes. *Journal of Clinical Neuroscience, 62*, 636–649.
16. Igressa, A., Pechlivanis, I., Weber, F., Mahvash, M., Ayyad, A., Boutarbouch, M., et al. (2015). Endoscope-assisted keyhole surgery via an eyebrow incision for removal of large meningiomas of the anterior and middle cranial fossa. *Clinical Neurology and Neurosurgery, 129*, 27–33.
17. Kelly, D. F., Griffiths, C. F., Takasumi, Y., Rhee, J., Barkhoudarian, G., & Krauss, H. R. (2015). Role of endoscopic skull base and keyhole surgery for pituitary and parasellar tumors impacting vision. *Journal of Neuro-ophthalmology, 35*, 335–341.
18. Kim, Y., Yoo, C. J., Park, C. W., Kim, M. J., Choi, D. H., Kim, Y. J., et al. Modified supraorbital keyhole approach to anterior circulation aneurysms. *Journal of Cerebrovascular and Endovascular Neurosurgery, 18*, 5–11.
19. Klironomos, G., Mehan, N., & Dehdashti, A. R. (2018). Lateral supraorbital craniotomy for tuberculum sella meningioma resection. *Journal of Neurological Surgery Part B, Skull Base, 79*, S263–S264.
20. Louis, R. G., Eisenberg, A., Barkhoudarian, G., Griffiths, C., & Kelly, D. F. (2014). Evolution of minimally invasive approaches to the sella and parasellar region. *International Archives of Otorhinolaryngology, 18*, S136–S148.
21. Lucas, J. W., & Zada, G. (2016). Endoscopic endonasal and keyhole surgery for the management of skull base meningiomas. *Neurosurgery Clinics of North America, 27*, 207–214.
22. McLaughlin, N., Ditzel Filho, L. F., Shahlaie, K., Solari, D., Kassam, A. B., & Kelly, D. F. (2011). The supraorbital approach for recurrent or residual suprasellar tumors. *Minimally Invasive Neurosurgery, 54*, 155–161.
23. Prat-Acin, R., Galeano-Senabre, I., Pancucci, G., Evangelista, R., Ayuso-Sacido, A., & Botella, C. (2013). Supraorbital trans-eyebrow craniotomy and fluorescence-guided resection of fronto-basal high grade gliomas. *Clinical Neurology and Neurosurgery, 115*, 1586–1590.
24. Wilson, D. A., Duong, H., Teo, C., & Kelly, D. F. (2014). The supraorbital endoscopic approach for tumors. *World Neurosurgery, 82*, S72–S80.
25. Marx, S., Clemens, S., & Schroeder, H. W. S. (2018). The value of endoscope assistance during transcranial surgery for tuberculum sellae meningiomas. *Journal of Neurosurgery, 128*, 32–39.
26. Melamed, I., Merkin, V., Korn, A., & Nash, M. (2005). The supraorbital approach: An alternative to traditional exposure for the surgical management of anterior fossa and parasellar pathology. *Minimally Invasive Neurosurgery, 48*, 259–263.
27. Ormond, D. R., & Hadjipanayis, C. G. (2013). The supraorbital keyhole craniotomy through an eyebrow incision: Its origins and evolution. *Minimally Invasive Neurosurgery, 2013*, 296469.
28. Romani, R., Laakso, A., Kangasniemi, M., Lehecka, M., & Hernesniemi, J. (2011). Lateral supraorbital approach applied to anterior clinoidal meningiomas: Experience with 73 consecutive patients. *Neurosurgery, 68*, 1632–1647.

29. Salma, A., Alkandari, A., Sammet, S., & Ammirati, M. Lateral supraorbital approach vs pterional approach: An anatomic qualitative and quantitative evaluation. *Neurosurgery, 68,* 364–372.
30. Teo, C. (2010). The concept of minimally invasive neurosurgery. *Neurosurgery Clinics of North America, 21*, 583–584.
31. Cheng, C. M., Noguchi, A., Dogan, A., Anderson, G. J., Hsu, F. P., McMenomey, S. O., et al. (2013). Quantitative verification of the keyhole concept: A comparison of area of exposure in the parasellar region via supraorbital keyhole, frontotemporal pterional and supraorbital approaches. *Journal of Neurosurgery, 118*, 264–269.
32. de Divitiis, E., de Divitiis, O., & Elefante, A. (2014). Supraorbital craniotomy: Pro and cons of endoscopic assistance. *World Neurosurgery, 82*, e93–e96.
33. Perneczky, A., Fries, G. Endoscope-assisted brain surgery: Part 1—evolution, basic concept, and current technique. *Neurosurgery, 42,* 219–224.
34. Reisch, R., Marcus, H. J., Hugelshofer, M., Koechlin, N. O., Stadie, A., & Kockro, R. A. (2014). Patients' cosmetic satisfaction, pain, and functional outcomes after supraorbital craniotomy through an eyebrow incision. *Journal of Neurosurgery, 121*, 730–734.
35. Figueiredo, E. G., Deshmukh, P., Nakaji, P., Crusius, M. U., Crawford, N., Spetzler, R. F., et al. (2007). The minipterional craniotomy: Technical description and anatomic assessment. *Neurosurgery, 61*, 256–264.
36. Wong, J. H., Tymianski, R., Radovanovic, I., & Tymianski, M. (2015). Minimally invasive microsurgery for cerebral aneurysms. *Stroke, 46*, 2699–2706.
37. Ammirati, M., Spallone, A., Ma, J., Cheatham, M., & Becker, D. (1994). Preservation of the temporal branch of the facial nerve in pterional-transzygomatic craniotomy. *Acta Neurochirurgica, 128*, 163–165.

36

Endoscopic Endonasal Approaches to the Optic Apparatus: Technique and Pathology

CHANDALA CHITGUPPI, MD, JUDD H. FASTENBERG, MD, GURSTON G. NYQUIST, MD, MARC R. ROSEN, MD, JAMES J. EVANS, MD, AND MINDY R. RABINOWITZ, MD

The optic apparatus includes the optic nerves, chiasm, and optic tracts. Lesions affecting this region vary widely with respect to histologic type, site, extent, and clinicopathologic behavior. Treatment of these lesions therefore requires a comprehensive multidisciplinary approach with a team consisting of skull base neurosurgeons, otolaryngologists, and ophthalmologists, as well as radiation and medical oncologists. Although observation and radiotherapy may play important roles, surgical treatment represents the mainstay of therapy, with a relatively recent shift from traditional open approaches to less invasive endoscopic endonasal approaches (EEAs).

Pathology

Some of the common pathologies affecting the optic apparatus are discussed in the following text. Pituitary macroadenomas and meningiomas represent the most common lesions in adults, whereas craniopharyngioma is the most common in children.[1]

Pituitary Adenoma

Pituitary adenomas represent the most frequent type of sellar mass[2] with a prevalence of 77 to 100 cases per 100,000 population.[3-5] These tumors can be classified into nonfunctional or functional (hormone-secreting) subtypes.

Among the pituitary tumors that are associated with visual dysfunction, nonfunctioning adenomas are the most common (58%).[6] Superior extension of tumors may compress the optic chiasm and lead to visual field deficits, most commonly bitemporal hemianopia.[7,8] Other visual symptoms may include loss of visual acuity and diplopia.[9] The progression of visual loss is typically slow (50%); however, rapid (27%) and intermittent progression (12.5%) have also been reported.[10] Importantly, although 75% of patients with pituitary adenomas have visual field defects, fewer than half report these visual changes subjectively.[11] This underscores the importance of obligatory visual field testing in all patients with pituitary adenomas irrespective of whether they report visual impairment.

Treatment of pituitary tumors is individualized and is based on tumor type, size, anatomic location relative to surrounding critical structures (optic apparatus, carotid arteries, third ventricle) and the degree of visual and/or hormonal impairment. Surgical resection is first-line treatment for most tumors except prolactinomas, which typically respond well to medical management with a dopamine agonist. Today at most academic medical centers, the overwhelming majority of surgical resections are performed through an endoscopic transsphenoidal approach.[12,13]

Meningioma

Meningiomas arising from the optic nerve sheath or in proximity to the optic chiasm in the suprasellar region may affect the optic apparatus. Optic nerve sheath meningiomas, which arise from cap cells of the arachnoid surrounding the optic nerve and spread through subarachnoid spaces,[14] are the most common optic nerve sheath tumors[15] and account for one-third of intrinsic optic nerve tumors.[16] Involvement of the extraorbital portion of the optic nerve without (49%) or with involvement of optic chiasm (40%) is common.[17] These tumors usually present with unilateral symptoms[16] and are frequently seen in middle-aged women.[14] Prognosis depends largely on the size and extent of the tumor and less so on histopathologic features.[18]

Suprasellar meningiomas may arise from the tuberculum sellae (TS), diaphragma sellae (DS), or planum sphenoidale (PS).[19] The majority (50%) arise from the TS[19] and are most commonly seen in women in their fifth decade.[19-21] Identification of the anatomic subtype is important in selecting the type of surgical approach for resection, which is often challenging. The relative displacement of the optic apparatus, however, can help in distinguishing one subtype from another. For example, TS meningiomas lead to posterior or superoposterior displacement of the optic chiasm, whereas DS meningiomas lead to superior displacement, and PS meningiomas lead to posterior and inferior displacement.[19] The nuances of surgical approach can then be based on these anatomic distinctions. Although TS meningiomas can be resected using a purely supradiaphragmatic approach, a combined supradiaphragmatic and infradiaphragmatic approach is necessary for DS meningiomas.[19]

GTR of tumor (at least Simpson grade I/II) with improvement or stabilization of visual function are the goals of surgical treatment. Surgical treatment is also a viable option for radiation-resistant meningiomas.

Craniopharyngioma

Craniopharyngiomas are the most common suprasellar tumor found in children, accounting for 50% of masses in this region.[22] These tumors arise from remnants of the Rathke pouch[23] and demonstrate a bimodal age distribution, most commonly affecting children 5 to 14 years and adults 65 to 74 years.[24]

Although a benign tumor, craniopharyngiomas are associated with significant mortality among all sellar and suprasellar tumors, with a standardized overall mortality rate ranging from 2.88% to 9.28%.[25] In pediatric patients, symptoms of elevated intracranial pressure (ICP) are commonly seen, whereas in adults, visual disturbance and hypopituitarism are also noted.[25,26] Hypothalamic involvement is frequently seen in pediatric patients. Gross total resection (GTR) of the tumor with maintenance of hypothalamic functionality should be the goal of treatment; however, in patients in whom maintaining hypothalamic functionality is challenging owing to unfavorable tumor localization, subtotal resection followed by adjuvant radiotherapy should be performed.[27] Additionally, adjuvant radiotherapy improves local control[28,29] and helps prevent permanent endocrine and neurocognitive sequelae, as well as injury to critical neurovascular structures in difficult tumors.[25,30] If GTR is not possible, our preference is to preserve the pituitary stalk. In addition to visual dysfunction, long-term morbidity associated with craniopharyngiomas includes hypopituitarism, hypothalamic injury, detrimental cardiovascular effects, reduced bone health, neurologic deficits, lower cognitive function, and poorer quality of life.[25]

Rare Pathologies Affecting Optic Apparatus

Other, less common lesions affecting the optic apparatus are listed in Table 36.1.[31-37]

TABLE 36.1 Rare Pathologies Affecting Optic Apparatus[1, 31–37]

Sub types	Tumors	Non-tumorous lesions
Benign	Chiasmatic/Hypothalamic glioma, Germ cell tumors (germinomas, non-germinomatous and teratomas), Hypothalamic hamartoma, Rathke cleft cysts, Yolk sac tumor, Pilocytic astrocytomas, Gangliocytomas	Langerhans cell histiocytosis and other granulomatous disorders, Arachnoid cysts, Lymphocytic hypophysistis, Pituitary apolexy, Opticochiasmatic arachnoiditis, Aneurysms of circle of Willis, Xanthogranuloma, Colloid cysts, Epidermoid cysts
Malignant/ Potentially malignant	Lymphoma, Paraganglioma Ependymal metastases in third ventricle, metastasis to optic chiasm and pituitary gland	–

Clinical Features

Lesions affecting the optic apparatus frequently cause significant visual morbidity and, given their anatomic location, may contribute to hypopituitarism and symptoms of elevated ICP. Specific visual complaints vary depending on the anatomic site, size, and extent of lesion. Gradual and painless visual loss is a common initial symptom,[14,15] although nonspecific symptoms such as headache and nausea (owing to elevated ICP) and weight disturbance may be present.[20,30,38,39] Other visual findings may include visual field defects, color vision disturbance, optic atrophy, afferent pupillary defect, choroidal folds, presence of opticociliary shunt vessels, and edema of the optic disc and macula.[14,3,40-42] Given the breadth of the possible visual symptoms and signs, a thorough ophthalmologic examination, including measurement of visual acuity, color vision, visual fields, and optic nerve examination, is obligatory in both the preoperative and postoperative setting.

Surgical Treatment

EEAs to the optic apparatus include both transsphenoidal and extended transsphenoidal approaches (ETSAs).[39,43-47] Transsphenoidal approaches are commonly used for lesions confined to the sella, whereas ETSAs, such as transplanar or transtubercular, may be necessary to access anatomic areas superior, posterior, or lateral to the sella.

Preoperative Planning

Preoperative assessment using magnetic resonance imaging and computed tomography is recommended. Anatomic ease of access (deviated nasal septum, concha bullosa, sphenoid sinus pneumatization, intrasphenoid and intersphenoid septae, and so on), tumor characteristics (consistency, extension, and so on), and surrounding critical structures (prefixed and postfixed chiasma, bony dehiscence, carotid artery position and encasement, location of the pituitary gland and its stalk, apoplexy, and so on) should be noted. Patient selection is of paramount importance for success of the procedure and hence should be done based on the surgeon's expertise.

Equipment

Technological advances in the form of computer-assisted surgical navigation, specialized instrumentation with long handles, suction irrigation, micro drills, and ultrasonic aspirators have improved the surgical precision in the EEA.[48] Rigid 18-cm endoscopes (Karl Storz, Tuttlingen, Germany) of size 4 mm (0-, 30-, and 45-degree) are used in adults, whereas smaller sized endoscopes (2.7 mm) are used in the pediatric age group.

Intraoperative Setup

Standard neurosurgical anesthetic practices are followed. Total intravenous anesthesia is recommended to maintain a hypotensive state to reduce bleeding (mean blood pressure maintained approximately 90-100 mm Hg and pulse rate approximately 55-60 beats/min). Paralytic agents should be avoided if intraoperative neurophysiologic monitoring with somatosensory evoked potentials is intended. Intraoperative somatosensory evoked potentials, electromyography for perfusion, electroencephalography, motor evoked potentials, and selective cranial nerve monitoring can be used as required to reduce the risk of injury to adjacent neurovascular structures, including the optic apparatus and carotid artery.[49] Corticosteroids may be administered if preoperative hypocortisolism or visual disturbance is suspected. ICP-lowering agents or lumbar drain are rarely required. Urinary catheterization is performed to monitor fluid balance during the surgery. At all times during the surgery, both suction and cautery are usually maintained at a lower setting to prevent mucosal injury.

The setup of the operating room is similar to other endoscopic neurosurgical procedures.[13] The right-handed surgeon usually stands on the right side of the patient and the monitor screen is set up behind the patient's head. The patient's head and body are elevated to 30 to 45 degrees from the horizontal plane to reduce ICP and venous bleeding. The bilateral nasal cavities are filled with cottonoids soaked in vasoconstrictive agents (oxymetazoline or diluted epinephrine) under endoscopic guidance to prevent inadvertent mucosal trauma. The patient is then prepped and draped. The nasal mucosa is injected medially into the posterior nasal septum and middle and inferior turbinates with local anesthesia (lidocaine 1% with epinephrine 1:100,000) using a spinal needle with the tip bent to 20 degrees.

Operative Technique

The Endonasal Stage

Creation of an adequately wide endonasal corridor is the first step and is imperative to any endoscopic procedure. Bilateral nasal endoscopy is performed to evaluate both the nasal airways and to identify anatomic entities, such as septal deviation, septal spurs, septal perforations, synechiae (from previous procedures), and turbinate hypertrophy, among others. Surgical procedures, such as septoplasty, turbinate reduction, or lysis of adhesions, may be performed to improve access and postoperative sinonasal function. Bilateral lateralization of the middle and superior turbinates is performed to expose the sphenoid face and natural os sphenoidale in a transnasal fashion. Resection of the middle turbinate is rarely required.

The Sphenoid Stage

To approach the sella, resection of the anterior face of the sphenoid is required, which may result in sacrifice of the pedicle for a nasoseptal flap (NSF). Traditionally, the NSF is raised at the beginning of the operation. However, the majority of cases do not incur an intraoperative cerebrospinal fluid (CSF) leak; even if leak is present, it is usually small and of a low-flow type that does not normally require an NSF for cranial base defect closure. In our center, we do not routinely use an NSF after excision of sellar or suprasellar tumors. Therefore an NSF preservation approach is used. A number of techniques have been described to preserve the NSF pedicle without raising an NSF, which include transseptal approach (tunnel), pushdown or rescue flap, or "1.5 with pushdown" techniques.[50-53]

We commonly us the 1.5 with pushdown technique that is described briefly. With the sphenoid face well visualized, the natural os on the right side is enlarged superiorly and bony septum is fractured off the rostrum. The mucosa is elevated off the face of the sphenoid on both the right and left sides, preserving the pedicle for a septal flap. The ipsilateral mucosa inferior to the os is then carefully displaced inferiorly to preserve the pedicle to the NSF. Through the contralateral naris, the mucosa is removed superior to the os, preserving the pedicle to the NSF (Fig 36.1). A small posterior septectomy is performed if necessary for exposure.

Alternatively, the ETSA for giant pituitary adenomas, meningiomas, and craniopharyngiomas where a large dural defect (high-flow leak) is expected and an NSF is used as part of the multilayer reconstruction of the cranial base, the NSF is harvested at the beginning of the procedure and is stored in the nasopharynx during the extirpative portion of the case.

The degree of pneumatization of the sphenoid sinus significantly influences the ease of access to the sella and optic apparatus. Presellar and conchal sellar types, such as in pediatric patients, may prevent identification of reliable anatomic landmarks.[48] Ultimately, the distance between the two opticocarotid recesses, the height of dorsum sella, and the size of posterior clinoids determine the dimensions of intrasphenoid corridor.[48,54] The intersinus septations are removed by either through-cutting hand instruments or a high-speed drill with diamond burr, being careful to identify any attachment to the carotid canals. The paramedian septum often leads to the carotid artery, and therefore it should be excised with particular care. The mucosa is removed from the sellar face to facilitate reconstruction and to avoid postoperative mucocele formation.

Cranial Base Stage

Several key anatomic landmarks can be identified along the cranial base (sellar face), including the sella, PS, TS, lateral opticocarotid recesses, optic canals, and clinoidal carotid protuberance

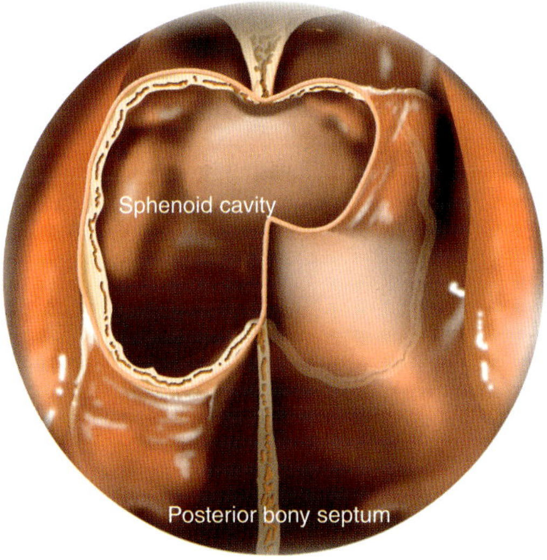

• **Fig. 36.1** The Sphenoid Stage. The 1.5 approach with pushdown wherein the right and left submucosal bony sphenoidotomy is shown. The mucosa on the right side is pushed down and the left side mucosa above the sphenoid os only is removed preserving the nasoseptal flap pedicle bilaterally. (Courtesy Paul Schiffmacher and Tawfiq Khoury, MD.)

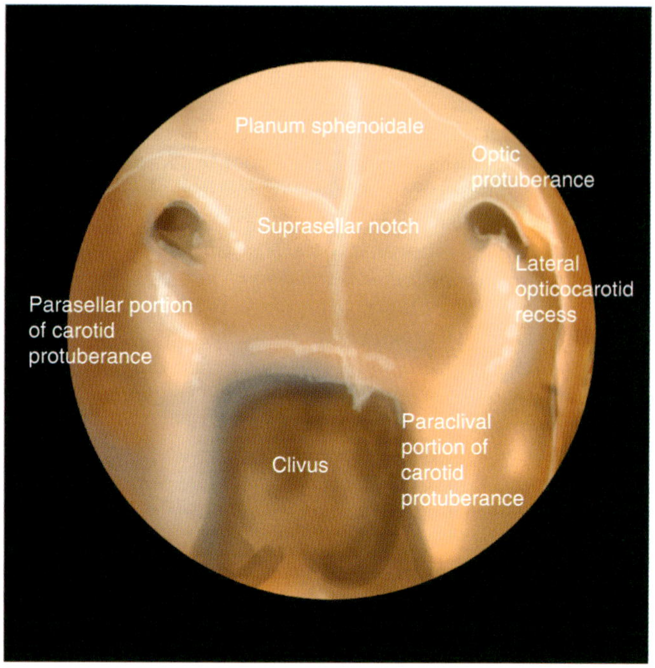

• **Fig. 36.2** The Cranial Base Stage. Key anatomic landmarks at the anterior cranial base (sellar face) are shown here. (Courtesy Paul Schiffmacher and Tawfiq Khoury, MD.)

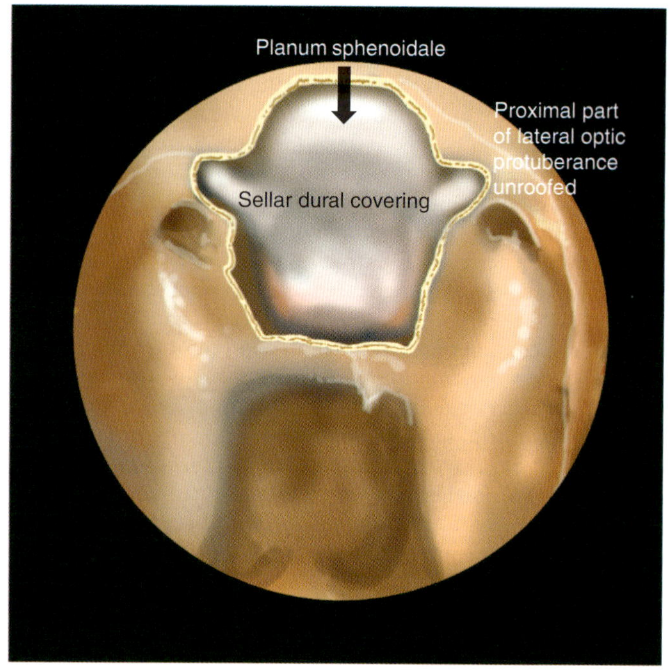

• **Fig. 36.3** The Cranial Base Stage. After removal of the bony sellar face (in a T-shirt shape), sellar dura is visualized. (Courtesy Paul Schiffmacher and Tawfiq Khoury, MD.)

(Fig 36.2). Neuronavigation and micro-Doppler monitoring may be used to confirm anatomic landmarks and to determine the extent of bony removal that is necessary to access the intradural lesion.

For the majority of pituitary tumors, the sellar face is then removed with either a Kerrison punch or high-powered drill from one cavernous carotid to the other, and inferiorly to the level of the sella floor. If a drill is used, copious irrigation is advised to prevent thermal injury. The internal carotid artery should be carefully identified; however, we prefer not to remove the bone over the internal carotid artery for most cases to prevent iatrogenic carotid injury. The caveat is that additional exposure is required for resection of tumor within the cavernous sinus.

For excision of meningiomas and craniopharyngiomas, the optic canal is unroofed using a diamond drill to a thin eggshell of bone that can be removed with a microdissector. The length of canal that needs to be unroofed depends on the extent of the lesion. However, proximal unroofing is performed for most cases to prevent injury to the optic nerve at the entrance to the optic canal during intradural dissection. Bony removal in the rostral direction along TS and PS is usually performed to expose the limbus sphenoidale. Again, the degree of planum drilling depends on the extent of tumor (Fig. 36.3). Removal of the lateral strut of the TS also allows for wider access to the opticocarotid cistern. If additional bone needs to be removed to expose this area, it should be done before opening the dura.

Dural Stage

The principles of intradural excision—namely, internal debulking followed by capsule mobilization, extracapsular dissection of neurovascular structures, focal coagulation, and capsule removal—are duly followed.[46] These maneuvers should be performed in a controlled, bimanual fashion. The site and extent of dural incision is tailored to the lesion. Usually a smaller incision is placed first, and upon confirmation of the arachnoid plane, the incision is extended using endoscopic microscissors. The dura may be opened in various methods—a vertical linear incision with crossed extensions, two lateral vertical incisions joined by a transverse one,[13] a set of four incisions to create a rectangular window, or a cruciate incision.[55] We usually prefer the cruciate incision, which is made using a retractable knife (Fig. 36.4). This opening must be precise and generally should not extend beyond the tumor margins initially, especially during the transplanum approach, because excessive exposure can place uninvolved structures at risk and can lead to brain herniation, which in turn limits the visualization. After this opening is made, a blunt nerve hook or microdissector is placed along the circumference of the opening to create a subdural, extraglandular, or extracapsular plane. Bleeding from superior intercavernous sinus is controlled using bipolar electrocautery and/or local hemostatic agents. The superior hypophyseal branches to the optic apparatus and infundibulum are carefully dissected and mobilized superolaterally to prevent inadvertent injury.

Tumor Excision Stage

The tumor can be removed en bloc after internal debulking or in piecemeal fashion.[13] Extracapsular dissection and complete resection is the goal whenever possible. Although these general principles are applicable for excision of most lesions, several more nuanced techniques are applicable in specific circumstances.

For instance, if the optic canal is found to be invaded, then the canal is decompressed in a retrograde manner from the lamina papyracea back to the orbital apex (270 degrees around the canal). The part of the canal adjacent to the carotid artery is completely unroofed, and the bone overlying the more superior and medial portions of the canal is also excised bilaterally for at least 1 to 2 cm distal to the orbital apex. Resection of a TS meningioma

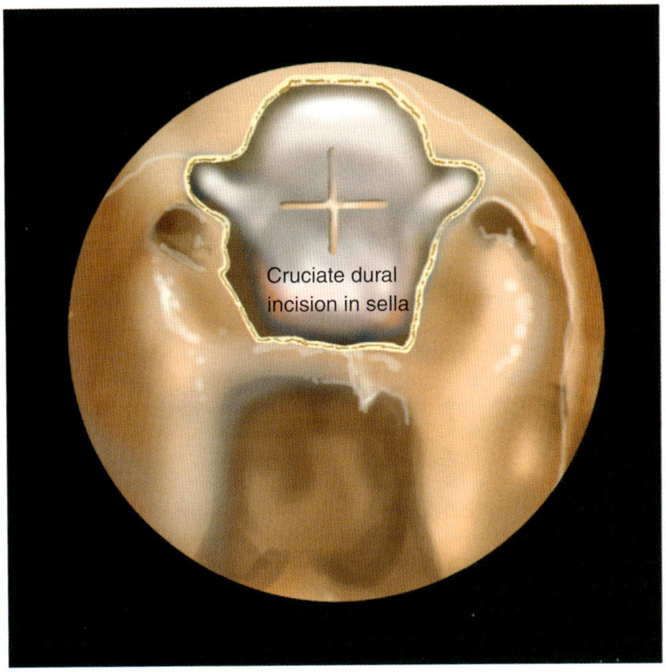

• **Fig. 36.4** The Dural Stage. Cruciate incision is perfomed on the sellar dura to access the pituitary gland. (Courtesy Paul Schiffmacher and Tawfiq Khoury, MD.)

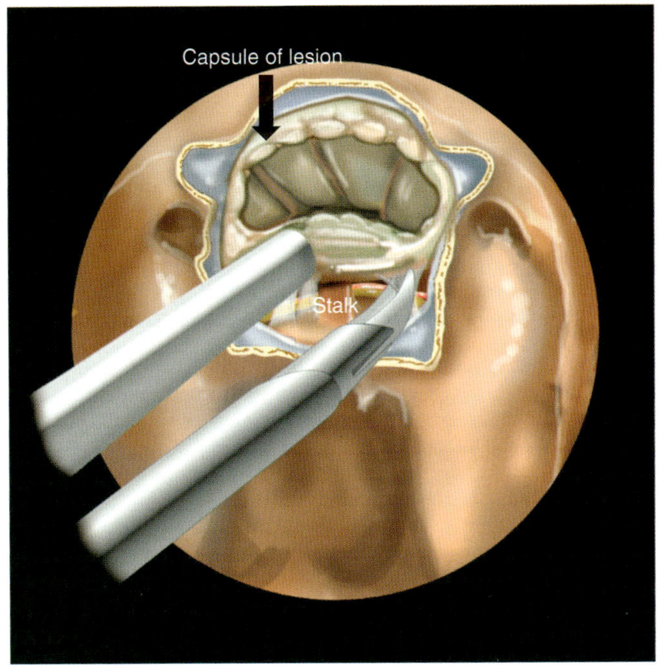

• **Fig. 36.5** The Tumor Excision Stage. Extracapsular dissection of the tumor. The tumor (*greenish structure*) and pituitary stalk are also seen. (Courtesy Paul Schiffmacher and Tawfiq Khoury, MD.)

may be particularly difficult if it has a firm and rubbery consistency; therefore, sharp dissection rather than simple suctioning may be necessary.[39,56] In close proximity to critical structures, internal decompression may be performed with a sharp and blunt manual dissection or with ultrasonic tumor aspiration. For craniopharyngiomas the cyst capsule may need to be coagulated before internal decompression to shrink the tumor and contain cyst content spillage. After adequate internal debulking, extracapsular dissection can then be performed (Figs. 36.5 and 36.6). Preservation of the infundibulum should be attempted whenever possible. However, if the stalk is invaded, it needs to be excised to prevent increased need for postoperative radiation and risk of tumor recurrence. At no point during the intradural excision should the lesion be blindly or indiscriminately pulled or retracted.

Inspection Stage

After resection the surgical field must be thoroughly examined with angled scopes (30 degrees and 45 degrees) to avoid leaving residual tumor tissue. Although complete excision of the lesion is an ideal scenario, this may not be realistically possible in some cases owing to the inability to separate the lesion from critical neurovascular structures.[57-59] In such cases, it is necessary to avoid overzealous excision at the cost of significant patient morbidity.

Dural Reconstruction Stage

A wide range of techniques for dural reconstruction have been described.[43,60-62] Reconstruction is typically tailored based on the extent of bony osteotomies at the cranial base, the integrity of the DS, and the presence of a low- or high-flow intraoperative CSF leak. All high-flow repair techniques begin with a primary dural repair, and most are followed by a vascularized mucosal flap.

Techniques of dural repair may involve the use of inlay or onlay grafts made of synthetic materials or autologous tissue, such as fat

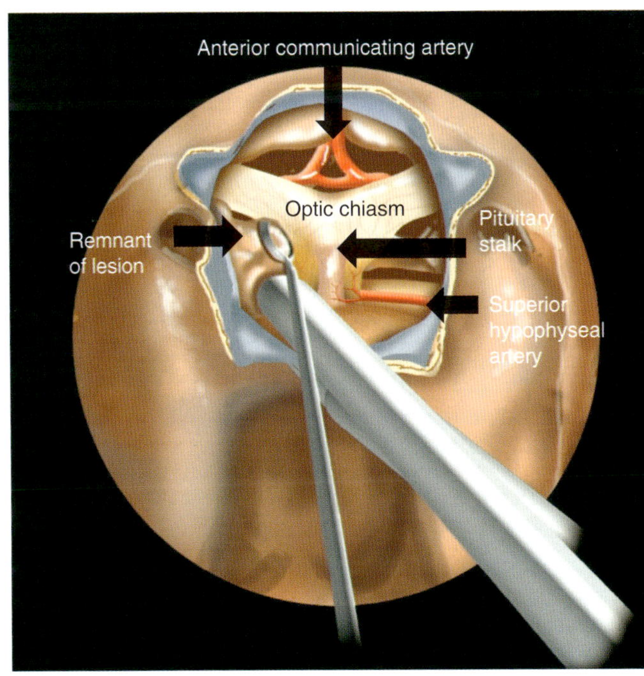

• **Fig. 36.6** The Tumor Excision Stage. After excision of tumor, critical structures can be clearly observed. Optic chiasm, pituitary stalk, anterior communicating artery, and superior hypophyseal vessels are shown. (Courtesy Paul Schiffmacher and Tawfiq Khoury, MD.)

or fascia lata. A number of repair techniques have been described, such as the bilayer button graft, gasket seal, and AlloDerm (LifeCell, Branchburg NJ) closure.[60,62-65] A bilayer button graft using fascia lata is particularly suited for complex defects[62] (Figs. 36.7 through 36.9). The bilayer graft prevents migration, can be used

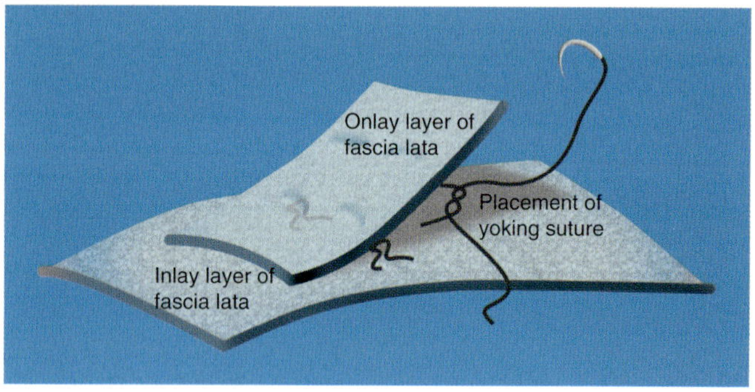

• **Fig. 36.7** The Dural Reconstruction Stage. Button graft made from two layers of fascia lata. The inlay layer is 25% larger in area than the onlay. Both layers are held together by a yoking suture. (Courtesy Paul Schiffmacher and Tawfiq Khoury, MD)

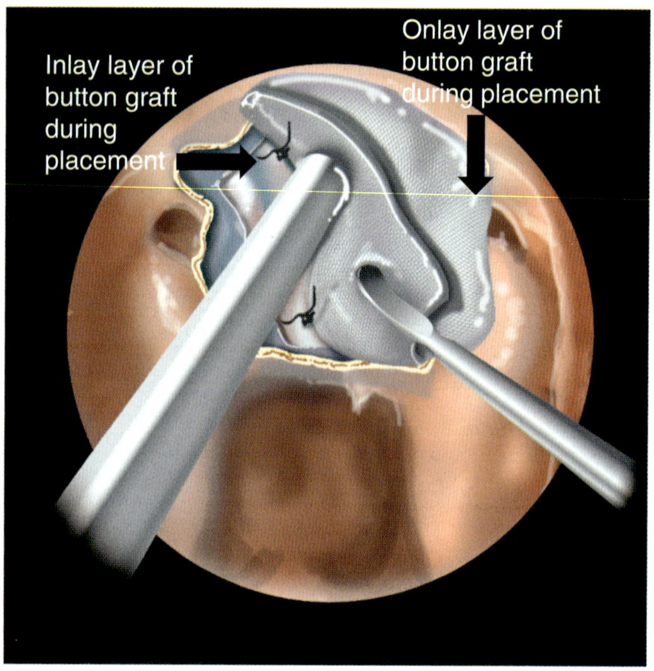

• **Fig. 36.8** The Dural Reconstruction Stage. In situ placement of button graft is shown. The inlay layer is neatly tucked along the dural edges while the onlay lays over the defect. It should be noted that the placement of sutures is such that they always lie inside the area of sellar defect. (Courtesy Paul Schiffmacher and Tawfiq Khoury, MD.)

in defects spanning more than one plane, and can be placed around delicate neurovascular structures without the need for a rigid buttress. When the graft is properly positioned, normal dural pulsations are clearly visible, thus confirming a watertight and stable primary dural repair. Bony cranial base reconstruction is not routinely needed or performed.

Closure

Closure is often individualized and may involve the use of either synthetic or autologous tissue. In cases of pituitary adenoma resection, there is often no intraoperative CSF leak and a simple closure with Surgicel (Johnson & Johnson, New Brunswick, NJ), fat, or a dural substitute is adequate. Use of a vascularized NSF is preferred in the setting of high-flow defects.

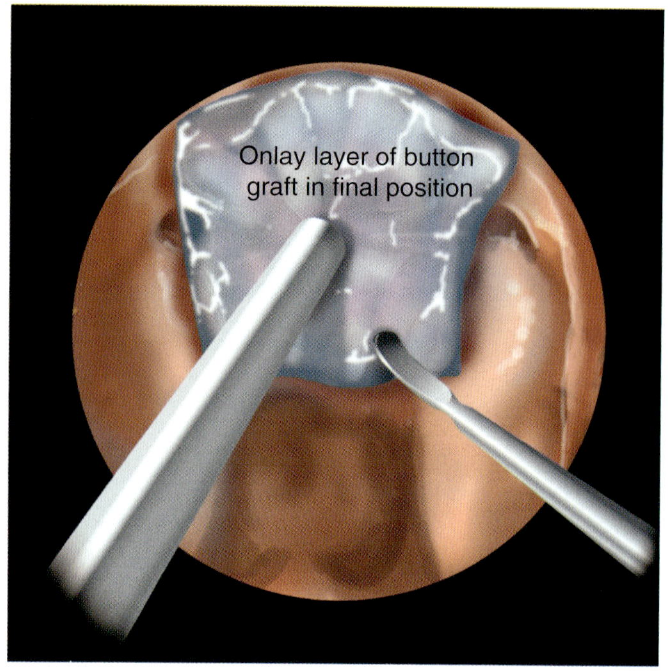

• **Fig. 36.9** The Dural Reconstruction Stage. Button graft after proper placement along the sellar defect. (Courtesy Paul Schiffmacher and Tawfiq Khoury, MD.)

Harvest of the NSF is performed by making cuts with either a scalpel or needle tip cautery under a low-power (5-7 W) setting.[50,66] The muscles of the soft palate are avoided. The width of the flap may be increased by extending the cuts beneath the inferior turbinate and up along the lateral nasal sidewall. The mucosal surface of the flap can be marked with a surgical pen to distinguish it from the perichondrial/periosteal surface. The flap is then carefully raised in a subperichondrial/subperiosteal plane and left pedicled on the septal branch of the sphenopalatine artery. The flap can then be placed into the nasopharynx, or less frequently the maxillary sinus, until it is needed for reconstruction. If an NSF was initially harvested but is not necessary for the repair, it may be returned to the septum and sutured back in place in a "raise and return" fashion.

Care should be taken to avoid inadvertent creation of dead space between the dural repair and vascularized tissue. Polyethylene glycol hydrogel glue or other sealants may then be applied to the flap edges to improve its adherence. Absorbable nasal packing can be used to buttress the flap if needed, but no removable packing is used. The turbinates are medialized and absorbable packing is placed bilaterally in the bilateral middle meatus.

Postoperative Management

The patient is ideally extubated at a moderate depth of anesthesia with spontaneous breathing to avoid positive pressure or coughing that could displace the reconstruction. Airway reflexes during emergence can be reduced by the use of topical or intravenous lidocaine, remifentanil, or dexmedetomidine.

Once the patient is awake, vision can be immediately tested to confirm the integrity of the optic apparatus before formal ophthalmic evaluation. Vision should be examined frequently for the first 24 to 48 hours; if there is deterioration, immediate imaging should be obtained to rule out postoperative hemorrhage. If postoperative hemorrhage or compression is detected, the patient should return to the operation room for immediate evacuation to preserve/restore vision.

Throughout the postoperative period, precautions are taken to reduce the chance of a CSF leak. This includes elevating the head of the bed to 45 degrees, use of stool softeners, restriction of nose blowing, and instructing the patient to sneeze with his or her mouth open. If a postoperative CSF leak develops, our preference is to return to the operating room for closure rather than placing a lumbar drain on the hospital floor. Furthermore, intake/output, electrolyte, and cortisol levels are monitored.

After discharge, visual function can be objectively documented (using a Snellen chart for visual acuity, Ishihara chart for color vision, and Humphrey or Goldmann chart for visual fields) during serial clinic visits. This may allow for documentation of progressive improvement or early identification of clinical deterioration. Postoperative follow-up visits at 1 to 2 weeks, 3 to 4 weeks, and 7 at 8 weeks are typically advised for nasal debridement. Use of topical nasal sprays and irrigation improves nasal hydration and facilitates mucosal healing of nasal cavity. Electrolyte and endocrine disturbances (diabetes insipidus, syndrome of inappropriate hormone secretion, and hypocortisolism) as well as CSF leaks are carefully monitored. In the circumstance of a postoperative CSF leak, early exploration and closure are recommended. Follow-up radiologic surveillance with magnetic resonance imaging is typically performed at 3 months postoperatively.

Postoperative Complications

One of the major surgical complications is CSF fistula and the associated risk of meningitis. Rates of postoperative CSF leak with the EEA vary widely (0-62%) depending on the site of lesion, the extent of osteotomies at cranial base, the type of dural repair, and the expertise of the surgical team. Use of an NSF has been demonstrated to effectively lower the incidence,[60,67,68] especially with increased surgeon experience.[68]

Other major perioperative complications include visual disturbance (transient/permanent), internal carotid artery injury, extraocular muscle palsy, facial hypesthesia, and hypopituitarism (diabetes insipidus, hypothyroidism, hypocortisolism, and panhypopituitarism).[9,20,30,43,44,60] Table 36.2 provides a brief description of surgical techniques to avoid these complications.

TABLE 36.2 Major Perioperative Complications and Their Respective Preventive Techniques

Perioperative complications	Intra-operative preventive technique/s
Olfactory disturbance	Minimal use of coagulation in upper one cm of nasal cavity
Epistaxis (Early/Delayed)	Adequate coagulation of bleeding sites
Sinusitis/Mucocele	Middle turbinate medialization at the end of surgery. Avoid trapping mucosa (adequate mucosal removal)
CSF leak/Meningitis/Pneumocephalus	Blind dissection and suctioning of tumor before adequate mobilization is avoided. "Flashlight effect" may be used to prevent arachnoid tear. If CSF leak is present intra-operatively, then immediate repair is advised.
Carotid Injury	Careful review of anatomical knowledge, preoperative imaging, use of intra-operative navigation and doppler.
Pituitary hormonal deficiencies	Always predict the position of pituitary gland and infundibulum in preoperative MRI. Prompt intra-operative recognition of the gland.
Apoplexy/bleed from the lesion	Ensure excision of complete lesion or at least maximum possible part of it.
Visual disturbance	Avoid overzealous sellar/suprasellar packing

(Adapted from Sharma BS 2016)

Visual Outcomes

Preservation or improvement of visual function is one of the main surgical goals. To date, the most reliable prognostic factor of postoperative visual outcome is the retinal nerve fiber layer, especially for inferior quadrant on optical coherence tomography. Thinning of the retinal nerve fiber layer on preoperative examination indicates optic atrophy and is associated with worse visual outcomes.[69]

In a majority of patients, restoration of visual function occurs in three distinct postoperative phases: early fast, early slow, and late. In the first postoperative month, a rapid improvement in *visual fields* is usually seen owing to a release of compression and associated conduction block. The second phase takes place from 1 to 4 months, during which *visual acuity* is restored in a majority of cases owing to restoration of axoplasmic flow and remyelination. The final phase, from 4 months to 3 years, is usually defined by mild improvements in *visual functioning* owing to the same mechanisms previously described, as well as possible neuronal plasticity effects seen within the anterior visual pathways.[70-72] The early slow phase is considered the most consistent phase of improvement.[71]

Various factors affect the postoperative visual outcomes. The duration of preoperative visual loss may also have an effect. Some studies have reported that a shorter duration of preoperative visual dysfunction is associated with better visual outcomes postoperatively.[73] In cases in which preoperative visual loss is present for less than 24 hours, improvement in visual function is observed in approximately 75% compared with 58% in those with visual loss for more than 24 hours.[36] Therefore prompt surgical treatment is necessary, especially for those with progressive visual deficits. Younger age, better preoperative visual acuity, and lack of optic nerve pallor (owing to a shorter duration of compression of anterior visual pathways) are associated with better postoperative recovery of visual function.[6,72,74] In addition to these factors, surgical treatment itself may contribute to visual dysfunction in some cases (0-11%) by various mechanisms including direct injury to optic apparatus or its vascular supply, vasospasm, orbital fracture, postoperative hematoma, scarring, traction, postoperative chiasmal prolapse, and overzealous sphenoid, sellar or suprasellar packing.[9,75] In some cases of postoperative chiasmal prolapse, chiasmapexy (surgical repositioning of optic chiasm to a more normal anatomic position) may be necessary to restore visual function.[9,76]

Currently objective documentation of visual function using standard testing, both preoperatively and postoperatively, is generally lacking in the literature.[77] This lack has limited meaningful comparison of visual outcomes among various surgical techniques. In general, EEA is associated with higher rates of postoperative visual improvement (50%-100%) compared with transcranial approach (TCRA) (25%-78%).[45,78] This may be related to increased ability to avoid chiasmal ischemia as the inferior perforators to optic apparatus may be identified early in the operation and preserved with EEA.[79]

Advantages of the Endoscopic Endonasal Approach

The EEA has several advantages over TCRA. It offers a more direct surgical pathway to lesions around the medial optic apparatus with excellent visualization, magnification,[80] illumination,[81] and panoramic view using angled telescopes.[81-83] Furthermore, EEA provides access between the optic chiasm, anterior communicating artery complex, and frontobasal perforators cranially, as well as the midbrain structures caudally. For lesions invading the optic canal, especially inferomedially, EEA readily allows early bilateral extradural optic nerve decompression.[56] Importantly, EEA is associated with a lower risk of frontal or temporal lobe retraction, seizures, sylvian fissure dissection, intracranial hemorrhage, injury to olfactory fibers, and other cranial neuropathies. Additionally, EEA does not place critical neurovascular structures between the surgeon and target pathology,[84] thus reducing the risk of neurovascular injury. It is also associated with a more complete and consistent excision of tumors with intracavernous sinus extension, and provides a possibility of preservation of the DS and basal arachnoid if needed.[45,48,79] Adhesions and scar tissue from previous TCRA also may be bypassed with reoperations using EEA. Lesions with ethmoid and sphenoid extension as well as hyperostotic bones can be easily resected. EEA also may reduce blood loss by allowing surgeons the ability to devascularize the blood supply from the skull base vessels before starting tumor resection.[46] EEA is also better tolerated by patients with multiple comorbidities given reduced blood loss and faster recovery time compared with craniotomy.[20,77] The extent of tumor resection with EEA has been found to be comparable or better than that in TCRA.[78]

Limitations of the Endoscopic Endonasal Approach

It is important to recognize the limitations of the EEA. For certain lesions, such as those with vascular encasement, dural attachment lateral to anterior clinoid process or midorbital roof, extensive cavernous sinus invasion, internal carotid artery encasement, lateral optic canal involvement, and relatively narrow endoscopic endonasal corridor, EEA may not be appropriate.[20,43] For many surgeons, EEA involves a steep learning curve[20] with respect to hand–eye coordination, nondominant hand dexterity, and two-handed dissection within relatively small corridors.[48] EEA may also be associated with reduced depth perception owing to use of two-dimensional digital images.[48] However, this has not been a major problem for experienced surgeons. Furthermore, vascular control in the setting of a major vascular injury is also more challenging in EEA compared with open TCRA; therefore careful avoidance of vascular injury in EEA is paramount.[48]

References

1. Warmuth-metz, M., Gnekow, A. K., Müller, H., & Solymosi, L. (2004). Differential diagnosis of suprasellar tumors in children. *Klinische Padiatrie, 216*(6), 323–330.
2. Freda. P. U., & Post K. D. (1000). Differential diagnosis of sellar masses. *Endocrinolology and Metabolism Clinics of North America, 28*(1), 81–117, vi.
3. Daly, A. F., Rixhon, M., Adam, C., Dempegioti, A., Tichomirowa, M. A., & Beckers, A. (2006). High prevalence of pituitary adenomas: A cross-sectional study in the province of Liege, Belgium. *Journal of Clinical Endocrinology and Metabolism, 91*(12), 4769–4775.
4. Fernandez, A., Karavitaki, N., & Wass, J. A. (2010). Prevalence of pituitary adenomas: A community-based, cross-sectional study in Banbury (Oxfordshire, UK). *Clinical Endocrinology, 72*(3), 377–382.
5. Raappana, A., Koivukangas, J., Ebeling, T., & Pirila, T. (2010). Incidence of pituitary adenomas in Northern Finland in 1992-2007. *Journal of Clinical Endocrinology and Metabolism, 95* (9), 4268–4275.
6. Cohen, A. R., Cooper, P. R., Kupersmith, M. J., Flamm, E. S., & Ransohoff, J. (1985). Visual recovery after transsphenoidal removal of pituitary adenomas. *Neurosurgery, 17*(3), 446–452.
7. Ogra, S., Nichols, A. D., Stylli, S., Kaye, A. H., Savino, P. J., & Danesh-Meyer, H. V. (2014). Visual acuity and pattern of visual field loss at presentation in pituitary adenoma. *Journal of Clinical Neuroscience, 21*(5), 735–740.
8. Vance, M. L. (2001). Diagnosis, management, and prognosis of pituitary tumors. In K. Thapar, K. Kovacs, B. W. Scheithauer, & R. V. Lloyd (Eds.), *Diagnosis and management of pituitary tumors* (pp. 165–172). Totowa, NJ: Humana Press.
9. Fraser, C. L., Biousse, V., & Newman, N. J. (2012). Visual outcomes after treatment of pituitary adenomas. *Neurosurgery Clinics of North America, 23*(4), 607–619.
10. Wilson, P., & Falconer, M. A. (1968). Patterns of visual failure with pituitary tumours: Clinical and radiological correlations. *British Journal of Ophthalmology, 52*(2), 94–110.
11. Hollenhorst, R., & Younge, R. (1973). Ocular manifestations produced by adenomas of the pituitary gland: 1000 cases. In P. Kohler & G. Ross (Eds.), *Diagnosis and treatment of pituitary tumours*. Amsterdam: Excerpta Medica.
12. Miller, B. A., Loachimescu, A. G., & Oyesiku, N. M. (2014). Contemporary indications for transsphenoidal pituitary surgery. *World Neurosurgery, 82*(6 Suppl), S147–S151.
13. Sharma, B. S., Sawarkar, D. P., & Suri, A. (2016). Endoscopic pituitary surgery: Techniques, tips and tricks, nuances, and complication avoidance. *Neurology India, 64*(4), 724–736.
14. Dutton, J. J. (1992). Optic nerve sheath meningiomas. *Survey of Ophthalmology, 37*, 167–183.
15. Miller, N. R. (2004). Primary tumours of the optic nerve and its sheath. *Eye, 18*, 1026–1037.
16. Cantore, W. A. (2000). Neural orbital tumors. *Current Opinion in Ophthalmology, 11*, 367–371.
17. Schick, U., Dott, U., & Hassler, W. (2004). Surgical management of meningiomas involving the optic nerve sheath. *Journal of Neurosurgery, 101*, 951–959.
18. Frosch, M. P., Anthony, D. C., & De Girolami, U. (2010). The central nervous system. In V. Kumar, A. K. Abbas, & J. C. Aster (Eds.), *Robbins and Cotran pathologic basis of disease* (pp. 1279–1344). Philadelphia, PA: Elsevier.
19. Ajlan, A. M., Choudhri, O., Hwang, P., & Harsh, G. (2015). Meningiomas of the tuberculum and diaphragma sellae. *Journal of Neurological Surgery Part B Skull Base, 76*(1), 74–79.
20. Bowers, C. A., Altay, T., & Couldwell, W. T. (2011). Surgical decision-making strategies in tuberculum sellae meningioma resection. *Neurosurgical Focu, 30*(5), E1.

21. Kwancharoen, R., Blitz, A. M., Tavares, F., Caturegli, P., Gallia, G. L., & Salvatori, R. (2014). Clinical features of sellar and suprasellar meningiomas. *Pituitary, 17*(4), 342–348.
22. Rossi, A., Cama, A., Consales, A., Gandolfo, C., Garrè, M. L., Milanaccio, C., et al. (2006). Neuroimaging of pediatric craniopharyngiomas: A pictorial essay. *Journal of Pediatric Endocrinolology & Metabolism, 19*(Suppl 1), 299–319.
23. Poretti, A., Grotzer, M. A., Ribi, K., Schönle, E., & Boltshauser, E. (2004). Outcome of craniopharyngioma in children: Long-term complications and quality of life. *Developmental Medicine and Child Neurology, 46*(220–229), 2004.
24. Bunin, G. R., Surawicz, T. S., Witman, P. A., Preston-Martin, S., Davis, F., & Bruner, J. M. (1998). The descriptive epidemiology of craniopharyngioma. *Journal of Neurosurgery, 89*, 547–551.
25. Erfurth, E. M., Holmer, H., & Fjalldal, S. B. (2013). Mortality and morbidity in adult craniopharyngioma. *Pituitary, 16*(1), 46–55.
26. Müller, H. L., Merchant, T. E., Puget, S., & Martinez-Barbera, J. P. (2017). New outlook on the diagnosis, treatment and follow-up of childhood-onset craniopharyngioma. *Nature Reviews Endocrinology, 13*(5), 299–312.
27. Müller, H. L. (2014). Childhood craniopharyngioma: Treatment strategies and outcomes. *Expert Review of Neurotherapeutics, 14*(2), 187–197.
28. Müller, H. L., Gebhardt, U., Schröder, S., Pohl, F., Kortmann, R. D., Faldum, A., et al. (2010). Analyses of treatment variables for patients with childhood craniopharyngioma—results of the multicenter prospective trial KRANIOPHARYNGEOM 2000 after three years of follow-up. *Hormone Research in Paediatrics, 73*(3), 175–180.
29. Stripp, D. C., Maity, A., Janss, A. J., Belasco, J. B., Tochner, Z. A., Goldwein, J. W., et al. (2004). Surgery with or without radiation therapy in the management of craniopharyngiomas in children and young adults. *International Journal of Radiation Oncology, Biology, Physics, 58*(3), 714–720.
30. Cohen, M., Bartels, U., Branson, H., Kulkarni, A. V., & Hamilton, J. (2013). Trends in treatment and outcomes of pediatric craniopharyngioma, 1975-2011. *Neuro-oncology, 15*(6), 767–774.
31. Arai, A., Morishita, A., Hanada, Y., & Aihara, H. (2010). Solitary metastatic tumor within the optic chiasm—case report. *Neurologia Medico-Chirurgica, 50*(2), 158–161.
32. Carreras, E. M., Lyons, C. J., & Cochrane, D. D. (2014). Delayed visual loss from optochiasmatic arachnoiditis after resection of craniopharyngioma. *Journal of Neurosurgery Pediatrics, 13*(5), 520–524.
33. Chaudhry, N. S., Ahmad, F., Blieden, C., & Morcos, J. J. (2013). Suprasellar and sellar paraganglioma presenting as a nonfunctioning pituitary macroadenoma. *Journal of Clinical Neuroscience, 20*(11), 1615–1618.
34. Kaptain, G. J., Vincent, D. A., & Laws, E. R. (2001). Cranial base reconstruction after transsphenoidal surgery with bio-absorbable implants. *Neurosurgery, 48*, 232–234.
35. Petrakakis, I., Pirayesh, A., Krauss, J. K., Raab, P., Hartmann, C., & Nakamura, M. (2016). The sellar and suprasellar region: A "hideaway" of rare lesions. Clinical aspects, imaging findings, surgical outcome and comparative analysis. *Clinical Neurology and Neurosurgery, 149*, 154–165.
36. Turgut, M., Ozsunar, Y., Başak, S., Güney, E., Kir, E., & Meteoğlu, I. (2010). Pituitary apoplexy: An overview of 186 cases published during the last century. *Acta Neurochirurgica, 152*(5), 749–761.
37. Vassal, F., Pommier, B., Boutet, C., Forest, F., Campolmi, N., & Nuti, C. (2014). Isolated primary central nervous system lymphoma arising from the optic chiasm. *Neurochirurgie, 60*(6), 312–315.
38. Müller, H. L., Emser, A., Faldum, A., Bruhnken, G., Etavard-Gorris, N., Gebhardt, U., et al. (2004). Longitudinal study on growth and body mass index before and after diagnosis of childhood craniopharyngioma. *Journal of Clinical Endocrinology and Metabolism, 89*(7), 3298–3305.
39. Wang, Q., Lu, X. J., Li, B., Ji, W. Y., & Chen, K. L. (2009). Extended endoscopic endonasal transsphenoidal removal of tuberculum sellae meningiomas: A preliminary report. *Journal of Clinical Neuroscience, 16*, 889–893.
40. Dutton, J. J. (1991). Optic nerve gliomas and meningiomas. *Neurology Clinics, 9*, 163–177.
41. Turbin, R. E., Thompson, C. R., Kenderell, J. S., Cockerham, K. P., & Kupersmith, M. J. (2002). A long-term visual outcome comparison in patients with optic nerve sheath meningioma managed with observation, surgery, radiotherapy or surgery and radiotherapy. *Ophthalmology, 9*, 890–900.
42. Wright, J. E., McNab, A. A., & McDonald, W. I. (1989). Primary optic nerve sheath meningioma. *British Journal of Ophthalmology, 73*, 960–966.
43. Couldwell, W. T., Weiss, M. H., Rabb, C., Liu, J. K., Apfelbaum, R. I., & Fukushima, T. (2004). Variations on the standard transsphenoidal approach to the sellar region, with emphasis on the extended approaches and parasellar approaches: surgical experience in 105 cases. *Neurosurgery, 55*, 539–550.
44. De Divitiis, E., Esposito, F., Cappabianca, P., Cavallo, L. M., de Divitiis, O., & Esposito, I. (2008). Endoscopic transnasal resection of anterior cranial fossa meningiomas. *Neurosurgical Focus, 25*(6), E8.
45. De Divitiis, E., Esposito, F., Cappabianca, P., Cavallo, L. M., & de Divitiis, O. (2008). Tuberculum sellae meningiomas: High route or low route? A series of 51 consecutive cases. *Neurosurgery, 62*, 556–563.
46. Gardner, P. A., Kassam, A. B., Thomas, A., Snyderman, C. H., Carrau, R. L., Mintz, A. H., et al. (2008). Endoscopic endonasal resection of anterior cranial base meningiomas. *Neurosurgery, 63*, 36–54.
47. Wang, Q., Lu, X. J., Ji, W. Y., Yan, Z. C., Xu, J., Ding, Y. S., et al. (2010). Visual outcome after extended endoscopic endonasal transsphenoidal surgery for tuberculum sellae meningiomas. *World Neurosurgery, 73*(6), 694–700.
48. De Divitiis, E. (2013). Endoscopic endonasal transsphenoidal surgery: From the pituitary fossa to the midline cranial base. *World Neurosurgery, 80*(5), e45–e51.
49. Singh, H., Vogel, R. W., Lober, R. M., Doan, A. T., Matsumoto, C. I., Kenning, T. J., et al. (2016). Intraoperative neurophysiological monitoring for endoscopic endonasal approaches to the skull base: A technical guide. *Scientifica, 2016*, 1751245.
50. Hadad, G., Bassagasteguy, L., Carrau, R. L., Mataza, J. C., Kassam, A., Snyderman, C. H., et al. (2006). A novel reconstructive technique after endoscopic expanded endonasal approaches: Vascular pedicle nasoseptal flap. *Laryngoscope, 116*, 1882–1886.
51. Otto, B. A., Bowe, S. N., Carrau, R. L., Prevedello, D. M., Ditzel Filho, L. F., & De lara, D. (2013). Transsphenoidal approach with nasoseptal flap pedicle transposition: Modified rescue flap technique. *Laryngoscope, 123*(12), 2976–2979.
52. Rivera-Serrano, C. M., Snyderman, C. H., Gardner, P., Prevedello, D., Wheless, S., Kassam, A. B., et al. (2011). Nasoseptal "rescue" flap: A novel modification of the nasoseptal flap technique for pituitary surgery. *Laryngoscope, 121*(5), 990–993.
53. Koszewski, I., Garcia, H., Parkes, W., Chitguppi, C., Rabinowitz, M., Nyquist, G., Evans, J., Rosen, M., et al. (2019). The endoscopic endonasal approach for pediatric craniopharyngiomas. *Operative Techniques in Otolaryngology—Head and Neck Surgery, 30*(1), 44–53.
54. Cavallo, L. M., Esposito, F., & Cappabianca, P. (2010). Surgical limits in transnasal approach to opticocarotid region and planum sphenoidale: An anatomic cadaveric study. *World Neurosurgery, 73*(4), 301–303.
55. Lucas, J. W., & Zada, G. (2012). Endoscopic surgery for pituitary tumors. *Neurosurgery Clinics of North America, 23*(4), 555–569.
56. Liu, J. K., Christiano, L. D., Patel, S. K., Tubbs, R. S., & Eloy, J. A. (2011). Surgical nuances for removal of tuberculum sellae meningiomas with optic canal involvement using the endoscopic endonasal extended transsphenoidal transplanum transtuberculum approach. *Neurosurgical Focus, 30*(5), E2.
57. Koutourousiou, M., Gardner, P. A., Fernandez-Miranda, J. C., TylerKabara, E. C., Wang, E. W., & Snyderman, C. H. (2013). Endoscopic endonasal surgery for craniopharyngiomas: Surgical outcome in 64 patients. *Journal of Neurosurgery, 119*, 1194–1207.

58. Koutourousiou, M., Fernandez-Miranda, J. C., Stefko, S. T., Wang, E. W., Snyderman, C. H., & Gardner, P. A. (2014). Endoscopic endonasal surgery for suprasellar meningiomas: Experience with 75 patients. *Journal of Neurosurgery, 120*(6), 1326–1339.
59. Weiner, H. L., Wisoff, J. H., Rosenberg, M. E., Kupersmith, M. J., Cohen, H., Zagzag, D., et al. (1994). Craniopharyngiomas: A clinicopathological analysis of factors predictive of recurrence and functional outcome. *Neurosurgery, 35*(6). 1001–1010.
60. Cavallo, L. M., Messina, A., Esposito, F., de Divitiis, O., Dal Fabbro, M., de Divitiis, E., et al. (2007). Skull base reconstruction in the extended endoscopic transsphenoidal approach for suprasellar lesions. *Journal of Neurosurgery, 107*(4), 713–720.
61. Kaptain, G. J., Vincent, D. A., Sheehan, J. P., & Laws, E. R. (2001). Transsphenoidal approaches for the extracapsular resection of midline suprasellar and anterior cranial base lesions. *Neurosurgery, 49*(1), 94–100.
62. Luginbuhl, A. J., Campbell, P. G., Evans, J., & Rosen, M. (2010). Endoscopic repair of high-flow cranial base defects using a bilayer button. *Laryngoscope, 120*(5), 876–880.
63. Kshettry, V. R., Nyquist, G., & Evans, J. J. (2018). Endoscopic endonasal resection of retrochiasmatic craniopharyngioma with fascia lata button and nasoseptal flap reconstruction. *Journal of Neurological Surgery Part B, Skull Base, 79*(2), S191–S193.
64. Takeuchi, K., Nagatani, T., & Wakabayashi, T. (2015). How I do it: Shoelace watertight dural closure in extended transsphenoidal surgery. *Acta Neurochirurgica 15, 157*(12), 2089–2092.
65. Wessell, A., Singh, A., & Litvack, Z. (2013). One-piece modified gasket seal technique. *Journal of Neurological Surgery Part B, Skull Base, 74*(5), 305–310.
66. Pinheiro-Neto, C. D., & Snyderman, C. H. (2013). Nasoseptal flap. *Advances in Oto-Rhino-Laryngology, 74*, 42–55.
67. Eloy, J. A., Choudhry, O. J., Shukla, P. A., Kuperan, A. B., Friedel, M. E., & Liu, J. K. (2012). Nasoseptal flap repair after endoscopic transsellar versus expanded endonasal approaches: Is there an increased risk of postoperative cerebrospinal fluid leak? *Laryngoscope, 122*, 1219–1225.
68. Kassam, A. B., Thomas, A., Carrau, R. L., Snyderman, C. H., Vescan, A., Prevedello, D., et al. (2008). Endoscopic reconstruction of the cranial base using a pedicled nasoseptal flap. *Neurosurgery, 63*(1 Suppl 1). In *ONS44–52.*
69. Jacob, M., Raverot, G., Jouanneau, E., Borson-Chazot, F., Perrin, G., Rabilloud, M., et al. (2009). Predicting visual outcome after treatment of pituitary adenomas with optical coherence tomography. *American Journal of Ophthalmology, 147*(1), 64–7000.
70. Kayan, A., & Earl, C. J. (1975). Compressive lesions of the optic nerves and chiasm: Pattern of recovery of vision following surgical treatment. *Brain, 98*(1), 13–28.
71. Kerrison, J. B., Lynn, M. J., Baer, C. A., Newman, S. A., Biousse, V., & Newman, N. J. (2000). Stages of improvement in visual fields after pituitary tumor resection. *American Journal of Ophthalmology, 130*(6), 813–820.
72. Marcus, M., Vitale, S., Calvert, P. C., & Miller, N. R. (1991). Visual parameters in patients with pituitary adenoma before and after transsphenoidal surgery. *Australian and New Zealand Journal of Ophthalmology, 19*(2), 111–118.
73. Gnanalingham, K. K., Bhattacharjee, S., Pennington, R., Ng, J., & Mendoza, N. (2005). The time course of visual field recovery following transphenoidal surgery for pituitary adenomas: Predictive factors for a good outcome. *Journal of Neurology, Neurosurgery, and Psychiatry, 76*(3), 415–419.
74. Fisher, P. G., Jenab, J., Goldthwaite, P. T., Tihan, T., Wharam, M. D., Foer, D. R., et al. (1998). Outcomes and failure patterns in childhood craniopharyngiomas. *Child's Nervous System, 14*, 558–563.
75. Barrow, D. L., & Tindall, G. T. (1990). Loss of vision after transsphenoidal surgery. *Neurosurgery, 27*, 60–68.
76. Welch, K., & Stears, J. C. (1971). Chiasmapexy for the correction of traction on the optic nerves and chiasm associated with their descent into an empty sella turcica: Case report. *Journal of Neurosurgery, 35*, 760–764.
77. Kitano, M., Taneda, M., & Nakao, Y. (2007). Postoperative improvement in visual function in patients with tuberculum sellae meningiomas: Results of the extended transsphenoidal and transcranial approaches. *Journal of Neurosurgery, 107*(2), 337–346.
78. Clark, A. J., Jahangiri, A., Garcia, R. M., George, J. R., Sughrue, M. E., McDermott, M. W., et al. (2013). Endoscopic surgery for tuberculum sellae meningiomas: A systematic review and metaanalysis. *Neurosurgical Review, 36*(3), 349–359.
79. Frank, G., & Pasquini, E. (2010). Tuberculum sellae meningioma: the extended transsphenoidal approach—for the virtuoso only? *World Neurosurgery, 73*, 625–626.
80. Snyderman, C. H., Carrau, R. L., Prevedello, D. M., Gardner, P., & Kassam, A. B. (2009). Technologic innovations in neuroendoscopic surgery. *Otolaryngologic Clinics of North America, 42*, 883–890.
81. Gopal, H. V. (2000). Endoscopic transnasal transsphenoid pituitary surgery. *Current Opinion in Otolaryngology & Head and Neck Surgery, 3*, 43–48.
82. Cappabianca, P., Cavallo, L. M., Colao, A., & de Divitiis, E. (2002). Surgical complications associated with the endoscopic endonasal transsphenoidal approach for pituitary adenomas. *Journal of Neurosurgery, 97*, 293–298.
83. Moses, R. L., & Keane, W. M. (1999). Endoscopic transseptal transsphenoid hypophysectomy with 3-D intraoperative localization technology. *Laryngoscope, 109*, 509–512.
84. Nyquist, G. G., Anand, V. K., & Schwartz, T. H. (2011). Transplanum transtuberculum approach to suprasellar lesions in transnasal endoscopic skull base and brain surgery: Tips and pearls. In: A. Stamm. *Endoscopic skull base and brain surgery* (pp. 193–200). New York, NY: Thieme Medical Publishers.

37

Reconstructive Techniques in Endoscopic Skull Base and Orbital Surgery

ZACHARY J. CAPPELLO, MD, CHRISTOPHER R. ROXBURY, MD, AND RAJ SINDWANI, MD, FACS, FRCS(C)

Advances in endoscopic surgical techniques and instrumentation have led to an expansion in the size and diversity of skull base lesions that are amenable to endoscopic resection. However, one of the stipulations for adopting an endoscopic approach for the removal of skull base lesions is the ability to repair the resultant defect, as failed reconstructions, and the subsequent cerebrospinal fluid (CSF) leak, add significant morbidity.[1] With this in mind, the ideal endoscopic skull base repair is technically feasible as part of the endoscopic procedure and provides a reliable and robust separation between the nasal and cranial cavities that will last over the long term.[2] In addition, the repair should reconstruct the natural tissue barriers of the skull base, minimally affect normal sinonasal and cranial physiology, and possibly obliterate the dead space after tumor removal.[2] The surgeon must also consider the anticipated location, size, and geometry of the bony and dural defects, as well as the anticipated volume of CSF leak.[3] Finally, the surgeon must also consider previous sinonasal surgery, previous or planned postoperative radiotherapy, and the extent of tumor involvement of nasal structures, such as the septum and turbinates, all of which may limit the available options for reconstruction.[4]

Endoscopic skull base reconstruction has shown excellent success rates with low perioperative and postoperative morbidity even when large defects are present.[5] In some cases of skull base surgery, when no or a low-flow CSF leak is encountered—for example, a simple reconstruction—may be all that is required using free grafts or even alloplastic materials. A large variety of local and regional vascularized pedicle flaps can be used to reconstruct more complex defects of the skull base. Both free grafts and vascularized flap repairs usually use a multilayered closure to establish a reliable barrier between the cranial and nasal cavities. The most common points of failure of flap repairs are the dependent parts, presumably owing to increased pressure, or the most superior parts, likely owing to flap migration or retraction.[6,7]

Pre-Reconstruction Considerations

Given the multitude of options available for reconstruction, an effort has been made to define the indications and utility for each type of repair. Likely the most important factor guiding the selection of a repair method is classifying the volume and flow of CSF leak (if any) as well as the size and complexity of the anticipated defect.[8-10] The CSF flow rate can be classified as no leak (no intracranial opening, or appreciable leak into the nose), a low-flow (intracranial opening but minimal flow observed or no direct communication with a cistern or ventricle), and a high-flow leak (intracranial opening, direct communication into a ventricle or cistern). Preoperative imaging can be used to predict the type of CSF leak likely to be encountered after resection of a given lesion.

When there is no CSF leak, the repair is at the surgeon's discretion and can range from simple onlay or epidural/subdural underlay placement of a synthetic graft or repair with packing and/or dural sealant at the level of the sella.[10] Skull base defects that are small with a low-flow CSF leak can be reconstructed with a wide variety of multilayered (or even monolayered) avascular free grafts or biosynthetic materials with high success rates and limited morbidity.[9,11] Larger and more complex skull base defects (>2–3 cm) and those that are associated with high-flow CSF leaks are best repaired with a multilayered technique using a vascularized flap of tissue (Table 37.1).[3,5,10]

In addition to leak type, other independent factors must be considered to help guide the reconstructive decision-making process. The extent of the skull base defect should be assessed because resections involving extended approaches often result in large and more complex defects with high-flow CSF leaks that are best managed with vascularized flaps.[9,10] Specific disorders also carry an increased potential for postoperative CSF leak, and as such, the use of a vascularized pedicled flap should be strongly considered in these unique instances. Among these are meningiomas (extensive bony and dural resection with intracranial disruption of the arachnoid plane), craniopharyngiomas (often requiring expanded approaches and involving arachnoid dissection), Cushing disease (reduced healing from hypercortisolemia), and morbid obesity (possible increased intracranial pressure, also potentially present with Cushing disease).[9,10] Furthermore, in patients who have had or will potentially need radiation therapy, vascularized flaps should be strongly considered, as they are more likely to withstand the effects of radiation therapy in providing a durable repair. Lastly, independent of CSF leak and radiation status, vascularized reconstructions may provide adequate coverage of exposed neurovital structures

TABLE 37.1 Endoscopic Reconstructive Ladder of Skull Base Defects by Type of Cerebrospinal Fluid Leak

No Leak	Low-Flow Leak	High-Flow Leak
Single layer	Multilayer	Multilayer
Synthetic dural replacement graft	Synthetic dural replacement graft	Synthetic dural replacement graft
Autograft (fat or mucosa)	Autograft (fascia lata or mucosa)	Autograft (fascia lata or fat)
No repair		Intranasal vascularized flaps
		Extranasal vascularized flaps
		Free tissue transfer

(e.g., internal carotid artery) that may be uncovered and mobilized during tumor resection.

The use of a lumbar drain as part of the reconstructive strategy deserves consideration as preoperative planning takes place. The placement of a perioperative lumbar drain has not been shown to positively affect postoperative leak rates when vascularized flaps are used. However, the use of a lumbar drain in the setting of a postoperative CSF leak has been shown to be effective as first-line therapy.[12] In our experience, lumbar drains can provide advantages in some high-risk clinical situations. In addition to potentially enhancing the success rate in some complex, high-flow CSF leak cases, the use of drains also provides the opportunity to (1) measure opening pressures before and after repair and (2) permit the intrathecal injection of fluorescein, which may be of value in some cases. The use of lumbar drains is associated with certain attendant risks that must be balanced in any given case.[12-14]

The Reconstructive Ladder

A thoughtful and systematic way to organize available options is to use the idea of a "reconstructive ladder" when considering skull base reconstruction.

No Reconstruction

When no CSF leak is encountered, no complicated reconstruction is required. It is worth mentioning that provocative testing by having the anesthesiologist raise intrathoracic pressure (simulating a Valsalva maneuver) is worthwhile to perform routinely at the end of every procedure in which a CSF leak is not obvious to ensure that a small or otherwise clinically occult leak is not present. The "no CSF leak" scenario is often encountered during routine transsellar approaches for pituitary lesions. A monolayer reconstruction aimed to simply cover the exposed diaphragm sella can be used with great success. In fact, very little is required by way of reconstruction in these cases, and some may prefer to only place a small amount of absorbable hemostatic agent into the sella at the conclusion of the procedure.

Some otherwise complex skull base procedures, including approaches to the craniovertebral junction, often do not require reconstruction of the resultant defect. As this is an entirely extradural procedure during which a CSF leak should not be encountered, an involved reconstruction is not required. When no obvious intraoperative CSF leak is encountered, hemostasis is obtained and the surgical field is thoroughly irrigated. Afterward, Valsalva maneuvers are undertaken to ensure a low-flow CSF leak has not been missed. A small amount of absorbable hemostatic agent may then be placed into the surgical defect, and the lateral aspects of the nasopharyngeal muscles and soft tissues may be approximated to the midline.[15,16]

Synthetic Dural Replacement Grafts

Fundamental to the endoscopic approach to intracranial lesions is the need to perform intradural dissection. The dura is typically reconstructed by some surgeons even in resections that do not result in a CSF leak (i.e., during a sellar approach without intraoperative CSF leak). When a low-flow or high-flow CSF leak is encountered, a multilayered reconstruction is used. In either case, a synthetic dural replacement graft is often used to reapproximate the dural defect. A variety of grafts are available depending on surgeon preference; however, grafts that can be sutured offer a sturdier repair substrate and are more pliant, making them easier to place and secure.[10] A major advantage of the use of such synthetic materials is that they are readily available and do not require additional donor site morbidity for the patient.

Free Autografts

Autograft choices typically include free mucosa, fat, and fascia lata. These tissues were some of the first reconstructive materials described for skull base reconstruction and are still excellent options.[17] Fascia lata grafts are harvested from an incision on the lateral thigh and offer a durable inlay or onlay material. The major drawbacks to the use of fascia lata are the presence of a permanent scar on the leg and wound-related issues, especially in young physically active patients.

Autologous fat grafts also provide a suitable inlay graft that can serve to occupy dead space and also to "cork" the defect opening. These grafts are typically harvested from the abdomen but may also be harvested from the thigh, particularly when the surgeon has already decided to harvest a fascia lata graft. Abdominal fat harvest is usually performed through a periumbilical incision to permit a less obvious scar as well as to avoid confusion with an appendectomy scar. Autologous fat grafts do not necessarily provide a watertight seal by themselves but are useful for filling large cavities left behind by resection or removal of a tumor.

Free grafts may also be harvested locally from multiple sites within the nasal cavity. Free mucosal grafts may be harvested from the septum, inferior turbinate, middle turbinate, or the nasal floor. If the middle turbinate is removed during the initial approach to the skull base, use of this mucosa for a free graft may negate further donor site morbidity.[18] The nasal floor graft is an attractive option owing to both its ease of harvest and very low donor site morbidity (Fig. 37.1).[19] Regardless of the donor site of the free mucosal graft, it is then applied with the mucosal side toward the nasal cavity to prevent development of a mucocele and is secured in place with a tissue sealant/glue of the surgeon's choice.

Local Pedicled Flaps

The principal workhorse of contemporary endoscopic skull base repair techniques is the Hadad-Bassagasteguy flap, or the pedicled nasoseptal flap (NSF) (Fig. 37.2). First described in 2006, it has proven to significantly reduce postoperative CSF leak rates.[6, 9] This flap has consistent vascularity (posterior septal branch of the

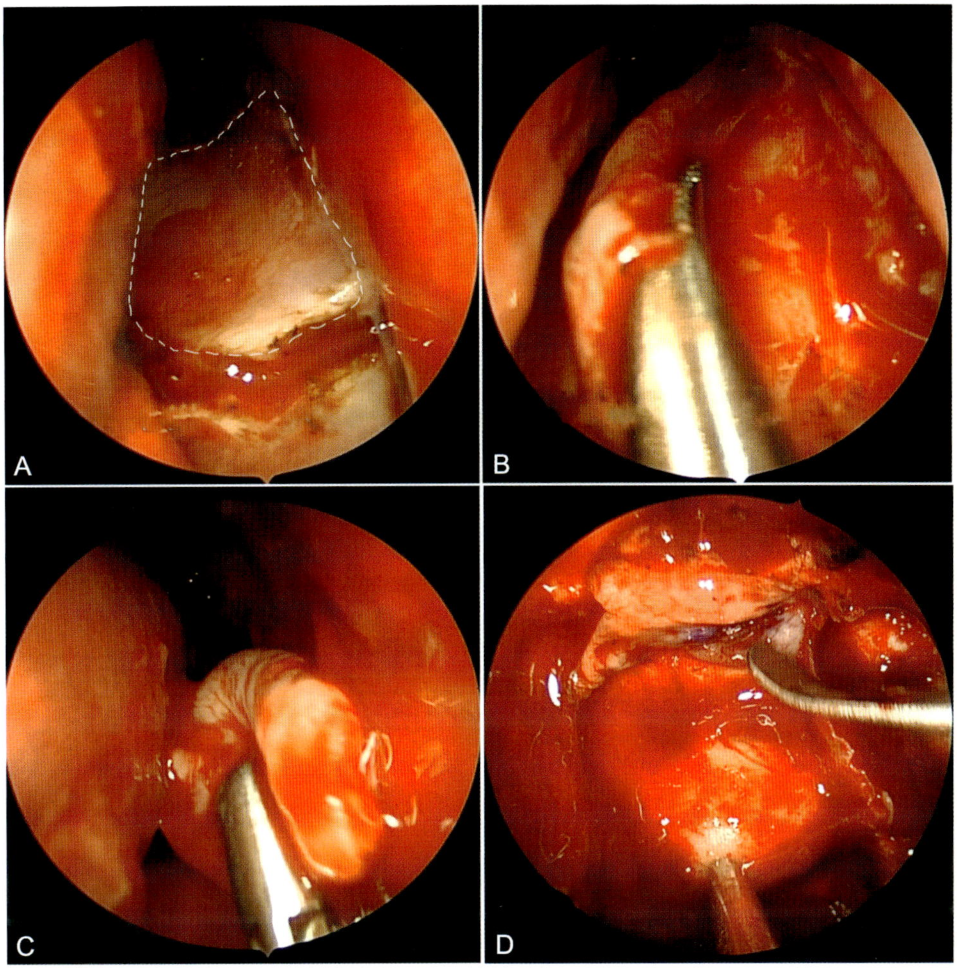

• **Fig. 37.1** Nasal floor free mucosal graft. A, A Colorado-tipped monopolar electrocautery (Stryker Corporation, Kalamazoo, MI) is used to outline a mucosal graft on the right nasal floor (*dashed lines*). B, A Cottle elevator (Karl Storz, Tuttlingen, Germany) is used to elevated the graft from the nasal floor in a submucoperiosteal plane. C, Once the graft is free from any attachments, a grasping forceps is used to remove the graft from the nasal cavity. D, The mucosal surface of the graft is then inked and placed over the skull base defect, in this case a small planum sphenoidale defect resulting from reduction of a meningoencephalocele.

sphenopalatine artery), a long and robust pedicle, is easy to harvest, and offers customizability/adaptability.[17] The flap is made by making three incisions in the nasal septal mucosa using needle-tip monopolar cautery. The first cut starts superiorly just inferior to the level of the sphenoid os and extends along the septum anteriorly, keeping 1 to 2 cm below the cribriform plate to preserve olfactory neuroepithelium. Next, an inferior cut starts from the superior margin of the choana, then extends across to the posterior margin of the vomer, and proceeds along the junction of the septum and the nasal floor over the maxillary crest. This inferior incision can be extended laterally to include the nasal floor and even the lateral nasal wall for coverage of wider defects. When this inferior incision is carried laterally, care must be taken to not incise over the soft palate. The superior limb of the NSF can be extended anteriorly as far as the junction between the septal mucosa and the vestibular skin. The two incisions are joined anteriorly by a vertical incision. Once these three incisions are completed, the flap is carefully elevated from the underlying cartilage and bone with care to preserve the posterior vascular pedicle. When elevating the flap off the face of the sphenoid sinus posteriorly, the surgeon must take care to not shear or tear the flap at this point, as this would likely injure the vascular pedicle. Once sufficiently elevated, the flap is then pushed into the nasopharynx or into a large maxillary antrostomy for more inferior approaches to avoid inadvertent damage during the remainder of the procedure.

Although the NSF is the workhorse of vascularized skull base repair options, in some instances the NSF is not an option (e.g., tissue is not available, septum is involved with tumor), and other local flaps may need to be considered. Both a posterior pedicled inferior turbinate flap and posterior pedicled middle turbinate flap have been described.[20] The inferior turbinate flap is best suited to sellar, suprasellar, and midclival defects.[17] The flap is supplied by the inferior turbinate artery, which is a terminal branch of the posterior lateral nasal artery arising from the sphenopalatine artery. The blood supply must be carefully delineated by first identifying the sphenopalatine artery as it leaves its foramen and then following it to identify the posterior lateral nasal artery. Once identified, parallel incisions are made as far rostral in the middle meatus and inferiorly along the medial margin of the inferior turbinate. A vertical incision is then made connecting the two incisions, and the flap is carefully elevated in an anterior to posterior direction. This flap is typically useful for small clival defects because of its limited arc of rotation and may also be used for repair of oroantral fistulas or oronasal fistulas.[3,21]

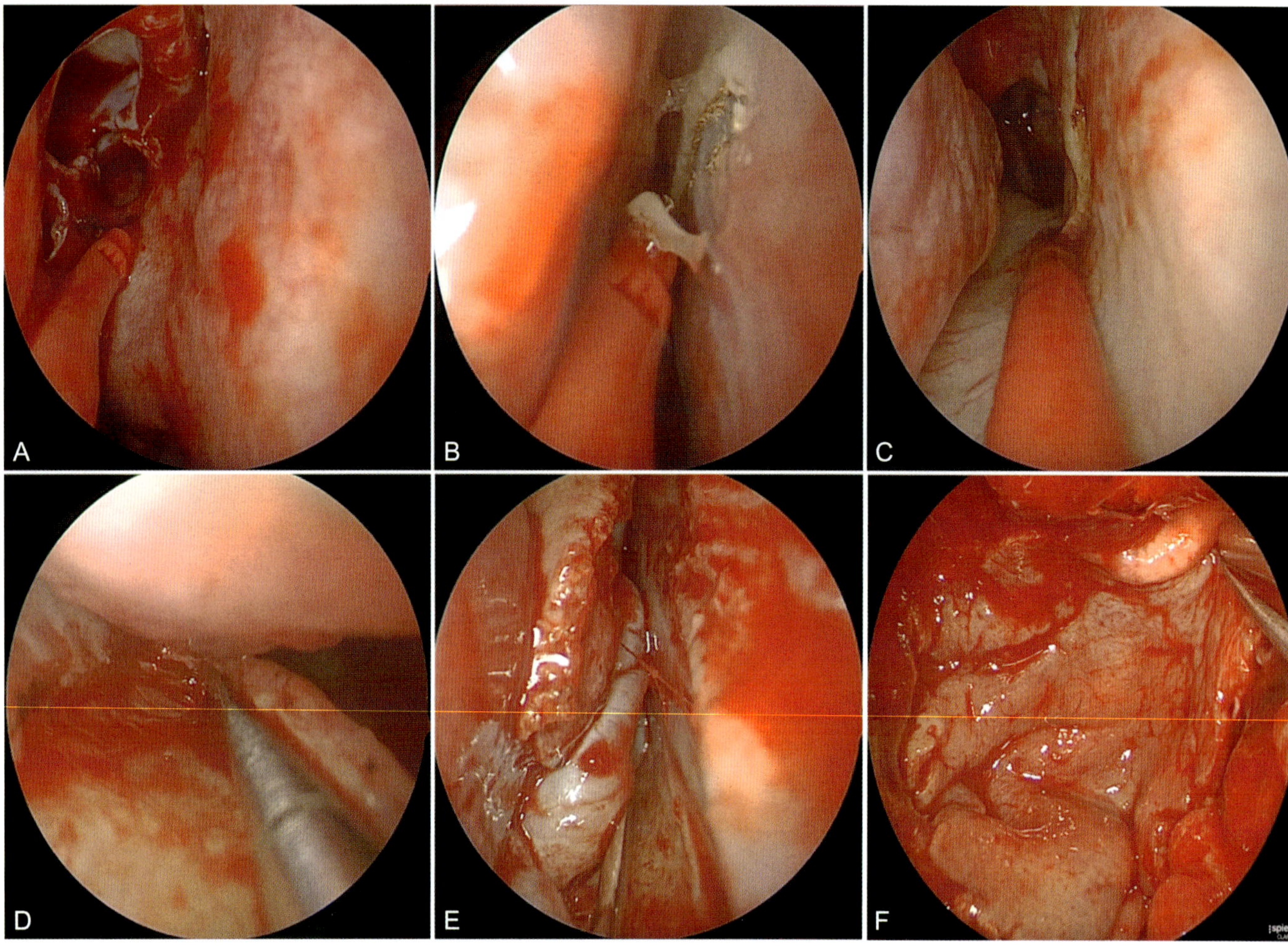

• **Fig. 37.2** Nasoseptal flap. A, After gentle outfracture of the middle and superior turbinates, the inferior aspect of the superior turbinate is resected, a limited posterior ethmoidectomy is performed, and the natural ostium of the sphenoid sinus is widened. A Colorado-tipped monopolar electrocautery is used to start the superior flap incision just inferior to the sphenoidotomy. B, The incision is carried onto the superior septum at the level of the middle turbinate. The olfactory neuroepithelium above the attachment of the middle turbinate is preserved. C, Once the superior incision is carried anteriorly and a descending limb is created on the septum at the level of the inferior turbinate head, the posterior choanal cut is carried down onto the nasal floor. D, Flap elevation is performed from lateral to medial along the nasal floor. E, The flap is then elevated from anterior to posterior and is tucked into the nasopharynx or a maxillary antrostomy for protection during the extirpative portion of the case. F, Once tumor resection is complete, the flap can be rotated to cover the resultant skull base defect.

The posterior pedicled middle turbinate flap is a pedicled flap that is suitable for limited defects of the planum sphenoidale, cribiform plate, or the sella.[3] Like the other flaps, the blood supply is derived from branches of the sphenopalatine artery. In this case, the flap is supplied by a branch of the sphenopalatine artery at the posterior attachment of the middle turbinate. The use of this flap is limited by its small surface area, restricted arc of rotation, and difficulty of flap harvest. To make harvest even more difficult, there are often anatomic variations of the middle turbinate that make flap elevation even more challenging for the surgeon, including paradoxical middle turbinate and concha bullosa.

Regional Pedicled Flaps

When the resection of a skull base lesion results in a large defect, or the defect is at the most anterior extent of the skull base, the NSF or other local pedicled flaps may not be available or suitable for reconstruction. In this case an extranasal or regional flap may be required. The endoscopic-assisted pericranial flap (PCF) is an example of a regional pedicled flap often used in such reconstructions, especially for midline defects (Fig. 37.3).[20,22,23] The PCF blood supply is derived from the supraorbital and supratrochlear arteries and is often used for anterior fossa reconstruction when accessed through open approaches. The endoscopic-assisted flap harvest is a modification of this robust and large pedicled repair option. The flap is harvested by first making a 1-cm glabellar incision and a larger 2- to 3-cm lateral pretrichial incision along the coronal plane of the scalp. Landmarks with or without a Doppler monitor are then used to identify both the supraorbital and supratrochlear arteries. Endoscopic browlift instrumentation can be useful in raising this flap. A subgaleal elevation is performed from the posterior incisions to the level of the pedicle anteriorly. The flap is then divided laterally and posteriorly using an angled monopolar cautery and then elevated off the calvarium under endoscopic

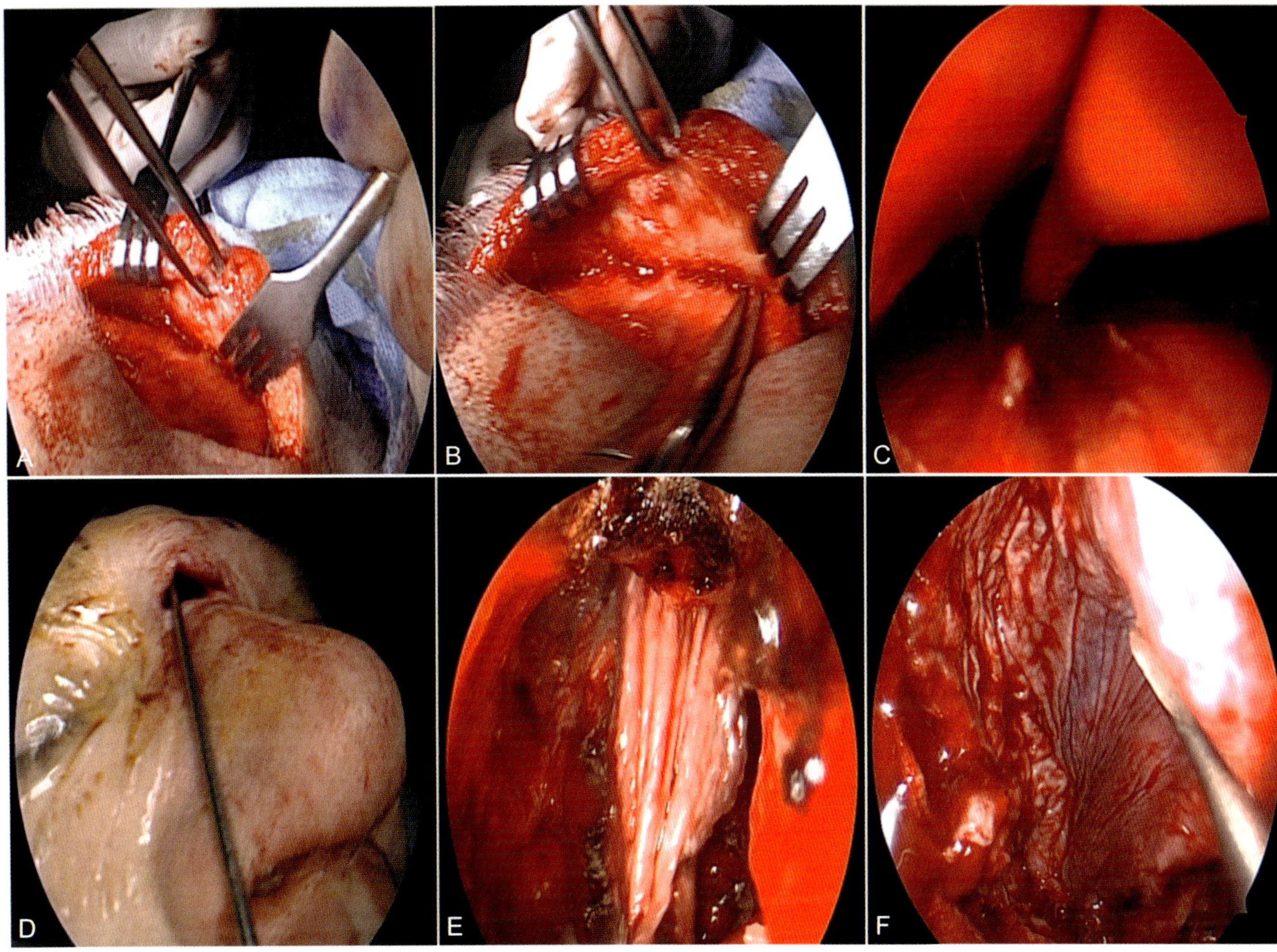

• **Fig. 37.3** Pericranial flap. A, A hemicoronal incision is created and dissection is carried through the subcutaneous tissue to expose the pericranium. B, Subgaleal elevation is performed from the posterior incisions to the level of the supraorbital and suptratrochlear arterial pedicles anteriorly. C, A Colorado-tipped monopolar electrocautery is then used to create lateral and posterior incisions, and the flap is elevated off the calvarium. D, An incision is made over the nasion and a coarse diamond drill is used to create a 1- to 2-cm port through which the elevated pericranial flap may be transposed. E, The pericranial flap is transposed through the port in the nasion, visualized endoscopically, and pulled into the nasal cavity using endoscopic grasping instruments. F, The flap is then manipulated into position endonasally to cover the defect, taking care not to twist the flap pedicle.

guidance using a variety of periosteal elevators. Next, a skin incision is made over the nasion and a subperiosteal plane is developed and extended to the pedicle of the flap superiorly. The flap is rotated into the nasal cavity using a bony conduit drilled through the nasion, making sure not to twist the flap as it enters into the nasal cavity.[10] Its passage into the nose is facilitated by performing an endoscopic-modified Lothrop procedure.

Another regional pedicled flap option is the temporoparietal fascia flap. This flap is familiar to the otolaryngologist, as it has been used extensively in head and neck reconstructions. This flap is supplied by the superficial temporal artery (STA).[10,24] The harvest begins with an anterior and posterior ethmoidectomy and a large maxillary antrostomy followed by clipping of the sphenopalatine artery and the posterior nasal artery at the level of the sphenopalatine foramen. The sphenopalatine artery is then dissected and followed, permitting exposure of the pterygopalatine fossa by removal of the posterior wall of the maxillary sinus. A portion of the lateral wall of the maxillary sinus is then removed, opening the infratemporal fossa and identifying the descending palatine artery. The contents of the pterygopalatine fossa are displaced inferiorly and laterally to expose the pterygoid plates. The pterygopalatine ganglion can be preserved by dividing the vidian nerve to permit displacement of the ganglion. The anterior pterygoid plates are reduced via high-speed drill, permitting a space large enough for tunneling the flap. A hemicoronal scalp incision can be made with care to preserve the STA within the subcutaneous tissue. The flap can be fashioned by incising the fascia laterally (the flap width can be determined based on the size or extent of the defect) followed by separation from the underlying muscle and deep fascia. The deep fascia is then incised and removed from the calvarial surface, permitting a passage for tunneling the flap.[10] The soft-tissue tunnel is sequentially dilated by passage of a guidewire into the nose under endonasal endoscopic guidance and then advancement of percutaneous tracheotomy dilators over the wire. After an adequate tunnel is created, the dilators are removed, the flap is tied to the external end of the guidewire, and the nasal end of the guidewire is pulled out through the nostril, with the flap proceeding through the tunnel intranasally. The flap is assisted through the tunnel with careful external manipulation carefully to avoid rotation of the flap and to maintain its blood supply.[10]

Another option that can be considered is the buccal fat pad flap. This is a very technically challenging flap to raise and is suited for repair of defects involving the greater sphenoid wing, inferior and superior clivus, sella, planum, and bilateral ethmoid cavities.[25] The blood supply is from the internal maxillary artery (IMA), suggesting a robust blood supply. The harvest is begun with removal of the posterior and lateral maxillary walls. The periosteum posteriorly is then incised to expose the buccal lobe of the buccal fat pad. The posterior lobe of the fat pad is dissected off the underlying masseter muscle. All three lobes of the buccal fat pad are then dissected free of the surrounding structures and advanced from within the space between the medial and lateral pterygoid muscles into the sinonasal cavity.[25]

A drawback of the previously described regional pedicled flaps is the added effort in harvesting them and often the requirement for skin incisions. In addition, the temporoparietal fascia flap places the frontotemporal branches of the facial nerve at risk. Because of the axis of rotation the temporoparietal fascia flap is limited to defects involving more lateral clival and parasellar regions. Conversely, the PCF is most suitable for defects anterior to the sella extending along the ventral skull base up to the posterior table of the frontal sinus.

Free Tissue Transfer

The majority of skull base defects and CSF leaks can be successfully managed with the NSF and other pedicled flap techniques. However, it is worth noting that in very rare recalcitrant cases, free tissue flaps can be called upon to repair especially difficult CSF leaks or massive skull base defects not amenable to conventional techniques. Thus, free tissue transfer represents the "top rung" of the reconstructive ladder in skull base surgery. A variety of distant tissue sources may be used, including the pedicled fascia lata free flap, with which we have success placing into the defect through minimally invasive approaches.

Special Considerations for Reconstruction of the Orbit

Defects associated with transnasal endoscopic surgery (typically targeting the medial orbit as far as approach) often do not require reconstruction. Resection of the floor of the orbit is associated with greater morbidity, however, and often necessitates reconstruction to avoid enophthalmos and associated diplopia. Exposed orbital fat in the sinonasal cavity is readily mucosalized with minimal patient morbidity. One must ensure that prolapsing orbital fat does not obstruct the maxillary antrostomy or frontal recess, which may result in chronic rhinosinusitis or mucocele formation. These are lessons learned from endoscopic orbital decompression surgery performed for years in patients with Graves disease who have thyroid eye disease.[26]

Although our ability to resect orbital tumors in the intraconal space such as hemangiomas through endoscopic approaches has improved significantly, there is still debate as to when reconstruction of the lamina papyracea is necessary in these cases.[27] The goal of orbital reconstruction is to prevent postoperative loss of orbital volume with resultant enophthalmos and/or diplopia.[28] Immediate reconstruction of the lamina papyracea with porous polyethylene mesh has been described.[29] However, a large multinational review of orbital cavernous hemangioma resections performed by experienced orbital surgeons suggested that surgeons did not reconstruct the orbit after resection of extraconal lesions, while reconstruction rates increased after intraconal lesion resection.[27] Some have advocated reconstruction of the medial orbit with a NSF after resection of intraconal cavernous hemangiomas, with the hypothesis that the flap provides coverage of the defect and may contract around the orbit over time while allowing time for adequate reduction in swelling and transudation in fluid that could potentially lead to an orbital compartment syndrome if a rigid reconstruction were undertaken.[30]

Therefore the surgeon should consider deferring reconstruction or performing a reconstruction without rigid materials during the primary surgery. A secondary or delayed reconstruction may then be planned at a later date once extraocular muscular edema and orbital transudation have ceased. In our experience, the small and even moderate-sized openings into the medial orbit that are typically required for the endoscopic resection of the majority of posteriorly located intraconal lesions rarely necessitate any reconstruction. The periorbita reforms over this area and the expected (often severe) diplopia, which typically ensues immediately postoperatively, is usually temporary. Patients do need to be counseled during the informed consent process about the expected diplopia and the possible need for strabismus surgery if it persists. In cases requiring significant intraconal dissection, we routinely now treat patients postoperatively with a short course of oral steroids and send them home with an eye patch if the diplopia is debilitating.

Outcomes

Endoscopic endonasal approaches for resection of lesions of the anterior skull base have proved as effective as open approaches. With the evolution of reconstructive techniques, postoperative CSF leak rates have been shown to be comparable to open repair techniques. A review of the literature yields a rate of postoperative CSF leak of 8.9%.[7,31-35] This success rate was confirmed in study by Soudry and colleagues that showed in a review of a total of 673 patients from 22 case series that the postoperative CSF leak rate was 8.5%.[18] Repair with vascularized flaps yielded a success rate of 94% regardless of the materials used in conjunction with the flap, whereas free grafts achieved successful closure in 82% of patients in the review. The study also assessed the operative site/extent of the skull base defect. The anterior skull base exhibited successful reconstruction in 92% of patients, with a higher success rate achieved when vascularized flaps were used. Sellar defects had an overall successful closure rate of 93%, with vascularized flaps achieving a closure rate of 94% to 100% for both high-flow and low-flow leaks, and free grafts yielding a success rate of 87% to 100% for low-flow leaks alone.[36] Similarly, in a large systematic review, an overall CSF leak rate of 11.5% was noted after reconstruction of large dural defects. Upon further classification of reconstruction, a 15.6% postoperative leak rate was noted for free grafts compared with a 6.7% leak rate for vascularized reconstructions.[8]

As endoscopic endonasal techniques continue to expand, our understanding of the key risk factors necessary to successfully repairing complex skull base defects also needs to expand. The thoughtful approach to reconstruction can be facilitated by considering the goals of repair and stratifying relevant options using the concept of the reconstructive ladder.

Conclusion

Endoscopic endonasal approaches to resection of skull base tumors have become the gold standard for appropriately selected lesions. Methods for endoscopically reconstructing the skull base have also advanced significantly, and now multiple techniques are in the armamentarium of the skull base team. Selection of the best repair method should be based on a graduated approach, factoring in the specific factors, including the degree of intraoperative CSF leak, extent of skull base defect, specific disorder involved, and comorbidities present in each case.

References

1. Shahangian, A., Soler, Z. M., Baker, A., Wise, S. K., Rereddy, S. K., Patel, Z. M., et al. (2017). Successful repair of intraoperative cerebrospinal fluid leaks improves outcomes in endoscopic skull base surgery. *International Forum of Allergy & Rhinology, 7*, 80–86.
2. Sansoni, E. R., & Harvery, R. J. (2019). Large skull base defect reconstruction with and without pedicled flaps. In A. G. Chiu, J. N. Palmer, & N. D. Adappa (Eds.), *Atlas of endoscopic sinus and skull base surgery* (pp. 285–298). Philadelphia: Elsevier.
3. Patel, M. R., Stadler, M. E., Snyderman, C. H., Carrau, R. L., Kassam, A. B., Germanwala, A. V., et al. (2010). How to choose? Endoscopic skull base reconstructive options and limitations. *Skull Base, 20*, 397–404.
4. Hachem, R. A., Elkhatib, A., Beer-Furlan, A., Prevedello, D., & Carrau, R. (2016). Reconstructive techniques in skull base surgery after resection of malignant lesions: A wide array of choices. *Current Opinion in Otolaryngology & Head and Neck Surgery, 24*, 91–97.
5. Harvey, R. J., Smith, J. E., Wise, S. K., Patel, S. J., Frankel, B. M., & Schlosser, R. J. (2008). Intracranial complications before and after endoscopic skull base reconstruction. *American Journal of Rhinology, 22*, 516–521.
6. Hadad, G., Bassagasteguy, L., Carrau, R. L., Mataza, J. C., Kassam, A., Snyderman, C. H., et al. (2006). A novel reconstructive technique after endoscopic expanded endonasal approaches: Vascular pedicle nasoseptal flap. *Laryngoscope, 116*, 1882–1886.
7. Thorp, B. D., Sreenath, S. B., Ebert, C. S., & Zanation, A. M. (2014). Endoscopic skull base reconstruction: A review and clinical case series of 152 vascularized flaps used for surgical skull base defects in the setting of intraoperative cerebrospinal fluid leak. *Neurosurgical Focus, 37*, E4.
8. Harvey, R. J., Parmar, P., Sacks, R., & Zanation, A. M. (2012). Endoscopic skull base reconstruction of large dural defects: A systematic review of published evidence. *Laryngoscope, 122*, 452–459.
9. Zanation, A. M., Thorp, B. D., Parmar, P., & Harvey, R. J. (2011). Reconstructive options for endoscopic skull base surgery. *Otolaryngologic Clinics of North America, 44*, 1201–1222.
10. Sigler, A. C., D'Anza, B., Lobo, B. C., Woodard, T. D., Recinos, P. F., & Sindwani, R. (2017). Endoscopic skull base reconstruction: An evolution of materials and methods. *Otolaryngologic Clinics of North America, 50*, 643–653.
11. Roxbury, C. R., Saavedra, T., Ramanathan, M., Jr., Lim, M., Ishii, M., Gallia, G. L., et al. (2016). Layered sellar reconstruction with avascular free grafts: Acceptable alternative to the nasoseptal flap for repair of low-volume intraoperative cerebrospinal fluid leak. *American Journal of Rhinology & Allergy, 30*, 367–371.
12. D'Anza, B., Tien, D., Stokken, J. L., Recinos, P. F., Woodard, T. R., & Sindwani, R. (2016). Role of lumbar drains in contemporary endonasal skull base surgery: Meta-analysis and systematic review. *American Journal of Rhinology & Allergy, 30*(6), 430–435.
13. Tien, D., Stokken, J. L., Recinos, P. F., Woodard, T. D., & Sindwani, R. (2006). Cerebrospinal fluid diversion in endoscopic skull base reconstruction: An evidence-based approach to the use of lumbar drains. *Otolaryngologic Clinics of North America, 49*(1), 119–129.
14. Stokken, J. L., Recinos, P. F., Woodard, T., & Sindwnai, R. (2015). The utility of lumbar drains in modern endoscopic skull base surgery. *Current Opinion in Otolaryngology & Head and Neck Surgery, 23*(1), 78–82.
15. Tang, D., Roxbury, C., D'Anza, B., Kshettry, V., Woodard, T., Recinos, P., et al. (2018). Technical notes on the endoscopic endonasal approach to the craniovertebral junction for odontoidectomy. *American Journal of Rhinology & Allergy, 32*(2), 85–86.
16. Kshettry, V. R., Thorp, B. D., Shriver, M. F., Zanation, A. M., Woodard, T. D., Sindwani, R., et al. (2016). Endoscopic approaches to the craniovertebral junction. *Otolaryngologic Clinics of North America, 49*(1), 213–226.
17. Esposito, F., Dusick, J. R., Fatemi, N., & Kelly, D. F. (2007). Graded repair of cranial base defects and cerebrospinal fluid leaks in transsphenoidal surgery. *Neurosurgery, 60*, 295–303.
18. Marks, S. C. (1998). Middle turbinate graft for repair of cerebral spinal fluid leaks. *American Journal of Rhinology, 12*, 417–419.
19. Dadgostar, A., Okpaleke, C., Al-Asousi, F., & Javer, A. (2017). The application of a free nasal floor mucoperiosteal graft in endoscopic sinus surgery. *American Journal of Rhinology & Allergy, 31*(3), 196–199.
20. Clavenna, M. J., Turner, J. H., & Chandra, R. K. (2015). Pedicled flaps in endoscopic skull base reconstruction: Review of current techniques. *Current Opinion in Otolaryngology & Head and Neck Surgery, 23*, 71–77.
21. Fortes, F. S., Carrau, R. L., Snyderman, C. H., Prevedello, D., Vescan, A., Mintz, A., et al. (2007). The posterior pedicle inferior turbinate flap: A new vascularized flap for skull base reconstruction. *Laryngoscope, 117*(8), 1329–1332.
22. Kim, G. G., Hang, A. X., Mitchell, C., & Zanation, A. M. (2013). Pedicled extranasal flaps in skull base reconstruction. *Advances in Oto-Rhino-Laryngology, 74*, 71–80.
23. Zanation, A. M., Snyderman, C. H., Carrau, R. L., Kassam, A. B., Gardner, P. A., Prevedello, D. M., et al. (2009). Minimally invasive endoscopic pericranial flap: A new method for endonasal skull base reconstruction. *Laryngoscope, 119*(1), 13–18.
24. Patel, R., Shah, R. N., Snyderman, C. H., Carrau, R. L., Germanwala, A. V., Kassam, A. B., et al. (2010). Pericranial flap for endoscopic anterior skull-base reconstruction: Clinical outcomes and radioanatomic analysis of preoperative planning. *Neurosurgery, 66*, 506–512.
25. Markey, J., Benet, A., & El-Sayed, I. H. (2015). The endonasal endoscopic harvest and anatomy of the buccal fat pad flap for closure of skull base defects. *Laryngoscope, 125*, 2247–2252.
26. Stokken, J. L., Gumber, D., Antisdel, J., & Sindwani, R. (2016). Endoscopic surgery of the orbital apex: Outcomes and emerging techniques. *Laryngoscope, 128*(1), 20–24.
27. Bleier, B. S., Castelnuovo, P., Battaglia, P., Turri-Zanoni, M., Dallan, I., Metson, R., et al. (2016). Endoscopic endonasal orbital cavernous hemangioma resection: Global experience in techniques and outcomes. *International Forum of Allergy & Rhinology, 6*, 156–161.
28. Miyake, M. M., & Bleier, B. S. (2019). Endoscopic approach and removal of orbital tumors. In A. G. Chiu, J. N. Palmer, & N. D. Adappa (Eds.), *Atlas of endoscopic sinus and skull base surgery* (pp. 165–170). Philadelphia, PA: Elsevier.
29. Colletti, G., Saibene, A. M., Pessina, F., Duvina, M., Allevi, F., Felisati, G., et al. (2017). A shift in the orbit: Immediate endoscopic reconstruction after transnasal orbital tumors resection. *Journal of Craniofacial Surgery, 28*, 2027–2029.
30. Chhabra, N., Healy, D. Y., Freitag, S. K., & Bleier, B. S. (2014). The nasoseptal flap for reconstruction of the medial and inferior orbit. *International Forum of Allergy & Rhinology, 4*, 763–766.
31. Zuniga, M. G., Turner, J. H., & Chandra, R. K. (2016). Updates in anterior skull base reconstruction. *Current Opinion in Otolaryngology & Head and Neck Surgery, 24*, 75–82.

32. Borg, A., Kirkman, M., & Choi, D. (2016). Endoscopic endonasal anterior skull base surgery: A systematic review of complications over the past 65 years. *World Neurosurgery*, *95*, 383–391.
33. Dehdashti, A. R., Ganna, A., Karabatsou, K., & Gentili, F. (2008). Pure endoscopic endonasal approach for pituitary adenomas: Early surgical results in 200 patients and comparison with previous microsurgical series. *Neurosurgery, 62,* 1006–1017.
34. Zhang, M., Singh, H., Almodovar-Mercado, G. J., Anand, V. K., & Schwartz, T. H. (2016). Required reading: The most impactful articles in endoscopic endonasal skull base surgery. *World Neurosurgery*, *92*, 499–512.e2.
35. Choby, G. W., Mattos, J. L., Hughes, M. A., Fernandez-Miranda, J. C., Gardner, P. A., Snyderman, C. H., et al. (2015). Delayed nasoseptal flaps for endoscopic skull base reconstruction: Proof of concept and evaluation of outcomes. *Otolaryngology–Head and Neck Surgery*, *152*, 255–259.
36. Soudry, E., Turner, J. H., Nayak, J. V., & Hwang, P. J. (2014). Endoscopic reconstruction of surgically created skull base defects: A systematic review. *Otolaryngology–Head and Neck Surgery*, *150*, 730–738.

38

Transorbital Endoscopic and Neuroendoscopic Surgery

KRIS S. MOE, MD, FACS AND RAJEEV D. SEN, MD

The development of transnasal endoscopic approaches to skull base pathology significantly decreased the surgical disruption and collateral damage relative to their open predecessors, such as the craniofacial[1] and subcranial[2] approaches. In addition, the improved illumination, magnification, and visualization on a high-quality monitor afforded by endoscopes provided surgeons with major technologic improvements.

Although transnasal approaches are the most common endoscopic pathways in use today, drawbacks to these procedures remain largely because of the presence of the orbits. The orbits occupy approximately 80% of the anterior cranial fossa (ACF) and a significant portion of the middle cranial fossa (MCF).[3] They obstruct transnasal access to these locations or force the use of angled endoscopy and instrumentation. Another drawback to transnasal approaches is the *narrow funnel effect*—again, because of obstruction by the orbits—in which access to the ACF narrows significantly in the superior aspects, making simultaneous visualization and instrumentation a challenge. In addition, when accessing the ACF, particularly intracranially, it is necessary to approach with upward angulation and then progress parallel to the floor of ACF. We refer to this as the *attic effect*—when the surgeon is required to reach up into another space and work within that plane. The opposite of this is when the surgeon can visualize and use instruments in the same plane as the entry portal, or what we call *coplanar* surgery.

In 2005, we began to investigate whether the orbit could be transformed from an obstruction into a portal. The orbital bone is among the thinnest in the body; the orbit is adjacent to the paranasal sinuses (maxillary, ethmoid, sphenoid, and frontal). The roof of the orbit is composed of the ACF; the deep extension of the orbit abuts the MCF; and the lateral wall is adjacent to the infratemporal fossa (ITF) and MCF through the greater wing of the sphenoid. These observations suggested that the orbit could provide a direct pathway to these regions. After extensive study in the cadaver laboratory, we developed four primary routes to targets within the orbit and regions adjacent to the orbit (Fig. 38.1). In 2010, we reported our initial clinical experience and outcomes using these approaches.[3] In that consecutive series, all procedures were successfully achieved, and there were no complications related to the surgical approaches. We subsequently published multiple reports on further applications, experience, and outcomes using these procedures, the means of combining them with other approaches in multiportal technique (Fig. 38.2), strategies for preoperative panning, techniques in reconstruction, feasibility for use in robotic surgery, and pediatric applications.[4-19] Groups from Italy,[20-23] South Africa,[24] and the United States[25-28] have added significantly to this literature.

We found that transorbital approaches allow ample access to targets without the narrow funnel effect. And because the entry portal and surgical target are usually with in the same plane, the attic effect is avoided and coplanar surgery is possible. By approaching targets from the orbit, endoscopic access to the ACF, MCF, and ITF is no longer obstructed.

As noted previously, numerous groups have also published their international experience with these procedures. In a particularly important work, Locatelli et al.[22] published their experience as well as an excellent meta-analysis of the literature in 2016. They identified 38 clinical articles in the literature from 2010 to 2015, as well as multiple nonclinical studies, with no significant complications reported. They concluded that "transorbital endoscopic skull base surgery appears to be a safe and effective technique with complications lower than traditional external approaches and comparable with or even better than those published for transnasal or transmaxillary approaches."

At the time of writing, a PubMed search of transorbital endoscopic procedures yielded more than 90 publications, and we are aware of others in press. Endoscopic orbital surgery has thus received a significant amount of attention given the relatively short duration of its use, with rapid adoption and highly favorable reports in the literature. This chapter outlines our techniques for endoscopic orbital and transorbital surgery, as well as our surgical outcomes, and provides references for further education.

Indications and Contraindications

Endoscopic orbital and transorbital surgery may be indicated to treat pathology involving the orbit and related structures, as well as structures adjacent to the orbit in the frontal sinus, ACF, and MCF. These approaches may be used alone, in multiportal combination with other approaches, or in hybrid techniques combining endoscopic and open approaches. At times we use these approaches bilaterally[29] or approach a target from the contralateral side for improved approach and instrumentation angles.[3,9]

We have treated patients ranging in age from 18 months[8] to 92 years for a full range of pathologic conditions, including benign

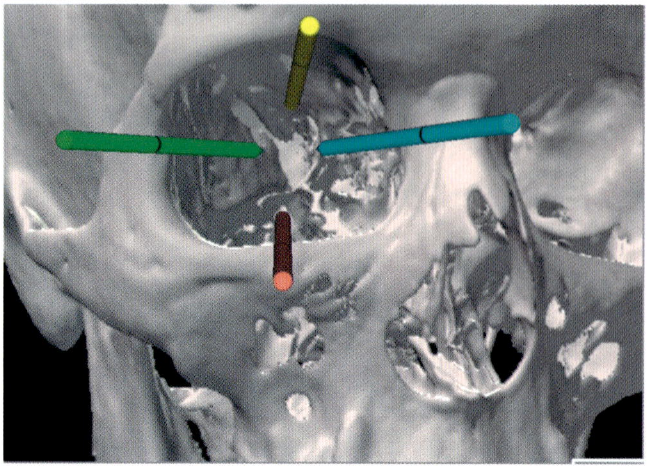

• **Fig. 38.1** Schematic of four transorbital endoscopic approaches: superior (*yellow*), medial (*blue*), inferior (*orange*), and lateral (*green*). Vectors demonstrate some of the regions of the orbit that can be accessed, relative to the adjacent orbital bone.

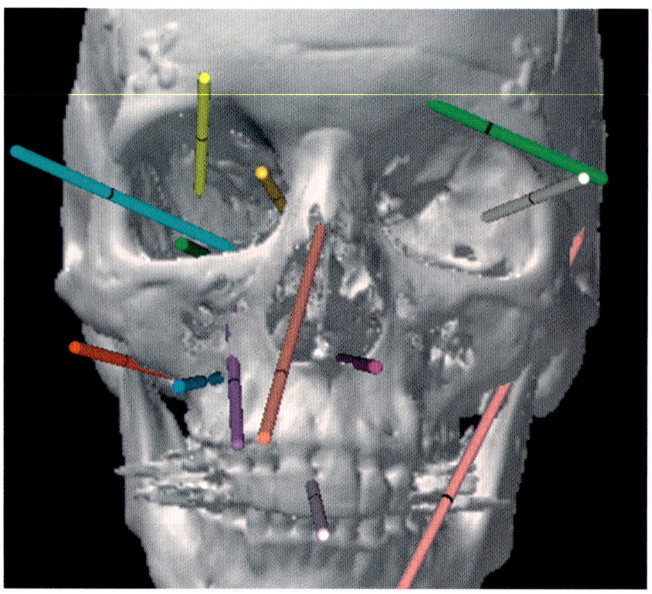

• **Fig. 38.2** Schematic of multiportal endoscopic surgery. Colored vector diagrams indicate some of the many transorbital, transnasal, transmaxillary, paramaxillary, and transoral approaches that can be used in combination to improve access, visualization, and manipulation of surgical targets.

and malignant tumors, infection (epidural, orbital, sinogenic), vascular/hemorrhage, trauma, cerebrospinal fluid (CSF) leak, and endocrine disorders.[3,5,6,19]

Contraindications to endoscopic orbital and transorbital procedures are somewhat theoretical at this point, given that relatively few complications have been reported in the literature. Primary concerns would be a history of recent ophthalmologic issues, such as a ruptured globe, hyphema, or infection. Relative contraindications would include a history of ocular surgery within the past 6 months, conditions of increased intraocular pressure (inflammatory processes), and prior LASIK surgery (a potential cause of decreased corneal sensation). These conditions, along with glaucoma or dry eye symptoms, should be evaluated by an ophthalmologist before proceeding with surgery.

Surgical Planning

Meticulous preoperative planning is critical in skull base surgery owing to the complexity of the anatomy, with multiple critical structures in highly close proximity encased in bone.[10,11,28] Planning must include a global analysis of the pathology and its proximity to, or involvement of, adjacent structures. Once it is determined that a lesion can and should be resected, the ideal minimally disruptive technique is determined.

The choice of a surgical technique can be quite complex but may be simplified when broken down into its key components: the *portal* (an incision or natural orifice), the *pathway* (a dissection route within tissue planes or a preexisting corridor), and the *target* (the pathology).[30] A portal should be created to prevent scarring or loss of function and to provide ample access to the pathway. A natural orifice such as a nostril can be excellent for this purpose. A pathway should provide the shortest possible distance from the portal to the target in the least disruptive manner possible. It must (1) allow the repeated passage of multiple instruments without the production of excessive secretions or blood and (2) provide adequate volume for an endoscope and/or instrument. In addition, reconstruction of the pathway, if needed, must be possible.

The type of instruments to be used is important in planning. Although it has been emphasized that four-handed surgery should be possible during a procedure, with contemporary instruments consideration of the number of functions required may be more important than the number of hands to activate them. For example, a surgical bone aspirator provides suction, irrigation, and ablation in one instrument. In addition to these functions, illumination and visualization (two functions provided by one instrument) are needed. Thus two instruments operated by two hands may provide five functions. Typically, we aim to perform four to six functions synchronously through a given pathway.

Additional factors important in the choice of pathway are the angles of approach, instrumentation, and visualization. Although angled endoscopy may provide the ability to view a target, available instrumentation may not be adequate for resection of a target that is poorly angled from the approach. The angle between instruments used simultaneously must also be sufficient to prevent collisions (approximately 18 degrees for pituitary surgery).[9] Likewise, the volume of the approach must be adequate for the manipulation of instruments and endoscope, yet small enough that adjacent structures are not endangered (approximately 3 mL^3).[11] The geometry of the pathway is also very important. As determined by digital tracking and analysis of instrument motion during endoscopic surgery,[31-35] instruments may not pass from the portal to target in a linear fashion, but may actually traverse a biconical or other shape.[36] The pathway shape must therefore allow the natural geometry of unimpeded instrument motion. Finally, the experience and abilities of the surgical team, as well as the desires of the patient, must be considered.

Surgical Technique

Detailed understanding of the anatomy of the orbit and structures contained therein (as outlined in Chapter 4) is critical before beginning to use these procedures.[37-39] Key landmarks to consider are the location of the superior orbital fissure and the cranial nerves that traverse it; the inferior orbital fissure; the ethmoid neurovascular bundles marking the location of the base of the ACF; and the optic foramen. The fascial condensations that surround the orbital

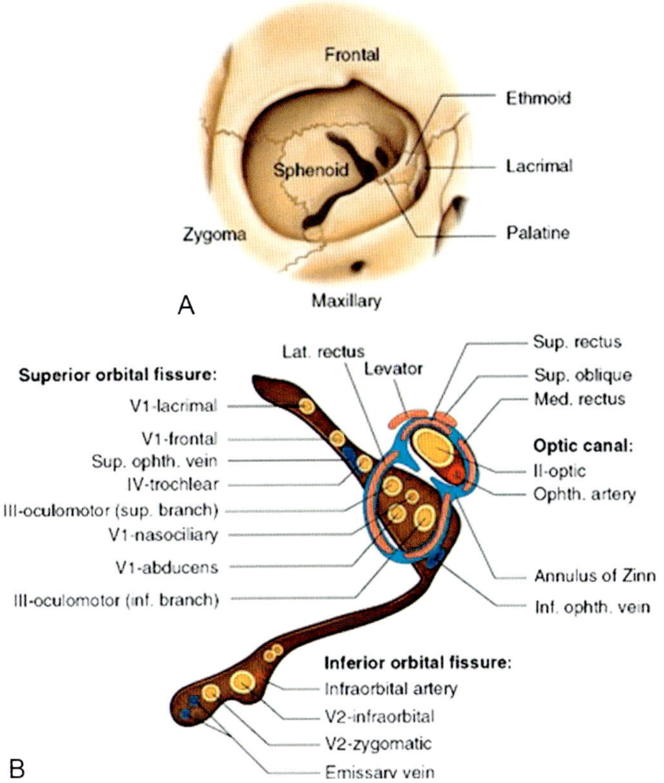

• **Fig. 38.3** Key orbital anatomy. A, Osseous anatomy of the fissures and foramina. B, neurovascular contents of the fissures and foramina. (From Bevans, S. E., & Moe, K. S. [2017]. Advances in the reconstruction of orbital fractures. *Facial Plastic Surgery Clinics of North America, 25*[4], 513–535.)

fissures and optic foramen are important in protecting these structures during endoscopic surgery within the orbit (Fig. 38.3).

The patient is placed in the supine position, and general anesthesia is administered. The patient is given dexamethasone, appropriate antibiotic therapy, and for intracranial procedures acetazolamide may also be given. The head is rotated slightly toward the surgeon, and the neck is extended approximately 15 degrees to allow the brain to retract from the skull base if an intracranial procedure is anticipated. The head of the bed is elevated to minimize bleeding. The surgical navigation system is applied and registered, and accuracy is confirmed. Both eyes, the nose, and any other relevant anatomy are prepped and draped in the usual sterile fashion. The pupils are checked for baseline size and symmetry, the eyes are rinsed, and lubricant is applied. We do not typically use corneal protectors, as we regularly check the pupils for size, shape, and symmetry during the procedure. However, the use of corneal protectors may be desired until the surgeon has gained confidence with the procedures. Before beginning, surgical navigation is used to analyze the vector from the planned entry portal to the surgical target, and the appropriate surgical pathway is confirmed. The appearance of a typical approach is demonstrated in (Fig. 38.4) The equipment is arranged as described earlier.[38]

The basic instrumentation required is similar to that for other endoscopic skull base approaches. In addition, a Gorney suction elevator (JedMed), fine scissors (NovoSurgical), and range of malleable brain retractors (Millenium Surgical) are needed. Powered instrumentation, including an ultrasonic bone aspirator, may also be of use.

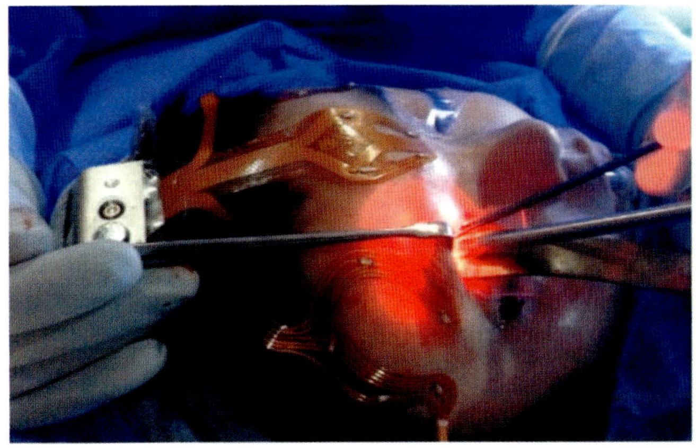

• **Fig. 38.4** Superior transorbital neuroendoscopic approach, right eye, 6-year-old boy. Note the silastic sheet protecting orbital contents and use of malleable brain retractor to gently create optical cavity.

During surgery the pupils are monitored regularly for change in size or shape. There is no set frequency for doing this, but the deeper within the orbit the dissection proceeds, particularly as the optic nerve is approached, the more often the pupils are checked. If the pupil begins to dilate or change shape (such enlargement or the occurrence of an oval shape in the vector of globe displacement), the instruments are removed from the orbit until the baseline shape returns—usually a brief period. Care should be taken to provide the minimal amount of globe displacement necessary for the procedure, without undue pressure behind the equator of the globe.

Superior Approach

The superior approach provides access to the frontal sinus, ACF, and frontal lobe of the brain. This approach can be used unilaterally, bilaterally, or contralaterally[29] as needed.

The superior approach is the only one of the four approaches that uses a skin incision, the same one used in upper blepharoplasty. A No. 15 blade or electrocautery on low voltage is used to make an incision in a dominant crease in the upper eye lid (Fig. 38.5). The incision is typically 2 to 3 cm, depending on the location and depth of the pathology; the position of the incision is chosen by vector analysis with the navigation system. After incising the skin and orbicularis muscle, dissection continues superiorly toward the superior orbital rim in the suborbicularis (preseptal) plane, using a fine scissors. When the superior orbital rim is reached, the periosteum is incised with care taken not to injure the supraorbital and supratrochlear neurovascular pedicles. The periosteum is then raised and the subperiosteal plane is entered. Dissection proceeds posteriorly in the subperiosteal (subperiorbital) plane into the orbit using a malleable brain retractor to gently displace the orbital contents, and a suction Freer elevator is used to lift the periorbita from the bone (see Fig. 38.4). A layer of silastic or other pathway protector may be placed between the orbital contents and the malleable retractor. As dissection proceeds posteriorly, the ethmoid arteries will be encountered at the medial aspect where the orbital roof and lamina papyracea meet in the frontoethmoid suture. Following this suture posteriorly leads to the optic nerve, with the curvature of the orbit increasing as the apex is approached. As the orbital apex is approached, the superior orbital fissure will be encountered at the lateral extent, and medial to this the optic nerve is encountered. These structures are heavily

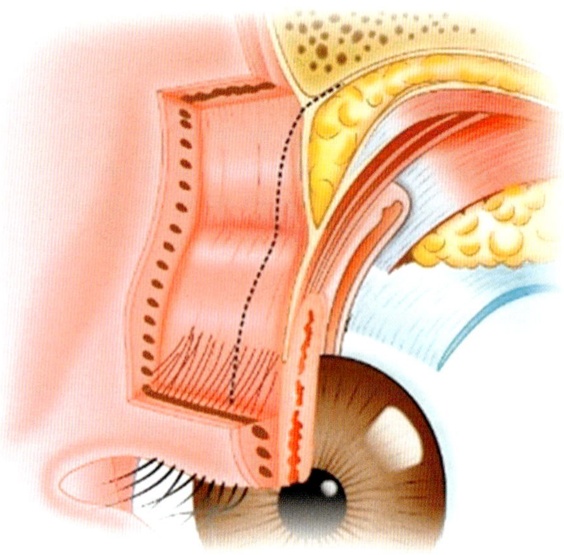

• **Fig. 38.5** Pathway of superior approach (upper eye lid blepharoplasty technique). The skin and orbicularis muscle are elevated off the orbital septum until the superior orbital rim is reached. Dissection then continues between the periosteum and orbital roof to the destination. The *dotted line* represents the path of dissection. (From Bevans, S. E., & Moe, K. S. [2017]. Advances in the reconstruction of orbital fractures. *Facial Plastic Surgery Clinics of North America, 25*[4], 513–535.)

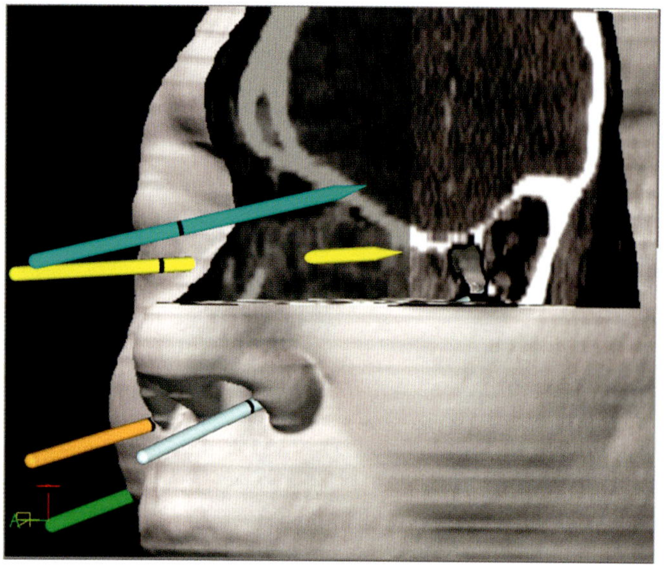

• **Fig. 38.6** Schematic of tumor surveillance and mapping. Surveillance of the orbital contents and intracranial inspection of dura is performed through a medial approach before beginning tumor resection. The *blue vector* shows dural surveillance; the *yellow vector* shows inspection of orbital contents. Additional multiportal vectors noted in assorted colors are used after tumor mapping and creation of the final surgical plan.

invested in fascial condensation, which provides an element of protection during the dissection.

Bone of the orbital roof is removed as needed to proceed along the surgical path. If the pathology is located within the frontal sinus or anterior aspect of the frontal lobe, the planned pathway may extend through the floor of the frontal sinus. Navigation is used to determine the site of bone removal. Although a diamond drill may be used with care, we prefer an ultrasonic bone aspirator, which is less likely to injure orbital contents.

At the conclusion of the procedure, significant bone defects may be spanned with a 0.25-mm polydioxanone (PDS) sheet if the periorbita was damaged or to keep orbital contents from herniating into the frontal sinus (see later text). The wound is then closed in two layers: the orbicularis muscle and then skin, using 5-0 or 6-0 dissolving suture.

Medial Approach

The medial approach is used to access the medial orbit, lamina papyracea, optic nerve, and superior nasal cavity. At times we use this as a bilateral or contralateral[38] medial approach to work across the skull base for improved instrumentation and visualization.[3,37] The medial approach is also highly effective for surveillance of tumors occupying the nasal cavity that are at risk for invasion of the orbital structures and/or dura (Fig. 38.6). In this case we begin with a medial approach (extending into an inferior approach as necessary). We explore the component of the tumor extending into the orbit, then dissect intracranially superior to the interorbital skull base to surveil the ACF dura. Having determined the involvement of the orbital structures and dura early in the procedure, we know what will be required for tumor resection and can place a protective barrier (PDS sheet) between these structures and the dura to prevent inadvertent damage during tumor resection.

The medial approach is accessed through a transconjunctival precaruncular incision,[40] located posterior to the lacrimal ducts and sac (Fig 38.7). An incision is made in the conjunctiva immediately medial to the caruncle using a fine scissor. This opens into the preseptal plane deep to the Horner muscle. Spreading the scissors in this plane will delineate a single artery that is cauterized with bipolar technique. The Horner muscle is then followed posteriorly to the posterior lacrimal crest, which is deep to the lacrimal sac. Here the periorbita of the lamina papyracea is incised and elevated, and dissection continues within this plane toward the orbital apex. Superiorly, the dissection continues to the anterior, middle (Berens artery), and posterior ethmoid arteries, using a bipolar to cauterize these as needed. The radius of curvature tightens posteriorly as the orbital apex is encountered, and navigation is used to confirm location as the optic nerve is approached. Inferiorly, the dissection can be taken to the orbital floor. Depending on the path of dissection, the lamina may be removed by gently fracturing into the ethmoid cavity, or with bone forceps. From this region the dissection may proceed intracranially over a tumor within the orbit and/or nasal cavity for surveillance of the dura before tumor resection.

Reconstruction of the medial orbit is achieved, when needed, with PDS alone or a titanium sheet lined with PDS as a glide layer[41] (see later text). The conjunctiva is not typically closed, although a single 6-0 fast-absorbing suture can be used to reposition the caruncle if edema causes displacement.

Inferior Approach

The inferior approach is used for access to the inferior orbital contents, orbital floor, and regions of the MCF. This transconjunctival incision is made directly onto the inferior orbital rim, using the technique common in lower eyelid blepharoplasty and fracture repair. We often using a lateral canthotomy and cantholysis, depending on the depth that the orbit is dissected. The incision is made in the conjunctiva of the inferior fornix directly above

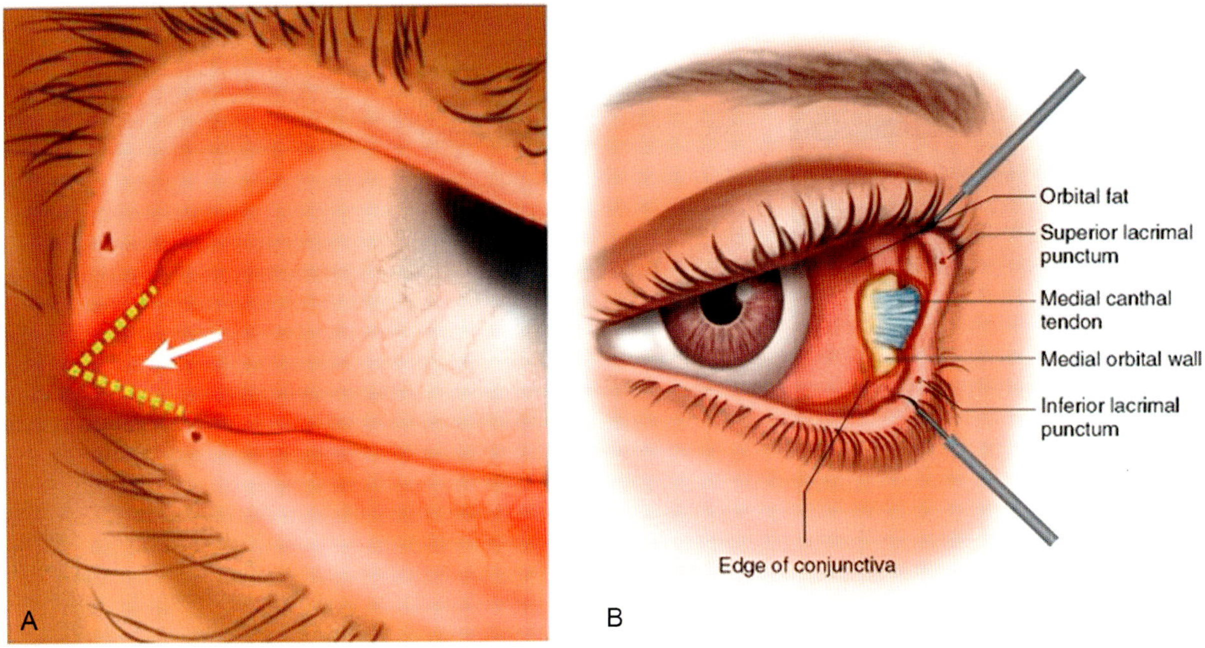

• **Fig. 38.7** A, precaruncular approach to the medial orbit. The *dotted lines* represent vectors of transconjunctival incision. B, the conjunctiva reflected, demonstrating the posterior limb of the medial canthal tendon leading to the posterior lacrimal crest, where the periosteum of the medial orbit is incised and elevated. (From Bevans, S. E., & Moe, K. S. [2017]. Advances in the reconstruction of orbital fractures. *Facial Plastic Surgery Clinics of North America, 25*[4], 513–535.)

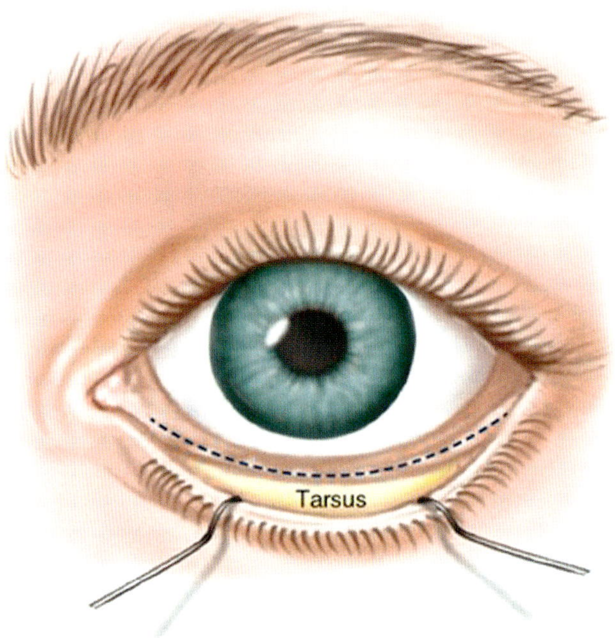

• **Fig. 38.8** Inferior approach. The lower eye lid is retracted anteriorly. An incision is made directly over the inferior orbital rim onto the periosteum, which is then incised and elevated to create the optical cavity for endoscopic dissection. (From Bevans, S. E., & Moe, K. S. [2017]. Advances in the reconstruction of orbital fractures. *Facial Plastic Surgery Clinics of North America, 25*[4], 513–535.)

the palpated location of the inferior orbital rim using a small scissors or low-power electrocautery (Fig. 38.8). When the periosteum of the inferior rim is reached, it is incised and lifted. Dissection is then continued into the orbit in the subperiorbital plane posteriorly toward the orbital apex. The infraorbital nerve may run on the deep aspect or within the bone of the orbital floor, where it is easily identified and dissected from the adjacent periorbita and orbital contents and left in situ. Medially the dissection can extend to the inferior aspect of the medial wall. If the contents of the inferior orbital fissure are cauterized with bipolar technique and divided, the dissection can extend partially up the lateral orbital wall. The inferior orbital fissure can be followed posteriorly and medially as it courses in the direction of the optic nerve.

If a significant amount of the orbital floor is removed and the adjacent periorbita is injured, reconstruction with titanium mesh lined with a PDS sheet is recommended. We do not suture the conjunctiva, but if canthotomy and cantholysis are performed, the canthus is reconstructed with a 5-0 PDS suture.

Lateral Approach

The lateral transorbital approach is used to access the ITF, lateral orbital contents, MCF, Meckel cave, and lateral aspect of the cavernous sinus.[3,11] The entry portal is created with a lateral retrocanthal approach.[42] It can be used with or without canthotomy and cantholysis, depending on the planned extent of dissection. A fine scissors or electrocautery is used to make a conjunctival incision approximately 3 mm deep to the orbital rim (Fig. 38.9). This is extended 4 to 5 mm superiorly, and then inferiorly as far as is desired into the inferior fornix as described previously. The periosteum of the lateral rim is incised and elevated, and the subperiorbital plane is entered. The dissection is continued inferiorly onto the orbital floor as desired, although the contents of the inferior fissure must be transected as noted earlier. Superiorly the dissection can continue to the orbital roof. Proceeding posteriorly, the ITF can be accessed, or the dissection can continue onto the greater wing of the sphenoid bone. In this region, as the dissection continues medially, the confines narrow, being limited inferiorly by

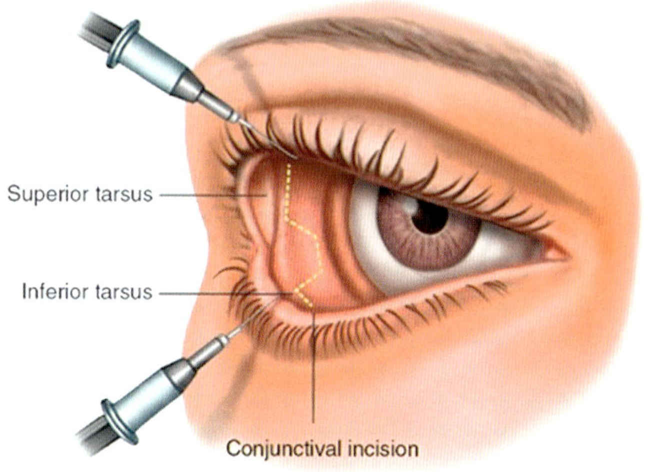

• **Fig. 38.9** Lateral retrocanthal approach. The *dotted line* indicates the conjunctival incision. The incision is made posterior to the medial canthus, 3 mm behind the lateral orbital rim. A canthotomy and cantholysis can be added if desired. (From Bevans, S. E., & Moe, K. S. [2017]. Advances in the reconstruction of orbital fractures. *Facial Plastic Surgery Clinics of North America, 25*[4], 513–535.)

the inferior orbital fissure and superiorly by the superior orbital fissure, which must be left undisturbed unless involved with pathology. Similar to the previous techniques, bone is removed as indicated by the surgical plan and delineated by navigation. Once the surgical goal is accomplished, a large defect in the bone is typically filled with a fat graft, and the bone is resurfaced with a PDS sheet to prevent impeding the function of the lateral rectus muscle directly or through scar formation. The conjunctival incision is not closed, but if a canthotomy was used, it is reconstructed as previously described.

For pathology located in the superior lateral orbit, a lateral blepharoplasty approach has been described that provides effective access to this region.[24] The choice of portal depends on location of the pathology and the ideal vector of approach, and we at times make the final decision based on analysis with the patient under general anesthesia at the beginning of the procedure.

Reconstruction of the Orbit and Adjacent Bone

The need for reconstruction of bone removed as part of an endoscopic orbital or transorbital procedure depends on the location and size of the defect. In general, orbital bone defects that are large enough to allow significant herniation of orbital contents resulting in enophthalmos, restrict extraocular muscle function, or cause adjacent sinus obstruction should be repaired. If the site is a load-bearing region, such as the orbital floor or medial orbit, consideration should be given to reconstruction with a permanent implant such as titanium mesh lined with a PDS sheet. For non–load-bearing areas, resorbable implants such as a PDS sheet alone may be a viable option. The condition of the periorbita is also important. The periorbita provides significant support to the orbital contents and may obviate the need for reconstruction of moderate bone defects if it is intact at the end of the procedure. We typically perform exophthalmometry (Hertel or Naugle) preoperatively, and this can be done intraoperatively at the conclusion of the procedure to help guide the decision on reconstruction (exophthalmometry is straightforward and rapid to learn and perform).

If it is known at the beginning of a procedure that there is high likelihood of requiring weight-bearing orbital reconstruction, we perform *preconstruction* of the implant—endoscopic placement and in situ shaping before removing the bone. This allows very precise fabrication of the implant, which can at times be left in place during the procedure to aid in tissue retraction and protect the orbital contents while working through another portal. An example of this is when multiportal resection of the medial orbit is anticipated; we place the implant during the transorbital component of the procedure to protect the orbital contents and dura, and leave it in place while the sinonasal component of the pathology is being addressed to prevent inadvertent injury to those structures.

If the defect is larger than anticipated at the end of the procedure or preconstruction was not feasible for other reasons, reconstruction of a significant defect can present challenges in recreating symmetry of the orbital structures. In these situations, we use navigation guidance and mirror-image overlay[10] as a reconstructive template. With this technique, the unaffected region of the craniofacial computed tomography (CT) image is copied, reversed (right-left), colored, and superimposed on the pathologic side (Fig. 38.10). Using this as a guide, a titanium three-dimensional mesh plate is then shaped and implanted using endoscopic technique. The entire surface of the implant is then navigated and checked against the mirror-image overlay template and adjusted as needed to match the premorbid contouring. The titanium mesh is then lined with a resorbable 0.25-mm PDS sheet that forms a glide layer to prevent restriction of muscular function while preventing herniation of fat through the mesh, which can also restrict muscle function. Although titanium implants covered with polyethylene can also be used, these can lead to chronic infection if exposed to the paranasal sinuses, and subsequent removal may provide a significant challenge.

Reconstruction of the orbital roof is a somewhat controversial topic. Major concerns include the development of postoperative pulsatile exophthalmos or contamination of the orbit from frontal sinus contents. Typically even large defects do not require

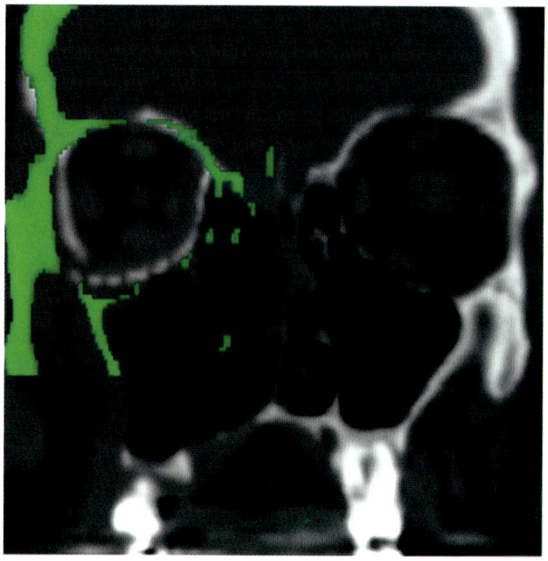

• **Fig. 38.10** Mirror image overlay orbital reconstruction. The contralateral (unaffected) orbit is colored *green* and superimposed over the pathologic (right) side. For purposes of illustration, a postoperative computed tomography scan shows the right orbital floor and medial wall implant and how it conforms to the surgical plan.

reconstruction. When pulsatile exophthalmos occurs, it generally resolves within 1 to 2 weeks. Exposure of the orbital contents to the frontal sinus is not in itself an indication for reconstruction, as the periorbita typically seals the defect and allows normal frontal sinus function. However, if the periorbita is not intact and there is significant prolapse of contents into the sinus, particularly in the region of the frontal outflow tract, reconstruction with PDS is indicated. If extraocular muscles are exposed to orbital bone or dura, consideration should be given to placing a layer of PDS to prevent adhesion. In addition, if the bone adjacent to the attachment of the trochlea of the superior oblique is removed, we typically reconstruct the defect with PDS to ensure normal relocation of the trochlea, although to date, studies confirming the need for this are lacking. A detailed review of these techniques is described elsewhere.[41]

Postoperative Care

On completion of the procedure, a head CT scan is obtained as indicated. Iced saline gauze is applied to the eye for 20 minutes each hour for 48 hours. Moisturizing ophthalmic ointment is applied twice daily for 7 days. If the patient is admitted to the hospital, intravenous steroid therapy is continued for 24 hours. Neurologic checks including pupil size and reactivity are performed per routine. Postoperative pain is typically minimal, typically less than after endoscopic sinus surgery; oral nonopioid management is often adequate. Significant, increasing pain, particularly in a retrobulbar distribution and accompanied by a decrease in vision, should raise concern for retrobulbar hemorrhage, a condition that warrants consultation with an ophthalmologist, as failure to recognize and treat this emergently could lead to permanent loss of vision. We have not had this occur, nor are we aware of reports of this in the literature to date.

Patients who have had CSF leak repair are treated in a fashion similar to those who have undergone transnasal endoscopic repair. If nonresorbable sutures were used to close a cutaneous incision, they are removed 5 to 7 days after surgery. We typically follow up with the patient at postoperative weeks 1, 2, and 4, and as indicated by the pathology thereafter. The majority of the surgical edema resolves during the first week after surgery. It is common for the patient to have a degree of diplopia postoperatively owing to retraction of the extraocular muscles and edema. If this occurs, it typically resolves gradually over 1 to 2 weeks but occasionally somewhat longer. Sensory disturbances in the forehead are common with the superior approach owing to retraction of the supraorbital and supratrochlear nerves. Even if one of these nerves is transected during the procedure, the sensation appears to return over time.

Outcomes and Safety

It is often notable to surgeons who are learning these procedures that the globes can be retracted without damage. There are two primary reasons for this; there is significant redundancy in the optic nerve (without this, the globe could not rotate), and there is the capacity to mildly decrease the volume of the orbital contents through gentle pressure by decreasing the amount of venous blood within the vasculature. In addition, as noted earlier, the volume of orbital retraction required for endoscopic procedures is fairly small, on the order of several cubic milliliters with approximately 1 cm of globe displacement.[11] The optic and other cranial nerves are surrounded by a thick condensation of the periorbita at the margins of the superior orbital fissure and optic canal, which provides an element of protection when operating in the subperiorbital plane.

Our experience to date has been highly successful without major complications. We reported the outcomes of our initial experience with these approaches, including a series of 107 consecutive patients without complications related to the surgical approach. In particular, there were no cases of blindness or decreased visual acuity, and no cases of permanent postoperative diplopia.[3,6] More recently, we reported our series of 45 consecutive transorbital procedures involving the skull base and brain. All of the procedures were successful, and the complications were limited to one case of ptosis that resolved spontaneously, and one case of delayed epiphora that occurred 1 month after surgery and resolved with dacryocystorhinostomy.[19] The most significant complication we have encountered to date is a postoperative CSF leak after treatment of a complex supraorbital frontal sinus mucocele, which was treated with a revision endoscopic approach.[17]

Locatelli et al. performed a survey of the literature on transorbital endoscopic surgery from 2000 to 2015.[22] They found 38 clinical articles dating back to 2010. Including their vast experience, they found no reports of significant neurologic or vascular complications, CSF leak, hemorrhage, postoperative infection, visual loss, permanent diplopia, or death. In addition, they found that "patient recovery is rapid, intensive care unit stays can be reduced or avoided, and the requirement for protracted use of pain medicine is reduced." They concluded that "the inclusion of transorbital endoscopic approaches in the surgical armamentarium of the skull base surgeon will become crucial in the future."

Conclusion

In our experience, endoscopic orbital and transorbital procedures have provided a highly effective and safe addition to the current armamentarium of approaches, whether used alone or in multiportal combination. With these procedures, the orbit has been transformed from an obstacle to an efficacious pathway that offers access to structures deep with the ACF, MCF, and ITF. The challenges of other single-vector approaches, such as the narrow funnel and attic effects, are surmounted, and coplanar manipulation of the pathology is readily achievable. As a result, many groups are reporting favorable experience with these techniques, and descriptions of new applications are rapidly appearing.

Although the published international experience results agree with our impressions, a word of caution should be added. Endoscopic surgery within the orbit represents a group of relatively new procedures, and many surgeons are learning them after completing their training programs. In addition, the skills used in these procedures have not been traditionally taught as part of a single surgical discipline. As a result, before beginning to use these procedures, we recommend detailed study of the available literature on the subject, as well as attending courses or national meetings where these procedures are taught. Rehearsal in a cadaver laboratory is recommended. A multidisciplinary team is important in planning, undertaking, and caring for these patients after surgery and will add to the success of building a surgical program.

References

1. Janecka, I. P., Nuss, D. W., & Sen, C. N. (1991). Facial translocation approach to the cranial base. *Acta Neurochirurgica Suppplementum*, *53*, 193–198.
2. Vuillemin, T., Lädrach, K., & Raveh, J. (1998). Craniofacial surgery. Advantages of subcranial procedures in craniofacial surgery. *Schweizer Monatsschrift für Zahnmedizin*, *98*(8), 859–869 (in German).
3. Moe, K. S., Bergeron, C. M., & Ellenbogen, R. G. (2010). Transorbital neuroendoscopic surgery. *Neurosurgery*, *67*(3 Suppl Operative), 16–28. ons.
4. Ciporen, J. N., Moe, K. S., Lopez, S., Ledesma, E., Ramanathan, D., Rostomily, R., et al. (2010). Multi-portal endoscopic approaches to the central skull base: A cadaveric study. *World Neurosurgery*, *73*(6), 705–712.
5. Moe, K. S., Kim, L. J., & Bergeron, C. M. (2011). Transorbital endoscopic repair of complex cerebrospinal fluid leaks. *Laryngoscope*, *121*, 13–30.
6. Balakrishnan, K., & Moe, K. S. (2011). Applications and outcomes of orbital and transorbital endoscopic surgery. *Otolaryngology–Head and Neck Surgery*, *144*(5), 815–820.
7. Lim, J. H., Sardesai, M., Ferreira, M., & Moe, K. S. (2012). Transorbital neuroendoscopic management of sinogenic complications involving the frontal sinus, orbit and anterior cranial fossa. *Journal of Neurological Surgery Part B, Skull Base*, *73*(6), 394–400.
8. Oxford, R., Bly, R., Kim, L., & Moe, K. S. (2012). Transorbital neuroendoscopic surgery of the middle cranial fossa by lateral retrocanthal approach. *Journal of Neurological Surgery Part B, Skull Base*, (73), A197.
9. Bly, R. A., Su, D., Hannaford, B., Ferreira, M., & Moe, K. S. (2012). Computer modeled multiportal approaches to the skull base. *Journal of Neurological Surgery Part B, Skull Base*, *73*(6), 415–423.
10. Bly, R., Liu, J., Cjudekova, M., Chang, S. H., & Moe, K. S. (2013). Computer-guided orbital reconstruction improves surgical outcomes. *JAMA Facial Plastic Surgery*, *15*(2), 113–120.
11. Bly, R., Ramakrishna, R., Ferreira, M., & Moe, K. S. (2014). Lateral transorbital neuroendoscopic approach to the lateral cavernous sinus. *Journal of Neurological Surgery Part B, Skull Base*, *75*(1), 11–17.
12. Bly, R., Su, D., Lendvay, T., Friedman, D., Hannaford, B., Ferreira, M., et al. (2013). Multiportal robotic access to the anterior cranial fossa: A surgical and engineering feasibility study. *Otolaryngology–Head and Neck Surgery*, *149*(6), 940–946.
13. Bhama, P., Manning, S., & Moe, K. S. (2012). Skull base myxoma. *International Journal of Pediatric Otorhinolaryngology*, *7*(1), 26–29.
14. Bly, R., Morton, R., Kim, L. J., & Moe, K. S. (2014). Tension pneumocephalus after endoscopic sinus surgery: A technical report of multiportal endoscopic skull. *Otolaryngology–Head and Neck Surgery*, *15*(6), 1081–1083.
15. Patel, S., Berens, A. M., Devarajan, K., Whipple, M. E., & Moe, K. S. (2017). Evaluation of a minimally disruptive treatment protocol for frontal sinus fracture. *JAMA Facial Plastic Surgery*, *19*(3), 225–231.
16. Moe, K. S., Bly, R. A., & Ciporen, J. (2020). Pediatric transorbital endoscopic skull base surgery. In H. Singh, H., J. P. Greenfield, V. K. Anand, & T. H. Schwartz (Eds.), *Pediatric endoscopic endonasal skull base surgery*. Stuttgart, Germany: Thieme.
17. Miller, C., Berens, A., Humphreys, I., & Moe, K. S. (2020). Transorbital approach for improved access in the management of paranasal sinus mucoceles. *Journal of Neurological Surgery Part B, Skull Base*, *80*(6), 593–598.
18. Kirkham, E., Perkins, J., & Moe, K. S. (2018). Juvenile nasopharyngeal angiofibroma. In J. A. Perkins & K. Balakrishnan (Eds.), *Evidence-based management of head & neck vascular anomalies* (pp. 67–72). Cham, Switzerland: Springer.
19. Ramakrishna, R., Kim, L. J., Bly, R., Moe, K. S., & Ferreira, M. J. (2016). Transorbital neuroendoscopic surgery for the treatment of skull base lesions. *Journal of Clinical Neuroscience*, *24*, 99–104.
20. Dallan, I., Castelnuovo, P., Locatelli, D., Turri-Zanoni, M., AlQahtani, A., Battaglia, P., et al. (2015). Multiportal combined transorbital transnasal endoscopic approach for the management of selected skull base lesions: Preliminary experience. *World Neurosurgery*, *84*(1), 97–107.
21. Alqahtani, A., Padoan, G., Segnini, G., Lepera, D., Fortunato, S., Dallan, I., et al. (2015). Transorbital transnasal endoscopic combined approach to the anterior and middle skull base: A laboratory investigation. *Acta Otorhinolaryngologica Italica*, *35*(3), 173–179.
22. Locatelli, D., Pozzi, F., Turri-Zanoni, M., Battaglia, P., Santi, L., Dallan, I., et al. (2016). Transorbital endoscopic approaches to the skull base: Current concepts and future perspectives. *Journal of Neurosurgical Sciences*, *60*(4), 514–525.
23. Dallan, I., Sellari-Franceschini, S., Turri-Zanoni, M., de Notaris, M., Fiacchini, G., Fiorini, F. R., et al. (2018). Endoscopic transorbital superior eyelid approach for the management of selected spheno-orbital meningiomas: Preliminary experience. *Operative Neurosurgery (Hagerstown, MD)*, *14*(3), 243–251.
24. Lubbe, D., Mustak, H., Taylor, A., & Fagan, J. (2017). Minimally invasive endo-orbital approach to sphenoid wing meningiomas improves visual outcomes—our experience with the first seven cases. *Clinical Otolaryngology*, *42*(4), 876–880.
25. Alves-Belo, J. T., Mangussi-Gomes, J., Truong, H. Q., Cohen, S., Gardner, P. A., Snyderman, C. H., et al. (2019). Lateral transorbital versus endonasal transpterygoid approach to the lateral recess of the sphenoid sinus-a comparative anatomic study. *Operative Neurosurgery (Hagerstown, MD)*, *16*(5), 600–606.
26. Chabot, J. D., Gardner, P. A., Stefko, S. T., Zwagerman, N. T., & Fernandez-Miranda, J. C. (2017). Lateral orbitotomy approach for lesions involving the middle fossa: A retrospective review of thirteen patients. *Neurosurgery*, *1*, *80*(2), 309–322.
27. Noiphithak, R., Yanez-Siller, J. C., Revuelta Barbero, J. M., Otto, B. A., Carrau, R. L., & Prevedello, D. M. (2019). Comparative analysis between lateral orbital rim preservation and osteotomy for transorbital endoscopic approaches to the cavernous sinus: an anatomic study. *Operative Neurosurgery (Hagerstown, MD)*, *16*(1), 86–93.
28. Priddy, B. H., Nunes, C. F., Beer-Furlan, A., Carrau, R., Dallan, I., & Prevedello, D. M. (2017). A side door to Meckel's cave: anatomic feasibility study for the lateral transorbital approach. *Operative Neurosurgery (Hagerstown, MD)*, *13*(5), 614–621.
29. Humphreys, I., Hicks, K. L., & Moe, K. S. (2018). Bilateral transorbital and transnasal endoscopic resection of a frontal sinus osteoblastoma and orbital mucocele: A case report and review of the literature. *Annals of Otology, Rhinology & Laryngology*, *127*(11), 864–869.
30. Lubbe, D., & Moe, K. S. (2020). Transorbital approaches to the sinuses, skull base, and intracranial space. In B. S. Bleier (Ed.), *Endoscopic surgery of the orbit*. New York: Thieme.
31. Harbison, R. A., Berens, A. M., Li, Y., Bly, R. A., Hannaford, B., & Moe, K. S. (2017). Region-specific objective signatures of endoscopic surgical instrument motion: A cadaveric exploratory analysis. *Journal of Neurological Surgery Part B, Skull Base*, *78*(1), 99–104.
32. Yangming, L., Bly, R. A., Harbison, R. A., Humphreys, I. M., Whipple, M. E., Hannaford, B., & Moe, K. S. (2017). Anatomical region segmentation for objective surgical skill assessment with operating room motion data. *Journal of Neurological Surgery Part B, Skull Base*, *78*(6), 490–496.
33. Harbison, R. A., Li, Y., Berens, A. M., Bly, R. A., Hannaford, B., & Moe, K. S. (2017). An automated methodology for assessing anatomy-specific instrument motion during endoscopic endonasal skull base surgery. *Journal of Neurological Surgery Part B, Skull Base*, *78*(3), 222–226.
34. Berens, A. M., Li, Y., Aghdasi, N., Hannaford, B., & Moe, K. S. (2017). Quantitative analysis of transnasal anterior skull base approach: Report of technology for intraoperative assessment of instrument motion. *Surgical Innovation*, *24*(4), 405–410.
35. Li, Y., Bly, R. A., Harbison, A., Humphreys, I., Whipple, M., Hannaford, B., et al. (2017). Anatomical region segmentation for objective surgical skill assessment with operating room motion data. *Journal of Neurological Surgery Part B, Skull Base*, *78*(6), 490–496.

36. Moe, K. S., & Bly, R. (2019). Commentary: Comparative analysis of the exposure and surgical freedom of the endoscopic extended mini-pterional craniotomy and the transorbital endoscopic approach to the anterior and middle cranial fossae: A cadaveric investigation. *Operative Neurosurgery, 17*(2), E47–E49.
37. Ellenbogen, R. G., & Moe, K. S. (2015). Transorbital neuroendoscopic approaches to the anterior cranial fossa. In C. H. Snyderman (Ed.), *Master techniques in otolaryngology–head and neck surgery: Skull base surgery* (pp. 151–164). Philadelphia, PA: Wolters Kluwer.
38. Moe, K. S., & Ellenbogen, R. G. (2015). Transorbital neuroendoscopic approaches to the middle cranial fossa. In C. H. Snyderman (Ed.), *Master techniques in otolaryngology–head & neck surgery: Skull base surgery* (pp. 343–356). Philadelphia: Wolters Kluwer.
39. Berens, A., & Moe, K. S. (2017). Transorbital neuroendoscopic approaches. In M. Bernal-Sprekelsen, & I. Alobid (Eds.), *Endoscopic approaches to the paranasal sinuses and the skull base: A step-by-step anatomic dissection guide* (pp. 156–162). Stuttgart, Germany: Thieme.
40. Moe, K. S. (2003). The precaruncular approach to the medial orbit. *JAMA Facial Plastic Surgery, 5*, 483–487.
41. Bevans, S., & Moe, K. S. (2017). Orbital reconstruction. In K. S. Moe (Ed.), Trauma in facial plastic surgery. *Facial Plastic Surgery Clinics of North America,* 25(4):513–535.
42. Moe, K. S., Jothi, S., Stern, R., & Gassner, H. G. (2007). Lateral retrocanthal orbitotomy; a minimally invasive canthus-sparing approach. *JAMA Facial Plastic Surgery, 9*(6), 419–426.

39 Complications in Endoscopic Skull Base Surgery

KYLE K. VANKOEVERING, MD, DANIEL M. PREVEDELLO, MD, AND RICARDO L. CARRAU, MD

With continued advancements in endoscopic approaches for skull base surgery, understanding the risks and potential complications of these techniques is critical in planning surgical access and counseling patients. Extensive transclival operations, coronal plan approaches lateral to the carotid artery, and endoscopic orbital approaches have allowed more lesions to be accessed through less-invasive approaches. But each of these techniques is associated with an evolving risk profile. We discuss general considerations in minor and major complications[1] for endoscopic skull base surgery, with a subsequent focus on orbital complications and endoscopic orbital surgery.

Minor Complications in Skull Base Surgery

Endonasal surgery uses the sinonasal corridors to access the skull base. Access through the nasal cavity allows for a minimally invasive approach, but it also comes with an associated cost to the normal function of the sinonasal cavity.

Postoperative sinusitis and synechia formation are perhaps the most common minor complications from endonasal skull base surgery. After a comprehensive disruption of the normal sinonasal anatomy, some degree of postoperative crusting develops in many patients. This crusting is frequently debrided in the clinic to prevent sinusitis and synechia formation. A literature review of skull base sinonasal outcomes demonstrated a 50% incidence of significant postoperative crusting, with 40% of patients demonstrating sinusitis symptoms of nasal drainage and obstructive symptoms.[2] Although these symptoms can be relatively benign, they can significantly affect quality of life.[3] Synechia formation after endonasal sinus surgery has been reported in 5% to 28% of patients, and results from skull base surgery would presumably be similar.[3-5] Notably, delayed mucocele formation can occur when a sinus becomes obstructed from scarring of the outflow tract postoperatively and has been reported in 3% to 8% of cases.[2,6]

Postoperative epistaxis is a relatively common consideration after endoscopic sinonasal surgery. And although most postoperative epistaxis is mild, severe hemorrhage requiring operative control is well defined and typically stems from an arterial source.[7] Classically nasal epistaxis can be managed with nasal packing; however, in the fresh postoperative setting, particularly after a skull base resection, aggressive packing must be approached cautiously to avoid intracranial complications from improperly placed packs. Furthermore, it is worth noting that the majority of reported epistaxis events occur 2 to 4 weeks postoperatively.[7] In a recent review, Zimmer and Andaluz reviewed more than 400 endoscopic pituitary surgeries, demonstrating a 4.1% rate of postoperative epistaxis.[8] They noted that of the 18 patients, 11 were treated with in-office cauterization, packing, or intranasal hemostatic agents, whereas 5 required a return to the operating room and 2 required embolization. Similarly, Thompson et al. reported a 3% incidence of postoperative epistaxis in their single-institution cohort.[9] Although the majority of episodes of epistaxis were controlled with packing, 5 of 14 events required control in the operating room. These data confirm that, overall, postoperative epistaxis is relatively uncommon after endoscopic skull base surgery and frequently can be managed with conservative measures. However, some patients require operative control, particularly in cases of arterial hemorrhage.

Nasal deformities such as saddle nose have been reported after skull base surgery. This is particularly identified after nasoseptal flap and subsequent septectomy. In one major report on these nasal deformities, the authors highlight a nearly 6% overall incidence of nasal dorsal collapse.[10] The authors noted these deformities were associated with nasoseptal flap use (15% of patients who underwent nasoseptal flap) and highlight several potential explanations, including electrocautery, contracture scar forces, overaggressive septectomy, and postoperative radiation as potential implicating factors. Soudry et al. performed a retrospective review demonstrating a less than 1% rate of saddle deformity.[11] Although these nasal deformities are not life threatening, they are challenging to repair and can have significant impacts on the patient's social and functional status. We speculate that preservation of the entire septal attachments to the anterior premaxilla may help prevent this complication.

Using the sinonasal corridor for access to the skull base has several advantages, but one notable disadvantage is the potential disruption to the olfactory system. Postoperative hyposmia has been well documented and evaluated by several studies. Several technical concepts have been suggested to potentially improve olfaction outcomes, including the preservation of the septal olfactory strip and preservation of the middle turbinates when possible.[2,12,13] Results from a variety of studies demonstrate a wide variety of results, ranging from no significant dysfunction,[14] to temporary impairment,[13,15] to significant permanent olfactory disturbance.[16] Some studies have reported rates of long-term olfactory disturbance up to nearly 30%.[2,17] A prospective study of 42 patients who underwent baseline and periodic postoperative testing

(University of Pennsylvania Smell Identification Test) demonstrated that patients undergoing pituitary surgery with rescue flap elevation showed no evidence of olfactory dysfunction, whereas patients with a nasoseptal flap showed temporary dysfunction.[13] A recent evidence-based review and recommendation on olfactory function after endonasal skull base surgery was published by Greig et al.[18] They concluded that the body of evidence was heterogeneous, but routine transsphenoidal surgery with rescue flaps and at least one middle turbinate preserved likely leads to limited long-term olfactory dysfunction. However, they also concluded that nasoseptal flap harvest and potentially electrocautery likely lead to increased olfactory dysfunction.

Major Complications in Skull Base Surgery

The most common major complication after endoscopic skull base surgery is postoperative cerebrospinal fluid (CSF) leak. Breaching the dural layer of the skull base (and underlying arachnoid) typically results in a visible CSF Leak. Definitive reconstruction after surgical extirpation is critical to separate the intracranial contents from the sinonasal space and prevent infectious complications. Although various reconstructive approaches have been proposed, the nasoseptal flap has emerged as the workhorse, vascularized reconstructive tool for multilayered reconstruction (Fig. 39.1).[19,20] Consensus retrospective data have generally agreed that, intraoperatively, small, low-flow CSF leaks can be repaired with layered free graft approaches, whereas large, high-flow leaks should be repaired with a vascularized flap.[21,22] Postoperatively the patient must be observed for CSF rhinorrhea. The incidence of postoperative CSF leak after endonasal skull base surgery ranges significantly based on the surgical subsite. In general, data suggest sellar defects have the lowest incidence, followed by cribriform, suprasellar, and then clival defects, which are generally regarded as the most difficult to repair.[23]

Identification of a postoperative CSF leak is typically signified by clear rhinorrhea with challenge (leaning forward) or increasing pneumocephalus on computed tomography scanning. When this is identified, several strategies exist for management. For very low-flow, small persistent postoperative CSF leaks, bedrest and pressure reduction with acetazolamide (Diamox; Zydus Pharmaceuticals) can be considered. However, CSF diversion, typically with a lumbar drain, is often added to a conservative regimen for several days to allow the leak to scar and heal. Nevertheless, the majority of postoperative CSF leaks require surgical re-exploration with revision reconstruction. Often this requires minimal adjusting of the existing reconstruction, but the team needs to be prepared for a complete revision. Unfortunately, there is not an abundance of consensus data on when to choose a conservative versus operative approach, but one systematic review highlighted that the majority of cases (62%) required operative revision.[21]

The critical importance of successful skull base reconstruction after endonasal approaches cannot be overemphasized. Postoperative meningitis is highly correlated with reconstructive failure and persistent postoperative CSF leak. Lai et al. showed the risk of meningitis is directly related to postoperative CSF leaks with an odds ratio of 92. In the absence of a CSF leak, the risk of meningitis and intracranial infectious complications approached zero.[24] Persistent CSF leaks have been associated with up to a 21% incidence of meningitis and increased rates of reoperations and major complications.[25]

Postoperative meningitis or other infections sequelae are potentially devastating complications of endonasal skull base surgery. Fortunately, rates of postoperative meningitis and other intracranial infections are low, ranging from 0 to 10% depending on the study evaluated.[26] However, the complications of meningitis can be devastating, with studies highlighting up to 13% associated mortality.[27]

As the field of endoscopic skull base surgery has evolved and new surgical approaches and techniques have developed, the major limit in the extent of dissection remains the cranial nerves. Postoperative cranial neuropathy is typically associated with significant morbidity. An exquisite knowledge of the anatomic structures, high-resolution preoperative cross-sectional imaging, intraoperative stereotactic navigation, and neurophysiologic monitoring are critical components of safe endonasal surgery and limiting risk to the cranial nerves. Fortunately, cranial nerve injuries are rare and highly correlate with the anatomic location of the target lesion and the aggressiveness of the lesion. For example, in one study of cavernous sinus tumors, new postoperative cranial neuropathies developed in nearly 12% of patients with nonpituitary adenoma pathologies, while none of patients with the adenomas had this complication.[28] Another study highlighted an 8.7% incidence of postoperative cranial neuropathy after resection of clival chordoma.[29] Although data are limited, experience suggests malignant pathologies that require more aggressive resection, and tumors invading the cavernous sinus along the course of VI cranial nerve VI, or those invading the optic canal appear to have increased risk profiles. There are limited options for treatment of postoperative cranial nerve deficits. Many palsies are transient

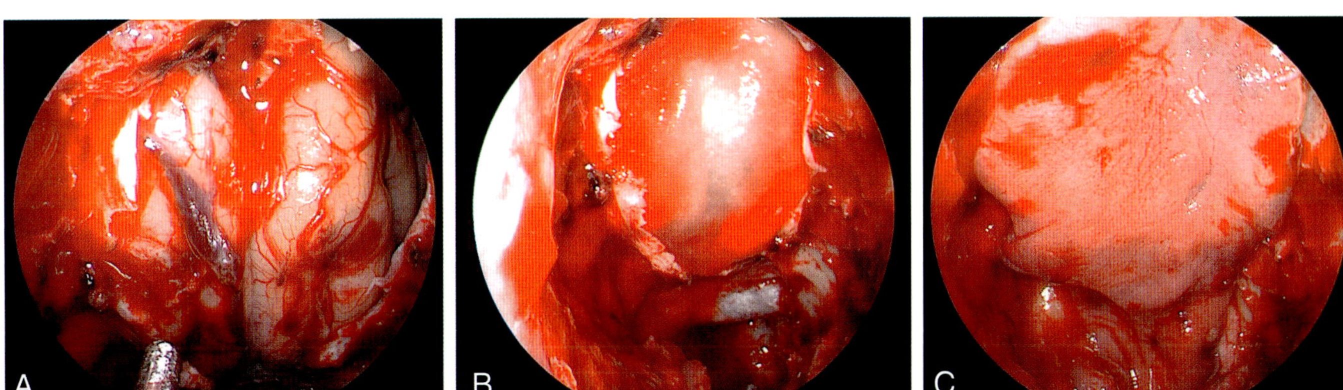

• **Fig. 39.1** Multilayered Endoscopic Skull Base Reconstruction. A, Endoscopic view of frontal lobes after resection of the cribriform plate with cerebrospinal fluid (CSF) leak. B, Synthetic collagen inlay for reconstruction. C Nasoseptal flap onlay completes a multilayered reconstruction to prevent postoperative CSF leak.

and may respond to steroids. There are a variety of surgical and corrective prism options for ophthalmoplegia, and consultation with a neurophthalmologist is often beneficial. For trigeminal dysfunction, symptomatic patients may require consultation with a neurologist to discuss medical management including anticonvulsants. For lower cranial neuropathies, involvement of the speech and language pathologist can help rehabilitate a functional swallow and speech.

Although cranial neuropathies result in significant morbidity for our patients, the most feared complication in endonasal surgery is a vascular injury of the carotid or basilar system. As with the cranial nerves, exquisite knowledge of the surgical anatomy and preoperative imaging are critical to prevent these catastrophic events. Vascular injuries remain uncommon in experienced surgical hands, and a recent literature review highlighted a 0.34% rate of arterial injury.[30] In the event of an arterial injury (Fig. 39.2A), the surgical team must act fast. Controlling the bleeding with pressure and packing intraoperatively are critical to prevent exsanguination. A crushed muscle patch has been proven to expedite hemostasis (Fig. 39.2B).[31] These injuries are high-stress situations for which there are several proposed training models, including live, synthetic, and cadaveric, that allow the participant to practice the surgical and psychomotor skills needed to control these catastrophic complications.[31-33] Once the bleeding is controlled intraoperatively, the patient is typically taken straight to the angio-interventional suite where, if feasible, carotid stenting can be performed. However, frequently carotid sacrifice must be performed for definitive control (Fig. 39-2C, D).[30]

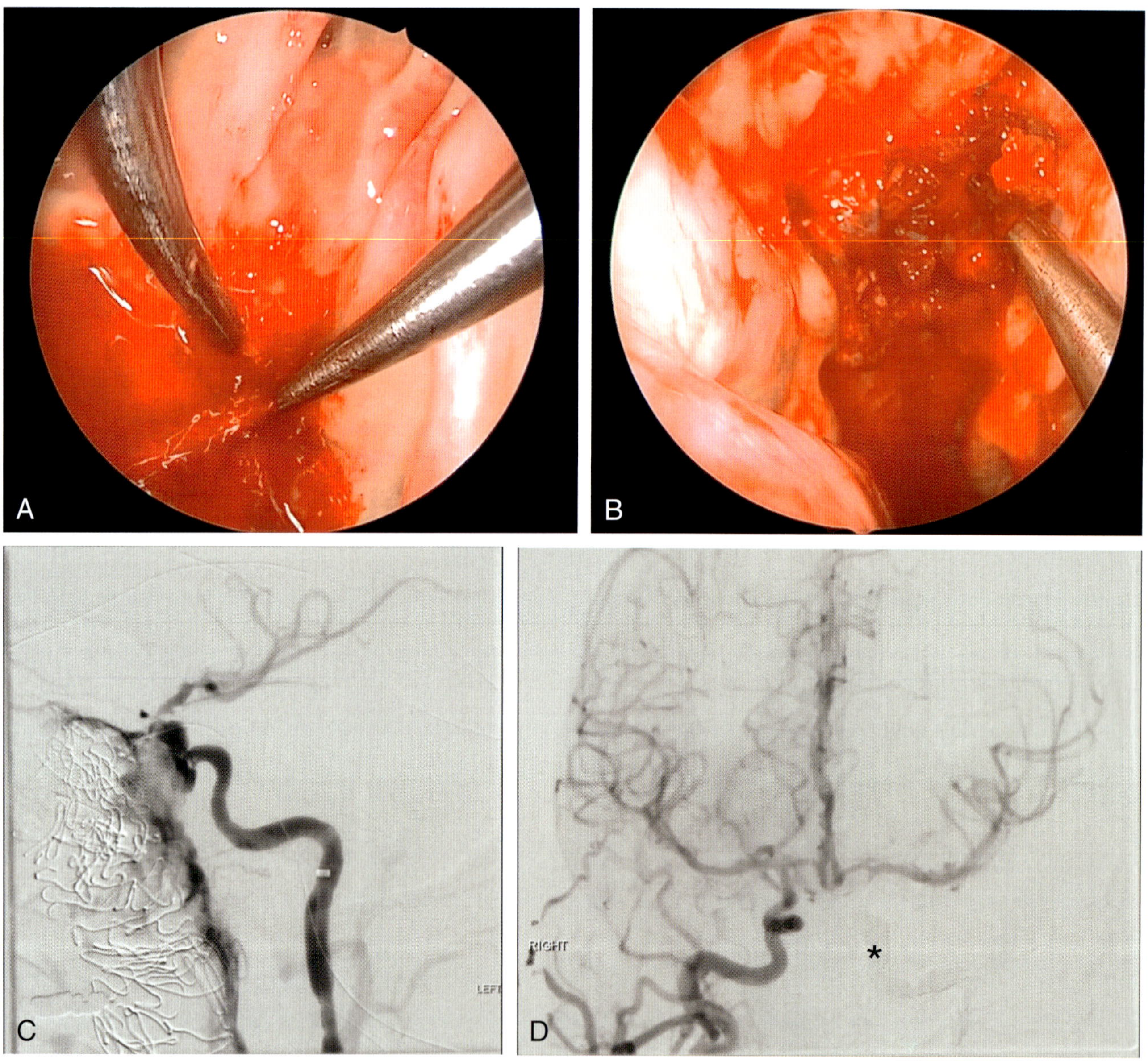

• **Fig. 39.2** Endoscopic Left Carotid Artery Injury With Coil Embolization. A, Endoscopic rupture of the left carotid artery in a patient with prior proton irradiation for chordoma. B, Crushed muscle patch secured in place to expedite hemostasis. C, Initial angiogram demonstrates carotid rupture with profuse extravasation. Note contrast filling the nasal cavity behind the nasal packing. D, Successful coil embolization (asterisk) and adequate cross-filling of the left hemisphere with right carotid angiography. The patient sustained no neurologic deficits.

Orbital Complications

With emerging techniques in endoscopic orbital surgery, complications of the orbit require separate discussion. In addition to endoscopic decompression techniques for Graves opthalmopathy,[34] the endoscope has been used for complex orbital apex and optic nerve decompression,[35] access to medial and inferior orbital apex lesions,[36] and now with transorbital neuroendoscopic surgery,[37] more lateral aspects of the anterior skull base can be accessed, providing minimally invasive options for otherwise complex lesions. These advanced orbital approaches also come with a new complication risk profile, including injury to the optic nerve, ophthalmoplegia, orbital hematoma, or extraocular muscle injury.

Orbital hematoma is a dreaded complication of any endoscopic skull base surgery, particularly those accessing the frontal outflow and cribriform. Transection of the ethmoid arteries as they exit the orbit can allow the proximal end to retract into the orbit, resulting in significant intraorbital hemorrhage and hematoma. This can, in turn, rapidly compromise vision as increased orbital pressure results in venous congestion and infarct of the optic nerve. Conversely, any disruption of the periorbita with uncontrolled venous oozing can result in a slower presentation of orbital hematoma. Fortunately, this complication is rare. A recent retrospective review highlighted 2 cases of orbital hematoma after more than 1600 endoscopic sinus cases (0.12%),[38] although this number may be higher for endoscopic orbital surgery. If the source is arterial, these hematomas present acutely with proptosis, ecchymosis, and increased pressure. If tonometry confirms an elevated pressure ($> \sim 20$ mm Hg), mannitol and dexamethasone may be used to reduce pressure and edema. However, if the pressures continue to climb or progressive vision loss is noted, a lateral canthotomy and cantholysis are required.[39] This procedure reduces the orbital compartment syndrome by allowing the globe to prolapse further out of the orbit. If symptoms or pressure continue to worsen, formal orbital exploration and hemorrhage control with or without endoscopic decompression is required.

Diplopia is a reasonably common complication of endoscopic orbital surgery. This is often speculated to result from edema within the orbit or prolapse of fat and muscle after decompression. In the literature, temporary diplopia has been reported in 15% to 64% of patients after endoscopic decompression.[40,41] However many of these patients have preexisting diplopia, and most symptoms are transient and self-limited. A systematic review noted that diplopia was present in 19.9% of patients after combined endoscopic lateral canthotomy decompression.[42] Maintaining an inferomedial bony strut during decompression may further reduce the diplopia risk.[41] However more permanent diplopia can occur after endoscopic orbital surgery related to extraocular muscle injury.[43] Although it is difficult to characterize the incidence of these more permanent injuries, this is likely directly related to the degree of orbital involvement of the lesion. When strabismus does not improve postoperatively, consultation with an ophthalmologist and cross-sectional imaging are important measures. Corrective lenses and surgical reconstruction of the rectus muscles may be indicated.

Injury to the optic nerve, globe, and retina are uncommon complications of most endoscopic orbital surgery. However, surgery at the orbital apex and optic nerve, such as that for medial apex lesions, would be associated with an obvious increased risk. Stokken et al. noted a 3.7% incidence of vision loss in a series of 27 patients undergoing endoscopic surgery of the orbital apex.[36] Again, the surgical exposure and degree of intraorbital extension likely are key in the risk profile. Meticulous microsurgical technique with delicate two-handed dissection and judicious use of the bipolar electrocautery are key concepts to limit cranial nerve injuries when working at the orbital apex.

Transorbital neuroendoscopic surgery brings even further access to the skull base by using the orbital corridor. With these techniques, typically a lid crease or transcaruncular approach are used to access the orbit, and subperiosteal dissection is typically used to access a variety of regions to the anterolateral skull base.[44] In addition to the earlier complication profile, the anterior orbital incisions also lead to risks of ptosis and epiphora. Ramakrishna et al. reported a 2.5% incidence of each of these complications, which may be related to the access chosen.[44] Proper closure of the levator aponeurosis is critical after a lid crease incision if the levator is breached.

Conclusion

Endoscopic endonasal and orbital surgery have greatly advanced over the past two decades with a variety of new approaches and techniques. Even though they provide innovative approaches to the skull base through minimally invasive corridors, advanced endoscopic orbital and skull base approaches carry with them a significant potential risk profile. These shared complications can have potentially devastating sequelae, but an exquisite knowledge of the surgical anatomy and preoperative imaging can help mitigate these risks.

References

1. Stankiewicz, J. A. (1989). Complications of endoscopic sinus surgery. *Otolaryngologic Clinics of North America, 22*(4), 749–758.
2. Awad, A. J., Mohyeldin, A., El-Sayed, I. H., & Aghi, M. K. (2015). Sinonasal morbidity following endoscopic endonasal skull base surgery. *Clinical Neurology and Neurosurgery, 130*, 162–167.
3. Henriquez, O. A., Schlosser, R. J., Mace, J. C., Smith, T. L., & Soler, Z. M. (2013). Impact of synechiae after endoscopic sinus surgery on long-term outcomes in chronic rhinosinusitis. *Laryngoscope, 123*(11), 2615–2619.
4. Fong, E., Garcia, M., Woods, C. M., & Ooi, E. (2017). Hyaluronic acid for post sinus surgery care: Systematic review and meta-analysis. *Journal of Laryngology and Otology, 131*(S1), S2–S11.
5. Xu, J. J., Busato, G. M., McKnight, C., & Lee, J. M. (2016). Absorbable steroid-impregnated spacer after endoscopic sinus surgery to reduce synechiae formation. *Annals of Otolology, Rhinolology & Laryngology, 125*(3), 195–198.
6. Bleier, B. S., Wang, E. W., Vandergrift, W. A., 3rd, & Schlosser, R. J. (2011). Mucocele rate after endoscopic skull base reconstruction using vascularized pedicled flaps. *American Journal of Rhinology & Allergy, 25*(3), 186–187.
7. Halderman, A. A., Sindwani, R., & Woodard, T. D. (2015). Hemorrhagic complications of endoscopic sinus surgery. *Otolaryngologic Clinics of North America, 48*(5), 783–793.
8. Zimmer, L. A., & Andaluz, N. (2018). Incidence of epistaxis after endoscopic pituitary surgery: Proposed treatment algorithm. *Ear, Nose & Throat Journal, 97*(3), E44–E48.
9. Thompson, C. F., Wang, M. B., Kim, B. J., Bergsneider, M., & Suh, J. D. (2012). Incidence and management of epistaxis after endoscopic skull base surgery. *ORL Journal for Oto-rhino-laryngology and Its Related Specialties, 74*(6), 315–319.
10. Rowan, N. R., Wang, E. W., Gardner, P. A., Fernandez-Miranda, J. C., & Snyderman, C. H. (2016). Nasal deformities following nasoseptal flap reconstruction of skull base defects. *Journal of Neurological Surgery Part B, Skull Base, 77*(1), 14–18.

11. Soudry, E., Psaltis, A. J., Lee, K. H., Vaezafshar, R., Nayak, J. V., & Hwang, P. H. (2015). Complications associated with the pedicled nasoseptal flap for skull base reconstruction. *Laryngoscope*, *125*(1), 80–85.
12. Thompson, C. F., Kern, R. C., & Conley, D. B. (2015). Olfaction in endoscopic sinus and skull base surgery. *Otolaryngologic Clinics of North America*, *48*(5), 795–804.
13. Upadhyay, S., Buohliqah, L., Dolci, R. L. L., Otto, B. A., Prevedello, D. M., & Carrau, R. L. (2017). Periodic olfactory assessment in patients undergoing skull base surgery with preservation of the olfactory strip. *Laryngoscope*, *127*(9), 1970–1975.
14. Griffiths, C. F., Cutler, A. R., Duong, H. T., Bardo, G., Karimi, K., Barkhoudarian, G., et al. (2014). Avoidance of postoperative epistaxis and anosmia in endonasal endoscopic skull base surgery: A technical note. *Acta Neurochirurgica*, *156*(7), 1393–1401.
15. Kahilogullari, G., Beton, S., Al-Beyati, E. S., Kantarcioglu, O., Bozkurt, M., Kantarcioglu, E., et al. (2013). Olfactory functions after transsphenoidal pituitary surgery: Endoscopic versus microscopic approach. *Laryngoscope*, *123*(9), 2112–2119.
16. Soyka, M. B., Serra, C., Regli, L., Meier, E., & Holzmann, D. (2017). Long-term olfactory outcome after nasoseptal flap reconstructions in midline skull base surgery. *American Journal of Rhinology & Allergy*, *31*(5), 334–337.
17. Gallagher, M. J., Durnford, A. J., Wahab, S. S., Nair, S., Rokade, A., & Mathad, N. (2014). Patient-reported nasal morbidity following endoscopic endonasal skull base surgery. *British Journal of Neurosurgery*, *28*(5), 622–625.
18. Greig, S. R., Cooper, T. J., Sommer, D. D., Nair, S., & Wright, E. D. (2016). Objective sinonasal functional outcomes in endoscopic anterior skull-base surgery: An evidence-based review with recommendations. *International Forum of Allergy & Rhinology*, *6*(10), 1040–1046.
19. Hadad, G., Bassagasteguy, L., Carrau, R. L., Mataza, J. C., Kassam, A., Snyderman, C. H., et al. (2006). A novel reconstructive technique after endoscopic expanded endonasal approaches: Vascular pedicle nasoseptal flap. *Laryngoscope*, *116*(10), 1882–1886.
20. van Koevering, K., Prevedello, D. M., & Carrau, R. L. (2018). Endoscopic endonasal approaches for the management of cranial base malignancies: Histologically guided treatment and clinical outcomes. *Journal of Neurosurgical Sciences*, *62*(6), 667–681.
21. Soudry, E., Turner, J. H., Nayak, J. V., & Hwang, P. H. (2014). Endoscopic reconstruction of surgically created skull base defects: A systematic review. *Otolaryngology–Head and Neck Surgery*, *150*(5), 730–738.
22. Oakley, G. M., Orlandi, R. R., Woodworth, B. A., Batra, P. S., & Alt, J. A. (2016). Management of cerebrospinal fluid rhinorrhea: An evidence-based review with recommendations. *International Forum of Allergy & Rhinology*, *6*(1), 17–24.
23. Fraser, S., Gardner, P. A., Koutourousiou, M., Kubik, M., Fernandez-Miranda, J. C., Snyderman, C. H., et al. (2018). Risk factors associated with postoperative cerebrospinal fluid leak after endoscopic endonasal skull base surgery. *Journal of Neurosurgery*, *128*(4), 1066–1071.
24. Lai, L. T., Trooboff, S., Morgan, M. K., & Harvey, R. J. (2014). The risk of meningitis following expanded endoscopic endonasal skull base surgery: A systematic review. *Journal of Neurological Surgery Part B, Skull Base*, *75*(1), 18–26.
25. Shahangian, A., Soler, Z. M., Baker, A., Wise, S. K., Rereddy, S. K., Patel, Z. M., et al. (2017). Successful repair of intraoperative cerebrospinal fluid leaks improves outcomes in endoscopic skull base surgery. *International Forum of Allergy & Rhinology*, *7*(1), 80–86.
26. Rosen, S. A., Getz, A. E., Kingdom, T., Youssef, A. S., & Ramakrishnan, V. R. (2016). Systematic review of the effectiveness of perioperative prophylactic antibiotics for skull base surgeries. *American Journal of Rhinology & Allergy*, *30*(2), e10–e16.
27. Proulx, N., Frechette, D., Toye, B., Chan, J., & Kravcik, S. (2005). Delays in the administration of antibiotics are associated with mortality from adult acute bacterial meningitis. *QJM*, *98*(4), 291–298.
28. Koutourousiou, M., Vaz Guimaraes Filho, F., Fernandez-Miranda, J. C., Wang, E. W., Stefko, S. T., Snyderman, C. H., et al. (2017). Endoscopic endonasal surgery for tumors of the cavernous sinus: A series of 234 patients. *World Neurosurgery*, *103*, 713–732.
29. Zoli, M., Milanese, L., Bonfatti, R., Faustini-Fustini, M., Marucci, G., Tallini, G., et al. (2018). Clival chordomas: Considerations after 16 years of endoscopic endonasal surgery. *Journal of Neurosurgery*, *128*(2), 329–338.
30. Romero, A., Lal Gangadharan, J., Bander, E. D., Gobin, Y. P., Anand, V. K., & Schwartz, T. H. (2017). Managing arterial injury in endoscopic skull base surgery: Case series and review of the literature. *Opererative Neurosurgery (Hagerstown, MD)*, *13*(1), 138–149.
31. Valentine, R., Boase, S., Jervis-Bardy, J., Dones Cabral, J. D., Robinson, S., & Wormald, P. J. (2011). The efficacy of hemostatic techniques in the sheep model of carotid artery injury. *International Forum of Allergy & Rhinology*, *1*(2), 118–122.
32. Maza, G., VanKoevering, K. K., Yanez-Siller, J. C., Baglam, T., Otto, B. A., Prevedello, D. M., et al. (2019). Surgical simulation of a catastrophic internal carotid artery injury: A laser-sintered model. *International Forum of Allergy & Rhinology*, *9*(1), 53–59.
33. Pham, M., Kale, A., Marquez, Y., Winer, J., Lee, B., Harris, B., et al. (2014). A perfusion-based human cadaveric model for management of carotid artery injury during endoscopic endonasal skull base surgery. *Journal of Neurological Surgery Part B, Skull Base*, *75*(5), 309–313.
34. Metson, R., Dallow, R. L., & Shore, J. W. (1994). Endoscopic orbital decompression. *Laryngoscope*, *104*(8 Pt 1), 950–957.
35. Mesquita Filho, P. M., Prevedello, D. M., Prevedello, L. M., Ditzel Filho, L. F., Fiore, M. E., Dolci, R. L., et al. (2017). Optic canal decompression: Comparison of 2 surgical techniques. *World Neurosurgery*, *104*, 745–751.
36. Stokken, J., Gumber, D., Antisdel, J., & Sindwani, R. (2016). Endoscopic surgery of the orbital apex: Outcomes and emerging techniques. *Laryngoscope*, *126*(1), 20–24.
37. Moe, K. S., Bergeron, C. M., & Ellenbogen, R. G. (2010). Transorbital neuroendoscopic surgery. *Neurosurgery*, *67*(3 Suppl Operative), 16–28.
38. Seredyka-Burduk, M., Burduk, P. K., Wierzchowska, M., Kaluzny, B., & Malukiewicz, G. (2017). Ophthalmic complications of endoscopic sinus surgery. *Brazilian Journal of Otorhinolaryngology*, *83*(3), 318–323.
39. Welch, K. C., & Palmer, J. N. (2008). Intraoperative emergencies during endoscopic sinus surgery: CSF leak and orbital hematoma. *Otolaryngologic Clinics of North America*, *41*(3), 581–596. ix–x.
40. Antisdel, J. L., Gumber, D., Holmes, J., & Sindwani, R. (2013). Management of sinonasal complications after endoscopic orbital decompression for Graves' orbitopathy. *Laryngoscope*, *123*(9), 2094–2098.
41. Pletcher, S. D., Sindwani, R., & Metson, R. (2006). Endoscopic orbital and optic nerve decompression. *Otolaryngologic Clinics of North America*, *39*(5), 943–958.
42. Leong, S. C., Karkos, P. D., Macewen, C. J., & White, P. S. (2009). A systematic review of outcomes following surgical decompression for dysthyroid orbitopathy. *Laryngoscope*, *119*(6), 1106–1115.
43. Huang, C. M., Meyer, D. R., Patrinely, J. R., Soparkar, C. N., Dailey, R. A., Maus, M., et al. (2003). Medial rectus muscle injuries associated with functional endoscopic sinus surgery: Characterization and management. *Ophthalmic Plastic and Reconstructive Surgery*, *19*(1), 25–37.
44. Ramakrishna, R., Kim, L. J., Bly, R. A., Moe, K., & Ferreira, M. Jr. (2016). Transorbital neuroendoscopic surgery for the treatment of skull base lesions. *Journal of Clinical Neuroscience*, *6*, 99–104.

40

Neuromonitoring in Endoscopic Skull Base Surgery

SOUMYA SAGAR, MBBS, HAMID BORGHEI-RAVAZI, MD, PABLO F. RECINOS, MD, RAJ SINDWANI, MD, FACS, FRCS(C), CHRISTOPHER R. ROXBURY, MD, MATTHEW CASSIDY, CNIM, DILEEP NAIR, MD, AND VARUN R. KSHETTRY, MD

Introduction

Endoscopic surgery of the cranial base is frequently utilized for pathologies such as pituitary adenoma, craniopharyngioma, chordoma, and chondrosarcoma. Such operations involve working in close proximity to critical neurovascular structures. Insult to these vital structures can result in postoperative neurological deficits that drastically impact the patient's quality of life. It becomes imperative for the neurosurgeon to not only perform optimum resection of the lesion but also preserve the structural and functional integrity of surrounding neurovascular structures.

Cranial nerves are routinely encountered during cranial base surgeries. They are delicate, meandering, and lack an epineurium; factors that make them susceptible to injury. Intraoperative neurophysiologic monitoring of cranial nerves enables the surgeon to confidently operate on offending lesions with continuous feedback on the integrity of cranial nerves. Depending on the location of the lesion and the cranial nerves involved, the choice of neuromonitoring techniques can vary. Here we present discussions of neuromonitoring techniques most commonly used in endoscopic endonasal skull base surgery. Particular focus will be made on the use of triggered and free-running electromyography (EMG) of extraocular muscles for lesions around the cavernous sinus and superior orbital fissure.

Neuromonitoring Modalities

Electromyography (EMG)

EMG was first used intraoperatively in the 1960s for the monitoring of facial nerve function during exploratory parotid surgery.[1] During endoscopic skull base surgery, EMG can be used for monitoring of any cranial nerve with motor function including cranial nerves III-VII and X-XII. The pathologies involving the cavernous sinus and/or superior orbital fissure often threaten cranial nerves III, IV, & VI. They are monitored by performing an EMG of the extraocular muscles. Because of their relative frequency of use in endoscopic skull base surgery, EMG monitoring of the extraocular muscles will be a particular focus of this chapter. For transclival approaches to prepontine or cerebellopontine angle pathologies, the facial nerve, vagal nerve, accessory nerve, and hypoglossal nerve may additionally be monitored.[2] The functional status of the facial nerve is monitored by recording EMG of the orbicularis oris and orbicularis oculi muscles. Similarly for the monitoring of glossopharyngeal, vagus, accessory, and hypoglossal nerves, EMGs of stylopharyngeus, laryngeal muscles, trapezius, and tongue are recorded, respectively.

Two types of EMG activity are recorded: free running and triggered EMG. Free running EMG continuously records the motor unit potentials (MUP) of the muscle fibers. It has high specificity and negative predictive value regarding postoperative cranial nerve deficits.[3] This provides some degree of confidence to the surgeon that these cranial nerves are not being disrupted during tumor exposure and removal. Based on the amplitude and frequency of discharges, the free running EMG signals can be classified into spikes, bursts, trains and neurotonic discharges. A single MUP wave is called a "spike." A short chain of MUPs firing at 30–100 Hz and less than 200 ms in duration is called a "burst." When a persistent chain of MUPs is recorded, it is referred to as a "train." Bursts and spikes are typically triggered by touching, rubbing, or other mechanical manipulations of the nerve[4–6] with no correlation to nerve injury. Trains are elicited by mechanical stimuli, saline irrigation, and possibly nerve ischemia.[7]

The neurotonic discharges are of primary interest to the neuromonitoring technician. They were first described in the 1980s[7] and are defined as a train of MUPs at high frequency (>30 Hz)[8] recorded from a muscle in response to mechanical or metabolic stimulation. Since neurotonic discharges are triggered by mechanical stimulation of motor axons, they act as sensitive indicators of nerve injury.[7] But absence of neurotonic discharges doesn't necessarily exclude nerve injury and presence of neurotonic discharge doesn't always signify nerve injury. Sharp transection of a nerve elicits negligible neurotonic discharges as compared to mechanical irritation or manipulation.[4] The signal voltage is set between 50 and 200 μV, the frequency filter between 30 Hz to 20 kHz, and the sweep speed is at 100 ms per division for recording the responses.

Triggered EMG activity is seen when the cranial nerve is electrically stimulated. This leads to recording of compound muscle action potentials (CMAPs) from the muscle fibers. Triggered EMGs are needed to check the integrity of peripheral motor axons.

CMAPs can be produced by either bipolar or monopolar stimulation. In bipolar stimulation both the cathode and anode are directly on the nerve, which reduces current spread to adjacent nerves leading to localized flow of current. But the localized flow of current may lead to submaximal stimulation if fluid causes current shunting.[9] In monopolar stimulation the cathode is directly on the nerve and the anode is kept away from the nerve by at least several centimeters. This lowers the chances of current shunting but increases the probability of activating nearby neural structures by current spread. Nevertheless, monopolar stimulation is mostly preferred as it is easier to use in confined spaces of the brain.[9] A current of very low intensity (0–2 mA) and duration (0.05– 0.1 ms) is typically used for cranial nerve stimulation during surgery. Higher intensities may be needed if the nerve is less responsive due to damage, insulated by tissue or fluid, or at a distance from the stimulating electrodes. Intensities stronger than 5 mA can spread and lead to unintended activation of nerves. The anesthetic regimen has to be optimized before recording intraoperative EMG. After the induction of anesthesia, muscle relaxants (e.g., vecuronium or pancuronium) are ceased once intubation has been performed, and a train of four should be performed to confirm absence of physiologic muscle relaxant.

Somatosensory Evoked Potentials (SSEP)

Intraoperative monitoring of somatosensory evoked potentials (SSEPs) is one of the most commonly used modalities for predicting and preventing postoperative neurological deficits. SSEPs have been reported to detect the presence of cortical ischemia during cerebrovascular procedures,[10,11] and their utility during skull base procedures is well recognized.[12,13] In endoscopic skull base surgery, SSEPs are most commonly utilized when working very closely on the carotid artery. In the event of a carotid artery injury, SSEPs can notify the surgeon if cerebral ischemia is occurring during use of temporary clipping or if too much packing or compression has been performed. SSEPs monitor the integrity of the spinal cord dorsal columns, medial lemniscus pathways to the thalamus, and its connections to the primary sensory cortex by detecting a stimulus—administered to a peripheral nerve—at the somatosensory cortex.

After the induction of anesthesia, baseline SSEPs are recorded. It can be recorded prior to patient positioning[12] or after positioning when lateral, three-quarter, or prone positioning is used.[3] Recording baseline before positioning is preferable, as pressure on the brachial plexus or peripheral nervous system can be detected and corrected.[14] For upper extremity SSEP recording, bilateral stimulation of the median or ulnar nerve is performed in an alternate fashion at the wrist with a pair of subdermal needle electrodes. For the lower extremities, bilateral alternate stimulation of the tibial nerve is performed. In case one cannot elicit a reliable tibial nerve response, the peroneal nerve can be stimulated. The stimulation of the tibial nerve is performed by a pair of subdermal needle electrodes placed at the medial malleolus of the ankle with a proximal cathode and distal anode separated by a gap of 1 cm. The stimulation of the peroneal nerve is carried out by a pair of subdermal needle electrodes placed at the head of the fibula and medially in the popliteal fossa.

The SSEPs resulting from the stimulation of ulnar or median nerves are recorded by P4/Fz and P3/Fz scalp electrodes (cortical) and a cervical electrode localized at the C7 spinous process (subcortical) and referenced to Fz. The SSEPs resulting from the stimulation of peroneal or tibial nerve are recorded by Pz/Fz and P4/P3 scalp electrodes, and a cervical electrode is localized at the C7 spinous process and referenced to Fz. Band-pass filters set at 30 to 300 Hz are used for cortical recordings, and band-pass filters set at 30 to 1000 Hz are used for subcortical (cervical) recordings. The alarm threshold is a sustained 50% decrease in primary somatosensory cortical amplitude or an increase in response latency by >10% from baseline.[12] Changes in amplitude or latency of SSEPs in >2 averaged trials qualify as sustained changes. SSEPs have certain limitations including their inability to detect subcortical ischemia and lack of information about the integrity of motor pathways.

Brainstem Auditory Evoked Potentials (BAEP)

BAEPs were first described by Jewett and Williston in 1971[15] and have increasingly assumed an important role in modern neurosurgery. BAEPs are more commonly used in lateral skull base surgery for posterior fossa lesions such as meningiomas, vestibular schwannomas, and microvascular decompression for hemifacial spasm and trigeminal neuralgia. Intraoperative monitoring of brainstem auditory evoked potentials (BAEPs) has greatly reduced the risk of hearing loss during the aforementioned surgeries.[16,17] BAEP is used much less commonly in endoscopic skull base surgery. The normal BAEP in humans comprises seven vertex positive submicrovolt waves originating within 10 milliseconds of an auditory stimulus. The first five components of the BAEP are designated waves I through V, out of which wave V is of primary interest for monitoring BAEPs. After induction of anesthesia and positioning the patient, the baseline BAEP is established. The right and left ears are independently stimulated throughout the surgery by delivering a click stimulus of 85 decibels (dB). The rate of the click stimulus is 17.5 Hz. White noise of 65 dB hearing level is applied to the contralateral ear. The observation duration is 12 milliseconds, averaging at least 256 responses. Subdermal needle electrodes are used for BAEP recording and are inserted at vertex to left ear mastoid (Cz/A1); vertex to right ear mastoid (Cz/A2); and vertex to cervical C2 (Cz/Cv2). The amplifier bandpass is 100 to 1000 Hz. The alarm criteria that mandate warning to the surgeon are >50% decrease in wave V amplitude or prolongation of wave V latency to 0.5 or 1.0 millisecond.[18] Loss of wave V is usually synonymous with postoperative hearing loss. BAEP has been shown to be a reliable and effective modality to prevent postoperative hearing loss.[18]

Visual Evoked Potentials (VEP)

Endoscopic skull base surgeries often involve exploration and dissection around the optic nerve, chiasm, and tracts. Common pathologies that occur adjacent to the optic nerves include pituitary adenomas, craniopharyngiomas, and tuberculum sella meningiomas.[19] Due to close proximity, many patients with these pathologies present with visual disturbances. Although the goal of surgery is visual preservation and restoration, there is a real risk of new or worsened postoperative visual impairment. Thus an important goal of the surgery is to also prevent postoperative visual deterioration. Intraoperative monitoring of visual evoked potentials (VEPs) was designed as a way to try and monitor optic function during surgeries around the cisternal and intracanalicular segments of the optic nerve and the optic chiasm and tracts.

Intraoperative monitoring of VEPs was pioneered in the 1970s[20–22] and has been through refinements and critical evaluations.[23–26] Although its use has increased among some centers, overall its use is uncommon due to concerns about reliability.[19,27,28] Prior to the recording of VEPs, total intravenous anesthesia is induced and maintained throughout the surgery. The technical aspects of the anesthetic regimen have been laid out by Wiedemayer *et al.*[23] Flash VEPs have been recommended as the best method for the intraoperative monitoring of VEPs.[19,28,29] Once the anesthesia is induced, the closed eyes are covered with transparent eye patches. Then the light-stimulating device is placed on the eyelids and they are covered with another transparent eye patch. Obviously, the setup of VEP precludes its use in transorbital surgery. The light stimulating device is usually an array of high-luminosity LEDs (light-emitting diodes) set in goggles or soft round silicone discs.[28,29] The color of the LEDs can have an influence on the recordings. The red LEDs stimulate only the cones of the macula whereas using white LEDs will stimulate both rods and cones, thus leading to larger activation of optic pathways and occipital cortex and enabling more comprehensive neuromonitoring. The electrodes for measurement of VEPs are needle electrodes that are placed subcutaneously at Oz, O1, O2, and the ground electrodes are placed subcutaneously in the mastoid process bilaterally (A1 and A2). These locations are according to the international 10/20 EEG system.[28] Band pass filters of 2 to 500 Hz are employed and can be streamlined according to the stimulation artifact. The LEDs deliver a stimulus at the rate of 1 Hz with each stimulus having duration of 8 msec to 20 msec. The signals are averaged over typically 50 to 100 sweeps to record a single VEP. Braiding of the recording wires improves the signal-to-noise ratios of recordings and maintenance of interhemispheric symmetry with reference to electrode impedance (≤ 5 kΩ) and ensures a better quality of recordings. A decrease in amplitude from baseline by 50% or more initiates the alarm. Appearance of these signs alert the surgeon to potential functional damage to the optic pathways. A limitation of using the cutoff of 50% decrease in amplitude is that though it can detect postoperative hemianopsia, it frequently cannot detect a new quadrantanopsia. This can be overcome by redefining the alarm criteria as "reproducible and permanent change of 20% or more" in the amplitude of the baseline.[28] A major factor that limits the use of VEPs for predicting postoperative visual impairment is that its response varies with stimulus delivery and the anesthetic regimen used.[30]

Extraocular Muscle Monitoring

Anatomy

The extraocular muscles comprise the superior oblique, inferior oblique, and four rectus muscles. As the periorbita thickens posteriorly, it gives rise to the common tendinous ring or the annulus of Zinn. It is this annulus that serves as the origin of the four rectus muscles. The superior oblique also arises from this ring, but it loops via the trochlea on the medial side of the orbital roof before terminating on the globe. The extraocular muscles are supplied by three cranial nerves: oculomotor (CN III), trochlear (CN IV), and abducens (CN VI). The oculomotor nerve is a pure motor nerve that arises from the rostral midbrain near the cerebral peduncle and innervates all the extraocular muscles except the superior oblique and lateral rectus and also supplies the sphincter pupillae and ciliary muscles. The trochlear nerve is the thinnest and longest cranial nerve, and the only cranial nerve to originate from the dorsum of the brainstem. It arises immediately lateral to the inferior colliculus and then exits on the contralateral side, coursing around the cerebral peduncle, and ends in the superior oblique muscle. The abducens nerve arises from the pontomedullary sulcus and supplies the lateral rectus. Since these nerves are purely motor, free running EMG for monitoring plus direct stimulation is the preferred intraoperative monitoring (IOM) technique.

Intraoperative Technique

There are three types of electrodes that are used to record EMG activity: surface, subcutaneous, or intramuscular. Surface and subcutaneous electrodes are generally not preferred because these electrodes do not come in close contact with the muscle fibers and thus miss out on many distant MUPs (motor unit potentials). Intramuscular electrodes are the electrodes of choice. They are of two types: needle electrodes and ring electrodes. Ring electrodes are cumbersome as well as more invasive to use, as they need to be sutured epiconjunctivally to the corresponding muscle while a surgical adhesive tape robustly secures its other ends.[4] They are also limited by lower-specificity EMG recordings. For intraoperative monitoring, the needle electrodes are inserted into the superior rectus/inferior rectus (CN III), superior oblique (CN IV), and lateral rectus (CN VI) muscles, and the signals are recorded (Figure 40.1). Before placing electrodes, a corneal eye shield with ophthalmic ointment are first placed. The needle electrodes are placed in the direction of their targets through the eyelid while simultaneously displacing the globe in the opposite direction with the contralateral hand. A reference electrode can be placed near the vertex. The recording and interpretation is performed as described in the section on EMG.

Clinical Evidence

There are many studies that have highlighted the clear advantage of intraoperative monitoring of cranial nerves in preventing

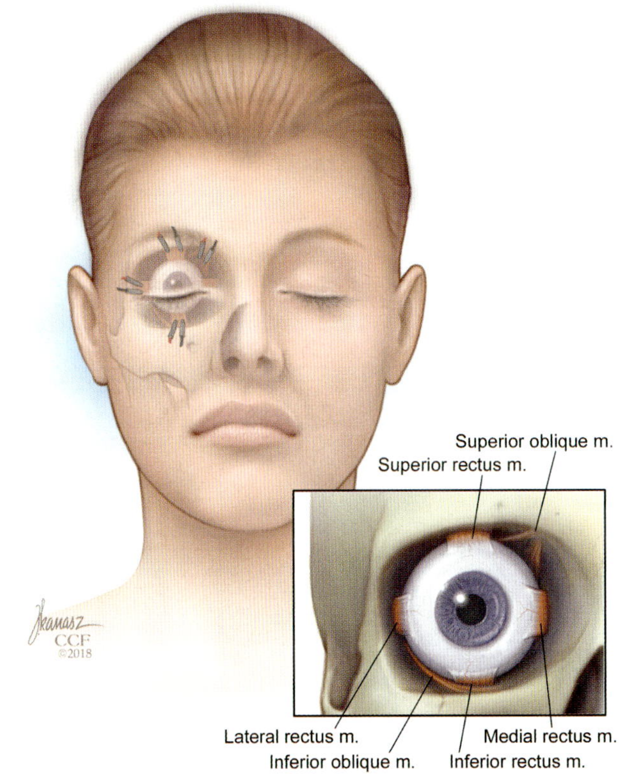

• **Fig. 40.1** Placement of needle electrodes. Needle electrodes are placed through the eyelid while depressing the globe in the opposite direction. The final position of the electrodes is depicted, with needles in the superior oblique, superior rectus, lateral rectus, and inferior rectus. Reprinted with permission, Cleveland Clinic Center for Medical Art & Photography © 2019. All Rights Reserved.

postoperative neurological deficits. In 1995, Kawaguchi *et al.* recorded triggered EMGs of the third to seventh cranial motor nerves in 15 patients undergoing cranial base surgery and recorded compound muscle action potentials in 23 individual muscles.[31] They found that complete loss of triggered EMG of motor cranial nerves had a predictive role for postoperative nerve function. A study by Schlake *et al* recorded free running and triggered EMGs after stimulating CN III (in 5 out 7 cases) and VI (12 out of 18 cases).[32] They determined that EMG was valuable in localizing the position of these nerves intraoperatively, but free running or triggered EMG did not correlate with functional outcome of the nerve. However, they note that this may have been related to their specific neuromonitoring technique. Elangovan *et al* recorded triggered and free run EMGs in pediatric patients underlying endoscopic endonasal skull base surgery.[3] Out of 321 monitored cranial nerves only 9 cranial nerves demonstrated a postoperative deficit. The authors found that there was a significant increase in the risk of a postoperative cranial nerve deficit when there was significant intraoperative free running EMG firing of the corresponding cranial nerve (9% vs 1.5%). In order to predict oculomotor nerve function after clipping of posterior communicating artery aneurysm, Zhou *et al*[9] inserted a needle electrode in the levator palpebrae superioris intraoperatively. They recorded triggered EMGs and found that the amplitude of the evoked CMAPs could reliably predict oculomotor nerve function. In another study done by Kaspera *et al* the advantage offered by intraoperative neuromonitoring of CN III and VI was clearly evident. In patients with cavernous sinus meningiomas, they compared cases with and without EMG neuromonitoring and found a statistically significant increase in the ability to identify the oculomotor nerve (89% vs. 32%) and abducens nerve (80% vs. 20%) when neuromonitoring was used.[5]

Case Example #1

A 50 year-old man with history of left cavernous sinus epidermoid tumor with prior resection 18 years prior to presentation came to our clinic with progressive double vision. The MRI demonstrated a recurrent epidermoid tumor in the ventral aspect of the left cavernous sinus and left superior orbital fissure (Figure 40.2). The neurological exam showed left trochlear nerve palsy and horizontal nystagmus toward the left. The tumor was initially observed but demonstrated growth at 6-month follow-up. Given growth and progressive symptoms, surgical options were discussed and an endonasal route was recommended given multiple prior cranial surgeries. Resection of the epidermoid cyst in the cavernous sinus was performed via an endoscopic endonasal transpterygoid approach. CN III, IV, and VI were monitored using free running EMG and direct stimulation technique. At the end of resection, all the cranial nerves were at their baseline except CN IV, which demonstrated persistent spontaneous discharges. Postop neurological exam showed baseline left side CN IV nerve palsy and partial left CN VI palsy, which had improved at 3-month postop follow-up. Immediate postop MRI demonstrated complete resection of the left cavernous sinus and superior orbital fissure epidermoid cyst (Figure 40.3).

Case Example #2

A 50-year-old man presented with right-sided headache, facial tingling, and burning sensation. MRI demonstrated an extra-axial mass lesion inside the right Meckel's cave (Figure 40.4). Given intractable facial pain associated with the mass, surgery was recommended. Needle electrodes were placed to monitor the right-sided CN III, IV, and VI. The tumor was resected via an endoscopic endonasal transpterygoid approach. The abducens nerve, as it curves around the paraclival ICA, runs along the medial aspect of V1, and therefore is on the superior aspect of the entrance into Meckel's cave from the endonasal perspective. The region around the entrance was stimulated to avoid injury. The lesion was eventually identified deep within Meckel's cave and medial to the V2 branch of the trigeminal nerve. Here, free running EMG and stimulation were utilized. Specifically, given the proximity of the lesion to the lateral wall of the cavernous sinus, direct stimulation was used to ensure that there was no injury to CN III, IV, or VI. Pathology was consistent with cavernous malformation. The patient had expected V2 numbness given that division of V2 fibers was necessary for access, but otherwise had no other neurologic deficits postoperatively. The postop MRI demonstrated gross total resection of the extra-axial lesion along the course of the trigeminal nerve (Figure 40.5).

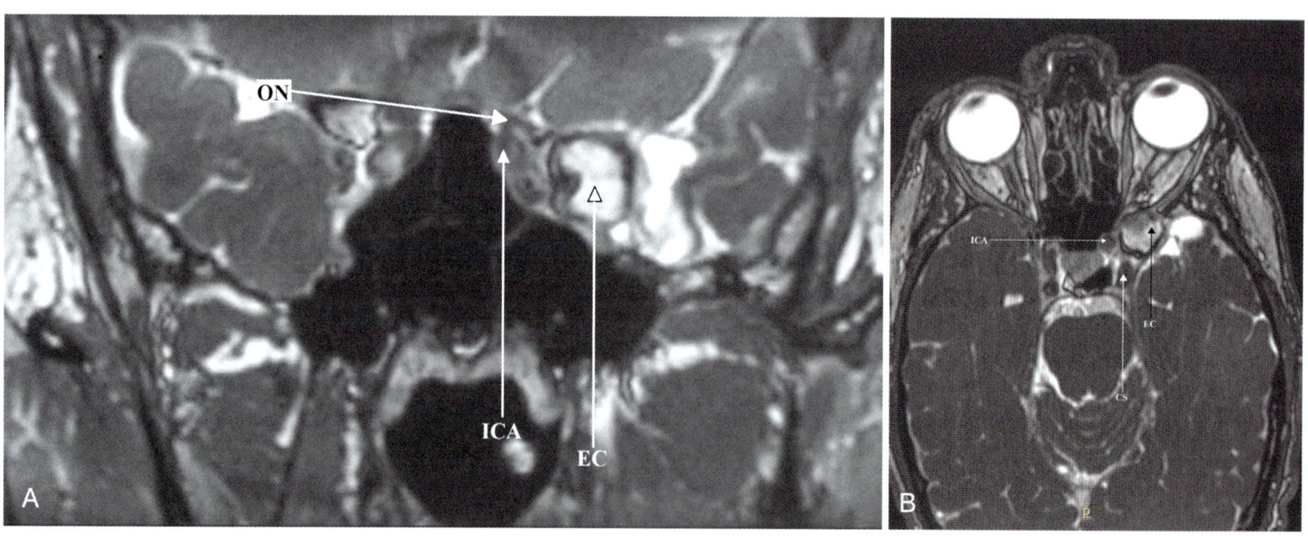

• **Fig. 40.2** Preoperative coronal (A) and axial (B) MRI constructive interference steady-state (CISS) sequence shows epidermoid tumor in ventro-lateral aspect of the left cavernous sinus extending into the left superior orbital fissure. ***ON***: *Optic nerve;* ***ICA***: *internal carotid artery;* ***EC***: *epidermoid cyst;* ***CS***: *Cavernous sinus.*

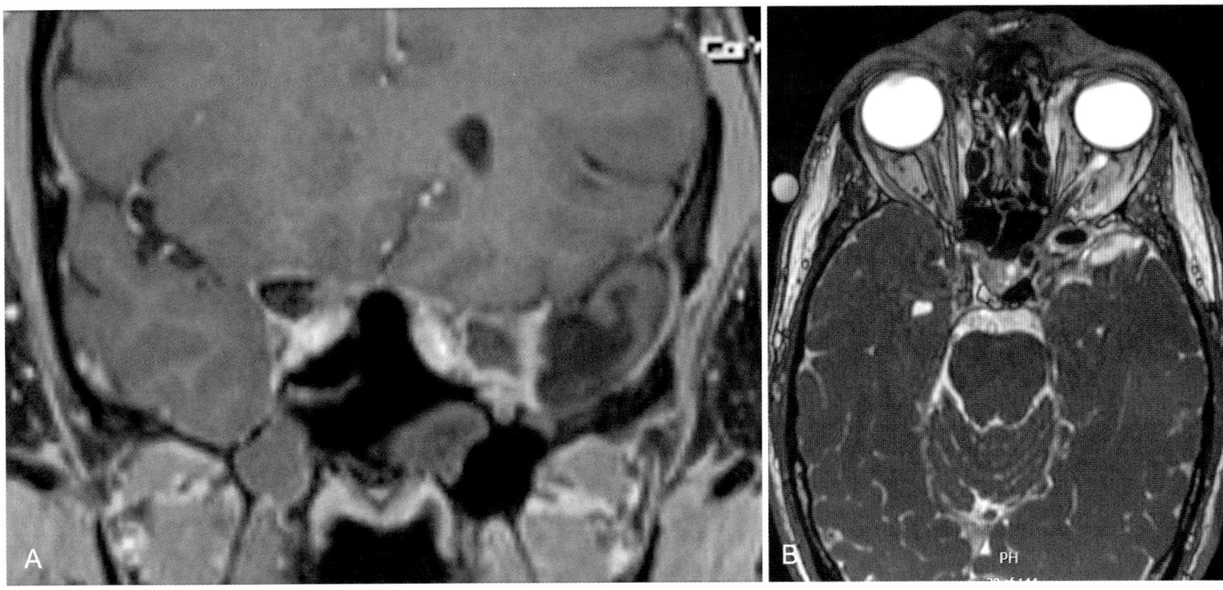

• **Fig. 40.3** Postoperative coronal MRI T1 with contrast (A) and axial CISS (B) demonstrating complete tumor resection.

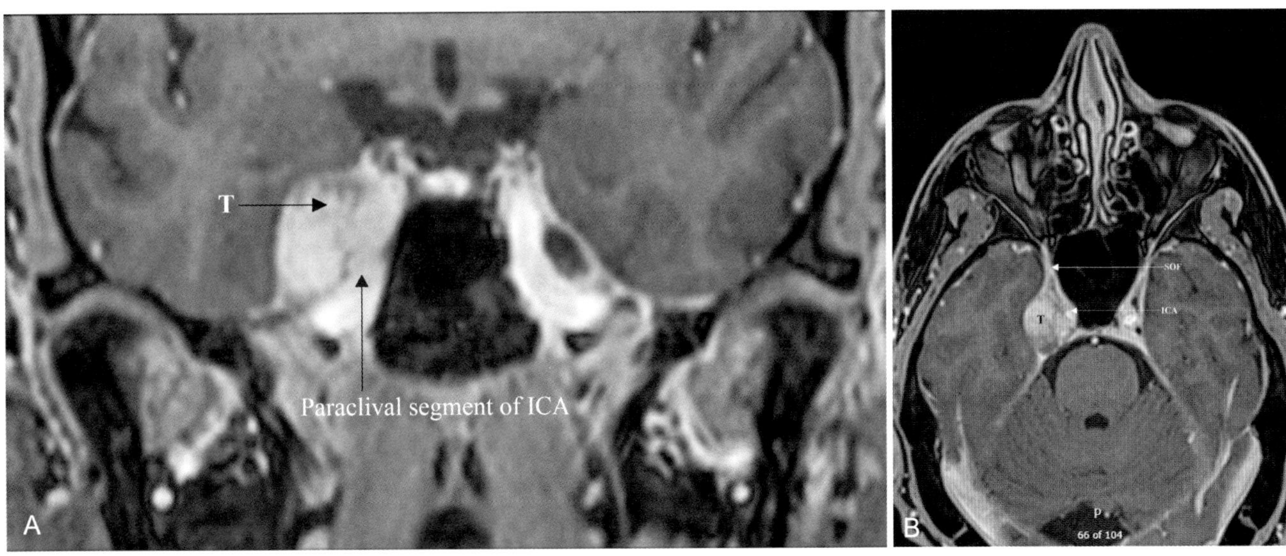

• **Fig. 40.4** Preoperative coronal (A) and axial (B) T1 MRI with contrast demonstrating an enhancing mass within Meckel's cave. ***T****: Tumor; ICA: internal carotid artery;* ***SOF: Superior orbital fissure***.

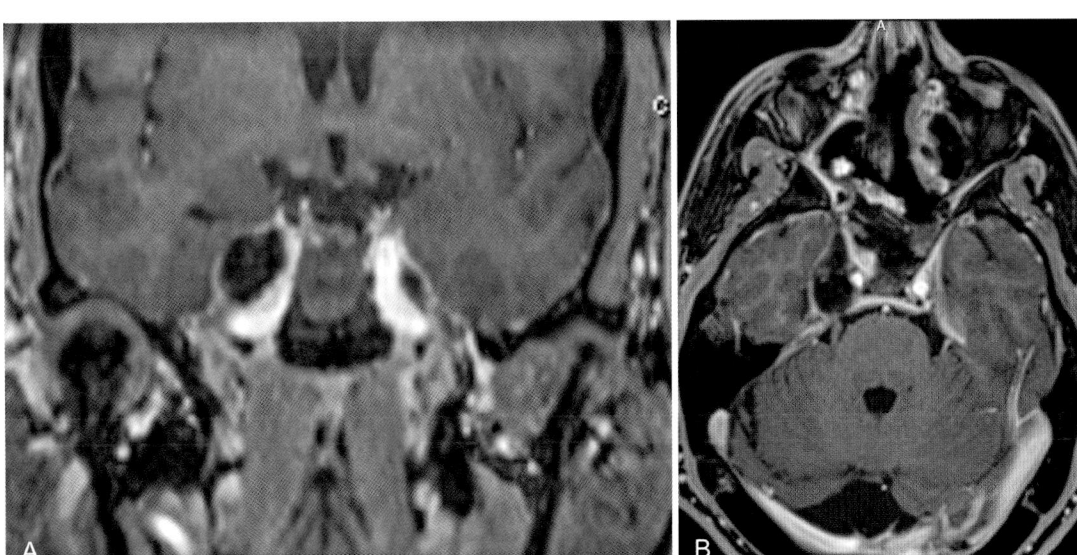

• **Fig. 40.5** Postoperative coronal (A) and axial (B) T1 MRI with contrast demonstrating complete resection of the cavernous malformation.

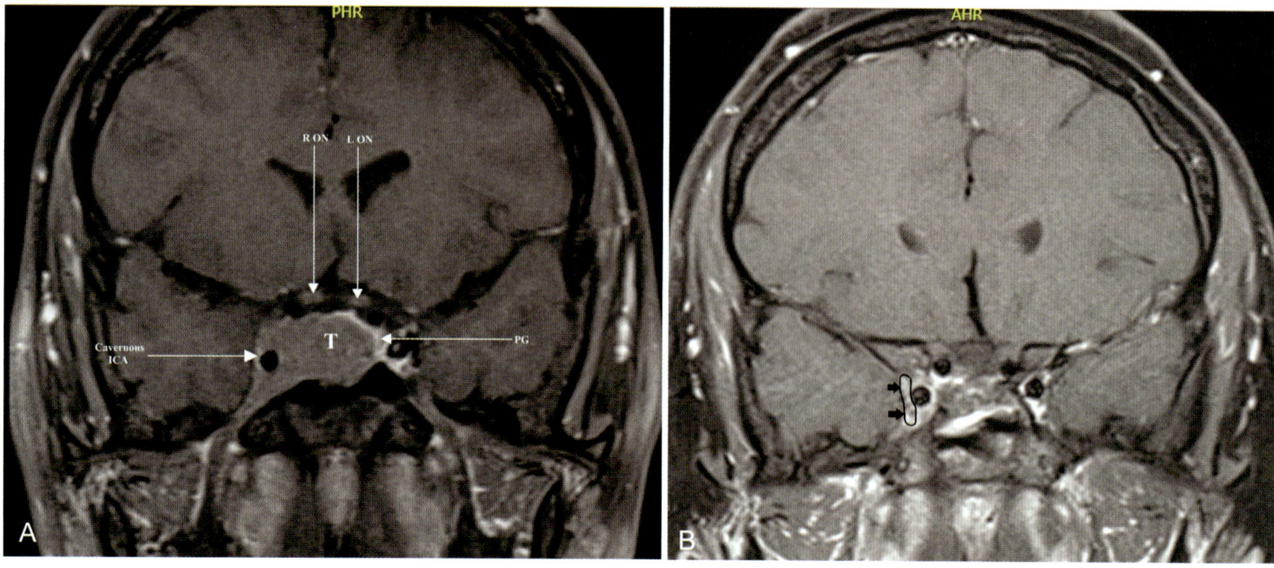

• **Fig. 40.6** (A) Preoperative coronal T1 MRI with contrast demonstrates a sellar lesion with extension to the right cavernous sinus and complete encasement of the cavernous ICA. (B) Postoperative coronal T1 MRI with contrast demonstrates a near-total resection with small residual tumor in the lateral wall of the right cavernous sinus. ***ON***: *Optic nerve,* ***ICA***: *internal carotid artery,* ***PG***: *Pituitary gland;* ***T***: *Tumor*

Case Example #3

A 16-year-old man with history of Ehlers–Danlos syndrome presented with gigantism and markedly elevated IGF-1 (Insulin-like Growth Factor). MRI showed a large sellar mass extending into the right cavernous sinus (Figure 40.6A). Clinical history, lab reports, and imaging were all consistent with acromegaly. Endoscopic transsellar, transpterygoid, transcavernous approach was utilized for tumor resection. Free running EMG of CN III, IV, and VI and direct stimulation techniques were used. When working medial and superior to the cavernous ICA, free running EMG was primarily utilized with intermittent stimulation to detect CN VI. When working lateral to the ICA, direct stimulation was consistently used and CN III, IV, and VI. All nerves stimulated at low stimulus at the end of tumor resection. Postoperatively, the patient experienced a partial CN VI palsy on the right side, which completely resolved by postoperative day 4. Postoperative MRI showed near complete resection of tumor with small residual in the lateral wall of the right cavernous sinus (Figure 40.6B).

Conclusion

Intraoperative neuromonitoring of cranial nerves has emerged as a vital tool for endoscopic skull base surgery. Depending on the type of surgery, area being operated, and nerves at risk, the surgeon can choose the most appropriate form of neuromonitoring. For endoscopic skull base surgery in and around the cavernous sinus and superior orbital fissure, EMG of extraocular muscles has helped tremendously in identifying the position and verifying the functional integrity of cranial nerves III, IV, and VI. Thoughtful collaboration between the surgeon and neurophysiology team can help maximize surgical outcomes.

References

1. Parsons, R. C. (1968). Electrical nerve stimulation at surgery. *Laryngoscope*, *78*, 742–748.
2. Minahan, R. E., & Mandir, A. S. (2011). Neurophysiologic intraoperative monitoring of trigeminal and facial nerves. *Journal of Clinical Neurophysiology*, *28*, 551–565.
3. Elangovan, C., Singh, S. P., Gardner, P., et al. (2016). Intraoperative neurophysiological monitoring during endoscopic endonasal surgery for pediatric skull base tumors. *Journal of Neurosurgery Pediatrics*, *17*, 147–155.
4. Hariharan, P., Balzer, J. R., Anetakis, K., Crammond, D. J., & Thirumala, P. D. (2018). Electrophysiology of extraocular cranial nerves: Oculomotor, trochlear, and abducens nerve. *J Clin Neurophysiol*, *35*, 11–15.
5. Kaspera, W., Adamczyk, P., Slaska-Kaspera, A., & Ladzinski, P. (2015). Usefulness of intraoperative monitoring of oculomotor and abducens nerves during surgical treatment of the cavernous sinus meningiomas. *Advances in Medical Sciences*, *60*, 25–30.
6. Sekhar, L. N., Pranatartiharan, R., Chanda, A., & Wright, D. C. (2001). Chordomas and chondrosarcomas of the skull base: Results and complications of surgical management. *Neurosurgical Focus*, *10*, E2.
7. Harper, C. M. (2004). Intraoperative cranial nerve monitoring. *Muscle & Nerve*, *29*, 339–351.
8. Oh, T., Nagasawa, D. T., Fong, B. M., et al. (2012). Intraoperative neuromonitoring techniques in the surgical management of acoustic neuromas. *Neurosurgical Focus*, *33*, E6.
9. Zhou, Q., Zhang, M., & Jiang, Y. (2012). Intraoperative oculomotor nerve monitoring predicts outcome following clipping of posterior communicating artery aneurysms. *Journal of Clinical Neuroscience: Official Journal of the Neurosurgical Society of Australasia*, *19*, 706–711.
10. Wicks, R. T., Pradilla, G., Raza, S. M., et al. (2012). Impact of changes in intraoperative somatosensory evoked potentials on stroke rates after clipping of intracranial aneurysms. *Neurosurgery*, *70*, 1114–1124. discussion 24.
11. Xu, B. N., Sun, Z. H., Romani, R., et al. (2010). Microsurgical management of large and giant paraclinoid aneurysms. *World Neurosurgery*, 73, 137–146. discussion e17, e19.
12. Thirumala, P. D., Kassasm, A. B., Habeych, M., et al. (2011). Somatosensory evoked potential monitoring during endoscopic endonasal approach to skull base surgery: Analysis of observed changes. *Neurosurgery*, *69*, 64–76.
13. Bejjani, G. K., Nora, P. C., Vera, P. L., Broemling, L., & Sekhar, L. N. (1998). The predictive value of intraoperative somatosensory evoked potential monitoring: Review of 244 procedures. *Neurosurgery*, *43*, 491–498.
14. Singh, H., Vogel, R. W., Lober, R. M., et al. (2016). Intraoperative neurophysiological monitoring for endoscopic endonasal approaches to the skull base: A technical guide. *Scientifica*, *2016*. 1751245.

15. Jewett, D. L., & Williston, J. S. (1971). Auditory-evoked far fields averaged from the scalp of humans. *Brain: a Journal of Neurology, 94*, 681–696.
16. Grundy, B. L., Jannetta, P. J., Procopio, P. T., Lina, A., Boston, J. R., & Doyle, E. (1982). Intraoperative monitoring of brain-stem auditory evoked potentials. *Journal of Neurosurgery, 57*, 674–681.
17. Lee, S. H., Song, D. G., Kim, S., Lee, J. H., & Kang, D. G. (2009). Results of auditory brainstem response monitoring of microvascular decompression: A prospective study of 22 patients with hemifacial spasm. *Laryngoscope, 119*, 1887–1892.
18. Thirumala, P. D., Carnovale, G., Habeych, M. E., Crammond, D. J., & Balzer, J. R. (2014). Diagnostic accuracy of brainstem auditory evoked potentials during microvascular decompression. *Neurology, 83*, 1747–1752.
19. Kodama, K., Goto, T., Sato, A., Sakai, K., Tanaka, Y., & Hongo, K. (2010). Standard and limitation of intraoperative monitoring of the visual evoked potential. *Acta Neurochir (Wien), 152*, 643–648.
20. Feinsod, M., Selhorst, J. B., Hoyt, W. F., & Wilson, C. B. (1976). Monitoring optic nerve function during craniotomy. *Journal of Neurosurgery, 44*, 29–31.
21. Wright, J. E., Arden, G., & Jones, B. R. (1973). Continuous monitoring of the visually evoked response during intra-orbital surgery. *Transactions of the Ophthalmology Society of the United Kingdom, 93*, 311–314.
22. Wilson, W. B., Kirsch, W. M., Neville, H., Stears, J., Feinsod, M., & Lehman, R. A. (1976). Monitoring of visual function during parasellar surgery. *Surgery in Neurology, 5*, 323–329.
23. Wiedemayer, H., Fauser, B., Armbruster, W., Gasser, T., & Stolke, D. (2003). Visual evoked potentials for intraoperative neurophysiologic monitoring using total intravenous anesthesia. *Journal of Neurosurgery and Anesthesiology, 15*, 19–24.
24. Cedzich, C., Schramm, J., & Fahlbusch, R. (1987). Are flash-evoked visual potentials useful for intraoperative monitoring of visual pathway function? *Neurosurgery, 21*, 709–715.
25. Cedzich, C., & Schramm, J. (1990). Monitoring of flash visual evoked potentials during neurosurgical operations. *International Anesthesiology Clinician, 28*, 165–169.
26. Chung, S. B., Park, C. W., Seo, D. W., Kong, D. S., & Park, S. K. (2012). Intraoperative visual evoked potential has no association with postoperative visual outcomes in transsphenoidal surgery. *Acta Neurochir (Wien), 154*, 1505–1510.
27. Goto, T., Tanaka, Y., Kodama, K., Kusano, Y., Sakai, K., & Hongo, K. (2007). Loss of visual evoked potential following temporary occlusion of the superior hypophyseal artery during aneurysm clip placement surgery: Case report. *Journal of Neurosurgery, 107*, 865–867.
28. Gutzwiller, E. M., Cabrilo, I., Radovanovic, I., Schaller, K., & Boex, C. (2018). Intraoperative monitoring with visual evoked potentials for brain surgeries. *Journal of Neurosurgery*, 1–7.
29. Sasaki, T., Itakura, T., Suzuki, K., et al. (2010). Intraoperative monitoring of visual evoked potential: Introduction of a clinically useful method. *Journal of Neurosurgery, 112*, 273–284.
30. Thirumala, P. D., Habeych, M. E., Crammond, D. J., & Balzer, J. R. (2011). Neurophysiologic intraoperative monitoring of olfactory and optic nerves. *Journal of Clinical Neurophysiology, 28*, 538–542.
31. Kawaguchi, M., Ohnishi, H., Sakamoto, T., et al. (1995). Intraoperative electrophysiologic monitoring of cranial motor nerves in skull base surgery. *Surgical Neurology, 43*, 177–181.
32. Schlake, H. P., Goldbrunner, R., Siebert, M., Behr, R., & Roosen, K. (2001). Intra-operative electromyographic monitoring of extra-ocular motor nerves (Nn. III, VI) in skull base surgery. *Acta Neurochir (Wien), 143*, 251–261.

Index

Note: Page numbers followed by *f* indicate figures, *t* indicate tables, and *b* indicate boxes.

P

Q

R